EARLY PHASE DRUG EVALUATION
IN MAN

Early Phase Drug Evaluation in Man

Edited by

John O'Grady, MD, FRCP

Medical Director
May and Baker Pharmaceuticals
Rhône-Poulenc Ltd
Dagenham RM10 7XS, UK
and Visiting Professor of Clinical Pharmacology
University of Vienna, Austria

and

Otto I. Linet, MD, PhD

Director of Clinical Development Unit 1
The Upjohn Company
Kalamazoo, MI 49001, USA

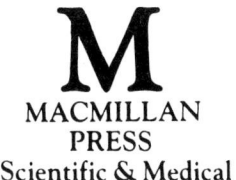

MACMILLAN
PRESS
Scientific & Medical

First published 1990

Published by
THE MACMILLAN PRESS LTD
Houndmills, Basingstoke, Hampshire RG21 2XS
and London
Companies and representatives
throughout the world

Filmset by Wearside Tradespools,
Fulwell, Sunderland

Printed in Great Britain by Billings & Son, Worcester

British Library Cataloguing in Publication Data
Early phase drug evaluation in man.
1. Man. Effects of drugs
I. O'Grady, John II. Linet, Otto I.
615′.7
ISBN 0–333–48732–X

The mention of a product is not an endorsement, and
the contributors, editors and publishers will
not be held liable for any dosages or
treatments mentioned in the text.

Contents

Foreword

Regrettably, there is ample evidence that the time taken for the development of a drug from discovery to marketing is lengthening. Ten to twelve years is now quoted as the norm but I am aware of at least one instance where it has taken more than seventeen years. In part, this disappointing trend is attributable to an increased demand for information on the safety and efficacy of a compound before it can be registered for sale. Clearly, there is a need, long perceived by the basic scientists, to conduct the early evaluation of drugs in man more effectively and more rapidly. The management of the industry has not sufficiently appreciated that there is a great deal of difference between the approach needed for the investigative first testing of a new chemical entity in man and that needed to organise large-scale phase III clinical trial programmes.

This book is to be welcomed because it is unique in concentrating on the initial investigations of the properties of new drugs in man and in bringing together, on an international basis, contributors from both industry and academia. It will have served its purpose well if it encourages the clinical scientist to use the most appropriate methods in an expeditious way to provide information necessary for decision making in drug development. This is indeed an area where months, if not years, could be saved by more imaginative management.

It is pleasing to see the comprehensive approach that John O'Grady and Otto Linet have adopted for this book. Not only does it describe in detail the essential animal tests needed before testing a drug in man, but it also discusses organisation and decision making as well as medical and legal considerations. However, the majority of the book deals with the assessment of drug activity in man and has drawn on the experience of many internationally recognised clinical pharmacologists.

I feel sure that the expertise provided in this comprehensive book will enable the early phases of drug testing in man to be speeded up. Thereafter one would hope that the clinical scientists responsible for phase III studies might be persuaded to pick up the ball and run with it as fast as their colleagues in the earlier stages of drug discovery.

London, August, 1989   Sir John Vane

ix

Preface

There are several books available which well describe how to conduct the large-scale clinical trial programmes needed before registration for sale of a new drug. However, there has not previously been available a single comprehensive volume which deals with the critical early phases of drug evaluation in man. These phases are the first testing in healthy non-patient volunteer subjects and the early trials in patients, which provide the evidence of efficacy and relative safety which allow a decision to be made to progress to the later, comprehensive, stages of drug development.

Increasingly there is concern about the time delays in developing modern drugs and debate about ethical aspects of clinical trials. Both topics focus attention on the need to use the optimum methods to provide as rapidly as possible information of maximum predictive value for drug safety and efficacy. We have tried to ensure that this volume describes in particular the clinical pharmacological methods which may be applied to assessment of drug safety and efficacy in man. We have deliberately confined the scope of the book to what is commonly known as 'phases I and II of clinical development', that is the earlier stages of human testing up to demonstration of efficacy and relative safety such that a decision to proceed with extended-scale phase III development can be made. The book is intended to be a practical guide for those concerned with evaluation of drugs in all the major classes of activity. Early clinical development cannot, however, be divorced from the preclinical studies which provide essential and often predictive information in relation to clinical safety and efficacy. We have dealt with selected aspects of these in the first part of the book, although we make no apology for not making this section exhaustive, as to do so would require a volume on its own.

The editors may choose the aim of the book and provide the concept and a framework. We are in debt to the contributors who have written this volume and are also grateful to them for accepting with good grace the confines of space within which to discuss their own particular important areas.

We are grateful to many, but in particular to Professor Paul Turner who encouraged us to pursue the original idea, to Dr Susan Boobis for excellent editorial and administrative assistance, to David Grist of The Macmillan Press for his unfailing guidance and support, and to Cindy Shattuck, Hazel Gunn and Jacqueline Smith for skilful secretarial assistance.

London and Kalamazoo, August, 1989   J.O'G.
                                                          O.I.L.

I
Preliminaries to Testing
of Drugs in Man

1
The Pharmaceutical Background

Shri C. Valvani

Director, Drug Delivery Systems Research, The Upjohn Company, 7000 Portage Rd, Kalamazoo, MI 49001, USA

INTRODUCTION

For medicine today, the ultimate goal of most research-based pharmaceutical and allied health care organisations around the world is to discover, develop and procure necessary regulatory approvals for marketing new drugs for treatment or prevention of diseases in humans and animals. Drug discovery and development involves a complex process from early discovery of a chemical entity to demonstration of its safety and effectiveness for specific therapeutic indication(s). Introduction of new drugs either could be in the form of new chemical entities, or from regulatory perspectives a drug might be considered 'new' because of changes in its composition, route of administration, recommended dosage or dosage form. This chapter will deal primarily with pharmaceutical considerations for development of new chemical entities only, which usually require the greatest amount of investigation for safety and clinical evaluation to demonstrate their effectiveness. A comprehensive discussion of all pharmaceutical considerations in the design and development of all dosage forms or drug delivery systems for all routes of administration is beyond the scope of this chapter. An overview of critical pharmaceutical considerations for dosage forms generally developed for preclinical and early human testing will be covered.

BACKGROUND

The discovery phase of new chemical or molecular entities usually involves chemical synthesis or isolation from natural sources. With the advent of genetic and protein engineering, a new generation of drugs, protein or polypeptide molecules, is beginning to be introduced as well as being under development. Since most protein drugs and large peptides cannot be synthesised, they are produced via genetic engineering or recombinant DNA techniques, fermentation or cell culture, isolation and purification steps. A decision to develop new drugs often depends on the results of 'screening', which involve testing of new drugs using whole animals or *in vitro* techniques to determine the pharmacological response which reflects potential therapeutic benefit(s).

Once the new drug has been shown to possess the desirable therapeutic or pharmacological promise through animal models or *in vitro* techniques during initial screening, it must undergo preclinical safety, pharmacokinetics or biopharmaceutics testing, followed by extensive generation of other scientific information, before early testing in humans can begin, usually after regulatory review and permission in most countries in the western world.

When the decision is made to develop a compound, usually the first step is to prepare a reasonable quantity of drug substance so that multidisciplinary approach to early investigation and development can begin.

In order for a new drug to be evaluated for preclinical safety assessment, often in several animal species, it must be formulated in a dosage form or a delivery system which will deliver the drug in a way that maximises the 'availability' of drug at the site of action. The development of early dosage forms for preclinical testing and eventually for early testing in humans requires an interplay of physicochemical, biological and dosage form considerations.

PREFORMULATION CONSIDERATIONS

The development process usually begins with preformulation characterisation of drug substance. Preformulation is the study of physicochemical properties which could affect the drug performance, processing and design and the development of an efficacious dosage form. Table 1.1 lists some of the important parameters which may be evaluated during the preformulation investigation stage. Most of these are molecular properties of the drug and provide a sort of 'finger-print' of the drug. Preformulation characteristics are critical to successful formulation design and development.

Some of the preformulation parameters may be affected by processing, e.g. solubility or surface area of the drug may be affected by micronisation, milling or manipulation of crystallisation procedures. Development of formulations for toxicology testing, for early human evaluation or for eventual marketing may not require extensive evaluation of all of these parameters. It often depends on the type of drug, the dosage form or the route of administration. For example, for solid dosage forms, stability of the drug in the solid state should be investigated in depth, while for solution formulations (parenteral or oral), degradation and kinetics of solution stability may require critical evaluation. Likewise, for aerosol delivery systems for inhalation, particle size and surface characterisation, solubility and compatibility with vehicle and propellants are some of the important considerations. For proteins and polypeptide macromolecular drugs, conformational stability, including denaturation and aggregation, must be addressed for formulation development. For targeted or site-specific drug delivery systems, e.g. monoclonal antibodies, consideration of biochemical and transcellular events at the cellular level is important.

Table 1.1 Preformulation characterisation of bulk drug substances

Chemical structure and molecular weight
Organoleptic properties:
  colour, odour
Chemical purity:
  level and identification of impurities
  spectral properties (infrared, ultraviolet)
Physical properties:
  particle size (distribution) and shape
  bulk density
  microscopic characterisation
  surface area
  surface activity
  effect of milling/micronisation
Aqueous solubility:
  pH solubility profile
  effect of temperature
  effect of solubilising agents
  effect of buffers, ionic strength
Non-aqueous solubility:
  pure solvents
  mixed cosolvents
Dissolution rate:
  bulk drug and pure drug compact
  effect of particle size, surface area
Partition coefficient:
  octanol/water
  alkane/water
Ionisation constants (pK_a):
  aqueous and non-aqueous systems
Biopharmaceutics properties:
  In vitro absorption/transport properties
Crystalline properties:
  melting point
  polymorphism (effect on bioavailability)
  thermal analysis (DSC, TGA, etc.)
  isomerism
Mechanical properties:
  viscoelastic properties
  compressibility
  flowability
Solution stability:
  pH rate profile
  degradation rate and mechanism
  effect of temperature
  photolytic degradation
  oxidation/hydrolysis
  presence of metal
  non-aqueous solution stability
  effect of additives
Solid state stability:
  effect of temperature
  effect of humidity
  effect of light
  effect of oxygen/nitrogen
  effect of additives

Preformulation investigation usually commences with complete analytical characterisation of the drug with regard to chemical purity, including the level and nature of impurities. For proteins and peptides, drugs derived from recombinant technology, evaluation of trace contaminants, such as viral, nucleic acid, pyrogens, antigens, foreign proteins and microbial contamination may be carried out as part of characterisation in addition to several other specific tests for purity and identity. For organic drug molecules, early chemical synthesis is often directed towards maximising chemical purity of the drug, while minimising the impurities. Isolation and identification of impurities which may be present in the drug beyond a desired level is often required by most regulatory agencies world-wide. Chemical purity and impurities characterisation ensures that drug with no additional or higher level of impurities as compared with what has been used for toxicology or safety testing in animals will be used in the formulations for early human testing. In addition to analytical characterisation, determination of important physicochemical properties, such as melting point or boiling point, ionisation constant(s) for electrolyte drugs, isoelectric point for protein drugs, spectroscopic properties and polymorphic characterisation are critical to establishing identity and purity of the drug molecule.

From a physical standpoint, the goal of the pharmaceutical scientist is to design and develop a dosage form that is stable (usually for about 2 years), is elegant, contains the precise amount of drug which will deliver the drug in the most available form and can be manufactured on a large scale in an economic manner to meet market needs after regulatory approvals.

DOSAGE FORM CONSIDERATIONS

A review of pharmaceutical dosage forms available in most major markets around the globe would indicate that tablets and capsules are by far the most widely used dosage form, primarily because of advances in the technology of manufacture, flexibility in dosing, stability, elegance and ease of ingestion, etc. Table 1.2 provides a listing of major pharmaceutical dosage forms and drug delivery systems in use today. A comprehensive listing of different types of tablet dosage forms appears in the table. Similar variety is usually available for each of other dosage forms. However, for brevity, other dosage forms are listed in their simplest form.

Since administration of high concentrations of doses of formulations for preclinical safety testing in animals is usually required for early stages, solution or suspension formulations of drug are often developed for toxicological testing. For early metabolic or bioavailability studies in animals, and for early clinical studies in humans, a parenteral solution, particularly for intravenous administrations, is quite often required in order to assess drug disposition and clinical pharmacology. Other dosage forms, such as tablets, capsules, topicals and other delivery systems, may also be used for early and late toxicology testing and for other animal and human studies. One of the key requirements for these formulations is that they must present the drug in

Table 1.2   Dosage form or drug delivery system considerations

Tablets:
   compressed
   layered
   sugar-coated
   film-coated
   enteric-coated
   chewable
   controlled-release
   sublingual
   buccal
   effervescent
Hard-filled capsules
Soft gelatin capsules
Suppositories
Emulsions
Gels/creams/ointments
Oral solutions
Parenteral solutions
Ophthalmic solutions
Aerosols
Suspensions
Lyophilised powders
Ready-to-use injections
Liposomes
Transdermals
Biodegradable polymer systems
Bioerodible polymer systems
Insoluble (swellable) polymer matrix systems
Microspheres
Nanoparticles
Surgical foams
Edible foams
Softgels/hydrogels
Micellar solutions
Monoclonal antibodies
Implants/pumps
Microsponges

the most bioavailable form and they must be stable for the duration of investigational studies. Isotonicity and physiological pH are important considerations for parenteral formulations for toxicology testing. Suspensions must possess good homogeneity to deliver uniform dosing and should demonstrate acceptable physical stability, especially minimal settling tendency with good resuspendibility. The US regulations require that the formulations for toxicology testing must be manufactured in accordance with good laboratory practices (GLPs).

BIOLOGICAL CONSIDERATIONS

The ultimate goal in the drug design and development process is to improve or optimise the biological performance of drugs. Biological performance can be regarded as the most efficient delivery of drug substance to the site at which it is needed the most, and at such a rate of delivery that it elicits the most beneficial therapeutic response while minimising undesirable side-effects.

It is generally recognised that physicochemical properties of the drug and pharmaceutical considerations with regard to route of administration play an important role in governing the overall biological performance of drugs. Some of the important parameters influencing the biological performance are the absorption and transport processes across biological barriers. The nature of these biological barriers and enzymatic, metabolic or biochemical events associated with these barriers generally depend on the route of administration. For example, endothelial barriers are important in targeting specific delivery to liver, lungs or reticular endothelial system; cellular barriers are important for targeting to tumour and other specific cells; and epithelial barriers are dominant for oral, topical and transdermal delivery, etc. Since a majority of the drugs are administered by the oral route, we shall critically examine the factors influencing the gastrointestinal process for drug absorption and transport. These factors involve consideration from biological and physicochemical perspectives.

Table 1.3 shows some of the important biological considerations which govern the absorption process by the oral route. The absorption process depends on the complex interplay of some or most of these factors. Drug absorption, whether it is through the gastrointestinal tract, the nasal cavity, the buccal mucosa or other barriers, requires that the drug be transported in a molecular form across the barrier membrane. Biological membranes are composed of small amphipathic molecules, phospholipids and cholesterol, association of which creates lipoidal bilayers in an aqueous environment. Embedded in the matrix of lipid molecules are proteins which are generally hydrophobic in nature. It is generally thought that most lipid-soluble drugs can pass by passive diffusion through the lipid membrane from regions of high concentration to regions of low concentration. A few drugs can pass through by active transport, often by special mechanisms.

Similarly, the pH of the intestinal contents in various segments, the presence of bile salts and enzymes, the type and nature of food, the intestinal flora and the disease state will all influence the drug absorption process. It is generally thought that the presence of enzymes, e.g. proteolytic enzymes and other specific enzymes, inhibits or limits the absorption of large peptide or protein drugs.

Most solid dosage forms for oral administration (tablets, capsules and powders) must first undergo disintegration, followed by dissolution of drug particles and transport of drug molecules into the gut. Some controlled-release solid dosage forms may release the drug by a variety of mechanisms. Active drug molecules then diffuse across the gut mucosa into the systemic circulation, either by active transport or by passive diffusion. The drug may

Table 1.3 Biological considerations for oral drug delivery

Membrane transport mechanism:
  active transport
  passive diffusion
  facilitated diffusion
Gastrointestinal pH:
  stomach
  duodenum
  jejunum
  ileum
  colon
  surface and bulk pH
Stomach emptying and gastrointestinal motility:
  fasting
  non-fasting
  hydrodynamics
  type of food
Enzymes of the gastrointestinal tract:
  lumenal enzymes
  surface-bound enzymes
  intercellular enzymes
  specificity and distribution of enzymes
Bile acid secretions
Intestinal flora
Malabsorption due to disease state
Pharmacological drug effects

undergo a variety of enzymatic and/or metabolic conversions, transport and deposition into several organs, possible biotransformation, and finally excretion by one or more specific routes. A small fraction or most of the drug entity may eventually reach the receptor site, where the desired therapeutic response is achieved.

PHYSICOCHEMICAL CONSIDERATIONS

Table 1.4 shows some of the physicochemical properties involved in drug absorption and transport processes. Lipophilicity of the drug or the membrane–water partition coefficient and solubility are two of the most important properties of the drug molecule which have profound influence on these processes.

The parameters listed in Table 1.4 are extremely important in formulation design and development for preclinical testing or for evaluation in humans. For example, for parenteral administration, especially via the intravenous route, drugs must be formulated in solution form. Solubility of the drug in a particular solvent or a mixed solvent system will determine the limitation within which the drug may be formulated. Often, during the preclinical investigation phase, high concentrations or doses of drugs must be adminis-

Table 1.4   Physicochemical considerations for drug delivery

Drug molecular properties:
  lipophilicity
  molecular weight/size
  pK_a of the weak acid/base
  chemical stability
  enzymatic stability
Solubility:
  crystal form
  polymorphism
  coprecipitates
  particle size
  dissolution
  micellar solubilisation
  cosolvent solubilisation
  polymer complexation
  in vitro precipitation
  haemolysis
Molecular interactions:
  drug–drug complexation
  drug–drug interactions
  drug–mucoid polysaccharides
  drug–heavy metal ions
  protein binding
  adsorption

tered to determine the toxicological response. This creates a challenge for the pharmaceutical scientist, who must develop a formulation which not only will be in the solution form, but also must remain so without precipitation at the site of injection and in the body tissues and fluids. Furthermore, the drug or the formulation intended for intravenous route should not cause haemolysis or incompatibility with blood components. *In vitro* techniques for studying precipitation potential upon injection and haemolysis potential have been reported and are employed in the drug developement (Schroeder and Deluca, 1974; Yalkowsky *et al.*, 1983; Reed and Yalkowsky, 1985).

In whatever form the drug is presented or administered in the body, it must be available in the solution form, often after dissolution of solid dosage forms, before absorption across biological barriers can occur. Even when solutions with limited aqueous solubility are given via the oral route, they may precipitate in the stomach or intestinal region, because of either pH changes or solubility limitation, and then they must redissolve before absorption can occur. Drugs with low solubility usually dissolve slowly in the gastrointestinal tract. The rate of dissolution may be the rate-determining step in the absorption process. Drugs with poor or low aqueous solubility often present the greatest challenge for pharmaceutical scientists and frequently may be associated with bioavailability problems. For example, digitoxin, griseofulvin, some steroids, indomethacin, chlorpropamide and other drugs with low solubility are considered to have large variation in biological availability. Recently, the US Food and Drug Administration has stated that *in vivo* bioequivalency studies for drugs with bioavailability problems will be required whenever changes in formulation or manufacturing site occur (Dighe, 1988).

Because of limitations in aqueous solubility, various solubilisation techniques may be investigated to increase the apparent solubility and achieve the desired formulation goal. Solubilisation techniques, including the use of surface-active agents, e.g. polysorbates, sorbitan esters, quaternary ammonium compounds, sodium lauryl sulphates, etc., are often valuable tools in overcoming the limitations in aqueous solubility. These techniques have been successfully used for formulations of pharmaceutical compounds (Florence, 1981). However, the use of surface-active agents often presents toxicology problems and cannot be used for certain routes of administration.

Cosolvents such as polyethylene glycols, propylene glycol, glycerin and alcohol are often employed to improve the solubility behaviour of drugs with low solubility or poor stability in aqueous solutions. The solubility of drugs increases exponentially as a function of cosolvent concentration. In general, the lower the aqueous solubility, the greater the solubilising capacity of these cosolvents. Of course, some of these and other cosolvents have toxicological implications and constraints on the route of administration. Several drugs, such as digoxin, phenytoin sodium, diazepam, chlordiazepoxide, etc., are formulated in a variety of cosolvent systems (Wang and Korwal, 1980; Yalkowsky *et al.*, 1983). These types of drugs are often injected slowly in order to avoid precipitation or pain on injection (Yalkowsky and Valvani, 1977; Morris, 1978).

For drugs with weak ionisable groups, an improvement in solubility for drug formulation can be achieved by controlling the pH within reasonable bounds, depending on the ionisation constant (pK_a) of the drug molecule. Alternatively, an improvement in solubility can be accomplished by formation of a salt by chemical modification, complexation, coprecipitate formation and a variety of other techniques.

While low aqueous solubility may be a problem or limitation for the above situations, it is often desirable for most controlled-release or sustained-release delivery systems development. Often prodrugs or other chemical modification efforts are undertaken to reduce the solubility or improve solution stability (Anderson *et al.*, 1985a–c). The taste of organic drug molecules has been shown to be a function of aqueous solubility. For example, increasing the chain length of clindamycin esters, thus reducing aqueous solubility, dramatically improves the taste (Sinkula *et al.*, 1973).

For poorly absorbed drugs, which do not undergo significant degradation or first-pass metabolism, membrane permeability and the dose-to-solubility ratio are the key parameters controlling drug absorption (Amidon *et al.*, 1988). The membrane permeability for drugs absorbed by passive diffusion depends on the membrane–water or oil–water partition coefficient (a measure of lipophilicity). While solubility is one of the most important limiting factors in governing the flux across biological membranes, it is the combination of solubility and partition coefficient that influences the absorption and transport processes. It can be shown that biological activity may be dependent on concentration or dose and partition coefficient, concentration alone, solubility alone, or the product of solubility and partition coefficient.

Because of interdependence of solubility and partition coefficient, no single value for either parameters can be assigned. For example, an aqueous solubility of several micrograms/ml for a very potent drug requiring a few milligrams dose for therapeutic dose may suffice, but inadequate bioavailability may result for a drug with similar solubility which requires a therapeutic dose of several hundred milligrams. Similarly, a highly lipophilic drug may have low bioavailability because of its poor solubility and dissolution characteristics, while a drug which is too polar will probably exhibit poor transport properties.

Chemical and physical decomposition and degradation continually occur for most drugs and formulations in liquid or solid form. When drug formulations lose their potency by chemical degradation, the chemical potency should not fall below 90% of the labelled storage condition. Physical appearance, including other performance characteristics, e.g. dissolution rate, hardness, pH, etc., should still be within acceptable limits, otherwise they are considered subpotent and may no longer produce the desired pharmacological response. Thus, chemical and physical stability of the drug substance in solid and solution state under a variety of environmental conditions, e.g. light, humidity, temperature, pH, buffers, oxidation, solvents and physical stress, etc., provide the limitations and opportunities for successful design and development of dosage forms. Similarly, investigations of stability of formulations under most of these conditions, including testing under accelerated conditions, is critical to successful development for early clinical evaluation as well as for ultimate marketing. Process development, optimisation of formulations and validation are other important activities that must be carried out in later stages for large-scale manufacturing required for continued clinical evaluation or for marketing after regulatory approvals.

SUMMARY

To summarise, the drug discovery and development process involves a complex interplay of physicochemical, biological, dosage form and route of administration considerations. These considerations have significant impact on the biological performance of drugs by governing transport across biological barriers. A combination of these factors may be regarded as critical pharmaceutical considerations for successful formulation design and development. A thorough understanding and comparison of these by pharmaceutical scientists, medicinal chemists, biologists, clinicians, toxicologists and others involved in the drug design and development process can significantly improve the rational selection or design of drug molecules for early evaluation in animals and humans.

REFERENCES

Amidon, G. L., Sinko, P. J. and Fleisher, D. (1988). Estimating human oral fraction dose absorbed: a correlation using rat intestinal membrane permeability for passive and carrier-mediated compounds. *Pharm. Res.*, **5**, 651–4

Anderson, B. D., Conradi, R. A. and Knuth, K. E. (1985a). Strategies in the design of solution-stable, water-soluble prodrugs. I. A physical-organic approach to promoiety selection for 21-esters of corticosteroids. *J. Pharm. Sci.*, **74**, 365–74

Anderson, B. D., Conradi, R. A., Knuth, K. E. and Nail, S. L. (1985b). Strategies in the design of solution-stable, water-soluble prodrugs. II. Properties of micellar prodrugs of methylprednisolone. *J. Pharm. Sci.*, **74**, 375–81

Anderson, B. D., Conradi, R. A., Spillman, C. H. and Forbes, A. D. (1985c). Strategies in the design of solution-stable, water-soluble prodrugs. III. Influence of the promoiety on the bioconversion of 21-esters of corticosteroids. *J. Pharm. Sci.*, **74**, 382–7

Dighe, S. (1988). FDAs new policy on supplemental ANDAs for 'BP' rated products, requires *in vivo* bioequivalency data, may upgrade ratings to 'AB'. *FDC Reports*, **50**(39), 8

Florence, A. T. (1981). In Yalkowsky, S. H. (Ed.), *Techniques of Solubilization of Drugs*, Marcel Dekker, New York, pp. 15–89

Morris, M. E. (1978). Compatibility and stability of diazepam injection following dilution with intravenous fluids. *Am J. Hosp. Pharm.*, **35**, 669–72

Reed, K. W. and Yalkowsky, S. H. (1985). Lysis of human red blood cells in the presence of various cosolvents. *J. Parenteral Sci. Tech.*, **39**, 64–9

Schroeder, H. G. and DeLuca, P. P. (1974). A study on the *in vitro* precipitation of poorly soluble drugs from nonaqueous vehicles in human plasma. *Bull. Parenteral Drug Ass.*, **28**, 1–14

Sinkula, A. A., Morozowich, W. and Rowe, E. L. (1973). Chemical modification of clindamycin: synthesis and evaluation of selected esters. *J. Pharm. Sci.*, **62**, 1106

Wang, Y. J. and Korwal, R. R. (1980). Review of excipients and pHs for parenteral products used in the United States. *J. Parenteral Drug Ass.*, **34**, 452–62

Yalkowsky, S. H. and Valvani, S. C. (1977). Precipitation of solubilized drugs due to injection or dilution. *Drug Intell. Clin. Pharm.*, **11**, 417–19

Yalkowsky, S. H., Valvani, S. C. and Johnson B. W. (1983). *In vitro* method for detecting precipitation of parenteral formulations after injection. *J. Pharm. Sci.*, **72**, 1014–17

2
The Pharmacological Background

B. J. R. Whittle*, J. A. Salmon* and R. M. Ferris†

*Dept of Pharmacology, Wellcome Research Laboratories, Langley Court, Beckenham, Kent BR3 3BS, UK

†Burroughs Wellcome Co., Cornwallis Rd, Research Triangle Park, NC 27709, USA

INTRODUCTION

The pharmacological studies that must be conducted on a new chemical entity (NCE) to support the application for an CTX/IND or an MAA/NDA are not defined precisely by the regulatory authorities. Although most readers are probably familiar with the above abbreviations, they are defined here for clarification. Thus, the CTX is the exemption from the need to hold a full clinical trial certificate in UK and Europe; a similar stage of the development in the USA is an application to the Food and Drug Administration (FDA) for the Investigation of a New Drug (IND). At a later stage, a Marketing Authorisation Application (MAA; previously known as a Product Licence Application) and a New Drug Application (NDA) are submitted to the UK–European and USA agencies, respectively.

The toxicological data, as well as the absorption, metabolism, distribution and excretion (ADME) studies that are needed for submission, are identified, at least in general terms, by the Department of Health in the UK, by the European Drug Regulatory Authorities and by the FDA. The regulatory agencies also require for review suitable pharmacological–pharmacodynamic information about the NCE, although the nature and extent of the studies employed is largely the decision of the individual professional pharmacologist. The one exception is the regulatory authority in Japan. The Japanese Ministry of Health and Welfare, which is the Japanese regulatory and licensing authority, lists an extensive series of pharmacological tests which, by implication, are expected to be conducted and reported before permission for clinical study with the NCE will be granted. Since the requirements of the Japanese regulatory authority are also unique for the other preclinical disciplines, a separate chapter in this book is devoted to these specialised Japanese requirements, which are not, therefore, discussed further here.

In this chapter, primary consideration will be given to the development of pharmacological agents as therapeutic drugs, but a similar approach should be adopted for potential chemotherapeutic agents such as antiviral, anticancer or anti-parasitic drugs. In addition, products derived from biotechnological techniques should be evaluated in a comparable fashion, but since these agents may pose specific problems, investigators will have to apply their best scientific judgment.

REGULATORY REQUIREMENTS

Although the USA and European authorities differ in their specific requirements for toxicology and ADME studies, particularly at the CTX/IND stage, there are no significant variations in their general requirements for the pharmacological–pharmacodynamic information. Furthermore, the required format of the pharmacology reports for submission to the different regulatory authorities is similar. Although the regulatory agencies do not specify in detail the pharmacological tests which should be performed, they do provide guidance on the style and format for the reporting of the appropriate data.

Each of the regulatory authorities requires presentation of the pharmacological properties of the NCE in two separate sections: (1) the primary pharmacology, which should be concerned with the pharmacological actions relevant to the proposed therapeutic use; (2) the secondary pharmacology, which should describe other relevant activities of the NCE. These secondary tests are sometimes referred to as the 'safety pharmacology evaluation' but there is some concern about the use of the word 'safety' in this context. Thus, primary safety tests are conducted as part of the toxicological submission package and such studies must be conducted according to good laboratory practice (GLP) procedures. As will be discussed later, there are different opinions as to whether the pharmacological studies need to be performed according to GLP procedures. A third section on 'drug interactions', when appropriate to the NCE, is also required by the regulatory agencies.

ACTION RELEVANT TO THE PROPOSED THERAPEUTIC USE: PRIMARY PHARMACOLOGY

The term 'primary pharmacology' is employed in this section, although if the NCE is, for example, an antiviral or an antitumour agent, then the appropriate studies which support the primary activity for the proposed therapeutic utility of the compound should be reported. The authorities expect that the primary pharmacological properties of the NCE will be demonstrated by scientifically acceptable experimental techniques, and that these actions can be determined *in vivo* after administration by the route which will be used in the clinic.

The authorities expect to be able to review data which establish the mechanism of the principal pharmacological action. However, it may not be possible to explain fully the mechanism of action of some novel compounds. Indeed, this is particularly true of compounds that have been identified and selected by use of *in vivo* pharmacological models that assess the overall actions in a system rather than a precise pharmacological or biochemical effector mechanism. Although it is unlikely that a submission will fail if the pharmacological or biochemical mechanism of action is not fully elucidated, it is clearly desirable to establish the mode of action, if only for scientific and clinical reasons. Obviously the type and extent of these studies will depend on the particular NCE, and this is one reason why the regulatory authorities cannot, and do not, define the precise studies which should be performed.

The authorities do require appropriate validation of the experimental models and technical procedures employed in the studies. It would, therefore, be expedient to utilise procedures which are generally accepted by the scientific community as being appropriate and reliable, or to present information which illustrates the validity of the techniques and data. The guidelines published by the authorities also suggest that, where possible, the evaluation of the NCE should be performed in parallel with a standard drug of the same therapeutic class. As with most of the advice given by the authorities, this approach can be regarded as good scientific policy. However, if the NCE has a novel mode of action, it may not be possible or valid to undertake such comparisons, and, once again, it is anticipated that sound scientific judgement will be applied to the nature of the studies undertaken.

It is appropriate that the data should be expressed and presented in quantitative terms. The authorities not only expect to have the opportunity to review dose-related effects, but also would hope to assess the time-course of the activity. Thus, the relationship of the pharmacodynamics to the pharmacokinetic profile of the NCE should be considered. Indeed, there is a growing expectancy of the regulatory authorities that the pharmacological and pharmacodynamic studies should be linked closely to the pharmacokinetic evaluation, and, if possible, be conducted within the same series of experiments. When submitting data to the European authorities at the MAA stage, one has the opportunity to draw attention to the relationship of the pharmacodynamic findings to the pharmacokinetic profile in the 'Expert Report'.

OTHER ACTIONS DEMONSTRATED OR SOUGHT: SECONDARY PHARMACOLOGY

The primary safety evaluation of the NCE will be reported in the toxicology section of the application. However, a general pharmacological profile of the NCE is also required, with special attention to any effects additional to the primary pharmacological action. The aim of the secondary pharmacological studies should be to establish the effects on the major physiological systems by use of a variety of experimental models. Indeed, the Japanese authorities have suggested that another scientific reason for conducting the secondary pharmacological tests could be to explore whether the NCE has other potential clinical utilities. Data on the effects of the NCE on the cardiovascular and respiratory systems, and on the overall behaviour of laboratory animals, is expected. More extensive investigation is also required if the dose of the NCE that produces secondary effects approaches that producing the primary therapeutic effect.

The particular series of experiments conducted for the secondary pharmacological evaluation will, to some extent, depend on the research philosophy of the pharmaceutical house. An organisation which relies on random screening for discovery of drugs often includes in its submission of the NCE a large number of routine screens and tests which probably have no particular relevance to the proposed therapeutic utility. An example would be the determination of the anti-inflammatory properties of a new antihypertensive agent. In contrast, a company which has a focused drug discovery programme will probably only conduct selected experiments considered appropriate to these needs. Good scientific judgement is therefore required to decide on the nature and extent of these pharmacological studies. Thus, if the NCE which is to be used as an anti-inflammatory agent produces notable cardiovascular effects in experimental studies *in vivo*, it would be useful, and probably required, to establish the cause of such effects. In such cases, therefore, additional studies may be required—for example, by evaluation of the NCE in specific vascular beds *in vivo* or on isolated vascular tissues *in vitro*.

The guidelines published by the USA, the UK and the European authorities suggest that the secondary pharmacological activities of the NCE should be reported under the headings listed in Table 2.1. This list, therefore, gives an indication of the type of studies that the authorities expect to review. Although there are minor differences in the lists, principally in the terminology used to define the studies, it is probable that either list could be used as a general guide for writing reports on the NCE to be submitted to any of the drug regulatory agencies. Separate reporting on each facet of the various experimental studies on the NCE is encouraged for clarity and for ease of assimilation of the data.

The studies performed as part of the secondary pharmacology evaluation of

Table 2.1 Secondary pharmacological evaluation of new chemical entities

UK and Europe	USA
Central nervous system	Neuropharmacology
Autonomic system	Cardiovascular/respiratory
Cardiovascular system	Gastrointestinal
Respiratory system	Genitourinary
Gastrointestinal system	Endocrine
Other systems where relevant	Anti-inflammatory
	Immunoactive
	Chemotherapeutic
	Enzyme effects
	Other

These lists and terminologies are derived from the recommendations of the respective regulatory authorities, as laid out in the 'EEC Notice to Applicants. International Standard Book Number 92–825–9503 X' and the 'Guideline for the format and content of the nonclinical pharmacology/ toxicology section of an application. Centre for Drugs and Biologies, Food and Drug Administration, Department of Health and Human Services, Washington, USA, February 1987'.

the NCE can be classified according to those which are the essential or core studies and those which are necessary to define undesirable side-effects, observed in these core experiments. It is apparent that there is a reasonable agreement within the pharmaceutical industry about what constitutes the core pharmacological test package.

Central Nervous System

Almost without exception, the pharmaceutical industry assesses the overall behavioural effects of the NCE in mice (see Irwin, 1962, 1968). Behavioural changes induced by the NCE, such as hypoactivity and ataxia, are subjectively evaluated over a range of doses. Such studies in mice also serve to give an indication of the effect of the NCE on the autonomic nervous system; for example, any influence of the NCE on salivation, pupil size, penile erection, ear coloration or respiratory rate should be noted and reported. A few pharmacological laboratories do perform a similar series of tests in rats rather than in mice, yet in most instances there is no clear advantage.

Most companies monitor the interaction of the NCE with convulsant agents, as well as their effects on writhing induced by acetic acid, phenylbenzoquinone or acetylcholine in mice (Siegmund *et al.*, 1957; Koster *et al.*, 1959; Collier *et al.*, 1968; Follenfant *et al.*, 1988). The effect on barbiturate-induced sleeping time (Aston, 1966) is often included as part of the CNS evaluation. This latter study can also provide a valuable early indication of the effect of the NCE on liver metabolism, since liver enzyme induction or inhibition may be indicated by a decrease or increase in sleeping time, respectively.

Autonomic System

In addition to recording any effects resulting from autonomic interactions in the behavioural studies, it is usual to evaluate the *in vivo* effects of the NCE on the autonomic nervous system in more detail, using appropriate pharmacological techniques (see Davey and Reinert, 1965; Hughes and Chapple, 1976, 1981; Cavero *et al.*, 1978).

Cardiovascular System

The majority of pharmaceutical companies evaluate the cardiovascular profile of the NCE in some detail, including changes in heart rate and systemic arterial blood pressure, in both anaesthetised and conscious laboratory animals. Thus, a routine choice is to study the cardiovascular actions of these agents in both anaesthetised and conscious rats and dogs, using established experimental techniques (for example, see Cambridge *et al.*, 1988). However, other species may also be used, such as cats or monkeys (see Allan *et al.*, 1985), if it is considered appropriate or necessary to define the actions of that particular NCE in these species.

Respiratory System

The effects of the NCE on bronchopulmonary parameters, including respiratory rate and tidal flow minute volume, are usually determined in the conscious or anaesthetised cat or dog by use of standard experimental approaches (see Widdicombe, 1966). Occasionally these respiratory parameters are determined in the anaesthetised or conscious guinea-pig (Payne *et al.*, 1988). It can be useful to evaluate the respiratory effects in the same animals that are used to monitor the cardiovascular actions of the NCE.

Gastrointestinal System

As an overall index of gastrointestinal motility, most pharmaceutical companies investigate the effect of the NCE on the transit of a polyvinyl chloride or charcoal meal or of phenol red along the gastrointestinal tract following oral administration in mice or rats (Green, 1959; Scarpignato *et al.*, 1980).

ADDITIONAL SECONDARY PHARMACOLOGY

In addition to the core studies, a number of other studies are performed in some pharmacological laboratories, although these experiments often reflect the research interests and expertise available in the individual companies. Alternatively, they may be performed in response to particular observations made in the core studies. For example, an unexpected vascular response elicited during a cardiovascular study *in vivo* may be followed up with an assessment of the effects of the NCE on isolated preparations of heart or other organs *in vitro*, in order to establish the mechanism underlying such a response. Some of the additional studies that may be conducted are outlined below.

Central Nervous System

A few pharmaceutical companies consider that investigation of the effect of new compounds on the behaviour of cats or dogs is necessary for the secondary pharmacological evaluation, although it is a general experience that the regulatory authorities are satisfied if such behavioural studies on the NCE are only conducted in rodents. Other secondary tests that are conducted under rare circumstances include more detailed evaluation of the effects of the NCE on the EEG or on tetrabenazine-induced sedation and ptosis in rats (Vernier *et al.*, 1962).

Autonomic System

In addition to the core studies, the effect of the NCE on the autonomic nervous system may be evaluated further by use of suitable isolated tissue preparations *in vitro* and, occasionally, relevant ligand binding experiments. Such tests would not, however, be considered essential.

Cardiovascular System

The most pertinent cardiovascular studies will have been conducted as part of the core package. In addition, the arrhythmogenic or antiarrhythmic activity of the NCE may be determined in mouse, rat, cat or dog preparations (see Pool and Sonnenblick, 1967; Lawson, 1968; Wit *et al.*, 1970; Lubbe *et al.*, 1978). The evaluation of the NCE on isolated vascular smooth muscle is also sometimes included in the dossier submitted to the regulatory authorities.

Respiratory System

Occasionally, blood gas analysis following administration of the NCE to the rat or other species is reported in the submission.

Gastrointestinal System

The effects of new compounds on gastric acid secretion in anaesthetised rats or specific measurements of gastrointestinal motility in rats or rabbits are usually only reported if the NCE is expected to have a direct effect on these parameters by virtue of its pharmacological profile. Studies of the spasmogenic actions of the NCE on isolated gastrointestinal smooth muscle may also be reported.

Other Relevant Systems

Renal

Many companies monitor the effect of the NCE on diuresis in salt-loaded rats as part of the routine pharmacological profile. Other companies only include these studies if an effect is predicted or has been suggested from other studies, such as following cardiovascular evaluation in conscious dogs or rats. A more detailed evaluation of the effects of the NCE on renal function—for example, in conscious dogs—should be conducted if indicated in these preliminary tests.

Inflammation

The general anti-inflammatory activity of the NCE is sometimes included as part of the submissions of some pharmaceutical companies. These studies may include inhibition of adjuvant-induced arthritis (Curry and Ziff, 1968) and inhibition of carrageenan-induced hyperalgesia, pain or oedema in rats (Winter *et al.*, 1962; Vinegar *et al.*, 1973; Higgs *et al.*, 1988). However, this information probably does not serve any major purpose unless appropriate for the anticipated clinical utility. These data on the NCE are often generated in general screening schemes, and once they are available it is felt that they should be reported. If the compound exhibits proinflammatory reactions, clearly this property should be reported and, if possible, examined in more detail, as an indication of a potential side-effect of the NCE.

Platelet Function

If appropriate, the activity of the NCE on human platelet aggregation can readily be assessed *in vitro* (Born, 1962; Whittle, 1987) and such an evaluation may provide useful preclinical information. Studies on platelet function *ex vivo* following administration of the NCE can also be determined (Allan *et al.*, 1985). The effects on other haematological parameters are usually conducted as part of the toxicological investigation.

Drug Interactions

The regulatory agencies request that relevant pharmacological studies on the interaction of the NCE with other drugs that the patient is likely to receive be reported in a separate section of the submission. Furthermore, interaction studies may also be required with respect to anticipated excipients of the drug delivery system for the NCE.

ADDITIONAL COMMENTS

The regulatory requirements are, by necessity, constantly evolving and being refined but some trends that are emerging deserve some comment.

One important question is whether the pharmacological studies should be conducted according to GLP procedures. Clearly, all work submitted to the regulatory agencies is expected to be of a high scientific standard and fully validated. The regulatory agencies have not insisted, and do not yet insist, that pharmacological studies meet GLP requirements, although the guidelines on this aspect are vague and somewhat ambiguous. The decision to use GLP for these studies is left, at the present time, to the laboratory or company conducting the experiments, but whether this will eventually become a requirement is uncertain. There are obviously greater logistical problems in performing the primary pharmacological studies according to strict GLP procedures, and, therefore, it is less likely that these studies will attract such requirements.

Another question that is receiving considerable attention at the present time is how, or whether, a compound which is known to be a mixture of isomers should be developed and assessed. Obviously this is a debate of general interest which is not just confined to the pharmacological assessment of the NCE. However, it is clear that it will be important to determine whether the pharmacological activities, both primary and secondary, reside in one specific isomer. A similar question being actively discussed within the scientific and legislative community is how compounds with known impurities should be evaluated and developed.

The introduction of the Expert Report at the MAA stage will have a significant impact on the presentation of the submission to the European authorities, although there is no corresponding requirement of an 'expertise' for the US authorities. The European Expert Report should present a critical evaluation of the experimental studies and interpretation of the pharmacological data, with the relationship to the ADME and toxicological results adequately discussed. Thus, the Expert Report is a medium for justifying and explaining the preclinical development of the product. Much of the key experimental data will be expected to be included as appendices in appropriately designed tables. This may initially increase the editorial time needed to complete the dossier but the benefit of a standard presentation for the regulatory authorities should become apparent, and will eventually expedite the preparation of subsequent dossiers.

The FDA has started to consider the submission of data by electronic means—for example, the computer-assisted NDA (CANDA). It is anticipated that, as these systems evolve, such approaches will become an accepted method of transmitting data to regulatory agencies in the future. Therefore, it is apparent that industrial pharmacologists, as well as scientists from the other disciplines concerned with generating and submitting data for consideration by regulatory authorities, will need to keep abreast of developments in information technology.

BIBLIOGRAPHY

Allan, G., Follenfant, M. J., Lidbury, P., Oliver, P. L. and Whittle, B. J. R. (1985). The cardiovascular and platelet actions of 9β-methyl carbacyclin (ciprostene), a chemically stable analogue of prostacyclin, in the dog and monkey. *Br. J. Pharmacol.*, **85**, 547–55

Aston, R. (1966). Acute tolerance indices for pentobarbital in male and female rats. *J. Pharmacol. Exp. Ther.*, **152**, 350–3

Born, G. V. R. (1962). Aggregation of blood platelets by adenosine diphosphate and its reversal. *Nature*, Lond., **194**, 927–9

Cambridge, D., Whiting, M. V. and Allan, G. (1988). Cardiac and renovascular effects in the anaesthetised dog of BW A575C: a novel antiotensin converting enzyme inhibitor with β-adrenoceptor blocking properties. *Br. J. Pharmacol.*, **93**, 165–75

Cavero, I., Fenand, S., Gomeni, R., Lefevre, F. and Roach, A. G. (1978). Studies on the mechanism of the vasodilator effects of prazosin in dogs and rabbits. *Eur. J. Pharmacol.*, **49**, 259–70

Collier, H. O. J., Dinneen, L. C., Johnson, C. A. and Schneider, C. (1968). The abdominal constriction response and its suppression by analgesic drugs in the mouse. *Br. J. Pharmacol.*, **32**, 295–310

Currey, H. L. F. and Ziff, M. (1968). Suppression of adjuvant disease in the rat by heterologous antilymphocyte globulin. *J. Exp. Med.*, **127**, 185–203

Davey, M. J. and Reinert, H. (1965). Pharmacology of the antihypertensive, guanoxan. *Br. J. Pharmacol.*, **241**, 29–48

Follenfant, R. L., Hardy, G. W., Lowe, L. A., Schneider, C. and Smith, T. W. (1988). Antinociceptive effects of the novel opioid peptide BW 443C compared with classical opiates; peripheral versus central actions. *Br. J. Pharmacol.*, **93**, 85–92

Green, A. F. (1959). Comparative effects of analgesics on pain threshold, respiratory frequency and gastrointestinal propulsion. *Br. J. Pharmacol. Chemother.*, **14**, 26–34

Higgs, G. A., Follenfant, R. L. and Garland, L. G. (1988). Selective inhibition of arachidonate 5-lipoxygenase by novel acetohydroxamic acids: effects on acute inflammatory responses. *Br. J. Pharmacol.*, **94**, 547–51

Hughes, R. and Chapple, D. J. (1965). Effects of non-depolarising neuromuscular blocking agents on peripheral autonomic mechanisms in cats. *Br. J. Anaesth.*, **48**, 59–68

Hughes, R. and Chapple, D. J. (1981). The pharmacology of atracurium: a new competitive neuromuscular blocking agent. *Br. J. Anaesth.*, **53**, 31–44

Irwin, S. (1962). Drug screening and evaluative procedures. *Science, N.Y.*, **136**, 123–8

Irwin, S. (1968). Comprehensive Observational Assessment. Ia. A systemic, quantitative procedure for assessing the behavioural and physiologic state of the mouse. *Psychopharm. (Berlin)*, **13**, 222–57

Koster, R., Anderson, M. and de Beer, E. J. (1959). Acetic acid for analgesic screening. *Fed. Proc.*, **18**, 412

Lawson, J. W. (1968). Antiarrhythmic activity of some isoquinoline derivatives determined by a rapid screening procedure in the mouse. *J. Pharmacol. Exp. Ther.*, **160**, 22–31

Lubbe, W. F., Daries, P. S. and Opie, L. H. (1978). Ventricular arrhythmias associated with coronary artery occlusion and reperfusion in the isolated perfused rat heart: a model for assessement of antifibrillatory action of antiarrhythmic agents. *Cardiovascular Res.*, **12**, 212–20

Payne, A. N., Garland, L. G., Lees, I. W. and Salmon, J. A. (1988). Selective inhibition of arachidonate 5-lipoxygenase by novel acetohydroxamic acids: effects on bronchial anaphylaxis in anaesthetised guinea-pigs. *Br. J. Pharmacol.*, **94**, 540–6

Pool, P. E. and Sonnenblick, E. H. (1967). The mechanochemistry of cardiac muscle. I. The isometric contraction. *J. Gen. Physiol.*, **50**, 951–65

Scarpignato, C., Capovelle, T. and Bertaccini, G. (1980). Action of caerulein on gastric emptying of the conscious rat. *Arch. Int. Pharmacodyn.*, **246**, 286–94

Siegmund, E., Cadmus, R. and Lu, G. (1957). A method for evaluating both non-narcotic and narcotic analgesics. *Proc. Soc. Exp. Biol. Med.*, **95**, 729–31

Vernier, V. G., Hanson, H. M. and Stone, C. A. (1962). The pharmacodynamics of amitriptyline. In Nadine, J. H. and Moyer, J. H. (Eds.), *1st Hahnemann Symposium on Psychosomatic Medicine*. Lea and Febiger, Philadelphia, pp. 683–90

Vinegar, R., Truax, J. F. and Selph, J. L. (1973). Some quantitative temporal characteristics of carrageenan-induced pleurisy in the rat. *Proc. Soc. Exp. Biol. Med.*, **143**, 711–14

Whittle, B. J. R. (1987). Aggregometry techniques for prostanoid study and evaluation. In Benedetto, C., McDonald-Gibson, R. G., Nigan, S. and Slater, T. F. (Eds.), *Prostaglandins and Related Substances—A Practical Approach*. IRL Press, Oxford, pp. 151–66

Widdicombe, J. G. (1966). Action potentials in parasympathetic and sympathetic efferent fibres to the trachea and lungs of dogs and cats. *J. Physiol.*, **186**, 56–88

Winter, C. A., Risley, E. A. and Nuss, G. W. (1962). Carrageenan-induced oedema in hind paw of the rat as an assay for anti-inflammatory drugs. *Proc. Soc. Exp. Biol. Med.*, **111**, 544–7

Wit, A. L., Steiner, C. and Damato, A. N. (1970). Electrophysiologic effects of bretylium tosylate on single fibres of the canine specialised conducting system and ventricle. *J. Pharmacol. Exp. Ther.*, **173**, 344–56

3
The Metabolic Background

Wade J. Adams

Drug Metabolism Research, The Upjohn Company, 7000 Portage Road, Kalamazoo, MI 49001, USA

INTRODUCTION

Preclinical drug absorption, distribution, metabolism and excretion studies, collectively referred to as drug disposition studies, are of fundamental importance to the interpretation and rationalisation of animal pharmacology and toxicology data, and the extrapolation of these data to humans. An assessment of the exposure of animals and humans to a drug and its metabolites must be made on a more scientific basis than can be provided by simply comparing dosage levels. Dose alone is not a satisfactory index of exposure, especially when comparing across species, since the same dose may result in very different levels of exposure because of species variations in drug disposition, particularly variations in metabolism. Not only is the disposition of a drug species-dependent, but also a number of physiological, pathological, genetic and environmental factors are now known to influence the disposition of drugs in the same individual or population (Bousquet, 1970; Smith, 1988).

Early position papers (Drug Research Board, 1969) and regulatory statements (World Health Organization, 1966; Goldenthal, 1968) stressed the importance of using, in toxicology studies, animal species that have a metabolic pattern qualitatively similar to that of humans so that test animals are broadly exposed to the same array of metabolites as humans. Because of the lack of adequate basic animal pharmacology data for many species, only a few animal species can realistically be considered for safety testing, with the rat, dog or monkey, rabbit and mouse almost invariably used. Thus, the pronouncement to use animal species that have a metabolic pattern similar to that of humans must be regarded as a reminder to consider interspecies differences in metabolism in the interpretation and rationalisation of safety data, and to select from available animal species those that have metabolism most like that of humans. It has been suggested that it may be possible to take advantage of the marked strain differences in drug metabolism that exist within some species to find a strain that is more representative of the human situation (Smith, 1988).

More recently, the importance of obtaining comparative metabolic and pharmacokinetic data over the dosage range of the drug in animal species has been emphasised (EEC Commission, 1980; Glockin, 1982). Across-species assessments of exposure to drugs and their metabolites is best made on the basis of quantitative pharmacokinetic parameters such as maximum plasma concentration, area under plasma concentration–time curve (AUC), systemic clearance and terminal disposition half-life. These data allow an assessment of the extent and duration of exposure to the drug and indicate whether metabolic patterns change with dosage. High dose exposure may saturate major metabolic pathways and result in alternative pathway metabolism or metabolic switching. Metabolic switching can result in a different array of metabolites or, at the very least, in a change in the relative proportions of metabolites as compared with the low dose situation. High dose exposure may also lead to non-linear pharmacokinetics (i.e. AUC does not increase in proportion to drug dose), which may result in prolonged exposure and bioaccumulation in test species. The use of high doses in chronic safety studies where metabolic switching and/or non-linear pharmacokinetics can occur may confound the interpretation of data and cause major problems in safety assessment. Although high dose administration may reveal the toxic potential of drugs, particularly affected target organs, it is very difficult to use the results of such studies for safety assessment when therapeutic doses result in exposure that may be many orders of magnitude lower than where metabolic switching and/or non-linear pharmacokinetics do not occur. An additional concern in chronic dosing studies is the possibility of a drug inhibiting or inducing its own metabolism. Induction of drug metabolism with chronic exposure to a drug may result in the accelerated metabolism of the drug, thereby causing a lower than expected exposure.

Ideally, drug disposition studies should be conducted at an early enough stage of drug development to allow an assessment of the validity of the animal model in terms of qualitative and quantitative dispositional behaviour. The dosage and dosage regimen of the drug can then be appropriately adjusted to take into account interspecies differences in drug exposure. Comparative disposition studies may also provide insight into mechanisms of toxicity due to overexposure within particular species or to the formation of toxic or reactive metabolites. This information may provide a basis for a species-dependent toxic effect, and the relevance of this effect to the human situation can then be more readily assessed.

PRECLINICAL DRUG DISPOSITION STUDIES

Although *in vitro* studies are necessary to understand the intimate details of biological and biochemical processes and provide a great deal of insight into the disposition of drugs and their mechanism of action, they cannot replace *in vivo* studies. As is schematically depicted in Figure 3.1, the *in vivo* situation is infinitely more complex in that (1) the administered drug must traverse tissue barriers to reach its site of action; (2) a substantial fraction of the drug may be bound to blood components in the vascular system from which it may be slowly released; (3) the drug may be metabolised to active, inactive or reactive metabolites in a variety of tissues; (4) the drug must be distributed to tissues where it exerts its pharmacological effect, but will also be distributed along with its metabolites to other body tissues from which it may be slowly released or where it may react with macromolecules; and (5) the drug and/or its metabolites are eliminated from the body by excretion. Thus, the intensity and duration of action of drugs whose pharmacological and toxicological effects are dose-dependent and reversible are governed by the rates of drug input or absorption, distribution to tissues and elimination by metabolism or excretion (Ariens, 1966). For drugs that produce their effects indirectly by depletion of pharmacologically active endogenous substances, the intensity and duration of drug response are dependent on the rate of biosynthesis of the endogenous substance.

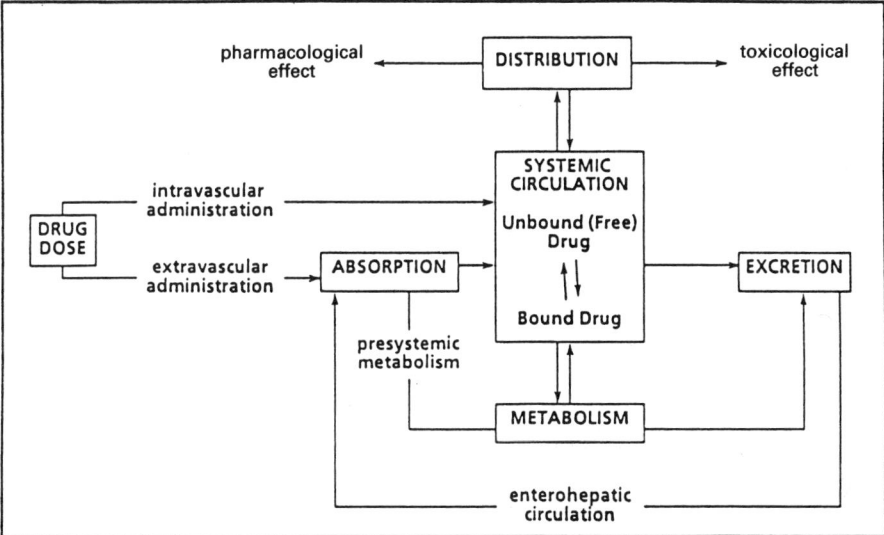

Figure 3.1 Schematic representation of *in vivo* absorption, distribution, metabolism and excretion

On the basis of the complexity of the *in vivo* situation, it is hardly surprising that the disposition of drugs is species-dependent and is affected by a broad range of physiological, pathological, genetic and environmental factors. As a consequence, it is critical to control these factors in disposition studies and, where appropriate, study their effects. A brief description of the preclinical drug disposition studies that may be relevant to the rational pharmacological and toxicological evaluation of drugs is presented below, along with a discussion of some of the factors that affect drug disposition.

GENERAL GUIDELINES

The conduct of *in vivo* drug disposition studies should be viewed as an essential adjunct to pharmacology and safety studies, and not as a regulatory exercise. The establishment of a 'checklist' or rigid protocol approach to the conduct of these studies is not appropriate, because of the diversity in the types of drugs under investigation and their novelty. Instead, a guidelines approach to drug development is preferred, in which studies are tailored to the specific drug and its intended clinical use (Glockin, 1982; Smith, 1988). The following general guidelines should be considered when conducting drug disposition studies.

(1) Disposition studies should be synchronised with acute and subchronic safety studies, prior to the initiation of chronic toxicology and carcinogenicity studies.

(2) The species, strain, sex and age of animals used in metabolism and disposition studies should be consistent with those used in safety studies; but information from animals of other species, strains, ages or altered physiological states may indicate important qualitative or quantitative differences in disposition which are important for the interpretation of pharmacological and toxicological data.

(3) Drug doses administered in disposition studies are dependent on the purpose of the study but should be representative of the range of doses used in pharmacology and safety studies.

(4) The routes of administration and dosage formulations used in disposition and safety studies should be comparable, except for disposition studies that are specifically conducted to evaluate the biopharmaceutical characteristics of the drug and its dosage formulations.

(5) Absolute (systemic) and/or relative bioavailability studies should be conducted to determine the absorption and pharmacokinetic characteristics of different forms and formulations of the drug used in definitive safety studies.

(6) Administration of drugs in safety studies as a bolus or as drug–diet mixtures should be based on the disposition characteristics of the drug, to ensure appropriate exposure to the drug.

(7) When safety tests have been conducted by one route of administration and studies by a new route are proposed, the disposition characteristics of the drug by both routes should be compared, to assess the extent of further safety testing required for the new route.

(8) Additional disposition studies may be required if absorption problems, unusual toxic dose–response relationships or notable species differences in toxicity are observed in safety studies.

It is important to remember that guidelines are intended to identify minimal criteria for producing consistent and comparable data. Guidelines should not suppress innovative research or the conduct of special studies beyond their specifications.

PRELUDE

Analytical Methodology

The development of suitable analytical methodology for the identification and quantification of parent drugs and their metabolites is an essential and highly challenging component of drug disposition studies. Furthermore, it frequently represents a challenge that may extend over the entire course of drug development, since new and more sensitive analyatical methodology is usually required as more is learned about the metabolism of drugs, and as ever-lower drug concentrations are encountered on progressing from acute animal toxicology studies to human efficacy studies.

The use of detection techniques that are highly sensitive and specific to the parent drug and its metabolites is preferred for quantitative studies. In this regard, the use of radioactive isotopes has been of inestimable value, because of the high sensitivity, specificity to parent drug and metabolites, and absolute unit of measurement they provide (Mertel, 1979). Radioisotopes most commonly used in metabolism and disposition studies are fairly long-lived weak β-emitters, namely ^{14}C and ^{3}H, with ^{14}C being the isotope of choice. An *in vivo* mass balance study should be conducted, usually in the rat, after the chemical stability of the radiolabelled drug has been established, to ensure that the drug has been labelled in a metabolically stable site. Loss of the radiolabel during the course of *in vivo* metabolism and disposition studies may confound the interpretation of these studies and result in excessive exposure of species to ionising radiation. On occasion, a test drug may have to be labelled in multiple sites with different label atoms to obtain a comprehensive assessment of its metabolism and disposition.

Chromatographic methods that use sensitive non-radiotracer detection techniques, particularly high-performance liquid chromatography and gas chromatography, are also widely used for the quantification of parent drugs and metabolites in biological specimens. Characterisation and identification of metabolites is usually accomplished by use of mass spectrometry and, on occasion, nuclear magnetic resonance spectroscopy.

Physicochemical Properties

Physicochemical properties such as molecular size and shape, lipid-to-water partition coefficient or lipophilicity, pK_a and solubility have a major effect on the disposition of drugs inasmuch as drugs must gain entry to the body and/or body tissues by penetration of a succession of lipoidal membranes. Ideally, the physicochemical properties of drugs should be evaluated prior to the selection of a drug candidate for development.

Drugs and their metabolites cross membranes in one of three ways: by filtration through pores, by specialised transport systems or by passive diffusion (Pang, 1983). Very small molecular species are filtered through small pores (70 Å) in the membrane. Larger molecular species that are chemically similar to endogenous cellular substrates may be transported across membranes by specialised transport systems such as facilitated diffusion or active transport. In both facilitated diffusion and active transport, the drug is transported across the membrane as a drug–carrier complex. Both of these processes can become saturated and both are competitively inhibited by substrates that utilise the same mechanism. Most drugs penetrate membranes by passive diffusion, which is dependent on the lipid-to-water partition coefficient or lipophilicity of the drug and the concentration gradient of the drug between the two phases that exist on opposite sides of the membrane. In the case of drugs that are protein-bound, only the free or unbound drug can passively diffuse across the membrane. The partition coefficient has been shown to have a parabolic effect on absorption rate, analogous to its effect on the biological activity of the compound (Hansch and Clayton, 1973). As the partition coefficient approaches zero, the compound will be so insoluble in lipid that it will not cross the membrane and will remain localised in the first aqueous phase that it contacts. Conversely, as the partition coefficient becomes very large, the compound will be so insoluble in the aqueous phase that it will tend to localise or accumulate in the lipoidal membrane.

Most drugs are weak organic electrolytes that may exist in the body in ionised or un-ionised form, depending on their pK_a and the pH of the medium. Since the un-ionised form of the drug is more soluble in lipoidal membranes, the un-ionised form of the drug is most readily transported across body membranes. Hence, the penetration of body membranes by these drugs can be predicted on the basis of their partition coefficient, their pK_a and the pH at the membrane surface.

Although it may not be feasible to ascertain the quantitative effect of aqueous solubility on the absorption of compounds following extravascular administration, it can provide insight into probable absorption difficulties, since a compound must be in solution before it can be transported through body membranes. As a general rule, aqueous solubilities greater than 1% (1 g/100 ml) would not be indicative of oral absorption problems due to solubility. It is important to recognise that the 1% solubility figure is arbitrary and does not represent a universal limitation on solubility. Other factors have to be considered in determining the influence of low aqueous solubility on drug absorption. These factors include the size of the therapeutic dose, the solubility and intrinsic dissolution rate as a function of pH within the physiological range, and the dissolution rate as a function of particle size or surface area of the compound (Kaplan, 1973). Even in the case of intravascular drug administration, adequate aqueous solubility is necessary so that the drug does not precipitate *in vivo*, and can be formulated in a vehicle that is well tolerated and does not cause the aggregation of vascular components.

ABSORPTION AND PHARMACOKINETICS

Absorption and pharmacokinetic studies should be conducted very early in the drug evaluation process in conjunction with pharmacology and toxicology studies to determine the temporal relationship between systemic drug levels and pharmacological and toxicological effects. These studies should be designed to gain insight into the rate and extent of absorption and to obtain a quantitative assessment of the extent and duration of systemic exposure to the drug. Pulmonary, intramuscular and subcutaneous routes of administration resemble the intravenous route, although the rate of delivery into the systemic circulation will be dependent on blood flow within the specific tissues. Administration by inhalation results in the delivery of drug via both the oral and pulmonary routes, with most of the dose (approximately 90%) being delivered orally. The intraperitoneal route is frequently used in animal studies on the basis of the assumption, which is not always valid (Pang, 1983), that the entire dose will be absorbed into the portal circulation and delivered to the liver, analogous to oral absorption from the gastrointestinal tract. The oral route is most commonly used in clinical situations; consequently, it will be the focus of discussion.

Biopharmaceutical as well as pharmacological and toxicological properties of drugs should be considered when evaluating the potential of a lead compound as a drug. In the case of orally administered drugs, the form of the drug having the greatest potential for absorption should be selected for development. After the biopharmaceutical properties of the drug have been defined, the effect of formulation variables can be determined. The formulation of the drug as a solution that can be administered intravenously is very desirable for the conduct of these studies, since a solution represents the most bioavailable formulation of the drug and is a suitable reference formulation with which all other formulations can be compared. A number of physiological factors influence oral absorption, including transit time, gastrointestinal pH, presence of food, microbial flora, and metabolic enzymes in the gut wall and liver (Kaplan, 1973). Control of these variables is important, when conducting absorption studies, to obtain consistent data. The effect of food on the rate and extent of absorption of lipophilic drugs should be evaluated, since food frequently improves the extent of their absorption. The dog represents the most convenient animal species for the conduct of biopharmaceutic studies, since unit dosage formulations can be administered, and serial blood specimens can be collected without difficulty. However, the monkey should be considered for these studies if the disposition of the drug class in dogs is known to differ from that in humans (Kaplan, 1973).

The most direct way of assessing drug absorption *in vivo* is to compare blood and, if possible, urinary levels of parent drug following administration of the drug by the intended route and by the intravenous route. If absorption is less than quantitative and/or presystemic metabolism of the drug occurs (e.g. in the gut wall or liver for an orally administered drug), then blood levels of intact drug will differ after extravascular and intravenous administration. The ratio between the areas under the concentration–time curves by the intended route and the intravenous route, normalised for drug dose, is defined as the systemic bioavailability and provides a quantitative measure of the extent to which the drug reaches the systemic circulation.

Assessment of drug absorption is greatly facilitated by the use of radiolabelled drug, since both the intact drug and metabolites can be readily measured in blood, urine, faeces or other excreta. These radiotracer studies are frequently referred to as mass balance or absorption and excretion studies, since they provide quantitative information about the rate and extent of drug absorption and the routes and extent to which the parent drug and its metabolites are excreted. Absorption and excretion studies are usually done sequentially in the rat and non-rodent (dog and/or monkey) prior to the administration of the drug to humans, and at dosage levels that are representative of the doses used in pharmacology and subchronic toxicity studies. These studies are also conducted in other species used in the toxicological evaluation of the drug. Human radiotracer studies are only conducted after mass balance and tissue distribution studies have been conducted in animals and the tolerance of humans to single doses of the drug has been established. This ensures that safe and appropriate doses of radiotracer are administered to humans after the need to do such studies has been established. The conduct of radiotracer studies in humans should not be considered if non-radiotracer analytical methodology is available that can quantitatively account for the excretion of parent drug and metabolites. Radiotracer studies in humans are not conducted in Japan, because of regulatory restrictions on the use of radioisotopes in human subjects.

Although concentration–time profiles of total radioactivity are useful for assessing the duration of exposure to drug-related material and for radiation dosimetry calculations, they are not useful for pharmacokinetic purposes. An understanding of the pharmacokinetics of a drug and its metabolites requires the specific measurement of each component, including any stereoisomers (Smith, 1988). Determination of maximum blood concentration, time at which the maximum blood concentration is achieved, area under the concentration–time curve, systemic clearance and terminal disposition half-life are important for a quantitative assessment of drug exposure. Information about the volume of distribution and rate and extent of elimination of the parent drug and metabolites is also of interest. Pharmacokinetic parameters should be determined over the range of doses used in pharmacology and safety studies, and following administration of single and multiple doses of the drug. The key pharmacokinetic information that is necessary for the interpretation of safety data and the design of subsequent studies is whether the extent of absorption and clearance of the drug is linear over the dosage range of pharmacology and toxicology studies, since changes in absorption and/or clearance affect the extent and duration of exposure; and whether the extent and duration of exposure change when multiple doses of the drug are administered.

DISTRIBUTION

The distribution of parent drug and metabolites and the factors that affect this distribution are of fundamental importance, since the intensity of a pharmacological response or the onset of toxic side-effects are, for most drugs, related to the concentration of the active component at the locus of action. As previously noted, the physiochemical properties of drugs have a major impact on their distribution and should be evaluated during the drug selection process. The apparent volume of distribution of drugs is highly dependent on their lipophilicity and the extent to which they are ionised at physiological pH (7.4). Thus, lipophilic drugs are extensively distributed, because they are readily transported by passive diffusion across cell membranes and have a high affinity for adipose tissue and lipid components of cells. Weak acids tend to be less extensively distributed than weak bases, because weak acids are ionised to a greater extent at physiological pH than are weak bases, which inhibits their transport across cell membranes. Polar compounds do not enter the brain readily, because of the endothelial lining that separates the brain from the circulation. Highly polar and ionised drugs are to a great extent restricted to the vascular system and tend to have low volumes of distribution.

The extent to which drugs bind to vascular components (e.g. plasma proteins and red blood cells), cellular components and tissues depends on the macromolecule involved in the binding and the drug, and has a major impact on the extent to which a drug is distributed, since the driving force for the distribution of passively transported drugs is the concentration of unbound drug. Albumin is the major plasma protein (59%) and is the predominant macromolecule involved in the reversible binding of most drugs, especially acidic or anionic molecular species. β-Lipoproteins are thought to play a major role in the binding of basic or cationic species. Binding to α- and γ-globulins is less important for most drugs (Pang, 1983).

The plasma-protein binding characteristics of drugs should be evaluated by standardised experimental procedures (e.g. ultrafiltration and equilibrium dialysis) (Chignell, 1977), to determine the binding capacity of plasma proteins and the affinity of drugs for binding sites on these proteins. The concentration dependence of protein binding should be evaluated over the range of drug concentrations observed in pharmacology and safety studies. Since highly significant species differences in protein binding have been observed (Davidson, 1971), these studies should be done on proteins from animals used in safety studies as well as from humans. In later stages of drug development, it may be useful to conduct competitive protein binding studies to assess the effects of other drugs on the protein binding of the investigational drug, particularly if protein binding studies have indicated that the drug is highly protein-bound. Drug interactions frequently have as their basis the competition of drugs for binding sites on proteins, some of which may be low-capacity binding sites.

The most comprehensive technique currently available for the semiquantitative determination of tissue distribution is that of whole-body autoradiography (Waddell and Marlowe, 1977). In this technique, animals are rapidly frozen in a suitable organic solvent at predetermined times after administration of radiolabelled drug, and embedded in a block of carboxymethylcellulose ice prior to being sectioned in a cryostatted microtome. Sagittal sections of the whole experimental animal are then placed against an X-ray film, to determine the distribution of radioactivity (parent drug and metabolites) in the entire animal. Although a variety of species have been used for this technique, the most widely used animals are the mouse and the rat. Use of pregnant and post-partum animals in these experiments allows an assessment of whether transplacental transfer of drug occurs and whether the drug is secreted into milk. Pigmented animal strains can also be used to evaluate binding to pigmented tissue. ^{14}C-labelled drug is ideal for nearly all autoradiography applications except those requiring high resolution, in which case ^{3}H is the isotope of choice.

Whole-body autoradiography has two unique advantages over classical tissue distribution studies, in which tissues are excised and homogenised before analysis for total radioactivity. First, tissues and fluids that ordinarily would not be sampled can be readily evaluated, and second, concentration gradients within a tissue can be detected. The latter advantage is particularly relevant to the toxicological evaluation of drugs, since highly localised concentrations of drugs in tissues may lead to tissue necrosis and toxicity. Classical tissue distribution studies and/or autoradiography studies in animals are conducted prior to the administration of radiolabelled drugs to humans, to assess the extent and duration of exposure of organs and tissues to the radiolabelled material.

METABOLISM

The duration and intensity of action of lipophilic drugs is highly dependent on their rate of metabolism or biotransformation, since the majority of these compounds are readily reabsorbed in the kidney tubule following glomerular filtration. The liver, replete with a variety of metabolising enzymes, cofactors and endogenous scavengers of reactive metabolites (e.g. reduced glutathione), is the principal organ mediating the biotransformation of drugs. However, other sites in the body may play a critical role in metabolism in certain situations. Thus, the skin, lung, small intestine and gastrointestinal flora may have a significant impact on biotransformation, depending on the drug, the drug dose and the route of exposure (Lake and Gangolli, 1981).

Many factors are now known that affect the metabolism and, consequently, the activity of drugs. A wide variety of xenobiotics, including drugs, have the ability to induce or inhibit metabolising enzymes, thereby altering not only their own metabolism but also that of other xenobiotics, drugs and endogenous substances. Other factors such as dose, route and frequency of administration, age, sex, genetic differences and diet may profoundly affect metabolism (Lake and Gangolli, 1981). Consequently, it is extremely important to carefully control experimental conditions in metabolism studies, and, where appropriate, study the effects of these factors on the disposition of the drug.

Although the general pattern of metabolism is common to all species, the initial phase usually consisting of functionalisation reactions (oxidations, reductions and hydrolyses) and the second phase consisting of synthesis reactions (conjugations), major species differences in drug metabolism exist. It is this diversity in metabolism among species that is the major difficulty in extrapolating animal pharmacology and toxicology data to humans (Williams, 1971). The prediction of species differences in qualitative patterns of metabolism is at best an inexact science or forecast. Particularly helpful in this regard is information that has been acquired concerning species defects with respect to particular metabolic pathways and substrates (Smith, 1988).

The physicochemical characteristics of drugs should be considered in evaluating preclinical metabolism study requirements. In general, drugs that have low lipid solubility at physiological pH are not metabolised but are eliminated by excretion. A number of antibiotics and quaternary ammonium drugs, among others, fall into this category (Renwick, 1983). The pharmacological and toxicological effects of these compounds in humans can often be predicted reasonably well on the basis of animal data. Furthermore, these drugs are not likely to be affected by a broad range of factors that may affect drugs that depend on biotransfusion for elimination (e.g. enzyme induction or inhibition). On the other hand, lipophilic drugs are often extensively metabolised, with the rate and extent of metabolism and pathways of metabolism species-dependent. In this situation, extensive effort will be required to characterise the metabolism and to investigate factors that may affect the metabolism of these drugs. Radioisotopically labelled drug is invariably used in these investigations to elucidate pathways of metabolism and detect low levels of potentially toxic metabolites or the reaction products of reactive metabolites.

In vitro metabolism studies, using tissue slices, isolated cell suspensions and homogenates of tissues and subcellular fractions (e.g. microsomes), or isolated liver perfusion studies can provide a wealth of information concerning the metabolism of the drug and potential reactive, toxic metabolites, and are a useful adjunct to *in vitro* toxicity studies. These techniques also represent a rapid means of isolating small quantities of metabolites for further testing. Metabolites that may be pharmacologically active should be isolated and characterised early in the drug evaluation process if comparative pharmacology and pharmacokinetic data suggest the presence of active metabolites. *In vivo* metabolism studies should be conducted in animal species and strains used in the toxicological evaluation of the drug, to elucidate metabolic patterns and to ensure that metabolic switching does not occur at high doses (Glockin, 1981). Pooled or individual specimens from mass balance studies can be used for this purpose. Elucidation of metabolic patterns during preclinical testing is essential for the expeditious interpretation and rationalisation of interspecies differences in toxicity that may affect the administration of the drug in humans. An investigation of a drug's potential to induce or inhibit metabolism should also be considered, since these attributes can have a major impact on drug interactions (Conney, 1971).

EXCRETION

An assessment of the rate and routes of excretion of intact drug and metabolites is an essential component of preclinical drug evaluation. The importance of determining the proportion of intact drug and metabolites excreted (i.e. metabolic pattern) in each animal species has already been emphasised. The rate and routes of excretion are best determined by mass balance studies using radioisotopically labelled drug, as previously described. In this manner, a rapid assessment can be made of the routes of excretion and the duration of exposure to intact drug or metabolites. These excretion studies also provide valuable insight concerning the potential for drug accumulation in patients with impaired renal or hepatic function.

Quantitatively, the kidney is the most important excretory organ for compounds of low molecular weight, and the vast majority of drugs and/or their metabolites appear in the urine to some extent (Levine, 1983). All unbound drugs or metabolites having molecular weights of approximately 5000 or less are filtered through the glomerulus, and some bound and unbound drugs and metabolites are secreted by active transport. Reabsorption of some drugs and metabolites occurs following glomerular filtration, mostly by passive diffusion and in some cases by active transport. The degree of reabsorption is dependent on lipophilicity, degree of plasma-protein binding and pK_a of the drug or its metabolites. Thus, the biotransformation of lipophilic drugs to polar metabolites enhances renal excretion. For drugs having a pK_a near the pH of urine, the rate of excretion can be increased or decreased by manipulation of urinary pH. The active transport systems for organic anions and cations are subject to competitive inhibition. For example, the half-life of a number of antibiotics can be extended by concomitant administration of probenecid, an organic anion that inhibits tubular secretion of other organic anions. Although there are notable differences in renal excretion between mammalian and non-mammalian species, tubular reabsorption appears to be a general phenomenon among common laboratory species (Trevor *et al.*, 1971).

Although fewer drugs are excreted by humans in the bile than in urine, the hepatobiliary system ranks next in importance to the kidney as an excretory organ. The function of the hepatobiliary system in the enterohepatic circulation is responsible for the persistence of some drugs and may result in prolonged pharmacological activity or toxicity. Conjugation, particularly conjugation with glucuronic acid, appears to facilitate biliary excretion (Plaa, 1971). A molecular weight threshold appears to exist for biliary secretion of organic anions, which varies among species, with approximate thresholds of 325, 475 and 500–700 for rats, rabbits and humans, respectively. The molecular weight threshold for organic cations is approximately 200, with little or no interspecies variation apparent. Renal ligation does not increase biliary excretion of compounds below the molecular weight threshold, and bile duct ligation does not increase urinary excretion of compounds well above the molecular weight threshold. Compounds of intermediate molecular weight are excreted in both urine and bile (Hirom *et al.*, 1976).

Drugs excreted in urine and bile are usually unbound; consequently, free drug concentrations in the urinary and biliary tract may be several orders of magnitude higher than in blood, accounting for the renal and hepatic toxicity of some highly protein-bound drugs (Clark and Smith, 1984). Furthermore, high drug and/or metabolite concentrations may be achieved in the renal cortex, even though little drug or metabolite ultimately appears in the urine. Consequently, it should not be assumed that the kidney is not exposed to high drug or metabolite concentrations simply because these compounds are not eliminated in the urine. Autoradiography or tissue distribution studies are required to reveal this phenomenon. The rate of drug administration also has an impact on renal and hepatic toxicity. Normally, bolus intravenous doses result in higher toxicity because of high drug concentrations in target organs (Clark and Smith, 1984).

Although quantitatively less important than urinary or biliary excretion, the excretion of drugs in expired air, sweat, saliva, faeces and milk may be of consequence for specific drugs and circumstances. The secretion of drugs into milk is of concern and should be examined in conjunction with reproductive toxicity studies and in humans before administration of drugs to nursing mothers.

CONCLUSIONS

Drug disposition studies should be conducted at an early enough stage of drug development to allow a biologically coherent evaluation of drug pharmacology and safety and to be of predictive value. The dosage and dosage regimen of the drug can then be appropriately adjusted to take into account interspecies differences in the extent and duration of drug exposure. These studies may also provide insight into mechanisms of toxicity due to overexposure within particular species or because of the formation of a toxic metabolite. This information may provide a basis for a species-dependent toxic effect, and the relevance of this effect to the human situation can be more readily assessed. Only too frequently disposition studies are done too late to be used in a beneficial manner. This may result in the development of a candidate with less than optimal properties that has a lower probability of ultimately receiving marketing approval, or in the rejection of drug candidates that might prove to be useful therapeutic agents. In the last analysis, what is required in terms of preclinical evaluation is a research programme that is scientifically appropriate to the drug under investigation and its intended clinical use. This evaluation should allow an assessment of the benefit: risk ratio of a new therapeutic agent which can be compared with similar ratios for already established drugs.

REFERENCES

Ariens, E. J. (1966). Receptor theory and structure–action relationships. *Adv. Drug Res.*, **3**, 235–85
Bousquet, W. F. (1970). In Swarbrick, J. (Ed.), *Current Concepts in the Pharmaceutical Sciences: Biopharmaceutics*. Lea and Febiger, Philadelphia, pp. 151–95
Clark, B. and Smith, D. A. (1984). Pharmacokinetics and toxicity testing. *CRC Crit. Rev. Toxicol.*, **12**, 343–85
Chignell, C. F. (1977). In Garrett, E. R. and Hirtz, J. L. (Eds.), *Drug Fate and Metabolism*, Volume 1. Marcel Dekker, New York, pp. 187–228

Conney, A. H. (1971). In LaDu, B. N., Mandel, H. G. and Way, E. L. (Eds.), *Fundamentals of Drug Metabolism and Drug Disposition*. Williams and Wilkins, Baltimore, pp. 253–78

Davidson, C. (1971). In LaDu, B. N., Mandel, H. G. and Way, E. L. (Eds.), *Fundamentals of Drug Metabolism and Drug Disposition*. Williams and Wilkins, Baltimore, pp. 63–75

Drug Research Board, National Academy of Sciences/National Research Council (1969). Application of metabolic data to the evaluation of drugs. *Clin. Pharmacol. Ther.*, **10**, 607–34

EEC Commission (1980). Proposal for a council recommendation concerning tests relating to the placing on the market of proprietary medicinal products, *Off. J. Eur. Communities*, No. C355/6-29

Glockin, V. C. (1982). General considerations for studies of the metabolism of drugs and other chemicals. *Drug Metab. Rev.*, **13**, 929–39

Goldenthal, E. I. (1968). FDA papers, May 3, 1968, U.S. Food and Drug Administration, Washington, D.C.

Hansch, C. and Clayton, J. M. (1973). Lipophilic character and biological activity of drugs. II. The parabolic case. *J. Pharm. Sci.*, **62**, 1–21

Hirom, P. C., Millburn, P. and Smith, R. L. (1976). Bile and urine as complementary pathways for the excretion of foreign organic compounds. *Xenobiotica*, **6**, 55–64

Kaplan, S. A. (1973). In Swarbrick, J. (Ed.), *Current Concepts in the Pharmaceutical Sciences: Dosage Form Design and Bioavailability*. Lea and Febiger, Philadelphia, pp. 1–30

Lake, B. G. and Gangolli, S. D. (1981). In Jenner, P. and Testa, B. (Eds.), *Concepts in Drug Metabolism*, Part B, Marcel Dekker, New York, pp. 167–218

Levine, W. G. (1983). In Caldwell, J. and Jakoby, W. B. (Eds.), *Biological Basis of Detoxication*. Academic Press, New York, pp. 251–85

Mertel, H. E. (1979). In Garrett, E. R. and Hirtz, J. L. (eds.), *Drug Fate and Metabolism*, Volume 3, Marcel Dekker, New York, pp. 133–91

Pang, K. S. (1983). In Caldwell, J. and Jakoby, W. B. (Eds.), *Biological Basis of Detoxication*. Academic Press, New York, pp. 213–50

Plaa, G. L. (1971). In LaDu, B. N., Mandel, H. G. and Way, E. L. (Eds.), *Fundamentals of Drug Metabolism and Drug Disposition*. Williams and Wilkins, Baltimore, pp. 131–45

Renwick, A. G. (1983). In Caldwell, J. and Jakoby, W. B. (Eds.), *Biological Basis of Detoxication*. Academic Press, New York, pp. 151–79

Smith, R. L. (1988). The role of metabolism and disposition studies in the safety assessment of pharmaceuticals. *Xenobiotica*, **18**, 89–96

Trevor, A., Rowland, M. and Way, E. L. (1971). In LaDu, B. N., Mandel, H. G. and Way, E. L. (Eds.), *Fundamentals of Drug Metabolism and Drug Disposition*, Williams and Wilkins, Baltimore, pp. 369–99

Waddell, W. J. and Marlowe, C. (1977). In Garrett, E. R. and Hirtz, J. L. (Eds.), *Drug Fate and Metabolism*, Volume 1, Marcel Dekker, New York, pp. 1–25

Williams, R. T. (1971). In LaDu, B. N., Mandel, H. G. and Way, E. L. (Eds.), *Fundamentals of Drug Metabolism and Drug Disposition*, Williams and Wilkins, Baltimore, pp. 187–205

World Health Organization (1966). Principles for pre-clinical testing of drug safety. *World Health Organization Technical Report Series*, 341

4

The Toxicological Background

Anthony Dayan

*Dept of Toxicology, St. Bartholomew's Hospital Medical College,
London EC1A 7EB, UK*

ROLE AND NATURE OF TOXICITY TESTING

Toxicity testing in the early phases of drug development has three main purposes: (1) to demonstrate toxic effects and the circumstances of their occurrence; (2) to show what toxic effects did not occur; (3) to suggest whenever possible the likely mechanisms of toxicity. From all these findings and analyses, a cautious prediction can be made of the possible nature and incidence of toxic effects in man, so that likely risks can be matched against anticipated benefits of treatment.

All these points require amplification, but they represent the basic classes of information which toxicologists produce, and from which risk and safety in man can be predicted. The extrapolation to clinical use requires the toxicologist to warn the physician about the possible nature, incidence or severity of toxic actions that may occur, and this implies pointing out hazards to be avoided as well as specific disorders to be monitored. Predictions of toxicity are rarely perfect, neither in kind nor in degree, so the intensity of some harmful actions may be overpredicted, while other unpleasant and even serious effects may not be modelled in experiments: for example, purely subjective complaints, such as headache, apathy or feeling unwell, cannot be directly predicted from laboratory studies, unlike most instances of target organ damage, such as hepatic toxicity, while the rat is more sensitive than man to the nephrotoxic effects of non-steroidal anti-inflammatory agents.

For ethical reasons, and because more extensive scientific investigation is possible, most toxicity testing is done in animals, and to a lesser extent in *in vitro* studies (Paton, 1984). It is only investigations in animals which can reveal the full range of integrated, indirect and secondary responses to a candidate drug, as well as its direct actions, and which permit the sometimes remote consequences of pharmcodynamic responses and metabolic handling of the substance to be observed. However, extrapolation from one species to another demands caution, because of the pharmacological, biochemical and metabolic differences that may exist between them. Equally, *in vitro* experiments employ artificially simplified, closed systems, are incapable of revealing more than a very limited range of responses and are devoid of many metabolic and excretory pathways. Results from them must be regarded with very considerable caution. The general nature of extrapolation between species and its problems are extensively discussed by Calabrese (1983) and Tardiff and Rodricks (1987).

The toxicity testing of a candidate medicine is not an exercise in pure science and logic. It represents a mobile, academic–practical balance between the scientific initiative of the toxicologist, concerned to do the best experiments to detect and explore the toxicity of a substance; the resources of his employer, anxious to advance compounds to study their actions in the target species—man; the standards and needs of the clinical investigators (who may take toxicological opinions on trust, without questioning their basis); and the specific requirements of regulatory authorities and ethical committees under whose jurisdiction the human investigations will come.

TYPES OF TOXICITY TESTS

The term 'toxicity' covers every adverse effect, ranging from acute local irritation to such long-term actions as the production of neoplasms, and even effects on succeeding generations—mutagenesis. Accordingly, different types of test have been pragmatically devised as reasonable means to display the disparate types of toxic potential. An equally important reason for subdividing the types of study is the scientific and practical importance of starting with brief, limited experiments to begin to uncover the toxic properties of a substance, and only extending to more costly and more prolonged investigations once there is sufficient understanding of the substance's actions to permit rational design and analysis of the experiments. A further reason for phasing toxicity work in this way is the importance of adapting later tests to pharmacokinetic and pharmacodynamic findings in man, and to the investigation of any new untoward responses found in the clinical studies. For all these reasons, our understanding of the toxicity testing of candidate pharmaceuticals has led to general agreement that it is both scientifically reasonable and ethically acceptable, in general, to perform a limited set of toxicity studies prior to any dosing of man, and then to extend the scope and nature of the preclinical work before more and different types of subjects are treated, e.g. the move from Phase I work in healthy volunteers to formal Phase II/III trials in patients, who may be male or female of any age, perhaps pregnant, certainly diseased, etc., and eventually for the toxicologist to investigate adverse effects discovered in those and Phase IV studies.

Specific, detailed regulations and professional requirements for toxicity data are discussed elsewhere in this book, and so are the principles of the pharmacokinetic investigations, but the nature of the procedures is sufficiently general for them to be described in reasonable detail, provided that the importance is understood of the zig-zag progress of a candidate drug between early preclinical studies, limited work in man, further nonclinical experimentation taking into account the findings in man, more extensive clinical investigations, and so on, including special studies to assess possible hazards in particular groups of patients.

In broad terms, the principal types of toxicity information required, and hence the necessary experiments, are as listed below, always bearing in mind how the types and detailed nature of the studies need adaptation to the specific properties and intended uses of the candidate medicine.

(1) To permit single dose studies in healthy volunteers:
general ('safety') pharmacology;
basic understanding of overall disposition in the species tested;
acute toxicity tests in two species;
subacute toxicity tests in two species (dosing for at least 14 days);
mutagenicity testing (at least an Ames test).
(2) To cover several doses, and perhaps treatment of patients for up to 7–10 days:
experiments listed above;
subacute tests in two species involving dosing for 30 days.
(3) For more general treatment in trials extending up to 6 months, or for a Product License:
all the above work, plus
chronic toxicity tests testing for 6 months (or 1 year in the USA);
carcinogenicity tests in two species;
further mutagenicity tests;
more detailed knowledge of pharmacokinetics, including metabolism;
reproduction toxicity tests comprising fertility, embryonic and fetal, perinatal and postnatal development;
if appropriate, topical irritancy and sensitisation tests to examine interactions between drugs that may be coadministered;
special studies to investigate particular adverse actions feared or seen in man, or to explore the consequences of disease, or to meet rules on the safety of workers in the manufacturing plant.

Administration of a drug by a particular route may entail additional studies to examine both the local and systemic consequences of use of that route, e.g. topical toxicity tests by inhalation or of the skin, eye, rectum or vagina. Similarly, parenteral administration will require testing by the chosen route, both for local and systemic effects, although the extent and nature of the studies may be modified if the substance has already been well studied after administration by the oral or some other route.

In general, the toxicologist will also need to examine the consequences of altered responsiveness or pharmacokinetics due to age or disease, and at least to consider the implications of physiological variation in metabolism and phenotype, e.g. could toxicity be greatly altered if the patient were a slow acctylator, or had a particular P 450 cytochrome isoform in the liver, or carried the sickle cell haemoglobin gene?

Since 1983 formal toxicity tests and the associated work (such as analyses of test materials, etc.) have been governed by a set of internationally agreed regulations, the *Principles of Good Laboratory Practice* (Department of Health and Social Security, 1986). The purpose of these rules is to ensure that there is a clear, permanent record of the complete experimental protocols, of the source and nature of the materials used in the tests, of the animals employed, and of all the raw results as they are obtained (e.g. clinical findings in individual animals by date, original biochemical measurements, including histological blocks and slides, etc.). As the purpose is to ensure a full record of what was done, it requires comprehensive, proven systems for record-keeping and secure storage of data and specimens, as well as full, written instructions to cover every procedure in tests (Standard Operating Procedures), ranging from maintenance of the environment in the animal house to use of computer systems for data collection and analysis. The OEDC agreement gives official agencies the right to inspect the procedures and records of laboratories that submit results supporting the licensure of medicines.

NATURE OF TOXICITY TESTS

General (Safety) Pharmacology

This type of work may well not be done by the toxicologist, but knowledge of the results is essential in predicting the hazards of use of a novel substance. It is reviewed in Zbinden and Gross (1979).

The need is for information about the range of acute, functional pharmacodynamic actions of the substance on major body systems, especially the cardiovascular, respiratory and nervous systems. In some countries it is customary also to include special studies of renal function and the blood clotting cascade, although they may well be assessed in the subacute and chronic experiments.

The general nature of these studies (Zbinden and Gross, 1979) relies on the classical, instrumented, anaesthetised animal and isolated tissue preparations of the pharmacologist to reveal the effects of various high parenteral doses of the test substance, and of its effects on a range of responses to standard agonists and antagonists of the autonomic nervous system and smooth muscle. There is no agreed set of observations that must be made, only acceptance of the importance of discovering any major functional activity that might affect humans.

The range of observations likely to be made on any substance, in addition to the essential information about its intended therapeutic activity, comprise the following.

Central nervous system   Open field test or Irwin screen on a small number of rodents. Clinical observations on rodents and non-rodents in acute toxicity and rising dose (non-lethal) tests, all done after several, single high doses.
Peripheral nervous system   Clinical observations during acute and more prolonged toxicity tests.
Autonomic nervous system   Changes in blood pressure and heart rate in anaesthetised animals induced by the substance, and in response to stimulation of the vagus and sympathetic nerve trunks, and on administration of

typical adrenergic, cholinergic and histaminergic agonists and antagonists.

Effects on isolated smooth muscle of the test material before and during exposure to conventional spasmogens and relaxants.

Cardiovascular system   Responses at least of blood pressure and heart rate (and perhaps of cardiac output), regional flow and dynamics to the new substance before and during administration of standard agonists and antagonists, and on stimulation of autonomic reflexes.

Actions on isolated strips of vascular smooth muscle are sometimes examined.

Respiratory system   At least respiratory activity and basic pulmonary mechanics should be followed after injection of the new material, as should any change in the response to autonomic agonists and antagonists.

Gastrointestinal system   Overall motor activity can be followed by timing the movement of a charcoal meal through the intestines. The pharmacological responses of the intestines in an organ-bath should also be investigated.

Other systems and responses   It is impossible to specify what is worth doing, but activities suggested by chemical structure or pharmacological class, or detected in some other study, should be investigated to determine their likely significance in clinical use. Similarly, specific experiments into local actions should always be considered for substances for local or parenteral administration.

The need for this broad assessment is shown, for example, by the clinical importance of the anticholinergic actions of the tricyclic antidepressants, and the endocrinological actions of many prostaglandin analogues, which should be known prior to treatment of man.

Interpretation of Findings

Results should be available for a range of doses, including those given parenterally, which will permit comparison of the dose or blood level producing the desired therapeutic effect, or a surrogate for it, and the other pharmacodynamic actions. The larger the 'therapeutic ratio' between the two values, the less likely it is that the general or secondary effects will be important in clinical practice. This type of judgement can be difficult, and sometimes no more than a cautious prediction can be given about probable lack of effect in man, plus a recommendation for clinical monitoring of a particular activity.

Acute Toxicity Testing

The objective is to administer to small numbers of animals a sufficiently high dose by the intended route of use, and a parenteral route that ensures absorption, to reveal the effects of acute poisoning, and perhaps non-immunologically-based 'sensitivity', and to help to guide dosage selection for other toxicity tests.

It is now agreed that the old-fashioned LD_{50} cannot be justified, except in a few, specialised circumstances (Dayan *et al.*, 1984; Brown, 1988). The favoured type of experiment involves administration either of a single, arbitrarily chosen high dose of the substance (limit test) or of two or three dose levels to groups of a few male and female mice and rats by, say, gavage and intravenously or intraperitoneally. The animals are then carefully followed by close clinical observations for up to 14 days. At the end of this period they are killed and an autopsy is done on them as well as on any that died prematurely. Sometimes, special additional investigations may help in investigating the actions of a specific compound, e.g. an open field test, or special studies of haematological or biochemical changes. It is also customary to administer a few high doses also to just one or two non-rodents, e.g. the dog, not to cause lethality but to gain an impression of the range of actions produced.

Interpretation of the findings depends on correlation of effects with doses, and their comparison with the likely circumstances of therapeutic use of the substance. Unless the lethal or severely toxic dose were found to be close to the anticipated therapeutic dose, results of this type of testing are likely to serve to guide and warn the clinician rather than to stop development of the substance.

SUBACUTE AND CHRONIC TOXICITY TESTING

These procedures have so much in common that they must be considered together. They form the basis of the most important attempts to define toxic risks in man and so underlie the ultimate risk–benefit analysis that determines the utility of a new medicine.

By convention they are done in the rat and the dog (or sometimes the primate) to gain the advantages of our extensive knowledge of responses and their causes in these species, and the availability of sufficient numbers of healthy, laboratory-bred animals for reasonable statistical power (Salsburg, 1988, includes a trenchant discussion of this and other aspects of statistical analysis). The importance of studies in two species is that it gives wider and therefore more secure coverage of likely effects and species differences in metabolism and responses. Valuable general accounts are given by Paget (1978), EHC6 (1976) and Wilson (1988). Several dose levels are administered over periods ranging from 14 days to 1 year (although there is no good evidence that useful additional findings are made between 6 months and 1 year: Dayan and Walker, 1987) and a very wide range of responses is sought during and at the end of dosing, and after a treatment-free recovery period related to the period of dosing.

The general nature of the protocols employed has become very constrained by customs and regulations specific to major countries, but it is still possible to incorporate limited flexibility in adapting the experiments to the particular properties and likely uses of the substance.

Species

For pharmacokinetic and sometimes pharmacodynamic reasons, the conventional outbred rat and dog may occasionally be inappropriate test species, and then the mouse, or a primate or mini-pig may be considered instead.

Route

The intended route in man should always be employed, but if absorption in animals were very limited relative to man, there might have to be an additional study of the effects of supplementary, parenteral treatment.

Administration by gavage can be well controlled, but may result in brief exposure to a short-lived substance, whereas dosing in the diet can give a more prolonged exposure, although the dose to individual animals is less well controlled.

Duration

The choice is arbitrary, but, in general, the more prolonged the animal study, the longer the acceptable period of treatment of man, because late and more slowly developing lesions will have been revealed.

For regulatory purposes, as already mentioned, the conventional requirements of regulatory agencies are as listed in Table 4.1.

Table 4.1 Duration of treatment

Animals	Permitted treatment of man
2 weeks	1 dose
1 month	up to 10 days
6 months	CEC and Japan—chronic[a]
1 year	USA—chronic[a]

[a]Carcinogenicity testing may also be required, as well as other investigations.

Following a 'recovery' group of animals left for a period without treatment is valuable, because it will show the reversibility of any toxic effects produced. Recoverable lesions may be regarded as less serious than permanent damage.

The frequency of dosing should be adjusted as far as possible to the duration of activity or the half-life of the compound in the test species.

Dose Levels

A logical way to settle dose levels is to choose multiples of the therapeutically active dose in either animals or man, or of that required to produce the corresponding blood or plasma level if it is known (and perhaps if it is closely related to the production of desired or undesired actions). In any case, the kinetics of the compound in animals must be considered and the frequency and magnitude of the doses must be adjusted in accordance with the half-life.

A common convention suggests that the low dose should be at least 3–5 × the anticipated human dose, that the top dose should be 100–200 × the latter value, and that the middle dose should be the geometric mean. Alternatively, the high dose may be set as the 'maximum tolerated dose' (MTD)—that which causes a clear but non-lethal effect, e.g. a 10% reduction in weight gain, with two convenient sub-multiples, depending on the steepness of the dose–response relationship.

In any case, three dose levels are normally employed to show the relationship between effects and dose and to demonstrate the 'no observed effect level' (NOEL). The latter helps to set a level of dose (or plasma concentration) which the treatment of man should not normally exceed.

Observations

(1) In life, at least the general appearance and clinical behaviour should always be monitored regularly, as well as ophthalmoscopic examination at intervals to study all the structures of the eye. In at least non-rodents the ECG, too, should be examined at regular intervals.

Special studies should be considered to follow any major pharmacodynamic action, especially the desired therapeutic effect, as the result will be some guide to whether clinical efficacy is likely to be sustained. Pharmacodynamic effects are also worth examining, because they may account for certain lesions of great toxicological concern, but now known not to be clinically important, such as the left venticular necrosis produced by high doses of β-agonists, which results from the profound hypotension induced by vasodilatation.

Body weight gain and food and water consumption should also be followed as a guide to general health.

(2) *Haematology* As a minimum, the measured and calculated variables recorded should include RBCs, haematocrit and haemoglobin level, white cell and differential count, platelet count and comments on a stained smear.

Such tests as the prothrombin time and the accelerated partial thrombo-plastin time can readily be incorporated as broad indicators of the clotting cascade.

These observations are best done before and at a few intervals during treatment, at its end and in the recovery group.

(3) *Clinical chemistry* A reasonably wide selection appropriate to the species being used should be made from the conventional tests for enzymes and other analytes in blood, to indicate damage to major organs, e.g. blood urea or creatinine, electrolytes, calcium, phosphate and uric acid, various enzymes and bilirubin, glucose, cholesterol and plasma proteins.

Urinalysis, too, may be used to test function (e.g. concentrating power or S.G.) as well as to reveal dysfunction, as shown by the presence of protein, casts, etc.

The specific biochemical and haematological tests done, and the urinalysis, and their frequency during the study should be adjusted to the activities of the test compound and the duration of the experiment, so that early, late and transient abnormalities are all detected, having regard to the samples that can reasonably be obtained. Such tests, and clinical and microbiological examinations, are often done even prior to dosing as a check on the health of the experimental animals.

(4) *Autopsy* All animals should undergo a full autopsy, whether they die prematurely or are killed according to a predetermined schedule. The procedure comprises external inspection and dissection to expose the major viscera and other tissues and any abnormalities, noting the appearances and weighing the principal organs. Representative samples are then taken from all tissues for histopathological examination by light microscopy, and, when necessary, by related techniques, such as electron microscopy and histo- and immunocytochemistry. Histological studies are important because they show the state of organs and tissues not otherwise readily open to examination and they are applicable both to discrete and diffuse structures.

Special Investigations

(1) It is important to monitor the plasma level or urinary excretion of the test substance, particularly in the higher dose groups and in prolonged studies, because a supralinear increase with dose, or the appearance of novel metabolites, may suggest that kinetics have become non-linear. In that case, handling of the compound by the body will have exceeded the normal metabolic capacity, and such unusual pathways or metabolites may be produced that there is a real risk that the resulting toxicity may not be a good guide to man (see Pharmacokinetics section of this book; Timbrell, 1984; Snell and Mullock, 1987).

Studying at least basic evidence about absorption and disposition in chronic toxicity tests may also be the first opportunity to show whether subtle physiological changes related to ageing can affect kinetics—information of real clinical value.

(2) It is also possible to incorporate almost any type of exploration of physiological or biochemical function, or of pharmacological response, but the value of doing so depends on what is known from other experiments about the activities of the substance, or whether information is required to understand the mechanism of an effect and, hence, more confidently to predict its importance for man.

As examples, consider an experiment in which there was nephrotoxicity. Doing renal function tests and measuring cells and appropriate enzymes in urine would show more clearly than routine procedures the relationship between dose and response, and, together with detailed histological studies, might well indicate the type of cell affected and even the organelle and toxic mechanism involved. Or, if a substance were found to depress spermatogenesis, assays of appropriate pituitary and steroid hormones in blood might help to show the site of action. Similarly, potent vasodilators, if they produce sustained hypotension and tachycardia, are associated with ECG changes, sometimes a rise in the plasma levels of certain enzymes, and a characteristic pattern of myocardial necrosis. But *proving* that association in a specific instance requires knowledge of the concurrent behaviour of BP, heart rate, blood enzyme levels and the pattern of cardiac damage.

Adverse effects first found in man are often studied by attempting to model them in the laboratory, so that their causes and significance can be assessed.

Interpretation of Results

This is the very essence of product-orientated toxicology. The objective is precise—what are the toxic effects produced in the laboratory (and not produced), what is their relation to dose and duration of treatment, and do the characteristics of the toxicity suggest a possible mechanism? Given that information, plus the known or likely dose or plasma level, or better formal pharmacokinetic data in man, what is the likelihood that toxicity will occur in humans and under what circumstances of dose and duration of therapy? How severe is the adverse effect likely to be at any given dose or blood level? Is it reversible? Assessment of the results of the preclinical studies will enable guidance to be given about the likely risk of clinical toxicity, which must be matched against the anticipated value of treatment in making the 'cost–benefit' analysis that determines whether development of the substance continues until it becomes a freely usable medicine or whether it fails as another abandoned prospect. The process is complex, it depends on co-operation between toxicologists and clinicians, and it is very dependent on experience.

There is an important difference here between what are sometimes termed 'biological' significance and 'statistical' significance. The latter is a summary of the results of formal statistical analysis, usually expressed as the 'p-value' of the null hypothesis. Given the complexity of toxicity tests and the mutiplicity of independent and interrelated variable assessed, it is not surprising that every test comes up with a number of 'significant' ($p < 0.05$) results. But the true biological importance of such a finding depends on normal background variation, the magnitude of the abnormality, its relation to dose and other features of toxicity (e.g. blood urea may rise because an unwell animal drinks less rather than as a feature of true nephrotoxicity), and whether the change is consistent with other findings in making up the pattern of disorders that represent a specific organ or tissue lesion. That is 'biological significance'. The latter may also represent a statistically non-significant but very rare finding that is suggestive of an action, e.g. occurrence of an unusual tumour even in a small number of animals.

From the toxicologist's viewpoint, in evaluating an effect in an experiment the most important questions to answer are: Did the experiment follow the intended design? What was the substance actually tested or could impurities or instability have influenced the results? Do the findings of toxicity make a consistent pattern, i.e. are there appropriate changes in multiple, overlapping investigations—for example, if hepatotoxicity is suspected, are there appropriate alterations in bilirubin and enzyme levels in plasma and urine, in prothrombin time, in the appearance and weight of the liver, and what are the histological findings? Having accepted that there is a real effect apparently associated with treatment, the next step is to consider historical and concurrent control data, to exclude the likelihood that the effect could have been due to biological variation or intercurrent disease in the animals. The next stage, now that there is reasonable assurance that there is a genuine effect of the compound, is to relate the frequency or intensity of toxicity to the dose or plasma level, and to assess the evidence of its reversibility, before the joint clinicotoxicological balancing of the circumstances of the toxic action against the therapeutic dose and benefit. Understanding pharmacokinetics and mechanism of action are very important here in improving extrapolation between the laboratory species and man in relative health and overt disease.

CARCINOGENICITY TESTING

Carcinogenicity testing resembles chronic toxicity testing but done over a much longer period, because tumorigenesis requires many months, even if potent compounds are involved (Grice and Ciminera, 1988). Current practice relies on tests in large numbers of rats and mice, or sometimes the Syrian hamster, given three dose levels ranging from the maximum tolerated dose, or 100–200 × the human dose, to a small multiple of the therapeutic dose. Treatment is commenced soon after weaning and is usually continued for 18 months in the mouse and hamster, and for 24 months in the rat. There are regular checks on general clinical state, especially for the development of swellings that could be tumours, and eventually a full autopsy and comprehensive histopathological survey. As in chronic studies, the blood level of the drug may be monitored, but few haematological and clinical chemistry tests are done, because senile changes tend to make the results too variable to be of much use. Care in the experimental design and in statistical analysis of the occurrence of tumours is essential in such prolonged and complex experiments, in order to minimise the influence of extraneous factors and to allow for intercurrent death of animals.

Interpreting the results requires care to avoid misleading impressions, e.g. the need to consider the background incidence of spontaneous tumours, the importance of distinguishing between a chance finding of just a numerically significant excess of tumours, and a biologically significant result, in which there may be supporting changes in function or other pathological findings in an affected organ, or in the type or time of onset of the tumours, to indicate their true importance. Species-specific responses and pharmacokinetics must be taken into account. This type of test will reveal the effects of genotoxic (see next section) and epigenetic (non-genotoxic) compounds; the latter may cause cancer in other ways than by directly affecting DNA, e.g. by disturbing normal growth control mechanisms (such as depression of the circulating thyroxine level, resulting in enhanced TSH production by the pituitary, and thence in hyperplasia and even neoplasia of the thyroid), or acting as a promotor, as described in the two-stage initiator–promotor theory of carcinogenesis. Supplementary experiments may be needed to separate these classes. The importance of doing that is because genotoxicants are believed not to have a threshold (i.e. any dose may carry some risk), whereas growth control disturbance and promotors probably do show thresholds, and their significance for human cancer is less certain. Thus, a genotoxicant is unlikely to be used as a medicine, except for the treatment of cancer and other fatal disorders, whereas the members of the other two classes may be used, e.g. sulphonamides (may affect thyroid function) and phenobarbital (promotes experimental but not human hepatic neoplasms).

MUTAGENICITY TESTING

Mutagenicity testing has been a fairly recent and rapid development, and its principles and problems have still not been completely integrated into general understanding of toxicity and its assessment. The basis of the importance of genotoxicity testing is twofold. First, as many tumours appear to arise by somatic mutation, and many carcinogens cause genetic damage, simple quick tests of genotoxic potential should also be an economical and speedy means of indicating at least some carcinogens. And second, the ability of a substance to cause mutations in germ cells, which are liable to be transmitted to the progeny, represents an independent toxic risk, true mutagenicity, as almost all mutations are harmful.

Most attention has been directed to the former use of genotoxicity data, in the hope that relatively inexpensive tests taking at the most 3 or 4 months, might be able to replace formal carcinogenicity experiments, which take about 3 years to complete and are very expensive in animals and other resources. The appearance of transmissible genetic harm in man due to a mutagen has been difficult to prove, even after mass exposure to such as potent mutagen as irradiation, e.g. at Hiroshima and Nagasaki.

If a substance or a metabolite is to cause genetic damage, it must do so by reacting chemically with somatic or germ cell DNA or chromosomes, and so interfering with translation and accurate replication. The purpose of genetic toxicity tests is to detect responses due to induced changes at the level of the gene, the chromosome or the genome, following exposure to the substance itself or to its metabolites.

Many types of test have been proposed, of which a few have been sufficiently well proven in practice to justify their acceptance as formal regulatory requirements (Parry and Arlett, 1984; Ashby *et al.*, 1988).

(1) Ames test   The oldest and best-known technique, in which four or five specially devised strains of the prokaryote *Salmonella typhimurium* are exposed to the substance with and without an S9 preparation of hepatic microsomes from rats previously treated with Aroclor (chlorinated biphenyls) to induce a range of activating, Phase I mixed function oxidases. The test strains have been constructed to depend on histidine in the medium for growth. After treatment they are plated on a histidine-deficient medium, on which only histidine-independent mutant auxotrophs will grow to produce visible colonies.

There are other analogous types of *in vitro* test employing strains of *E. coli* and various yeasts, but they are less often used. In the Ames test the bacterial DNA is exposed to the test chemical and any metabolites produced by the bacteria or the S9 microsomes. Point mutations can be detected in this way.

(2) In eukaryotic mammalian cells DNA is differently arranged in chromosomes.

A similar test for point mutations has been devised using CHO cells and a medium containing the cytotoxic nucleoside analogue 6-thioguanine. If the hypoxanthine guanine phosphoribosyl transferase (HGPRT) gene is functional in the selected, heterozygous cells, toxic metabolites are produced and the cells fail to grow. In the presence of a mutagen, that gene may be inactivated and the cells will grow into colonies. Metabolic activation is supplied with S9 mixture.

(3) At the level of chromosomes, a cytogenetic analysis can be done on many types of cells, especially human lymphocytes, cultured in the presence of the compound, and with and without S9, to produce putative active metabolites. Metaphases are examined for structural damage and numerical changes in the chromosomes.

(4) A very similar type of test can be done *in vivo* in dosed mice by collecting bone marrow cells for cytogenetic analysis, or by counting micronuclei, small fragments of DNA left behind in late-stage erythroblasts as a marker of damage to chromosomes.

(5) The dominant lethal test is the only simple method of looking for genetic damage to germ cells. In it male mice or rats are dosed and mated with undosed females over the period of one spermatogenic cycle. If there is major damage to DNA in sperm, there will be excess of early embryonic deaths.

(6) Other methods of some importance include directly measuring the chemical binding of radiolabelled compound to DNA *in vivo* or *in vitro*, and looking for DNA repair activity stimulated in response to a DNA-damaging chemical, the unscheduled DNA synthesis (UDS) test.

Choice of Tests

There is now sufficient understanding of genetic toxicity for agreement to have been reached that *in vitro* and *in vivo* and point mutation and chromosomal damage tests are required to survey the potential activities of a novel substance. This is reflected in scientific (Ashby and Tennant, 1988) and regulatory (see Chapters 6 and 7) requirements and is comprehensively reviewed by the Department of Health (1989).

In practice, because the Ames test is relatively cheap and quick, it would usually be done first, followed at a later stage in development by the HGPRT or similar test, cytogenetic studies on human lymphocytes *in vitro* and a micronucleus test in the mouse.

The Successful Test (UKEMS, 1984, 1985)

Certain inbuilt checks are essential, such as use of known positive controls (directly acting compounds and others requiring metabolic activation) and negative (vehicle only) preparations. The purity and stability of the test substance must be known, because the high concentrations used give impurities the opportunity to produce false-positive results.

A wide range of doses must be examined, because the genotoxic action may only be apparent over a narrow concentration band, sometimes close to the limit of toxicity to the organism or cell. There should always be a definite relationship between dose and toxicity.

Some exploration of the mechanism of generation of the electrophilic chemical species responsible for mutagenic activity *in vitro* should be considered, because it may be due to a metabolic pathway of no importance in man (e.g. *Salmonella* have an especially vigorous nitro-reductase that can be responsible for the powerful genotoxicity of organic nitrates in the Ames test, but is probably of little relevance to humans). Epoxidation of certain olefins can occur under the conditions of the Ames test *in vitro*, which is unimportant *in vivo*, because of the kinetics of epoxidation in mammals and the powerful protective activity of naturally occurring nucleophiles and the catabolic epoxide hydratase, which are largely absent from *in vitro* systems.

Interpretation of Results

A confirmed positive in any genetic toxicity test means that the substance or a metabolite is able to affect DNA in one way or another. Whether that means that there is a real risk of carcinogenicity and/or transmissible genetic damage depends on the strength of the evidence that the action is a true one and not an artefact, that it is due to the substance itself and not an impurity or artificial breakdown product, and that it is not due to an electrophilic chemical produced only in the closed system of an *in vitro* test owing to imbalance between metabolising system enriched in certain Phase I activating enzymes and largely devoid of Phase II catabolic enzymes and other protective nucleophilic substances and excretory mechanisms. At least as far as transmissible genetic damage is concerned, it is important to show whether the substance can penetrate the blood–testis barrier to reach germ cells.

If all these concerns are satisfied, then the substance should be regarded as a probable carcinogenic and mutagenic hazard (Ashby *et al.*, 1988; Shelby, 1988), which will sharply limit its possible utility.

A clear negative means that the compound can be regarded as not being genotoxic and so of not carrying that major class of carcinogenic hazard. It does not exclude the possibility that it might still act by an epigenetic mechanism, as discussed in the preceeding section.

REPRODUCTION TOXICITY TESTING

The technique must cover the entire reproductive process in the male and female, from successful production of sperm and ova, mating, fertilisation and development of the zygote into an embryo, birth and all aspects of postnatal growth and development to sexual maturity.

Three separate procedures have been devised to cover the major phases, the boundaries of which differ slightly between different regulatory authorities for arbitrary reasons.

Segment I or Fertility Testing

This test is normally done in the rat. Young adult males are given three dose levels of the test substance for 70 days, the duration of an entire spermatogenic cycle, before being mated to females dosed for 14 days in an attempt to reveal any major action on oestrus cycling (which can also be conveniently studied in subacute and chronic toxicity tests). Dosing of the females is stopped then or shortly afterwards, and they are followed for evidence of successful fertilisation and normal embryonic development to about day 13 or 15 of pregnancy. Assessment requires autopsy of the dams and examination of the embryos to demonstrate the normality of pregnancy and of the developing fetuses.

Segment II or 'Fetal Toxicity' Testing

Undosed male and female animals are mated. From day 6 to day 16 of gestation, the vulnerable period of organogenesis, pregnant dams are given one of three dose levels of the test substance. Some of them are killed immediately before parturition (to avoid cannibalism) and are examined at autopsy for the numbers of healthy-appearing embryos and the normality of their external, visceral and skeletal development. Litters born alive to the dams may be followed for up to 6 weeks for assessment of physical and neurological development.

These experiments are usually done in the rat (sometimes in the mouse) and the rabbit, a strain of the latter selected for susceptibility to thalidomide, to which rodents do not respond, being used.

Segment III: Perinatal and Postnatal Development

After mating undosed rats, pregnant dams are given three dose levels of test substance from about day 16 of gestation to the time of weaning on day 21 after parturition. This ensures exposure of the embryo *in utero* in the last phase of growth, followed by postnatal exposure of the young pup via the dam's milk until weaning, when the animals are normally killed and autopsied, after sequential examination of their physical and neurological development.

Test Details and Precautions

Full details are given in standard sources, including Wilson and Warkany (1965), Mattison (1983) and EHC 30 (1984).

The particularly important aspects of dose and route of administration are governed by much the same criteria as apply in subacute tests, modified by the need to check the extent to which pharmacokinetics may be altered in gestation. A prior pilot test and some measurements to indicate kinetics are valuable. It may be important, too, to check drug level in the testis, its passage across the placenta and its presence in maternal milk, as a guide to the dosing of suckling neonates.

The examinations made are basically for maternal and paternal well-being, as shown by appearance, behaviour and weight gain, and subsequently at autopsy. Fertilisation is best assessed by the number of viable embryos. Organogenesis is followed by careful internal and external examination of the offspring, and by following the growth and appearances at autopsy of those born alive. Finally, postnatal growth and development are studied by examining weight gain, the time after birth when certain developmental landmarks are achieved (opening of the eye, separation of the pinna, etc.) and the progress of neurological skills, e.g. balancing on a beam or a grid, recognising sound and light signals, and learning to run a maze.

The commonest sources of problems in interpreting results are administration of such high doses that maternal or paternal toxicity interfere secondarily with fetal development, and failure to check pharmacokinetics during gestation.

In reproduction toxicity tests, therefore, it is very important to show in a prior experiment that appropriate dose levels have been used. As reproduction is such a complex process, the health and well-being of the animals involved must also be checked with particular care. Secondary environmental factors that can disturb the interrelated endocrine mechanisms should be excluded by particularly careful control of lighting and temperature, noise and the proximity of other sexually mature animals, which may produce pheromones.

Interpretation of Results

The usual provisos apply about appropriate route of administration, doses and the chemical composition of the material tested. There is also the common need to take pharmacokinetics into account, especially any change during gestation.

The complexity of reproduction, especially the processes of organogenesis and fetal development, mean that they are likely to show some variation for unknown and incidental reasons. This variability makes it essential to compare treated groups with concurrent controls dosed with the vehicle alone to model the stress of the dosing procedure. It is also important to compare the incidence and nature of any abnormalities with the historical control values for that colony and laboratory. The anatomical abnormalities that may occur during embryonic development, and which may be manifest by or shortly after parturition, have been divided into minor and major classes. The former represent small variations from normal and do not carry any sinister significance, except that they may suggest that the dose was close to causing some maternal toxicity; examples include waviness of the ribs and delayed ossification of the skull bones. They must be sharply distinguished from major anatomical abnormalities, which show a true teratogenic effect of the treatment, e.g. the phocomelia caused by thalidomide, cleft palate, exencephaly, etc. A substance shown to produce such major abnormalities in embryos, or clear impairment of fertility by any means, must be considered with great caution before its administration to man. The examples of thalidomide and Vitamin A analogues as teratogens in patients show some of the possible consequences, and the sterility following treatment with certain cytotoxic agents is a comparable warning.

It is more difficult to assess the significance for man of embryolethality, or severe maternal toxicity, at a much lower dose in the pregnant than in the non-pregnant animal. The relative dose levels in the affected animals and human, and comparative pharmacokinetics, will be important in evaluation, and so is any available pointer to the mechanism of the effect. Beyond those aspects, it may be worth considering repetition of the study in a species with placentation and reproductive physiology closer to man—perhaps, e.g. the mini-pig or a primate—but such experimentation is difficult and may not give a conclusive answer regarding the reality of the hazard to man.

The assessment of effects on perinatal and postnatal development is even less certain. Such toxicants as lead, phenytoin and ethanol are known to be able to produce fetal and developmental defects in man and animals, so the general risk is a real one. However, except for a few compounds, there is no good background evidence from patients and animals for comparison, so the strength of the extrapolation is uncertain, particularly if the action concerned is a limited functional effect, not associated with a structural or biochemical abnormality. Prudence requires protection of man, but as aspirin, for example, can be a serious developmental teratogen in the rat, the prediction carries limited reliability.

SPECIAL ROUTES OF ADMINISTRATION

The preceding accounts, although biased towards the commonest method of administration, namely oral dosing, are generally applicable to other routes also, such as intravenous, intramuscular, subcutaneous, inhalation and percutaneous application, as well as per rectum, per vaginam, intraocular application and nasal drops.

In each of those instances, the toxicological investigations should attempt to answer two main questions, in addition to drawing on and adding to appropriate pharmacokinetic studies. The questions are: What is the local and what is the systemic toxicity? Answering them requires a mixture of experiments by local administration to animals, to explore topical effects (mainly local irritancy and, at least for the skin and lungs, the possibility of sensitisation) and systemic dosing by an appropriate route to reveal any general risks following absorption.

Local studies are self-evident; considerable technical skill is required, for example, to dose a laboratory animal intravenously (i.v.) or intraperitoneally (i.p.) for several months. It may sometimes be reasonable for particular substances to rely on brief local irritancy testing, probably a sensitisation study, and more prolonged systemic exposure by another, more convenient route (e.g. i.p. instead of i.v.), provided that absorption and metabolism are appropriate. If the latter condition is not met, more prolonged studies employing specialised routes of administration will be needed. However, if there are ample data about the oral toxicity of a substance, development of a suppository formulation, say, would, in general, not require more than a short-term rectal test in animals.

SPECIAL PROBLEMS

Certain problems are common in the development of new drugs.

Change in the Synthetic Route or Pattern of Impurities

If the change is quantitatively minor, and particularly if the novel contaminants do not differ much in their chemical structure, then no additional testing should be required. But if there were more major alteration in the final composition of the drug, say more than 0.5% total impurities, then a brief examination of one or two key pharmacodynamic actions, perhaps of pharmacokinetics, and possibly an Ames test or an acute or brief subacute toxicity test, might be required. The decision is best made empirically on the basis of all the analytical and pharmacological data.

Changes in Formulation

The development of a slow or accelerated release formulation should not entail additional toxicity testing unless the kinetics of the active ingredient so produced have not already been covered by completed experiments or the formulation ingredients have not previously been examined.

Change in Route of Administration

As noted above, whether extensive studies are required depends on the amount and quality of the available data and the magnitude of the change produced by the novel site of administration, especially in the kinetics and metabolism of the compound. In both the latter instances, there is a particular need for close co-ordination with clinical and laboratory observations in man.

SPECIAL TOXICOLOGICAL PROBLEMS

This section contains a pragmatic grouping of disparate themes that frequently cause difficulties to toxicologists.

Sensitisation

True immunologically based sensitisation or allergic reactions to drugs are uncommon, with certain exceptions (e.g. pencillins) and require careful distinction from pseudo-allergic responses, which may be a mixture of ill-defined direct pharmacological actions and ill-founded beliefs (Dewdney, 1983).

The allergies commonly present clinically as skin disorders or as tissue swelling, acute bronchoconstriction and even shock on challenge. They are rarely predictable from the results of conventional toxicity tests, and to produce them in animals for study may require special dosing and observational procedures not suited to general screening (van Loveren and Vos, 1989; see next sub-section on 'Immunotoxicity').

Cutaneous sensitisation can be predicted reasonably well by use of one or other of the skin sensitisation test procedures, such as the Magnusson–Kligman and Buehler techniques (Marzulli and Maibach, 1985).

Immunotoxicity

The notion that the immune system may be the target for an adverse drug action is still little explored and poorly understood, partly because much basic understanding of immunity and its mechanisms is new, and partly because analytical and experimental techniques have yet to be devised and validated (van Loveren and Vos, 1989).

It is theoretically possible for a drug to cause general or selective depression or enhancement of the immune system, resulting in specific or generalised immunosuppression, altered reactivity to self (auto-immunity) or heightened reactivity to foreign antigens (sensitisation). These actions may affect humoral, cellular or natural immunity (Berlin *et al.*, 1987).

It is not yet possible to recommend even a general scheme of investigation of adverse clinical reactions considered to be due to an effect on the immune system. Prediction in the laboratory of such actions is not yet possible with any reliability. Experimental investigations can only be planned pragmatically in relation to the substance in question and the actions it is suspected of producing.

Behavioural Toxicity

There is a belief founded in ignorance that adverse effects on human behaviour (e.g. addiction, hallucinations, amnesia) should be avoided by toxicologists and referred to the pharmacologist.

The combination of toxicological experimentation and neuropharmacological techniques can be very powerful, provided that there is foreknowledge of what actions are to be explored (Zbinden and Gross, 1979; Bondy, 1985).

Behavioural methods may be more capricious than simple biochemical techniques, and the detailed, specific procedures are not suited to routine application, but, given hints from appropriate pharmacodynamic actions in laboratory or man, or from chemical structure, a reasonable approach can be made in toxicological studies to defining much of the risk to man.

Biologicals and Recombinant DNA Products

The toxicity testing of old-fashioned vaccines and antisera, and of the products of the new biology, such as cytokines and monoclonal antibodies, does differ from the study of conventional chemicals. It is a large subject, too specialised to justify extensive discussion here; it is reviewed in Graham (1987) and Dayan *et al.* (1988).

The principle is to try to find a species responsive to the agent, so that pharmacological and toxicological actions can be monitored, and to dose and study animals until their likely but irrelevant immune response to a foreign protein overwhelms any effects of specific concern.

GENERAL PRINCIPLES OF TOXICITY TESTING

The purpose of toxicity testing is to obtain the information required to indicate the potential toxicity of a substance as it is likely to be used in clinical practice, and at least to indicate the most probable consequences if it is abused. The toxicologist should use those data with clinicians and others in a collaborative judgement about the relative risks and benefits of treatment with the material, which will indicate whether it should be used at all in man and, if so, the likely limits of dose and duration of therapy, the most probable adverse reactions and the circumstances under which they may occur (dose, associated illness, drug or disease interactions, physiological variability of patients, etc.).

The job of the toxicologist testing a novel product really covers two areas: (1) design and conduct of studies appropriate to the specific properties and intended uses of the particular compound; (2) interpreting the results as fully as possible, to define the toxic effects and their nature, and their probable significance for man. The former requirement, which has been described in this chapter, is largely concerned with scientific and medical questions, plus some concern for the efficiency and economics of the lengthy process of drug development. The procedures for pharmaceuticals are very close to those applied to industrial and agrochemicals and food additives, and toxicologists working in any of these industries can learn much from one another (EHC 6, 1978; Paget, 1978; Hayes, 1982). The second objective is a more difficult area, combining scientific understanding with professional judgement in making empirical extrapolations. It involves assessing the experimental findings to ensure that the most appropriate studies have been done; then considering their applicability in judgements directed to man; and finally making the cautious extrapolation from laboratory study to patient.

We shall consider each objective more fully.

Assessment of Experimental Findings

At one level, this means ensuring that the work has complied with the GLP regulations. In terms of pharmacological, biochemical and toxicological considerations, it requires adaptation of basic test designs to the specific properties of the substance being investigated and the circumstances of its use.

All these points together amount to determining the validity of the programme of toxicity experiments. It involves co-ordination of toxicological and the other biological studies that demonstrate what the substance does to living systems and how it acts.

Interpreting and Extrapolating Experimental Findings

Given that the toxicity experiments are valid because they have been properly done, the next, vital, question is whether they are appropriate for making decisions about clinical use. The answer requires a decision that appropriately responsive species or *in vitro* systems have been used and that a suitable range of observations has been made (hence the importance of negative as well as positive findings): Were the pharmacokinetics and metabolism in the test species appropriate to cover the range likely to occur in man? Were the doses in the experiments so high that the kinetics became non-linear, or a novel and irrelevant metabolic pathway became activated?

Having settled these and related concerns, the toxicologist must then answer a more difficult point—what is the value of each type of test and of each type of observation in predicting a risk to man? There has been relatively little attempt formally to examine this aspect until recently (Lumley and Walker, 1987a,b), as the value of toxicity tests in protecting us has been taken as self-evident, because of the rarity of serious predictable toxic reactions to new medicines (and other chemicals) and our ability to model most toxic events in the laboratory. From general experience, it appears reasonable to conclude that most toxic phenomena revealed in the laboratory would probably occur in man at some dose or blood level. The correlation is often not perfect, in the sense that the finding of nephrotoxicity in the rat, say, due to a novel anti-inflammatory agent does not always imply predominant nephrotoxicity in man to the exclusion of other effects, or even that the target organ in one species will always be affected in another. In fact, exceptions have been the sources of valuable ideas about toxic mechanisms and species differences, as discussed in general textbooks of toxicology (e.g. Dayan, 1986; Vilaassen *et al* 1986).

Where there can be most confidence is with a specific structural lesion in a target organ, e.g. peripheral neuropathy, and where there is less certainty is with functional changes in a diffuse system, e.g. a quantitative alteration in one compartment of the immune system, or some change in one component of behaviour. In such instances, standard toxicity tests may have succeeded in their screening role by indicating an effect, and proper evaluation of it will require further, more specific experimentation.

By this stage in assessment, the toxicologist should be able to suggest the validated and proven effects in man. This requires scientific understanding of the actions and their likely causes, and knowledge of whether the target species man can react similarly. There are no objective, scientifically based rules for extrapolation, only pragmatic professional judgements based on experience, and guidelines that generally correlate effects with dose in relation to body surface area or metabolic rate, or an arbitrary power factor derived from them (Calabrese, 1983; Tardiff and Rodricks, 1987). However, it is essential to realise that in most toxicity experiments effects are seen at much higher dose levels than those to which man will be exposed, so there should be a very considerable margin of safety. This is one reason why it is important to determine the NOEL in laboratory studies. The process of extrapolation must take into account differences in pharmacokinetics and any likely consequence of disease, drug interaction or natural variation in susceptibility or metabolic capacity in individual patients.

In almost all instances the occurrence of toxicity follows some form of dose–response curve, so that there is a threshold of exposure below which no effect will be seen, and then an increasingly marked response as the dose increases. This pattern fails in two important aspects—true immune (hypersensitivity) reactions, and carcinogenesis, at least that due to genotoxic carcinogens.

In the former, once sensitisation has occurred, even a very small trigger dose may suffice to excite a violent reaction, almost of the 'all or nothing' type. This affects any attempt at quantitative extrapolation to man. In the second instance, there is good evidence from animals and man that increasing exposure to a genotoxic carcinogen will increase the proportion of a population affected, and probably reduce the time taken for a tumour to appear. Accordingly, chemical carcinogenesis is regarded as a probabilistic (stochastic) effect, in which the important factor is how many individuals may be affected, and for which there is no practical threshold. For this reason, exposure to genotoxic carcinogens is strictly avoided, unless there is special justification for their use. On the other hand, non-genotoxic carcinogens, which include phenobarbital and other promoting agents, are known experimentally to show a threshold, so their cautious use may be considered permissible.

CONCLUSIONS

Toxicity testing comprises a broad range of empirical experimentation to reveal any detectable harmful effect of a compound. Its experiments require great care in design and conduct, because they have to cover many different types of actions, and because they are costly and prolonged. Interpreting the results needs much care to ensure that the findings are relevant to the circumstances of the intended use in man. The final stage of extrapolation to man from the laboratory findings involves more empirical guidelines and professional judgement than proven scientific rules.

Above all, toxicological assessment is marked by the breadth of knowledge required and the essential need to correlate its findings with related branches of experimental biology and clinical medicine in ensuring safe, usable medicines, and better understanding of bodily mechanisms of health and disease.

REFERENCES

Ashby, J. de Serres, F., Shelby, M. D., Margolin, B. H., Ishidate, M. and Becking, G. C. (1988). *Evaluation of Short-Term Tests for Carcinogens*, Volumes I, II. IPCS. Cambridge University Press

Ashby, J. and Tennant, R. W. (1988). Chemical structure, Salmonella mutagenicity and extent of carcinogenicity as indicators of genotoxic carcinogenesis among 222 chemicals tested in rodents by the U.S. NCI/NTP. *Mut. Res.*, **204**, 17–115

Berlin, A., Dean, J. H., Draper, M. H., Smith, E. M. B., Spreafico, F. (1987). *Immunotoxicology*. Martinmus Nijhoff, Dordrecht

Bondy, S. C. (1985). Neurobehavioural toxicology. *Crit. Rev. Toxicol.*, **14**, 381–402

Brown, V. (1988). *Acute Toxicity*, 2nd edn. John Wiley, Chichester

Calabrese, E. (1983). *Principles of Animal Extrapolation*. John Wiley, Chichester

Dayan, A. D. (1986). In Richardson, M. (Ed.), *Interpretation of Data in Toxic Risk Assessment of Chemicals*. Royal Society of Chemistry, London

Dayan, A. D., Campbell, P. N., Jukes, T. H. (Eds.) (1988). Hazards of biotechnology: Real or imaginary? *J. Chem. Technol. Biotechnol.*, **43**, No. 4, 1–138

Dayan, A. D., Clark, B., Jackson, M., Morgan, H., Charlesworth, F. A. (1984). Role of the LD_{50} test in the pharmaceutical industry. *Lancet*, **i**, 555–6

Dayan, A. D. and Walker, S.R. (1987). *Long-Term Animal Studies: Their Predictive Value for Man*. MTP Press, Lancaster

Dewdney, J. A. (1983). Clinical diagnosis of drug hypersensitivity in immunotoxicology. In Gibson, G. G., Hubbard, R. and Parke, D. V. (Eds.), *Immunotoxicology*. Academic Press, London, pp. 95–106

Department of Health (1989) *Guidelines for the Testing of Chemicals for Mutagenicity*. HMSO, London.

Department of Health and Social Security (1986). *Good Laboratory Practice*. DHSS, HMSO, London

EHC 6 (1978). *Principles and Methods for Evaluating the Toxicity of Chemicals*, Part I. IPCS/WHO, Geneva

EHC 30 (1984). *Principles for Evaluating Health Risks to Progeny Associated with Exposure to Chemicals During Pregnancy*. IPCS/WHO, Geneva

Graham, C. E. (1987). *Preclinical Safety Testing of Biotechnology Products Intended for Human Use*. Alan R. Liss, New York.

Grice, H. C. and Ciminera, J. L. (1989). *Carcinogenicity Testing*. Springer-Verlag, New York

Hayes, W. A. (1982). *Principles and Methods of Toxicology*. Raven Press, New York

Lumley, C. E. and Walker, S. R. (1987a). Predicting the safety of medicines from animal toxicity tests. I. Rodents alone. *Arch. Toxicol.*, **II**, Suppl., 295–99

Lumley, C. E. and Walker, S. R. (1987b). Predicting the safety of medicines from animal toxicity tests. II. Rodents and non-rodents. *Arch. Toxicol.*, **II**, Suppl., 300–4

Mattison, D. R. (1983). *Reproductive Toxicology*. Alan R. Liss, New York

Marzulli, F. and Maibach, H. (1985). *Dermatotoxicity*, 3rd edn. McGraw-Hill, New York

Paget, G. E. (1978). *Methods in Toxicology*, Blackwell, Oxford

Parry, J. and Arlett, C. F. (Eds.) (1984). *Comparative Genetic Toxicology*. Macmillan, London

Paton, W. (1984). *Man and Mouse*. Clarendon Press, Oxford

Salsburg, D. (1988). *Statistics for Toxicologists*. Marcel Dekker, New York

Shelby, M. D. (1988). The genetic toxicology of human carcinogens and its implications. *Mut. Res.*, **204**, 3–16

Snell, K. and Mullock, B. (1987). *Biochemical Toxicology*. IRL Press, Oxford

Tardiff, R. G. and Rodricks, J. V. (1987). *Toxic Substances and Human Risk: Principles of Data Interpretation*. Plenum Press, New York

Timbrell, J. A. (1984). *Introduction to Biochemical Toxicology*. Taylor and Francis, London

UKEMS (1984). *Report of the UKEMS Sub-committee on Guidelines for Mutagenicity Testing*, Part I: *Basic Test Battery*. UKEMS, Swansea

UKEMS (1985). *Report of the UKEMS Sub-committee on Guidelines for Mutagenicity Testing*, Part II: *Supplementary Tests*. UKEMS, Swansea

van Loveren, H. and Vos, J. G. (1989). Immunotoxicological considerations. In Dayan, A. D. and Paine, A. J. (Eds.), *Advances in Applied Toxicology*. Taylor and Francis, London, pp. 143–64

Vilaassen, C. D., Amour, M. O. and Doull, J. (1986). *Casarett and Doull's Toxicology*, 3rd edn. Macmillan Inc, New York

Wilson, A. B. (1988). Experimental design. In Anderson, D. and Conning, D. M. (Eds.), *Experimental Toxicology*. Royal Society of Chemistry, London, pp. 35–6

Wilson, J. and Warkany, J. (1965). *Teratology, Principles and Techniques*. University of Chicago Press, Chicago

Zbinden, G. and Gross, F. (Eds.) (1978). *Pharmacological Methods in Toxicology*. Pergamon Press, Oxford

5

Animal Tests as Predictors of Human Response

Peter I. Folb

Dept of Pharmacology, University of Cape Town Medical School, Observatory 7925, South Africa

INTRODUCTION

Many serious toxic reactions caused by new chemical entities may be detected reliably by routine toxicological testing. Experience has shown that predictable, 'dose- and time-dependent' reactions are likely to be revealed in animal experiments. It is the detail of these that forms the basis of the experimental toxicology that is applied to new drug development. Unpredictable idiosyncratic adverse effects, not related to time or dose, are considerably more difficult to identify in preclinical drug evaluation.

LIMITS TO EXTRAPOLATING ANIMAL DATA IN PREDICTION OF THE HUMAN RESPONSE

The limitations inherent in extrapolating animal toxicology data to prediction of the human response (Balazs, 1974; Zbinden, 1980) include the following.

(1) *Pharmacokinetic differences between test animals and humans* Considerable species differences exist in the plasma half-lives and metabolic disposition of a number of drugs. Rapid detoxification and excretion may account for the failure of a toxic effect to express itself. In the small number of animal species that are used in drug toxicity testing it is to be expected that quantitative and qualitative species differences in drug disposition and metabolism are the rule rather than the exception.

(2) Those adverse reactions in humans to drugs which are idiosyncratic, the mechanisms of which are poorly understood, are not normally demonstrable in animals by standard toxicological investigation.

(3) *Underlying pathological condition* Drugs may exacerbate underlying diseases in humans which do not exist in the healthy animals in which preclinical studies are usually conducted. Relationships that might exist between the drug and its metabolites on the one hand, and an underlying

disease on the other, cannot adequately be investigated or predicted from studies which have been conducted in healthy animals.

(4) *Species differences in anatomy and physiological functions* Numerous adverse reactions to drugs are connected with functional disturbances of the central nervous system and the autonomic nervous system, respectively. The symptomatology of such disturbances is likely to differ considerably between experimental animals and man. For example, postural hypotension, which is a common side-effect of drugs in man, is unlikely to be present in quadruped animals (Zbinden, 1980).

(5) *Tolerance and enzyme induction* Repeated administration of certain drugs (notably those with the capacity to induce the cytochrome P450 enzyme system) to experimental animals may result in auto-induction of their own metabolism. Following even a limited number of doses of such agents, peak blood levels may fall and excretion may be enhanced. As a result, toxic concentrations of the parent drug may not be reached, and concentrations that were potentially toxic initially may disappear. Kidney lesions may disappear despite the chronic administration of nephrotoxic substances such as mercuric chloride, salicylates and nephrotoxic antibiotics (Balazs, 1974).

(6) *Lack of appropriate assay methods* Adverse drug events that can only be communicated verbally by the patient are not normally recognised in animals, or at best are identified only with difficulty.

ACUTE TOXICITY TESTING

Acute exposure of experimental animals to a toxic agent may express itself either directly in one or more tissues or systemically following absorption from a local site (Brown, 1987). With certain toxicants both types of response may occur.

Direct Toxic Effects on Tissues

The skin, eyes, gastrointestinal mucosa, vagina and respiratory tract are at greatest risk of topical toxic effects of drugs. When a substance is known to be locally irritant or corrosive, it is not normally necessary for animal tests to be conducted in order to confirm what is already established. On the other hand, local irritation may be materially influenced by the conditions of exposure, such as local pH. Topical toxicity testing is required to determine this.

Skin

In order to evaluate the degree of skin irritation that may be exerted by a potentially toxic substance, it is necessary to examine the effect in human subjects. There is enormous variability in the response of the skin of different animal species to toxic chemicals, and major differences exist between animals and humans. Significant variation is also found between individuals, and between different anatomical sites in a particular person. For these reasons, there is little value in skin irritancy testing that requires extrapolation of findings from one species to another.

Eyes

As a general rule, any chemical with irritant or corrosive properties when applied to the skin is also likely to be irritant to the cornea and conjunctiva, and ocular irritancy tests need not be carried out. However, the correlation between the toxicity of chemicals on the skin and in the eye is not close. The most widely used predictive test for ophthalmological irritancy is still the Draize test in rabbits (Draize *et al.*, 1944), despite the widespread objection to the test. The obvious differences that exist between the eyes of rabbits and humans are not sufficient to invalidate the Draize test.

Mucosal Surfaces

Irritancy testing of mucosal surfaces is necessary when substances are designed for application to particular surfaces, such as the vagina, where local factors such as pH have to be considered.

There is comparatively little difference between species, and indeed between individuals, in mucosal responses to toxic injury.

The Lethal Dose 50 (LD$_{50}$) Test

The LD$_{50}$ test (Zbinden and Flury-Roversi, 1981; Paget, 1983; Rowan, 1983) is aimed at determining the dose of a toxic substance that kills 50% of the animals that receive it. It forms a traditional part of the early assessment of a new medicine, and it also makes it possible to study precisely the nature of the acute toxicity of a compound. Nevertheless, the concept of killing animals in this way has proved repugnant to many, and this has necessitated a critical review of the justification for the LD$_{50}$.

The Value of the LD$_{50}$ Test

The value of the LD$_{50}$ test in acute toxicity testing is as follows (Paget, 1983).

(1) *Biological standardisation of substances such as digitalis, agricultural toxins, hormones and synthetic chemicals* With improvements in assay systems this use of the LD$_{50}$ test will become obsolete.

(2) *Therapeutic margin* The margin between the effective dose and the toxic dose can be determined in this manner. Compounds may be compared, allowing for those with the widest margin of safety to be selected for further development. When significant species variation is found this is regarded as having serious implications for human use.

(3) *Toxokinetic evaluation* The LD$_{50}$ test makes it possible for lethal

effects to be compared with blood levels of the active principle, and with the findings obtained in repeated dosing studies.

In the past, the LD_{50} test has been used to compare the extent of absorption of a drug from different routes of administration. Precise methods of blood and tissue drug estimations have made the use of the LD_{50} test for this purpose less relevant.

Factors Influencing the LD_{50}

The following factors are known to influence the LD_{50}, and they need to be considered when acute toxicity data in animals are extrapolated to humans.

(1) *Species differences* LD_{50} values vary considerably between species.

(2) *Age* The metabolic activity of animals changes with age, and the differences between newborns and adult animals may be considerable. The LD_{50} value may vary by a factor of 500, or more, with age.

(3) Body weight differences may influence LD_{50} values.

(4) Sex differences in LD_{50} responses are sometimes encountered.

(5) *Strain* Marked differences in sensitivities have been reported between strains of a particular species.

(6) *Nutrition* The composition of the diet is known to influence LD_{50} values significantly. There may be synergistic toxicity due to contamination of food with traces of chemicals. The protein content of the diet may also influence the outcome. Food deprivation prior to testing has marked effects on the LD_{50} of a number of substances.

(7) *Environmental effects* Ambient temperature, housing conditions and chronological variations may all modify the LD_{50} of certain compounds. Factors such as air humidity, noise, acclimatisation and the technical skill of laboratory personnel are also important.

Since the various influences on LD_{50} results are so numerous, it follows that it is not feasible to standardise the test sufficiently for each to be taken into account.

Limits to Extrapolation

It is important that the objections that have been raised to the LD_{50} test, and the caveats to extrapolation of data derived from it, should be carefully considered (Zbinden and Flury-Roversi, 1981). Even when conducted with great care, the results of the LD_{50} test should be regarded as an isolated finding. The results need to be considered in conjunction with other findings from acute toxicity testing.

Zbinden has proposed the following guidelines for the use of the LD_{50} test, and these have been widely accepted.

(1) LD_{50} data should always be considered in conjunction with other relevant information, and not in isolation.

(2) Conduct of the LD_{50} test on large animals should be discontinued; a test on a limited number of small animals, including detailed recording of symptomatology and pathology, should be done instead.

(3) No LD_{50} test should be conducted with pharmacologically inert substances (a maximum dose of 5 g/kg for oral administration and 2 g/kg for parenteral administration should be sufficient if death or acute symptoms are not produced).

(4) The test should not be conducted in newborn animals.

In summary, it is important in acute toxicity testing of a new drug that full understanding be obtained of the nature of the acute toxic injury. In the foreseeable future it is unlikely that the whole animal will be replaced by simpler models. The LD_{50} test represents a comparatively small part of the information that can be gained from acute toxicity studies. If the test is carefully performed, with appropriate concern for the humane issues that are associated with it, it can provide valuable information about the biological and the toxicological properties of a new chemical entity.

Testing for Systemic Toxicity

Systemic effects resulting from short-term exposure to chemicals may develop either rapidly or after delayed onset, and the result may be transient, prolonged or irreversible.

The systemic toxicity of any substance is likely to be determined by the combined effects of the exposure, the route of administration and the physical presentation of the product to the target organ. For an animal model to provide meaningful results, it is necessary that it be comparable physiologically with humans, and that there should be toxokinetic similarities in the new chemical entity in the test animal and in humans.

CHRONIC (LONG-TERM) TOXICITY TESTING

The value of chronic toxicity testing in animals (Aldridge, 1976; Dayan, 1986; Frederick, 1986; Glocklin, 1986; Jackson, 1986; McLean, 1986; Rawlins, 1986; Worden, 1986; Worden and Walker, 1987) has been seriously questioned for many years, and it has been hoped that a more complete understanding of the relevant pharmacology, and of the physiological changes caused by acute exposure to a new drug, might provide sufficient information to anticipate adverse long-term effects. This has not been achieved, and there remains for the time being no better alternative for.

Dayan (1986) has pointed out that with repeated-dose testing most structural lesions that are likely to be produced should be identifiable, and that knowledge can also be gained of functional disturbances, although the latter are unlikely to be quantifiable. Long-term animal studies only partly reveal functional disorders, and the influence on toxicity of drugs of factors such as ageing, disease and diet remain uncertain.

Mechanisms of Long-term Drug Injury

In planning and evaluating long-term toxicity studies in animals, various mechanisms of drug injury are considered (McLean, 1986). These are as applicable to humans as they are to animals.

(1) Accumulation of the parent drug, and/or its metabolite(s), in the tissues, with consequent toxic injury. Pharmacokinetic considerations are important in assessing this category of risk. For example, evidence of slow accumulation in the body suggests the possibility of eventual toxic injury.

(2) Repeated or low-grade continuous injury may occur to DNA, or to the hereditable DNA expression which is found during cell differentiation. Carcinogenesis and cirrhosis are examples of this category of toxic injury. Damage to the retinal cells may also result from cumulative exposure (chloroquine).

(3) The adaptive synthesis of cell receptors may be disturbed, as is found with repeated exposure to the opiates.

(4) Damage to repair responses may occur in the experimental rat fed a low-protein diet, which as a result experiences difficulties in synthesising glutathione. Such an animal may be extremely sensitive to an additional toxic insult.

Dose Considerations

The normal practice is to employ a minimum of three treatment groups, divided according to dose, and one control group. An additional group may be added if it is necessary to examine a toxic effect in relation to a particular dose.

The lowest dose is conventionally set at the equivalent of five times the projected therapeutic dose, to establish a non-toxic dose level. The mid-dose usually represents the geometric mean between the low and high doses, but pharmacokinetic considerations have to be considered when selecting this. The high-dose level is calculated so as to identify toxic effects, but not to a degree that might jeopardise successful completion of the study.

Frequency of Administration

In general, adequate exposure of the experimental animal to a drug is achieved by once-daily dosing, 7 days a week, but more frequent administration may be necessary in the case of drugs with a very short half-life or brief duration of action. Inevitably in the experimental animal, peaks and troughs in drug levels occur which do not correspond with the effect of divided daily doses and the consistent therapeutic responses that are found in the clinical situation. It may be appropriate to administer long-acting drugs to experimental animals less frequently than once-daily, monitoring levels in the blood frequently.

Route of Administration

The route of administration in animal studies of an investigational new drug is normally the same as that which is proposed for clinical use (Jackson, 1986). Since the distribution of the drug and its metabolite(s), and the organ exposure that might result, are likely to vary with the route of administration, extrapolation is made with greater confidence if the method of administration is the same. This can be problematic if a high dose is required, which cannot be tolerated when given by a particular route. If use of an alternative route is inevitable, comparative pharmacokinetic data will be required. In inhalational or topical studies, when only low blood drug levels occur, it may be necessary to supplement by an additional route so as to characterise possible dose-related systemic toxicity.

Duration of the Study

In rodents, the number of incidental (spontaneous) lesions begins to rise from 15 to 18 months of age onwards (Dayan, 1986). This reduces the discriminative power of any study, because of the lesions themselves, and the impairment that they might cause to the normal response of the animals.

The metabolic consequences of ageing are considerable. The liver, kidneys and lungs are especially vulnerable, but other organs also might be affected. The time-scale differs, of course, between species. In the dog and primate, and other non-rodent species, an 18 month-old animal might not yet have reached the pubertal stage of development.

Glocklin (1986) has explained the USA Food and Drug Administration (FDA) requirement for 12 month long-term animal toxicity studies. This refers to rodent as well as non-rodent studies. The study should be extended beyond 12 months when warranted by a specific concern or by an unusual condition of use. Chronic studies conducted for less than 12 months are not accepted for registration purposes.

Lumley and Walker (1985b) and Worden (1986) have suggested that a 6 month study should be sufficient to establish the toxicity profile of new drugs, and that no-effect levels can also be predicted within that period. This is only true if reliance is not placed solely on histopathological changes.

United Kingdom Guidelines

Grahame-Smith (1986) has provided in broad outline the requirements of the UK authorities for the conduct of repeated-dose studies in animals, except for carcinogenicity and reproductive studies, for which the duration of testing is determined by the likely duration of treatment with the agent in humans.

Refinement of Existing Procedures

A number of recommendations have been made for refining the present procedures of long-term toxicity testing, and improving the data (Worden, 1987).

(1) Each individual study should be planned with pharmacologists, toxicologists and clinicians experienced in the field of medicine for which the new drug is intended.

(2) Observations should be conducted on live animals using non-invasive procedures, to assess the toxicological response *in vivo*.

(3) The chemistry and pharmacology of the active principle should be stated in detail, including the dose form, and absorption, distribution, metabolism and elimination data.

(4) Immunological techniques should be used where possible to examine antibody responses and other effects of the test substance on the immune system.

(5) Observations should be made of behavioural effects and of other complications, such as ocular and retinal injury.

(6) Histochemical and ultrastructural examination should be conducted on tissue obtained at the conclusion and also during the course of the study, to assess both cellular and subcellular changes.

CARCINOGENICITY TESTING

The majority of human carcinogens have also been shown to be carcinogenic in animals, and virtually all, when tested appropriately, induce cancer in several animal species (Gart *et al.*, 1979; Kodell *et al.*, 1982; Hoel *et al.*, 1983; IARC, 1984; Purchase, 1987; Weisburger, 1987). It is not unusual for 80–100% of the test animals to be affected, with a relatively short latent period of 12–18 months. Human carcinogens that are genotoxic (most are) also reliably display activity in the standard short-term *in vitro* mutagenicity tests.

Conversely, a chemical which (a) is consistently genotoxic in a number (not just one) of short-term *in vitro* tests, (b) is active in several *in vivo* bioassay systems (high yield of tumours, latent period less than 18 months), and (c) exhibits such activity over a range of dose levels, is a probable human cancer risk.

When an unknown test chemical is active only in a single bioassay system or in a small number of *in vitro* systems, its classification as a genotoxin requires careful analysis of the positive and negative data. It may be that in the intact mammalian system (i.e. the whole animal) biochemical defence systems adequately protect against reactive radicals, giving a negative test result, despite the evidence of genotoxicity that may be found with *in vitro* testing (Weisburger, 1987).

Database Required for Carcinogenicity Risk Assessment

The database required for carcinogenicity risk assessment of new chemical entities involves assessment of the following factors.

(1) The structure–activity relationships of the chemical, and its similarity to known carcinogens.
(2) The results of short-term genotoxicity tests.
(3) The outcome of *in vivo* studies in which evidence is sought in mice, rats and/or hamsters of a statistically significant incidence of cancer. (Whole animal studies are selected on the basis of comprehensive assessment of the probable mechanism(s) of action, whether genotoxic or promoting, of the chemical under consideration. Carcinogenesis is often organ-specific, as a result of the formation of locally produced reactive metabolites.)

It is most improbable that any human carcinogen will yield negative results for all three components of this screening procedure.

In Vivo Systems for Carcinogenicity Testing

The investigations that have proved most practical for predicting chemical carcinogenesis in humans are those in which mitotic lesions are induced in the livers of rats and mice, skin tumours in mice, mammary tumours in Sprague–Dawley female rats and pulmonary tumours in certain sensitive strains of mice. The majority of such tumours are induced in less than 1 year. The test compound is compared with a known positive control, if possible, at several dose levels, so as to provide an estimate of the dose–response relationship.

Agents which are thought to act as promoters are administered together with a genotoxic carcinogen appropriate for the relevant target organ. The test substance is administered in four or five dose levels. Comparison with the appropriate positive control will provide an indication of the relative potency of the test substance.

In all studies utilising *in vivo* bioassay systems, the same end points are considered: (a) the percentage of animals with histopathologically validated lesions, (b) the multiplicity and size of the neoplasms, and (c) the rate of development of the tumour. The latent period is normally expressed as the time taken for the experimental group to reach a 50% incidence of neoplasms or, alternatively, for all the animals to develop neoplasms.

Some workers (Gart *et al.*, 1979; Kodell *et al.*, 1982) have indicated how important it is in the evaluation of the data that there should be comprehensive pathological and toxicological assessment of individual animals in carcinogenicity testing, including comparison with controls, and evaluation of the 'case history'.

Squire (1981) has pointed out that extrapolation from animal data to potential carcinogenic risk in humans requires consideration of numerous factors. The response in intact experimental animals reflects at best a potential for human risk, but not an order of risk.

Principles Governing Dose Studies

The principles governing dose determination of the test substance in animal carcinogenicity studies are as follows (Weisburger, 1987).

(1) Carcinogens are different from other toxins in so far as the same total dose, when administered in small fractions over a prolonged period, may be more carcinogenic than when given in larger amounts over a shorter time.

(2) Potent genotoxic agents characteristically cause two dose-related effects: (a) an increasing percentage yield of neoplasms and multiplicity of tumours; and (b) an accelerated rate of development of the neoplasm(s).

(3) It has not been shown beyond reasonable doubt that for every carcinogen there is a threshold dose. However, from principles of drug metabolism, and considering the barriers to electrophiles from reaching critical targets in DNA, and the capacity of DNA repair processes, it does seem probable that a threshold may exist. This is likely to be low in the case of powerful carcinogens and high for weak carcinogens (Hoel *et al.*, 1983).

Special Issues in Extrapolating Carcinogenicity Data

Purchase (1987) found in a study of the carcinogenicity potential of 250 compounds that both the specificity (the prediction of carcinogenicity) and the sensitivity (the prediction of non-carcinogenicity) in rat and mouse studies were approximately 85%. Sixty-four per cent of the chemicals consistently produced cancer at the same site.

The chemical and the host are each involved in the expression of a carcinogen. The potency may vary between hosts, depending on tumour type, nutritional status, environmental conditions and other variables. This explains differences that are found between laboratories and in different test systems.

It is generally accepted that chemicals should be tested under constraints that minimise the number of false-negative results. The maximum dose chosen is usually larger than the dose that is likely to be given to humans. The group sizes are usually in the range of 50–100 animals. Results are extrapolated to humans on the (erroneous) assumption that the most sensitive outcome, from the most sensitive species, is appropriate to man, and that a simple quantitative correlation can be made. Animal data are neither quantitatively nor qualitatively reliable for such extrapolation, and the dose–response relationships cannot be assumed to be linear at low levels of exposure.

In general, evaluation of animal carcinogenicity data tends to be 'conservative', in that the result is commonly accepted which maximises the magnitude of the risk. For example: (a) the most toxic result is likely to be chosen, while negative results are disregarded; (b) data from experiments in which the maximum dose has compromised the general health and the immunological and hormonal responses of the animal are likely to be used; (c) benign and malignant neoplasms may be combined, which overestimates the risk, since in humans most benign neoplasms are not diagnosable; (d) a linear, non-threshold dose–response relationship is assumed, even for non-genotoxic carcinogens; (e) the upper confidence limit is selected, rather than the maximum likelihood estimate; and (f) the dose may be computed on the basis of surface area rather than on body weight.

If the aforementioned are indeed applied, assuming that each is more conservative than the real situation by a factor of 5, then the overall situation would be erroneous by a factor of $15\,625$ (5^6) (Purchase, 1987).

HYPERSENSITIVITY TESTING AND IMMUNOLOGICAL STUDIES

The assessment of the effect on immune function of a new chemical entity for human use seems to be a logical, and long overdue, part of new drug testing. A number of immunological assays are now available which make it possible to assess the degree of cellular injury and immune functional impairment resulting from drug toxicity (Dean *et al.*, 1982).

Miller (1987) has proposed a minimum screening panel for defining immune alteration after chemical exposure in rodents.

Pathotoxicology:	Haematology profile, complete blood count and differential; total body weight; organ weights— spleen, thymus, liver, kidney, brain.
Host resistance:	Susceptibility to transplantable syngeneic tumour.
Delayed cutaneous hypersensitivity:	T-cell-dependent antigen response.
Lymphocyte function:	Lymphocyte blastogenesis to phytohaemagglutinin or concanavolin A, lipopolysaccharide, and allogeneic lymphocytes (mixed lymphocyte culture).
Humoral immunity:	Immunoglobulin levels (IgG, IgM, IgA); antibody plaque response to sheep erythrocytes.

The study of the norms for each of the above parameters, and the biological significance of each when impaired by drugs, is an important development in the evaluation of drug toxicity. It has to be borne in mind that minor changes in immunological responsiveness may occur daily under the influence of environmental pathogens or drugs without there being undue susceptibility to infection. On the other hand, even mild immunosuppression may be a potential danger in a vulnerable population group. The ideal assessment of immunotoxicity in the whole animal, utilising a few selective assays in sequential fashion, is still being developed.

There is, at present, no suitable animal model for assessing the risk from inhaled, ingested or injected drugs of acute hypersensitivity reactions.

REPRODUCTIVE AND DEVELOPMENTAL TOXICITY TESTING

The consequences of human and animal exposure to teratogens depend on the extent, duration and time of exposure, and the chemical entity concerned. The results may be various: impaired ability of the female to conceive, abortion, dysmorphogenesis, premature birth, low birth weight, perinatal mortality and morbidity, cancer, and dysfunctional growth and development after birth (Wilson, 1959; Koeter, 1983; Lasagna, 1984; Miller *et al.*, 1985; Lansdown, 1987; Messite and Bond, 1988).

Hundreds of chemical agents are teratogenic to the experimental animal. These include poisons, therapeutic agents, and industrial and agricultural chemicals. However, proof of dysmorphogenic and other teratogenic effects on the human fetus has been shown for only a very small number of chemicals—thalidomide, androgens, virilising progestagens, cytotoxic drugs, antithyroid drugs and certain anticonvulsants.

Discrepancies between the Laboratory and the Clinic

For a number of reasons, reproductive toxicity data derived from animal experiments are not necessarily applicable to humans. These are as follows.

(1) Species differences in drug distribution and action, and in tissue and organ responses.

(2) Differences with regard to the method of dosing and the route and duration of administration. Selecting doses in teratological studies is not easy. Doses which are excessive may invalidate the test by killing the animals, while doses which are too low may give a misleading impression of safety. Demonstrating dose–response relationship is important, but not always realisable, and identifying a safe or threshold dose can be difficult. Even when there is concordance of results with humans, teratogenic doses are seldom comparable. Humans may be 2–50 times more sensitive than animals on a dose-per-weight basis.

(3) The epidemiological method is imprecise when applied to evaluation of human teratogenicity, compared with more exact animal experimental data. The effects of 'low-grade' human teratogens are frequently not discernible from the normal background incidence of major congenital malformations (2–3%). The problems of extrapolation are compounded by the lack of

accurate information commonly encountered when the time of exposure of the pregnant mother to the suspected teratogen is reported. The matter is further complicated by some agents that may act to enable expression of the primary offender (for example, cigarette smoking, alcohol and food additives).

(4) A variety of teratogens may produce the same malformation and, conversely, a variety of malformations may be produced by the same teratogen. Moreover, an established teratogen is not necessarily deleterious with every exposure. In such circumstances attribution of causation can be very complex.

(5) No clear relationship exists between a particular chemical or pharmacological class and specific effects on the embryo. For example, one sulphonylurea may cause a high percentage of malformations in animals, while another has little or no such effect.

Principles of Teratology Testing

The principles which govern the conduct of teratology testing, and which are considered in extrapolating data from animals to humans are as follows.

(1) There is no single vulnerable period in the development of the conceptus; each phase has its unique responses. The susceptibility of the fetus and the expression of toxicity usually depend upon the stage at which exposure takes place.

(2) The genotype influences the reaction of an animal to a teratogenic agent.

(3) Any dysmorphogenic agent is also likely to cause an increase in fetal mortality.

(4) Manifestations of abnormal development increase in extent and degree as the dose levels of the teratogenic agent increase, ranging from a no-effect threshold to lethal outcome.

Protocols for Teratogenicity Testing

It is assumed that teratogenic agents act at any time during the reproductive cycle to impair fertility, prenatal development or postnatal life. The expression of toxicity may be one of a number of these possible effects.

Single-generation studies are conducted to evaluate drugs and chemicals with short half-lives of elimination which are proposed for use by humans over brief periods of time. Drugs for long-term therapy, or which have long half-lives, are tested over more than one generation. It is generally accepted that two generations should be sufficient.

Teratology tests are normally performed in mammals in at least one rodent and one non-rodent species. In Phase 1 testing, general reproduction is examined, by exposure of males and females prior to mating, and dosing of females throughout gestation and weaning. Phase 2 testing involves treatment of pregnant animals during the organogenetic period of gestation. In Phase 3 studies, the effects on the latter period of gestation and on postnatal development are investigated. This investigation addresses problems of labour, delivery, lactation, neonatal viability and postnatal development of the newborn. Procedures for evaluation of postnatal behaviour may be included.

Preimplantation Toxicity Testing

Between conception and implantation the fertilised egg is actively dividing, but not differentiating. Toxic effects are likely to be devastating, with ablation of the embryo, or to have no significant teratogenic effect (the 'all-or-none' effect). However, such generalisations oversimplify the situation. Cellular differentiation may occur early in the developmental period, and drugs with a prolonged half-life may persist in the fetus for periods that extend into the period of organogenesis.

Fetal Toxicity after the First Trimester

The period of fetal development after the formation of the major organs has traditionally been considered to be one of low sensitivity to teratogenic effects. However, recently it has been realised that permanent defects in structure and function may result from drug exposure after the first trimester—for example, endocrine disorders, mental impairment, immunological defects, reproductive tract malformations and malignant tumours.

The rat and the mouse at birth are at an earlier stage of development compared with the human. The last third of gestation in the rat is more akin to the second trimester in humans (Miller *et al.*, 1985). The responses observed in rats during this period, namely tumour induction, disturbed central nervous system function, and immune and endocrine disturbances, can be compared with human responses more typical of exposure in the second trimester.

Preconception Toxicity

Exposure of male and female germ cells to mutagens before conception may result in cytogenetic damage. The result, in theory, may be impaired fertility, spontaneous abortion, birth defects or damage to the offspring of subsequent generations. (There are few substantiated reports of preconception germ cell exposure to toxins resulting in these outcomes.) Chemical exposure which results in a reduction in the total number of germ cells is likely to have a more obvious effect on the female, since the damaged oocytes are not replaced as readily as sperms are in the male (Kline *et al.*, 1977).

NEUROTOXICITY TESTING

Neurotoxicity evaluation (Silbergeld, 1982; Dewar, 1987) has become an important part of toxicology, with the recognition that the nervous system is a critical target for hazardous substances. This has been made possible by advances in the neurosciences, but limitations remain in techniques and methods of evaluation.

Limitations in Current Methods of Neurotoxicity Testing

Silbergeld (1982) has summarised the limitations in current methods of neurotoxicity as follows.

(1) Correlation of animal data with human results is limited by the problems inherent in assessing affect and intellectual function in an animal model.

(2) The difficulties experienced in obtaining premorbid material from animals.

(3) The limits to our understanding of the normal range of nervous system function, against which findings may be interpreted.

(4) Inadequate application of molecular biology and genetics to understanding the effects of toxins on the central nervous system.

Behavioural change is likely to be the earliest detectable expression of toxic injury to the nervous system, as adverse biochemical or pathological effects exceed the homoeostatic capacity of the central nervous system (Dewar, 1987). It may be very difficult, or impossible, to detect intellectual impairment (a common expression of neurotoxicity in man) by animal tests, particularly as distinctions are relative rather than absolute.

Age is another complicating issue in assessing toxic insult to the central nervous system. The immature and developing brain is especially susceptible to toxic injury at the time of active cellular proliferation, myelination and synaptogenesis. The ageing central nervous system is also very vulnerable.

STATISTICAL EVALUATION

(Schein *et al.*, 1970; Salsburg, 1979; Gart *et al.*, 1986; Glaister, 1986; Jackson, 1986.)

Mean versus Individual Evaluation

In toxicological analysis it is common for group values to be considered. The conventional level of significance is taken as $p = 0.05$. In long-term rodent studies it is not unusual for three or more group comparisons and numerous parameters to be evaluated on a number of occasions, and a comparison is made of mean values. This practice may be misleading. When the number in the group is small, mean values and other group statistics will not reflect early or isolated treatment effects (Jackson, 1986).

Group Size

The number of animals used in regulatory toxicology presents a major problem in statistical analysis. Tests on non-rodent species are often confined to 3–5 animals per sex per group, which obviously limits the power of statistical analysis; in short-term rodent studies there are usually not more than 10–20 animals per sex per group; and even in studies with 50 animals of each sex in a group, there may be difficulties in evaluation. When a background incidence of the abnormalities being sought as a result of the test exposure exists in control animals, a small group size is quite inadequate for detecting significance.

Pooling of Data

Data derived from both sexes within a species, or from different species and strains, should be analysed separately. The finding of an effect in more than one species or strain strengthens the association, particularly when the same organ or histological type is involved. If similar patterns of tumour or other organ disease are observed in multiple species, the results can be combined to provide a general quantification of risk.

Observer Drift

An individual observer may vary in his or her interpretation of findings when evaluating pathological or other toxicological material. This is known as observer drift. It may be the result of inexperience, poor working methods, fatigue or intermittent distraction. There are several ways of avoiding or minimising it. One is to examine the material without knowledge of the treatment that the animal has received. This is more commonly done in re-evaluation than initially. There has been increasing use of computer prompts. Many pathologists still believe in self-discipline, but this may weaken with strain and interruptions (Glaister, 1986).

CATEGORISING THE TOXICOLOGICAL RESPONSE

The outcome of a toxicological study in animals may fall into one of four categories (based on the International Agency for Research on Cancer, IARC, 1984).

(1) *Sufficient evidence exists of an association between the toxic agent and the purported outcome* This is based on findings in multiple species or strains, or in multiple experiments, preferably with different routes of administration, or different doses, or both; or the incidence of the finding is unusual in degree, site, type or age of onset. There may be additional data on dose–response effects, short-term studies and chemical structure.

(2) *Limited evidence* The data suggest a causative effect, but are insufficient because (a) only a single species or strain was examined, or the results were derived from a single experiment; or (b) the experiments were conducted with inadequate dosage levels, too brief duration of exposure, inadequate period of follow-up, poor animal survival and too few animals, or the reporting was inadequate; or (c) the lesions produced often occur spontaneously.

(3) *Inadequate evidence* Because of major qualitative or quantitative limitations the studies cannot be interpreted as showing either the presence or absence of an effect; or, within the limits of the test, the chemical has not been shown conclusively to produce the lesions concerned.

(4) No data are available.

The first two categories provide an indication only of the strength of the experimental evidence, and not of the extent of the activity of the chemical entity under review or the mechanism of its toxic effect. The classification may change as other information becomes available.

RECOMMENDATIONS FOR IMPROVING THE RELEVANCE OF TOXICOLOGY TESTING

A number of recommendations have been made for improving the relevance of toxicology testing in animals (Litchfield, 1962; Fletcher, 1978; Zbinden, 1980; Lumley and Walker, 1985; Zbinden, 1987a,b). These include:

(1) The establishment of data banks for collection of results, which could provide a valuable resource for analysis and for the design of future experiments (Lumley and Walker, 1985a).

(2) The methodology in experimental toxicology should develop to the extent that subjective effects in humans, such as hallucinations, dizziness, difficulty in concentrating and disturbance in memory, might be assessed in animals by behavioural testing (Zbinden, 1980).

(3) Improved systems of comparative evaluation of anatomical structure, physiological function and pathology, in test animals and in humans, including patients with the diseases for which the medicine is intended, should improve extrapolation and reduce the difficulties produced by species differences in metabolism, distribution and elimination.

REFERENCES

Aldridge, W. N. (1976). Chronic toxicity as an acute phenomenon: introduction to symposium. *Proc. Eur. Soc. Toxicol.*, **17**, 5–6

Balazs, T. (1974). Development of tissue resistance to toxic effects of chemicals. *Toxicology*, **2**, 247–55

Bolande, R. P. (1984). Models and concepts derived from human teratogenesis and oncogenesis in early life. *J. Histochem. Cytochem.*, **32**, 878–84

Brown, V. K. (1987). Animal models of responses resulting from short-term exposures. In Worden, A., Parke, D. and Marks, J. (Eds.), *The Future of Predictive Safety Evaluation*, Volume 2. MTP Press, Lancaster, pp. 47–55

Dayan, A. D. (1986). The scientific basis for long-term animal studies—what can and cannot be detected. In Walker, S. R. and Dayan, A. D. (Eds.), *Long-term Animal Studies: Their Predictive Value for Man*. MTP Press, Lancaster, pp. 3–7

Dean, J. H., Luster, M. I., Boorman, G. A. and Lauer, L. D. (1982). Procedures available to examine the immunotoxicity of chemicals and drugs. *Pharmacol. Rev.*, **34**, 137–48

Dewar, A. J. (1987). Neurotoxicity. In Worden, A., Parke, D. and Marks, J. (Eds.), *The Future of Predictive Safety Evaluation*, Volume 2. MTP Press, Lancaster, pp. 107–28

Draize, J. H., Woodard, G. and Calvery, H. O. (1944). Methods for the study of irritation and toxicity of substances applied topically to the skin and mucous membranes. *J. Pharmacol.*, **82**, 377–90

Fletcher, A. P. (1978). Drug safety tests and subsequent clinical experience. *J. Roy. Soc. Med.*, **71**, 693–6

Folb, P. I. (1981). *The Safety of Medicines: Evaluation and Prediction*. Springer-Verlag, Berlin

Frederick, G. L. (1986). The evidence supporting 18 month animal studies. In Walker, S. R. and Dayan, A. D. (Eds.), *Long-term Animal Studies: Their Predictive Value for Man*. MTP Press, Lancaster, pp. 65–76

Gart, J. J., Chu, K. C. and Tarone, R. E. (1979). Statistical issues in interpretation of chronic bioassay tests for carcinogenicity. *J. Natl Cancer Inst.*, **62**, 957–74

Gart, J. J., Krewski, D., Lee, P. N., Tarone, R. E. and Wahrendorf, J. (1986). General consideration on the evaluation of animal carcinogenesis experiments. In *Statistical Methods in Cancer Research*, Vol. III: *The Design and Analysis of Long-term Animal Experiments*, International Agency for Research on Cancer, Lyon, 6–20

Glaister, J. R. (1986). *Principles of Toxicological Pathology*. Taylor and Francis, London

Glocklin, V. C. (1986). Justification for 12 month animal studies. In Walker, S. R. and Dayan, A. D. (Eds.), *Long-term Animal Studies: Their Predictive Value for Man*. MTP Press, Lancaster, pp. 77–82

Grahame-Smith, D. (1986). What is expected from repeated-dose studies by the regulatory authorities. In Walker, S. R. and Dayan, A. D. (Eds.), *Long-term Animal Studies: Their Predictive Value for Man*. MTP Press, Lancaster, pp. 23–7

Griffin, J. P. (1986). Predictive value of animal toxicity studies. In Walker, S. R. and Dayan, A. D. (Eds.), *Long-term Animal Studies: Their Predictive Value for Man*. MTP Press, Lancaster, pp. 107–16

Hoel, D. G., Kaplan, N. L. and Anderson, M. W. (1983). Implication of nonlinear kinetics on risk estimation in carcinogenesis. *Science, N.Y.*, **219**, 1032–7

IARC Monographs on the Evaluation of the Carcinogenic Risk of Chemicals to Humans (1984). Supplement 4, *Chemicals, Industrial Processes and Industries*

Associated with Cancer in Humans. IARC Monographs, International Agency for Research on Cancer, Lyon, Volumes 1–29

Jackson, M. R. (1986). Conventional design of long-term toxicity studies in the pharmaceutical industry. In Walker, S. R. and Dayan, A. D. (Eds.), *Long-term Animal Studies: Their Predictive Value for Man.* MTP Press, Lancaster, pp. 35–44

Kodell, R. L., Farmer, J. H., Gaylor, D. W. and Cameron, A. M. (1982). Influence of cause of death assignment on time-to-tumor analyses in animal carcinogenesis studies. *J. Natl Cancer Inst.*, **69**, 659–64

Koeter, H. B. W. M. (1983). Relevance of parameters related to fertility and reproduction in toxicity testing. *Am J. Ind. Med.*, **4**, 81–6

Lansdown, A. B. G. (1987). Testing for reproductive toxicity. In Worden, A. N., Parke, D. V. and Marks, J. (Eds.), *The Future of Predictive Safety Evaluation*, Volume 2. MTP Press, Lancaster, pp. 77–106

Lasagna, L. (1984). Regulatory agencies, drugs and the pregnant patient. In Stern, L. (Ed.), *Drug Use in Pregnancy.* Adis Health Science Press, Sydney, pp. 12–16

Litchfield, J. T. (1962). Evaluation of the safety of new drugs by means of tests in animals. *Clin. Pharmacol. Ther.*, **3**, 665–81

Lumley, C. E. and Walker, S.R. (1985a). A toxicology databank based on animal safety evaluation studies of pharmaceutical compounds. *Hum. Toxicol.*, **4**, 447–60

Lumley, C. E. and Walker, S. R. (1985b). What is the value of animal toxicology studies beyond 6 months? *Br. J. Pharmacol.*, **84**, Suppl., 117P

McLean, A. E. M. (1986). The relationship between animal and human responses. In Walker, S. R. and Dayan, A. D. (Eds.), *Long-term Animal Studies: Their Predictive Value for Man.* MTP Press, Lancaster, pp. 99–104

Marzulli, F. and Maguire, H. C. (1982). Usefulness and limitation of various guinea-pig test methods in detecting human skin sensitizers—validation of guinea-pig tests for skin hypersensitivity. *Fd Chem. Toxicol.*, **20**, 67–74

Messite, J. and Bond, M. B. (1988). Reproductive toxicology and occupational exposure, In Zenz, C. (Ed.), *Occupational Medicine: Principles and Practical Applications*, Year Book Medical Publishers, Chicago, pp. 847–903

Miller, K., Maisey, J. and Malkovsky, M. (1984). Enhancement of contact sensitization in mice fed a diet enriched in vitamin A acetate. *Int. Arch. Allergy Appl. Immunol.*, **75**, 120–5

Miller, K. and Nicklin, S. (1987). Immunological aspects. In Worden, A., Parke, D. and Marks, J. (Eds.), *The Future of Predictive Safety Evaluation*, Volume 1. MTP Press, Lancaster, pp. 181–94

Miller, R. K., Mattison, D. R., Filler, R. S. and Rice, J. M. (1985). Reproductive and developmental toxicology. In Eskes, T. K. A. B. and Finster, M. (Eds.), *Drug Therapy During Pregnancy.* Butterworths, London, pp. 215–24

Paget, E. (1983). The LD_{50} test. *Acta Pharmacol. Toxicol.*, **52**, Suppl. 2, 6–19

Purchase, I. F. H. (1987). Carcinogenic risk assessment: Are animals good surrogates for man? In Bannasch, P. (Ed.), *Cancer Risks: Strategies for Elimination.* Springer-Verlag, Berlin, pp. 65–79

Rawlins, M. D. (1986). What is expected from repeated-dose studies by clinical pharmacologists. In Walker, S. R. and Dayan, A. D. (Eds.), *Long-term Animal Studies: Their Predictive Value for Man.* MTP Press, Lancaster, pp. 17–22

Rowan, A. (1983). Shortcomings of LD_{50} values and acute toxicity testing in animals. *Acta Pharmacol. Toxicol.*, **52**, 52–64

Salsburg, D. S. (1979). Research design from the statistician's viewpoint. *Clin. Toxicol.*, **15**, 559–69

Saxen, L. (1976). Mechanisms of teratogenesis. *J. Embryol. Exp. Morphol.*, **36**, 1–12

Schein, P. S., Davis, R. D., Carter, S., Newman, J., Schein, D. R. and Rall, D. P.

(1970). The evaluation of drugs in dogs and monkeys for the prediction of qualitative toxicities in man. *Clin. Pharmacol. Ther.*, **11**, 3–40

Silbergeld, E. K. (1982). Current status of neurotoxicology, basic and applied. *Trends Neurosci.*, **5**, 291–4

Squire, R. A. (1981). Ranking animal carcinogens: A proposed regulatory approach. *Science, N.Y.*, **214**, 877–80

Weil, C. S. and Scala, R. A. (1971). Study of intra- and interlaboratory variability in the results of rabbit eye and skin irritation tests. *Toxicol. Appl. Pharmacol.*, **19**, 276–360

Weisburger, J. H. (1987). Safety evaluation—carcinogenic risks. In Worden, A., Parke, D. and Marks, J. (Eds.), *The Future of Predictive Safety Evaluation*, Volume 2. MTP Press, Lancaster, pp. 129–52

Wilson, J. G. (1959). Experimental studies on congenital malformations. *J. Chron. Dis.*, **10**, 111–30

Worden, A. N. (1986). The evidence supporting 6-month animal studies. In Walker, S. R. and Dayan, A. D. (Eds.), *Long-term Animal Studies: Their Predictive Value for Man*. MTP Press, Lancaster, pp. 83–6

Worden, A. N. and Walker, S. R. (1987). Animal models for long term toxic effects. In Worden, A., Parke, D. and Marks, J. (Eds.), *The Future of Predictive Safety Evaluation*, Volume 2. MTP Press, Lancaster, pp. 57–64

Zbinden, G. (1980). Predictive value of pre-clinical drug safety evaluation. In Turner, P. (ed.), *Proceedings of Plenary Lectures Symposia and Therapeutic Sessions of the First World Conference on Clinical Pharmacology and Therapeutics*. Macmillan, London

Zbinden, G. (1987a) Risks predicted from animal studies. In Walker, S. R. and Asscher, A. W. (Eds.), *Medicines and Risk/Benefit Decision*. MTP Press, Lancaster, pp. 49–56

Zbinden, G. (1987b). Predictive value of animal studies in toxicology. Centre for Medicines Research, Carshalton

Zbinden, G. and Flury-Roversi, M. (1981). Significance of the LD_{50}-test for the toxicological evaluation of chemical substances. *Arch. Toxicol.*, **47**, 77–99

6
International Regulatory Requirements

F. W. Teather

Head, Product Registration Dept, Glaxo Group Research Ltd, Greenford Road, Greenford, Middx UB6 0HE, UK

INTRODUCTION

Over the past 4 years much progress has been made towards standardising the requirements for and the format of marketing applications. Probably the greatest changes have occurred in the European Community through the drive of the European Commission to achieve a unified procedure by 1992. The Nordic countries also have a 'group' procedure and these, like several other countries, accept application in a format very similar to that used in the European Community.

In contrast to this, with the exception of the Nordic countries, requirements for authorisation for clinical trials are very diverse, varying from no regulatory controls to controls which, with the obvious exception of the clinical section, are little less demanding than marketing applications. This diversity even occurs within the European Community and it will be interesting to see how this is dealt with in 1992 when either a 'mutual recognition' or 'single European Authority' procedure may be proposed for marketing applications.

Although there is great diversity between countries in regulatory controls applied to clinical trials, in most countries there is no distinction between the regulatory control of non-patient trials and early phase patient trials. The only exception to this is the United Kingdom, where, unlike trials in patients, non-patient trials are not included in regulatory controls.

Throughout the rest of this chapter, when reference is made to regulatory controls applied to clinical trials in the United Kingdom, such comment will apply only to early phase patient trials.

In Canada the regulatory authorities are particularly concerned with safeguards to protect healthy volunteers—e.g. to ensure that excessive blood sampling does not occur—but the administrative procedure does not differ from that followed for trials in patients.

A much more consistent requirement which must be met before undertaking clinical trials is the need to obtain the approval of an ethics committee. The interaction of ethical review and regulatory control will be examined during this review.

Rather than produce a catalogue on a country-by-country basis, this review will group together countries which have similar requirements for regulating clinical trials and highlight significant differences within these groups.

APPLICATION TO REGULATORY AUTHORITIES

When regulatory authorities are involved in reviewing the data which are submitted to support a proposed clinical trial, in the majority of cases they operate a negative vetting procedure. Thus, they raise 'no objections' to the proposed study rather than formally approving the study. The clinician and/or the sponsor must then accept liability for the study—although some support is provided by the lack of objections on the part of the regulatory authority. In certain circumstances, where an authority considers it appropriate to review data submitted in support of a study in more depth, they may then indicate their 'approval' of the study (for example, the issue of a Clinical Trial Certificate in the UK for a study considered inappropriate for progression through the Clinical Trial Exemption (CTX) procedure).

Among those countries where non-patient trials and early phase patient trials are carried out there are now only a few where there is no involvement of the regulatory authorities. Such countries are Holland, Switzerland and Portugal (see Group 1 in Table 6.1).

Table 6.1 Summary of regulatory controls for clinical trials

Group 1:	Countries where there is no regulatory action		
Holland	Switzerland	Portugal	France[a]
West Germany[a]			

Group 2:	Countries where regulatory authorities review summary data		
UK	Denmark	Norway	Ireland[b]
Sweden	Spain[b]	New Zealand[b]	Austria[b]
South Africa[b]	Belgium	Finland	

Group 3:	Countries where regulatory authorities review full reports	
United States	Canada	Australia
Italy[b]		

[a] Some documentation lodged with the authorities.
Note: When applications are reviewed (Groups 2 and 3) authorities indicate that they have 'no objections' to the proposed trials except those marked [b], which formally approve the studies.

In a few other countries involvement of the regulatory authorities tends to be only a formality. For instance, in France a document or letter of intent describing the basic data supporting the research and the opinion of an ethics committee (known as a Consultative Committee) is submitted, while in West Germany the reports of studies undertaken by or on behalf of the sponsor to support the proposed clinical studies are lodged with the authorities. Presumably, if any queries are subsequently raised as to the acceptability of the studies, the sponsors would have to justify their 'approval' on the basis of data available at the start of the clinical trial which will have been lodged with the regulatory authority.

In the majority of other countries the regulatory authorities review the safety and quality data presented to them in summary form and, if appropriate indicate, that they have 'no objections' to the proposed trial. This may be done positively by informing the applicant or negatively by failing to raise objections within a specified time period. Countries where regulatory authorities take this approach are listed under Group 2 in Table 6.1. These authorities usually reserve the right to ask for detailed reports if this is considered to be appropriate. It should be noted that in Belgium the regulatory authority is only involved to the extent of checking the quality of the product proposed for clinical trials (i.e. pharmacy aspects).

Some regulatory authorities still require full safety reports to be included in applications to undertake clinical trials. Countries where regulatory authorities adopt this approach are listed under Group 3 in Table 6.1. Until recently, in addition to requiring full safety reports, the Australian authorities also required extensive chemistry and pharmacy data. As a result of this, few early phase studies were undertaken in Australia. This requirement has now been relaxed and only abbreviated information on chemistry and pharmacy is required. A complicating factor in Canada is the requirement for animal safety studies to be of a longer duration than those required elsewhere to support dosing in man beyond 1 month.

When the authorities consider it is inappropriate that the clinical trial should proceed, more data may be requested and the application held until adequate data are provided. Alternatively, in the UK it may be suggested that the application should be routed through a formal approval procedure, i.e. an application for a Clinical Trial Certificate which passes through formal review by the advisory committee (Committee on Safety of Medicines) and is then 'approved' if appropriate.

In those countries where regulatory authorities are involved in reviewing clinical trial applications, there is usually a defined time period within which the authorities must respond to the application. This time period usually varies between 1 and 2 months. However, if the authorities raise queries on the application indicating that they have some concern about the data in the application, the specified time period no longer applies. Applications are then considered to be on 'hold' while further deliberations are under way. Such 'hold' periods are usually not covered by statutory time limits. Prolonged 'hold' periods are not allowed under the UK CTX scheme, where a decision has to be made within 35 days of receipt of the application with, at most, two additional extensions of 28 days.

When any of the details included in an application to undertake clinical studies are changed, the regulatory authorities have to be informed. If the proposed changes are not covered by the safety and quality data submitted with the original application, in most countries, the sponsor will be expected to await comment from the authorities. This is usually given within 1–3 months. In the USA the sponsor may proceed with the trials as soon as the data are filed with the FDA, but there is a risk that the FDA may require modifications to the changes.

REQUIREMENTS FOR ANIMAL SAFETY STUDIES

Most regulatory authorities will be satisfied if the standard 'European' requirements are followed for the duration of the acute/subacute animal safety studies (see Table 6.2). The requirements of the US FDA tend to be less demanding for early phase studies and the Scandinavian requirements are also slightly less demanding. In Canada animal studies of 12 months' duration are required to carry out clinical trials where the duration of dosing exceeds 1 month.

Table 6.2 Requirements for duration of toxicity studies

Duration of toxicity studies in animals	Intended duration of dosing in man
(1) European requirements	
14 days	Single dose or several doses on 1 day
28 days	Repeated up to 7 days
90 days	Repeated up to 30 days
180 days	Repeated beyond 30 days
(2) Nordic requirements	
14 days	Single dose to few people
28 days	Repeated for 1–2 weeks
90 days	Repeated for 1–3 months
180 days to 2 years	Repeated for 6 months or more
(3) US requirements (Phases I and II)	
14 days	1–3 days
28 days	Up to 4 weeks
90 days	Longer than 4 weeks

Note: In Canada, where dosing in man exceeds 1 month, 12 month toxicity studies in animals are required.

In addition to acute and subacute studies in animals, mutagenicity studies must also be carried out. If the clinical trials are to include women of child-bearing potential, teratogenicity studies must be completed. In most countries when the duration of dosing in clinical trials exceeds 1 year, carcinogenicity studies should also be completed. However, in West Germany such studies should be completed before clinical trials are extended beyond 6 months.

ETHICS COMMITTEE APPROVAL

Ethics committee approval is required before undertaking clinical trials in all countries (including those where there is no regulatory action).

Some regulatory authorities require ethics committee approval to be obtained before giving their 'approval'. Thus, this may cause a delay to the 'approval procedure', particularly where it may take up to 3 months to obtain ethics committee approval (e.g. Sweden, Canada). However, in most inst-ances approval is obtained within 1–2 months.

Usually the data required by an ethics committee for review are similar to those provided to clinicians who will be participating in the clinical studies, i.e. summary of animal safety studies and protocol of the trial. Thus, the clinician's manual is usually adequate for this purpose. If more detail is required, the summaries of animal safety studies as submitted to regulatory authorities are appropriate.

OVERALL COMMENT

In most countries where non-patient studies or early phase patient studies are carried out even if regulatory authorities are involved, significant delays are no longer a problem.

NOTE

The summary of international regulatory requirements relating to non-patient trials and early-phase patient trials presented in this chapter represents the current situation.

A bibliographical list is not presented here, since regulations and guidelines in this area are likely to change. Details of regulations and/or guidelines may be obtained from the relevant regulatory authority as appropriate.

Summaries of requirements for individual countries and currently available guidelines, together with the addresses of national regulatory authorities, are included in *The IFPMA Compendium on Regulation of Pharmaceuticals for Human Use*, 1987 edition, published by IFPMA, 67 rue de St Jean, 1201 Geneva, Switzerland.

The following guidelines should provide guidance to ensure that adequate data are available to meet the requirements in most countries:

Issued by Nordic Council of Medicines,
Box 607, S-751 25, Uppsala, Sweden:
Clinical Trials of Drugs
NLN Publication No. 11 June 1983

Issued by Department of Health and Social Security, United Kingdom
Printed in the UK for Her Majesty's Stationery Office:
Guidance Notes on Applications for Clinical Trial Certificates and Clinical Trial Exemptions, 1984
Supplement No. 1, 1985

Issued by Center for Drugs and Biologics, Food and Drug Administration, Department of Health and Human Services, Office of Drug Research and

Review (HFN-100), 5600 Fishers Lane, Rockville, Maryland 20857 (301-433-4330):

(a) *Guideline for the Format and Content of the Chemistry, Manufacturing and Controls Section of an Application*, February 1987

(b) *Guideline for Submitting Documentation for the Manufacture and Controls for Drug Products*, February 1987

(c) *Guideline for Submitting Documentation for the Manufacture of Drug Substances*, February 1987

(d) *Guideline for Submitting Documentation for the Stability of Human Drugs and Biologics*, February 1987

(e) *Guideline for the Format and Content of the Nonclinical Pharmacology/ Toxicology Section of an Application*, February 1987

7
Regulatory Requirements in Japan

Yasushi Yoshino

Head, Production Registration Group, Upjohn Pharmaceuticals Ltd, 17F Shinjuku Green Tower Building, 14-1 Nishi-Shinjuku 6-chome, Tokyo 160, Japan

INTRODUCTION

The Phase I clinical trial is the first clinical trial in which a drug is administered to human subjects. Accordingly, the most important aspect of carrying out the Phase I clinical trial is to ensure the safety of the human subjects. There are various views concerning the scope of animal tests to be performed before the start of Phase I clinical trials and decisions in this respect are important to doctors and drug manufacturers who perform them. Of course, biological differences between humans and animals must be taken into account when pharmaceuticals are being developed.

This chapter pertains to the requirements for tests to be conducted before the start of Phase I clinical trials in Japan as described in the Japanese Pharmaceutical Affairs Law, followed by Guidelines published by the Japanese Ministry of Health and Welfare. However, it must be realised that there are no guidelines specifying preclinical studies required before the start of Phase I clinical trials, nor specific data to be submitted with an IND in this regard. Nevertheless, one can see from the following discussion that a clear picture in regard to these requirements can be obtained from the Guidelines, Pharmaceutical Affairs Law and NDA requirements.

JAPANESE PHARMACEUTICAL AFFAIRS LAW[1-3]

The Japanese laws and regulations concerning drug standards and drug registration rank in the following order: (1) The Japanese Pharmaceutical Affairs Law, (2) The Enforcement Ordinance of the Pharmaceutical Affairs Law, (3) The Enforcement Regulations of the Pharmaceutical Affairs Law and (4) Notifications issued by the Japanese Ministry of Health and Welfare.

The purpose of the Japanese Pharmaceutical Affairs Law is to control and regulate matters related to drugs, quasi-drugs, cosmetics and medical devices, to assure their quality, efficacy and safety. This law stipulates the basic regulations. For example, its provisions are such that persons who want to manufacture or import drugs are required to obtain approval and a licence for each drug from the government, and persons who intend to commission clinical trials to outside institutions must submit a notification on each clinical trial programme to the government.

The Enforcement Ordinance of the Pharmaceutical Affairs Law ranks below the Japanese Pharmaceutical Affairs Law. This Ordinance chiefly specifies the fees which applicants for new drug registration have to pay.

The Japanese Pharmaceutical Affairs Law does not specify any detailed requirements such as data required for new drug registration applications and formats for notification on clinical trial programmes to be submitted to the Ministry of Health and Welfare. Therefore, the Ministry laid down the Enforcement Regulations of the Pharmaceutical Affairs Law, which stipulates regulatory requirements more concretely and in more detail.

Notifications issued by the Ministry of Health and Welfare are below the Enforcement Regulations of the Pharmaceutical Affairs Law. Detailed information concerning drug standards and drug registration, such as tests required for new drug registration applications and related guidelines, are given by the notifications. Since requirements for new drug registration applications should be reviewed in respect of the advances in medical and pharmaceutical sciences, the Ministry renews the notifications when necessary.

The most important regulatory requirements in regard to data needed for conducting clinical trials as specified in the Japanese Pharmaceutical Affairs Law, Enforcement Regulations of the Pharmaceutical Affairs Law and the government-issued Notifications are as follows.

The Pharmaceutical Affairs Law

Article 14 (3) (extracts): Persons who wish to obtain approvals for manufacture or import of new drugs as specified in Article 14 (1) shall submit data concerning results of clinical trials and other pertinent data to the Ministry along with the applications, in accordance with the Enforcement Regulations of the Pharmaceutical Affairs Law.

Article 80-2 (1) (extracts): Persons who commission clinical trials to outside institutions in order to collect clinical data as specified in Article 14 (3) of the Pharmaceutical Affairs Law shall ensure that the commissioned trials will be performed on the basis of the provisions laid down in the Enforcement Regulations of the Pharmaceutical Affairs Law.

The Enforcement Regulations of the Pharmaceutical Affairs Law

Article 67 (standards for requesting conduct of clinical trials): Persons who request clinical trials pursuant to Article 80-2, Paragraph 1 of the Law shall comply with the following standards:

(1) Tests on toxicity and pharmacological action, etc. of the drug required before requesting conduct of clinical trials shall be completed.

(1)-2 In order to take necessary measures to prevent the occurrence or spread of public health and sanitation hazards caused by the investigational drug, if a person requesting conduct of clinical trials does not reside in Japan, he shall select a person who resides in Japan (including the representative of the Japan office of a foreign corporation having such an office) to request conduct of clinical trials on behalf of him or her, and shall carry out the procedures relative to the request through this person (hereinafter called the in-country clinical trial administrator).

(2) The request shall be made in writing.

(3) The results of the tests specified in item (1) and other information required for the clinical trials shall be submitted to the clinical investigators.

(4) The request shall be made to medical or research institutions (hereinafter referred to as 'medical institutions') which are able to conduct the trials properly, provide adequate clinical observation and inspection, and take necessary measures in an emergency. In the case of clinical trials of Chinese medicines, medical institutions with sufficient clinical experience in the corresponding special fields shall be included among the institutions requested.

(5) Except in cases where the physician in charge deems it medically undesirable, the institution shall be requested to explain the details of the clinical trial to the subjects and obtain their consent (where subjects are not capable of giving their consent, the consent of those who can give it on behalf of the subjects).

(6) Necessary measures for compensation shall be taken in advance as a precaution against any public health hazard caused due to use of the investigational drug.

(7) The following shall be indicated in the Japanese language on the container or wrapper of the investigational drug.

(a) The drug is intended for clinical use.

(b) The name and address of the person requesting clinical trials (if the person does not reside in Japan, the name and country of the person requesting clinical trials and the name and address of the in-country clinical trial administrator).

(c) The chemical name or identifying symbol.

(d) The manufacturing number or symbol.

(e) Information relating to storage method and expiration date where applicable.

(8) The following shall not be indicated in documents attached to the investigational drug or on the drug or its container or wrapper (including the inner wrapper).

(a) The anticipated trade name.

(b) The anticipated indications, effects or properties.

(c) The anticipated dosage and administration.

(9) The investigational drug shall be delivered directly to the institutions and not through a third party such as a drug distributor.

(10) The following records concerning the investigational drug shall be kept. Provided that the person requesting conduct of clinical trials does not

reside in Japan, he shall have the in-country clinical trial administrator keep the records.

(a) Records on manufacture and tests of the investigational drug.

(b) The amount of the investigational drug which was delivered to the institutions and the date of delivery.

(11) Where the person who requests clinical trials does not reside in Japan, and when the Minister of Health and Welfare instructs cancellation or amendment of the trial request, or other measures deemed necessary in order to prevent the occurrence or spread of public health and sanitation hazards by the use of the investigational drug, the person requesting clinical trials shall have the in-country clinical trial administrator comply with the instruction.

The Notification No. 1330 Issued by the Ministry of Health and Welfare on 9 October 1980 (extracts)

Data mentioned in Article 67-(1) of the Enforcement Regulations of the Pharmaceutical Affairs Law are specified below.

Required before requesting conduct of clinical trials are the data related to the physicochemical properties, toxicity, pharmacology, absorption and excretion tests in animals of the investigational drug. The methodology should meet adequately the current level of science and reflect the scope of the clinical trials (phases of the clinical trials, the route of administration, administration period, selection of subjects).

GUIDELINES

In Japan information concerning tests required for new drug registration applications and related guidelines are given in the form of notifications from the Japanese Ministry of Health and Welfare. (Before 1987, however, such information and guidelines were officially given in the journal *Iyakuhin Kenkyu.*) To date, guidelines on clinical studies and toxicology studies have been issued in Japan. (Currently, the Japanese Ministry of Health and Welfare is considering issuing guidelines on general pharmacology, ADME and methods of statistical analysis as well.) These guidelines mainly concern requirements for NDA submission, but, as stated at the beginning of this chapter, there are no official guidelines for animal tests to be conducted before the start of Phase I clinical trials. The NDA requirements are summarised in Table 7.1.

Guidelines for Clinical Trials[4-13]

Several guidelines (and draft guidelines) for clinical development of drugs have so far been issued by the government notifications according to the therapeutic classes of drugs. Although these guidelines are not aimed at specifying the preclinical studies necessary for conduct of Phase I clinical

Table 7.1   Data required for NDA in Japan

A.	Origin and background of the discovery, conditions of use in foreign countries, etc.	(1) Origin and background of the discovery
		(2) Conditions of use in foreign countries
		(3) Properties and comparative studies with other drugs, etc.
B.	Physicochemical properties, standards and test methods, etc.	(1) Definition of structure
		(2) Physicochemical properties, etc.
		(3) Standards and test methods
C.	Stability	(1) Long-term storage test
		(2) Stress test
		(3) Acceleration test
D.	Acute, subacute and chronic toxicity, teratogenicity and other types of toxicity	(1) Acute toxicity (Table 7.3)
		(2) Subacute toxicity (Table 7.3)
		(3) Chronic toxicity (Table 7.3)
		(4) Effects on reproduction
		(5) Dependence
		(6) Antigenicity
		(7) Mutagenicity
		(8) Carcinogenicity
		(9) Local irritation
E.	Pharmacological action	(1) Tests supporting efficacy
		(2) General pharmacology
F.	Absorption, distribution, metabolism and excretion	(1) Absorption
		(2) Distribution
		(3) Metabolism
		(4) Excretion
		(5) Biological equivalence
G.	Results of clinical trials	Clinical trial results

trials, it is possible to understand from them to some extent what studies are required before the start of human trials. Table 7.2 specifies fundamental preclinical studies required for major therapeutic classes of drugs as described in these guidelines.

'The General Guidelines for Clinical Evaluation of New Drugs (Draft)' indicate that acute and subacute toxicity tests, reproduction toxicity tests (Segment I) and mutagenicity tests are necessary prior to conduct of Phase I clinical trials. Moreover, this draft mentions that specific toxicity tests (dependence test, antigenicity test and local irritation test) may be required, depending on the dosage form and characteristics of the drug. The pharmacology and pharmacokinetics are also required.

This draft guideline is currently being reviewed, and extensive opinions have been sought from various organisations in the Japanese pharmaceutical industry. The Ministry of Health and Welfare will publish the official guidelines in the near future after thorough investigation.

Other guidelines such as for immunotherapeutics for malignant tumours, antibacterial drugs, plasma fraction preparations, interferon preparations,

Table 7.2   Fundamental preclinical studies required before human trials

Drug	ADME — Pharmacology and Toxicology of Principal Metabolites	ADME — Drug Interaction	ADME — Bioavailability	ADME — ADME	Gen. Pharm. — Liver, Kidney, etc.	Gen. Pharm. — Smooth Muscles	Gen. Pharm. — Digestive Tract	Gen. Pharm. — Respiratory and Circulatory	Gen. Pharm. — Autonomic Nervous System	Gen. Pharm. — Animal Efficacy Pharmacology	Tox. — Others	Tox. — Carcinogenicity	Tox. — Mutagenicity	Tox. — Drug Dependency	Tox. — Reproduction	Tox. — General Toxicology
Hypnotic Agents	○	○	○	○				○	○	○	○	○		○	○	○
Antianxiety Drugs	○	○	○	○				○	○	○	○	○		○	○	○
Oral Contraceptive	○			○			○		○	○	○	○	○	○	○	○
Antihyperlipemics	○	○	○	○		○		○	○*3		○			○*2	○	○
Antiarrhythmic Agents	○			○				○	○*3		○			○*2	○	○
Antiangina Drugs	○			○				○	○*3		○			○*2	○	○
Analgesic-Anti-inflammatory Drugs	○			○				○	○*3		○			○*1	○	○
Anticardiac Insufficiency Drugs	○			○				○	○*3		○			○*2	○	○
Antiulcer Drugs (Draft)	○	○		○				○	○*3		○				○	○
Antihypertensive Drugs	○			○				○	○*3		○			○*1	○	○
General Guidelines for Clinical Evaluation (Draft)				○					○*3		○	○	○	○	○	○

○ Required

*1   Guidelines indicate that toxicity tests may be required prior to conduct of Phase I clinical trials, but the Guidelines do not give detailed explanation of the test required.

*2   Guidelines indicate that specific toxicity tests may be required prior to conduct of Phase I clinical trials, but the Guidelines do not give detailed explanation of the test required.

*3   Guidelines indicate that general pharmacology may be required prior to conduct of Phase I clinical trials, but the Guidelines do not give detailed explanation of the test required.

paediatric drugs and cerebral circulation and metabolism improvers are not mentioned in the preclinical studies required before the start of Phase I.

Guidelines for Toxicity Studies[14]

Some explanations are also given in the guidelines (and draft guidelines) for toxicology studies issued by the notification and notes of the Ministry of Health and Welfare. These guidelines refer to General Toxicology Studies single-dose and multiple-dose toxicity. Reproduction Studies (Segments I, II and III) and Specific Toxicity Studies (mutagenicity, carcinogenicity, skin sensitisation and skin photosensitisation). Table 7.3 specifies length of required toxicology studies for various lengths of dosing time in man.

Table 7.3   Length of dosing time in required toxicity studies based on length of dosing time in man

	Length of required toxicology studies		
Length of dosing time in man	*Single-dose toxicity*	*Multiple-dose toxicity*	*(Preliminary studies)*
Single dose	Single dose	1 month	
1 week or less	Single dose	1 month	
1 week and up to 4 weeks	Single dose	3 months	(1 month)
4 weeks and up to 6 months	Single dose	6 months	(1 month)
Over 6 months (or in the case of analogous drugs which develop delayed toxicity)	Single dose	12 months	(3 months)

CONCLUSION

The aim of the Phase I clinical trial is to examine the safety and pharmacokinetics of new drugs. However, the first consideration should be given to the safety of the subjects, and to ensure this, one must have data from preclinical testing.

Toxicity, pharmacology and pharmacokinetics are considered as fundamental tests in Japan, and before the start of human trials necessary testing should be carefully designed and selected on the basis of the characteristics of the new drug and the known properties of the analogous drugs, if available.

In Japan, before the start of Phase I clinical trials, at least acute and subacute toxicity tests, reproduction tests (Segment I and/or Segment II), mutagenicity tests, efficacy pharmacology tests, general pharmacology tests and ADME (blood level, urinary excretion) tests must be conducted, usually using several species of animals. Preclinical studies conducted in Japan are intended not only for ensuring safety in Phase I clinical trials, but also for safety in Phase II and III clinical trials. In addition, the data on preclinical studies are an important part of NDA documents.

REFERENCES

1. A collection of laws and regulations from the Japanese Pharmaceutical Affairs Law and Pharmacists Law. Yakumukohosha (1986)
2. Drug Approval and Licensing Procedures in Japan 1987 (compiled under the supervision of the MHW), Yakugyojiho Co., Ltd
3. Notification No. 1330, Pharmaceutical Affairs Bureau, Ministry of Health and Welfare (9 October 1980)
4. Guideline for Clinical Evaluation of Hypnotic Agents, Notification No. 18, First Evaluation and Registration Division, Pharmaceutical Affairs Bureau, Ministry of Health and Welfare (18 July 1988)
5. Guideline for Clinical Evaluation of Antianxiety Drugs, Notification No. 7, First Evaluation and Registration Division, Pharmaceutical Affairs Bureau, Ministry of Health and Welfare (16 March 1988)
6. Guideline for Clinical Evaluation of an Oral Contraceptive, Notification No. 10, First Evaluation and Registration Division, Pharmaceutical Affairs Bureau, Ministry of Health and Welfare (21 April 1987)
7. Guideline for the Clinical Evaluation of Antihyperlipemics, Notification No. 1, First Evaluation and Registration Division, Pharmaceutical Affairs Bureau, Ministry of Health and Welfare (5 January 1988)
8. Murakami, M. *et al.* (1979). Guideline for Clinical Evaluation of Antihypertensive drugs. *Iyakuhin Kenkyu*, **10**, 849–64
9. Harumi, K. *et al.* (1984). Guideline on Clinical Evaluation Methods for Anti-arrhythmic Agents. *Iyakuhin Kenkyu*, **15**, 497–503
10. Kato, K. *et al.* (1985). Guideline for Clinical Evaluation of Antiangina Drugs. *Iyakuhin Kenkyu*, **16**, 554–60
11. Horiuchi, Y. *et al.* (1985). Guideline Concerning Methods for Clinical Evaluation of Analgesic Anti-inflammatory Drugs. *Iyakuhin Kenkyu*, **16**, 544–53
12. Guideline for Clinical Evaluation of Anticardiac Insufficiency Drugs, Notification No. 84, First Evaluation and Registration Division, Pharmaceutical Affairs Bureau, Ministry of Health and Welfare (19 October 1988)
13. General Guideline for Clinical Evaluation of New Drugs (Draft), Note issued by First Evaluation and Registration Division, Pharmaceutical Affairs Bureau, Ministry of Health and Welfare (4 August 1988)
14. Information on the Guidelines of Toxicity Studies Required for Application for Approval to Manufacture (Import) Drugs, Notification No. 24, First Evaluation and Registration Division, Pharmaceutical Affairs Bureau, Ministry of Health and Welfare (11 September 1989)

II
Organisation and Decision Making

8
The Organisation of New Drug Evaluation in the Pharmaceutical Industry

Yves Champey

Vice President, Medical and Scientific Development, Rhône-Poulenc Santé, 20 Avenue Raymond Aron, 92165 Antony Cedex, France

INTRODUCTION

The pharmaceutical industry manufactures a consumer product: the drug. The production and sale of this consumer product are strictly regulated. There are, however, no such regulations governing research and development, with the exception of a few rules covering the methodology of toxicological studies and, in some countries, the methodology of clinical studies. Rules are, nevertheless, imposed upon the industrial researcher, and these are contained within two coexisting frames of reference which are a factor in all decision making. These frames of reference are those of medicine and of industry.

FOR EVERY CLINICAL DEVELOPMENT DECISION THERE ARE TWO FRAMES OF REFERENCE

The medical terms of reference concern quality of research and respect for patients. The industrial terms of reference are those in which management of the time and resources needed to introduce a new drug on to the market are essential elements.

Each of these frames of reference imposes upon the executive in the pharmaceutical industry a demand for clarity in the definition of objectives and in the determination of resources. The industrial executive cannot achieve these objectives or have control over the resources without impeccable organisation.

Medical and Scientific Imperatives

The medical terms of reference demand soundly based and clearly documented hypotheses as a basis for considering the potential administration of a new substance to man and a range of trials exposing several tens of

99

healthy volunteers and, sometimes, hundreds of patients. This demands, in terms of organisation, strategy for development and preparation of the necessary documentation to undertake these studies.

The medical terms of reference demand, in addition, that the quality of the data be indisputable: an intrinsic requirement of all scientific activity. In the case of clinical research activity, a supplementary element governs: this research and development involves asking healthy volunteers or patients to agree to participate. The minimum the industrial researcher owes to subjects agreeing to participate in the evaluation of therapeutic effects of a new substance is that the data collected be of very high quality so that they may actually serve a purpose. Besides these methodological aspects, the standard of personnel chosen to organise and follow through these programmes, the standard of investigators and the quality of the resources afforded in order to carry out this research are further organisational elements to which the industrial worker must pay close attention.

An organisational error which entails restarting a study is an event without glory. In general, the investigator, the Ethical Committee and—even more so—the patient who has agreed to take part in a clinical trial are unaware of the error. It is a classical situation caused by precipitate clinical research where personal conviction or the hope of saving time leads to the initiation of a programme of studies before the essential elements have been clearly established. Results reported orally, and guesses made on the basis of personal experience are common sources of this type of organisational error.

The Industrial Imperatives

Time saving is intrinsic to the needs of industry. A drug is an industrial consumer product which costs an enormous amount of money to introduce on the market. Very few drugs are sufficiently innovative to be developed without regard to industrial competition, and even in those rare cases, the life of a patent is limited. Each month wasted is a month's delay in getting a new drug on the market. The commercial success which leads to sales figures of 100 million dollars per year within 2 years after marketing is far from exceptional with a product having wide therapeutic applications. Each month of delay represents the failure to earn 8 million dollars. These figures incite the industrial executive to organise a plan so as to achieve this target as rapidly as possible. Good control of timetables is an inherent aspect of organisation, as is keeping within budgetary limits.

The pharmaceutical industry executive habitually organises more than one clinical development programme. Several programmes will be running concurrently, each one at a different stage. Besides organisational effort, allied to the design and realisation of a Phase I and Phase II programme with a new molecule, the researcher faces problems related to the utilisation of rare human resources: clinical pharmacologists of international repute, able to work effectively with investigators in different continents; all too few biostatisticians; medical editors with too large a workload. He also has to choose between, or organise, priorities within his budgetary limits, not only for the current year but also for subsequent years in a carefully thought out 3 or 5 year plan. The demands and fundamentals of good organisation will be described from two different but complementary angles: first, those related to balanced functioning of each major discipline within the enterprise, and second, those related to the accumulated data issuing from the clinical trials themselves.

COMPREHENSIVE DOCUMENTATON OF GOOD-QUALITY DATA IS ESSENTIAL TO THE DEVELOPMENT OF NEW DRUGS

Which Elements of Data?

Good internal organisation must ensure that all the elements of data and of decision are defined, known and taken account of. Good organisation should mean that all the appropriate members of staff are involved in the decision making. It is bad economics for a step backwards to be taken unless new facts demand it. The new facts are derived, above all, from the results of new studies. The reasons for organising a programme of Phase I and Phase II studies are simple and always the same. The organisation must allow for all the wheels to be set in motion which will ensure that the design and execution of the studies and collection of the data produced are both timely and of the highest quality.

The decision to organise a Phase I and Phase II programme is an important company decision. It will cause those responsible for the clinical disciplines to contact investigators and, later, to ask healthy volunteers or patients to participate in this programme. It involves expenditure over at least 2 years.

Is the information which must precede this decision to hand within the enterprise? The decision to organise the tests results from some 2 or 3 years' work or more for departments dealing with chemical synthesis, with in-process research and with pharmaceutical aspects of formulation.

This work generates a large amount of complex data, on the basis of which the hypothesis giving rise to the proposal of research in man is evaluated. The solidity of the pharmacological hypothesis must be established, particularly if the pharmacologists are claiming a new and original mechanism. This remains true, moreover, where the mechanism of action is not particularly original. The relevant documentation on the effect and its measurement must be placed at the disposal of those who have to take the decision to administer the new substance to humans.

The synthetic pathway must be known and assurance must be given that the various phases are or can be achieved in a cost-effective manner. The required quantities of raw material must be available and sufficiently stable. Subacute and acute toxicity studies must be carried out, the results presented and interpreted. A method of quantitative analysis in biological media must have been formulated and be available for use at the stage of the first tolerance studies. Precise data must have emanated from these years of work. These data are, indeed, mandatory for a certain number of Authorities, whose authorisation is required before starting a new compound administration to man or for a whole Phase I, Phase II clinical trial programme.

These points are mentioned here, without further detail, to underline the need for verification of all data, for the production of documents, for approval by all those responsible in the relevant disciplines and for interdisciplinary consultations at an early stage. Organisation is essential to the fulfilment of these needs.

Spontaneity and unorganised exchanges on their own can lead to important therapeutic innovations. Forecasting based only on spontaneous exchanges remains a hazard and is ultimately more time-consuming.

The Decisions Taken Should Be Adhered to without Continual Changes in Plan

The decision which must be taken is whether or not the enterprise will allocate the funds to determine, in man, the validity of the pharmacologists' hypothesis of therapeutic efficacy.

The decision involves several disciplines and several groups of workers, and affects several budgets. Since this same decision must be arrived at in the course of a year with regard to several propositions, coming from diverse research programmes, it follows that the section leader of each major discipline must participate, contribute and accept the decision, and not challenge it subsequently. This is done effectively if the organisation has a committee competent to make a decision on the basis of the recommendations made by each discipline. It is done most effectively if each member of the team recognises that the life and future of the company are greatly dependent upon the quality of decision making and pays it all the attention it deserves.

The elements which ensure that the decisions made will be solid ones, will be of good quality and will be adhered to by all concerned, are as follows: written proposals, regular and frequent meetings, clear and comprehensive minutes, assurance of the presence of all members of the committee at all meetings, the committee being composed of those responsible for major disciplines themselves and not of their representatives. These decisions will be made from a foundation of strength so as to withstand any attempts to challenge them. The only challenges and the only steps backwards which are valid are those generated by new results. No backward movement is acceptable if it comes as a result of an earlier precipitate decision.

Planning and Follow-up of Decisions

The decisions made before and during a Phase I and Phase II programme are: to initiate a new programme, to accelerate it, to review it, to terminate it, or to enrich it with new studies. These decisions must be translated in terms of a plan of campaign: i.e. a timed plan of execution and a plan of allocation of human and budgetary resources. Sophisticated logistic techniques now exist for the forecasting of time-scales for a clinical study programme, an anticipated chain of events, tracing of the critical pathway, lists of indispensable prerequisites, and of the tasks which are associated with the clinical activity: preparation of the protocol, choice of investigators, purchase of raw materials, supplies of finished product, printing of case record forms, data collection and treatment, verification of results, production of an interim or final analysis, production of the clinical report, internal approval, etc.

All these well-identified tasks must link up without any hiatus. Here only first-class organisation makes it possible to run a large number of studies set up for the realisation of 20–50 programmes running concurrently in the same enterprise, each programme being at a different stage and evolving on its own account.

Planning and progress-chasing are indispensable, but equally important is the following up of the execution of important decisions. Few decisions are made unanimously and without hesitation. There may be questions of the difficulty of producing the active substance, unacceptable toxicity results or prohibitive risks of intolerance. In many situations the decision to go ahead or to halt a programme of clinical studies is a source of frustration for one or more members of the team. The responsibility for decision maintenance consists of ensuring that the priorities are taken into account and that those of the enterprise take precedence over those of one or other discipline.

THE EXECUTION OF CLINICAL PROGRAMMES—THE ELEMENTS OF GOOD ORGANISATION NEEDED TO YIELD A HIGH-QUALITY PROGRAMME

To organise a Phase I and Phase II programme, and, subsequently, the weightier and most costly Phase III, involves taking the decision to amass data, in several tens of healthy volunteers and several tens of hundreds of patients, relating to the effect of the substance administered, its efficacy and its safety.

A programme on a given molecule will be carried out rapidly, smoothly, in an enthusiastic manner, when the pharmacological hypothesis is strong and innovative and when it is verifiable in a limited number of patients after a brief course of administration. This is unfortunately not always the case. Innovation is not always apparent and some hypotheses, such as, for example, that of a new mechanism of action for the basic treatment of rheumatoid arthritis, require a large number of patients and prolonged periods of administration.

Quality and Timing: The Two Imperatives

The complexity and dimensions of the problems of organisation differ, depending on whether the Phase is I or II. Nevertheless, they can all be reduced to one problem: how to ensure that the information sought and acquired at great expense is collected within the shortest time-scale and that its quality is as high as possible.

Phase I studies are, for the most part, carried out in specialist centres, their protocols are relatively standardised and they involve small numbers of subjects. The clinicians who carry them out, or the clinical research assistants who follow them up, cope fairly easily with the scheduled time-limits. The extent of the data collected on each volunteer is fairly limited. The processing of these data does not usually congest the biostatistics section.

Phase II studies, and particularly efficacy trials and those to determine the optimal dosage mode or levels, will involve several hundred patients when it concerns, for example, *an antihypertensive, an anxiolytic, an antidepressant or an antirheumatic agent*. The duration of treatment will vary from 1 week to 3 months, and the number of consultations and the number of data collected per consultation will be high. Each patient's case records, after administration of the prescribed treatment for the required duration, will represent between 1000 and 2000 individual items to be analysed. Only a precise and well-trained organisation can cope with such an influx of data within a specified time, having first determined that the data collected is authentic and verifiable.

The assurance of good quality data input must begin at the stage of study design, after consultation with pharmacologists and toxicologists, at least over the very first phases of the programme.

The organisation must provide a clear answer to three questions: Who is responsible in each study for meeting

the deadlines?

the budgets?

the standards of quality?

Then a series of time-honoured actions, familiar to all in industry, follows this first phase. These actions will not be studied in detail here. There is the choice of investigators and contact with them, and the preparation of a protocol and case record forms; there must be agreement between investigators in the case of a multicentre trial; the clinical trial samples must be manufactured and delivered on site; biological samples must be collected and transport organised; note must be made of unexpected side-effects, with the assurance of a rapid reaction in the case of a worrisome or severe effect; requests for authorisation to proceed with a clinical programme or trial must be prepared, if the legislation of the country in question requires it.

These different actions, already numerous and differing one from the other, must link up without loss of time from the outset. Good-quality organisation will afford the means to ensure regular visits, sometimes at frequent intervals, to the trial location: verification of the results *in situ*, data collection, organisation of the data in a database, programmed production of statistical analyses and of interim analyses if the nature of the trials demands them.

WHAT ORGANISATION?

How can good organisation facilitate the execution of these different tasks?

The dissemination of internal procedures, constantly updated, for the execution of these tasks is indispensable. It allows each of the executives in the enterprise to refer to the same set of practices and find in it the procedural answers to the question: how can it be done? The availability of clearly structured budgets is also indispensable. Each must know the cost limits imposed on a specific task. The availability of adequate human resources, in terms of quality and number, must be examined before trials commence. This question is predictable, a known element. If the problem only appears after the decision to carry out a programme of work has been made, it indicates that there has been a failure to foresee the problem of resources and a failure to tackle the essential problem: that of priorities and choices.

Human Resources

Among the human resources in question is the number of qualified clinicians required to devise the study, approach the investigators and come to an agreement with them on the best route to follow in order to gain an answer to the question posed. A further quota is the number of clinical research assistants, their geographical positioning and the reporting structure. This boils down, in fact, to one important question: who is responsible at each stage for budgetary control, for adherence to time-limits and for the quality of the data produced? There is no room for ambiguity in a well-organised plan. Ambiguity is a source of conflict, errors and delays.

Also among the human resources will figure the number and qualifications of those who will manage the database, carry out the statistical analyses and supervise part or all of these activities.

Therefore, human resources are represented by essential paper qualifications but also by the right mix of experience and imagination, of mobility and stasis, of strategic vision and a horizon fixed on the accomplishment of a precise task within a set time-limit.

The development of new pharmaceutical products is characterised by the large number of scientific disciplines which participate in the research, by the extent to which tasks are packaged so as to have little in common in their individual content while remaining interdependent in the chain of events. The sciences which participate in this research include the following.

Synthetic chemistry—here prediction is difficult, since new chemical structures are produced which may have an effect on a receptor, known or unknown. *Analytical chemistry* will establish the techniques for measuring the presence in man of a new chemical substance, its degradation over time, its presence and measurement in biological media. Then there are *pharmacology, toxicology, pharmaceutical chemistry, metabolism, biodynamics, clinical science* and *clinical pharmacology*, not to mention *production technology* and *market research*. This is a veritable catalogue of sciences and human abilities that must be capable of interacting effectively, each with its own tools, qualifications and predictive guidelines, if a new product is to be invented under the best possible competitive conditions.

The organisation of a programme of Phase I and Phase II studies on a new substance must not be confused with the organisation of the clinical trials themselves, but seen as an enterprise which will lead to the disciplines mentioned to work together. This means that these disciplines will accept a common objective and work to the timetable set.

How Can These Diverse Disciplines Work Together? How Can the Programme be Made to Evolve?

Several answers are usually proposed. Each is right, on condition that the enterprise has the will to make it work and to resolve, by clear decisions, by producing detailed progress charts and coherent procedures, a large number of questions: who does what? who is responsible to whom? This is a fact of life for every organisation requiring several hundred men and women to work together. The conflicts lie in the boundaries between each discipline, in the extent of agreement with decisions made and in arbitration over the allocation of resources. A definitive reply, now adopted by numerous enterprises, is illustrated in Figure 8.1.

Project Creation and Management Aspects

As soon as the decision is made to organise a programme of studies in man with a given molecule—and this decision is generally made at least 1 year before the first group of volunteers begins treatment with the substance—a project is created and a project leader is nominated.

The project leader gathers around him a group consisting of representatives of each of the disciplines which will contribute to the composition of a body of information justifying use of the substance in humans and also contribute to the administration of the Phase I and Phase II programme.

The group will work together for several years, at least as far as the major disciplines—clinical, toxicology, registration, marketing—are concerned. The first written document from the project leader, aided by this group, will be a proposal of a plan of action covering the non-clinical and clinical studies to be carried out, a timetable, a provisional budget and identification of the resources needed to carry the project right through to the end of Phase II.

This entails a succession of meetings, a willingness to work together on the part of the various members of the group and, above all, each of the members of the project group performing well within the group as a representative of a discipline. To this end, each representative must not only be selected by the project leader, but also be nominated by the head of that discipline. Another requirement is that the representative attend each meeting with the assurance that the head of his discipline is well aware of the questions posed and the solutions offered. The commitment of a given discipline to an action, a study or a series of studies will only take effect once the representative is assured that the necessary resources are available.

This system by project takes different forms in different companies, and the form will depend on the previous history of the laboratory, on the number of projects running concurrently and on geographical dimensions.

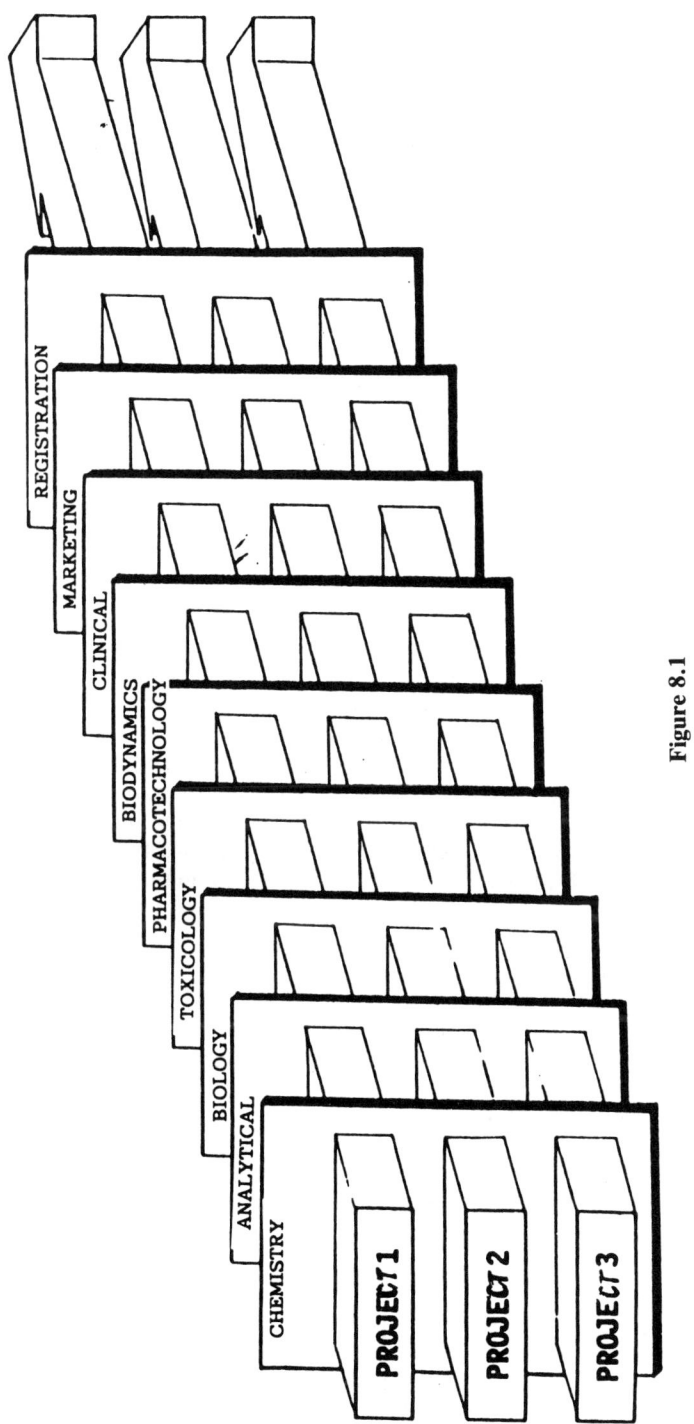

REGISTRATION

MARKETING

CLINICAL

BIODYNAMICS

PHARMACOTECHNOLOGY

TOXICOLOGY

BIOLOGY

ANALYTICAL

CHEMISTRY

PROJECT 1

PROJECT 2

PROJECT 3

Figure 8.1

A series of questions must be considered *a priori*: is the project leader a member of a well-defined hierarchy or does he simply come from one of the disciplines which contributes towards the progress of the project? In the first case, the project leader dedicates all his time to one or two projects; in the second, his responsibility as project leader is supplementary to the other responsibilities he will bear within a group of toxicologists, pharmacists or clinicians. How great are the powers of decision accorded to the project leader? Should he be answerable to a committee who will have the veto overall, or will he have the right to mobilise resources himself? In other words, does he reign over the molecule, an omnipotent decision-maker, or is he a professional co-ordinator who can ensure that each discipline makes its contribution under predetermined conditions agreed by the deciding group.

Who Makes the Decisions?

As with the previous question, this depends on the qualification of the project leader. Should he be a pharmacist, a clinician or a professional management executive? What grade is attributed to the project leader, particularly if decisions of importance have to be made by him?

The relevance of the answers to these questions is not insignificant, when one bears in mind that, from the moment the decision is taken to create a project for a particular molecule right up until the end of all the Phase III studies and completion of the final written synopsis, the number of projects running concurrently will amount to several tens, i.e. 20, 30, 40 or more.

Project leaders will need to tap the same resources of toxicology, of clinical departments, of clinical trial sample production, of marketing evaluation. Each of these project leaders will, quite legitimately, fight to obtain top priority for his or her project and demand that the industrial organisations be able to cope with conflict without causing disappointment or frustration to the individual.

Whatever the reply given to the above questions, no enterprise can afford to dispense with a committee, composed of the leader of each major discipline, i.e. of those given executive responsibility for the management of resources. The decisions and arbitration of this group must be maturely thought out, documented and elucidated so as to be clearly understood and adhered to by all concerned.

The organisation of a Phase I and Phase II programme cannot be summarised by the single acts of design and execution of 10 or 20 clinical studies which compose the programme. The realisation of these programmes has major implications for the enterprise. It concerns the preparation of products which will be marketed some 6–10 years after the decision has been made to initiate the Phase I and Phase II studies. The resources mobilised represent a very large part of the enterprise's expenditure. The success rate is low, since less than one molecule in ten administered in humans is likely to become a finished drug.

Competition is fierce and those who win the match, i.e. those who succeed in putting on the market a drug with a guaranteed, high level of return, are those who are capable of excellent applied science from a foundation of solid organisation and who promote the scientists' creative freedom around well-defined objectives.

BIBLIOGRAPHY

Booth, C. C. (1985). Clinical research today. *Trans. Med. Soc. Lond.*, **102**, 24–41

Feinstein, A. R. (1984). Current problems and future challenges in randomized clinical trials. *Circulation*, **70** (5), 767–74

IFPMA (1986). The impact of product registration. In *Symposium on Scientific Innovation in Drug Development*. IFPMA, Geneva

Meinert, C. L. (1988). Toward prospective registration of clinical trials. *Controlled Clin. Trials*, **9** (1), 1–5

Pinto, O. de S. (1986). Organisation and problems of drug evaluation in multicentre clinical trials. *Br. J. Clin. Pharmacol.*, **22**, suppl., 49S–53S

Rauch, L., Kranzler, J. and Chivis, A. Jr. (1988). The many faces of discovery: a managers' guide to research. *Pharmaceutical Executive*, April

Taylor, K. M., Shapiro, M. and Skinner, H. A. (1987). Some thoughts on the future of clinical trials groups in cancer [letter]. *Cancer Treat. Rep.*, **71** (4), 434–5

Walker, B. C. and Walker, S. R. (1986). Trends and changes in drug research and development. *Proc. Soc. Drug Res., London*, 26/09/1986, Kluwer Acad. Pub., London

9
The Role of Contract Research Units

A. P. Fletcher

Medical Director, IMS International, York House, 37 Queen Square, London WC1N 3BH, UK

SETTING THE SCENE

At a superficial level, the basic concepts of new drug research might appear to be fairly simple and straightforward. Once biological activity has been demonstrated in a number of experimental animal models, there follows a logical sequence of animal, human volunteer and patient testing to establish efficacy and safety, which, in the case of a successful compound, leads on to appraisal and marketing approval by national regulatory authorities. After this, the company relaxes, concentrates on selling the product and accumulates profits in order to develop more new compounds.

In the real world, this ideal situation is seldom, if ever, achieved, as numerous diversions, setbacks and other unanticipated events occur. The problems start right at the beginning with varying interpretations of the term 'new drug'. A brief consideration of some examples may help to show the kind of difficulties that are involved. A completely new chemical entity, which has never been used before, is, in principle, the least complicated developmental problem in that it is mandatory to conduct the full range of preclinical and clinical testing, as no existing data are available. The number of such pristine, new compounds is small in comparison with the very much larger number of compounds on which previously generated data are available.

Take the example of a recently introduced product, topical clindamycin (Delacin T) for the treatment of acne. Clindamycin is a highly effective, broad-spectrum antibiotic, first approved for marketing about 20 years ago for administration by the oral and parenteral route. In the intervening period, along with the even older and closely related lincomycin, it encountered serious problems because of its association with pseudomembranous colitis, which could, in certain cases, prove to be fatal. Successive bouts of activity, by national regulatory authorities in both Europe and the USA, led to restriction of its use to only the most serious infections. Now, applied topically as a solution, clindomycin is found to be effective in the treatment of acne, a common and distressing condition that is often very resistant to generally available treatments. The problem is clear. A large amount of data is already available on clindamycin, not all of it of good quality and not all of it reassuring. The company concerned will have closed down basic research involving animal toxicology and regulatory orientated clinical trials on the compound many years ago and will not be strongly motivated to start them up again. Nevertheless, the change in indications and route of administration requires certain additional information in order to meet regulatory demands. What studies have to be done and who is going to do them?

Another recent example involves the long-established bronchodilator compound salbutamol, which is generally regarded as a treatment of choice for many cases of asthma. In a new formulation, salbutamol is incorporated in a controlled-release tablet devised by the Alza Corporation which uses new technology based on osmotic diffusion through laser-drilled holes. Very similar technology was used for a new formulation of indomethacin (Osmosin) which ran into trouble because of associated gastrointestinal perforation. The cause was thought to be primarily due to the known ulcerogenic effect of indomethacin but also, in part, due to a potassium-driven osmotic pump. The new salbutamol formulation (Volmax) would not be expected to suffer this problem—first, because salbutamol is not known to be ulcerogenic, and second, because sodium ions are used instead of potassium for the osmotic pump. Even though salbutamol is an old and well-known drug, certain new studies are required for regulatory approval to be granted for such a new formulation, and achieving that objective may not be easy for a company whose main research resources are directed towards other newer development programmes.

The case of minoxidil, which started development as a potent vasodilator for the treatment of hypertension and has now been approved as a treatment for male pattern baldness, is a good example of a drug which has had a major change in indications many years after it was first introduced. Once again, new studies are required on a product that has long passed out of the basic research period, making unexpected demands on available resources.

Each of the above examples concerns an old drug presenting with a new problem of such a size that it has to be treated in much the same way as a new drug.

In recent years 'licensing in' of products originating in other companies has become a popular way in which the licensee company can add to its product range. The prolific discovery of new compounds by Japanese companies has led to many such licensing arrangements with the major multinational companies in Europe and the USA. In many cases the products are incompletely researched and require further studies in order to bring them up to the standards demanded by the major national regulatory authorities. In these circumstances a company which already has its research resources fully extended will have difficulty in meeting the additional requirements.

Even in the case of true new chemical entities, where it is possible, in principle, to design rational development programmes, the sequence of animal and human studies almost always gets out of phase, owing to unforseeable problems in earlier studies. As a consequence, important investigations, scheduled for early completion, may be further delayed because the available resources are already fully committed. In addition, the findings from earlier studies may raise questions that have to be answered by investigations that were not originally anticipated.

Thus, it can be seen that the process of new drug development is complex and difficult to schedule. Research resources in even the largest companies are limited and expensive, so it is essential that utilisation be maintained at a maximal level. This inevitably means that unscheduled investigations face delays while awaiting resource availability. The only alternatives are keeping in hand unused research resource (which is economically unacceptable) or using organisations which specialise in contract clinical research.

DECIDING FACTORS IN MAKING USE OF CONTRACT CLINICAL RESEARCH ORGANISATIONS

Although it is the purpose of this chapter to discuss early phase clinical development, it should be pointed out that much of what will be said is equally applicable to the later stages of clinical research, up to and beyond the granting of a licence to market the product. Early phase clinical investigations are commonly considered to be more suitable for conduct by contract companies because they tend to be relatively short-term, involve a small number of healthy volunteers or patients and are often conducted in a laboratory or hospital environment, whereas later phase studies tend to be larger-scale and longer-term. This distinction is probably not valid, but even so the contract organisations do tend to conduct predominantly small-scale, long-term studies.

The decision to make use of a contract clinical research company will have to take into consideration (a) the needs of the pharmaceutical company and (b) the facilities offered by the contract organisation.

THE NEEDS OF THE PHARMACEUTICAL COMPANY

A pharmaceutical company may consider using a contract organisation as a means of circumventing one or other of a number of internal problems or deficiencies. Even the largest multinational companies cannot cover all areas of clinical research, nor can they retain specialist personnel on a permanent basis if the demand for their skills is only intermittent. Although this is largely a matter of using available resources in the most cost-effective way, matters other than financial prudence have to be taken into account. Pharmaceutical companies may feel that longer-term benefit is to be gained by conducting major clinical studies themselves. Their scientific and medical personnel will come into close and frequent contact with the investigators and other people in the institution conducting the study, which, it is hoped, will foster good relationships between the company and the medical profession. Financial support for the studies may take the form of grants to teaching hospitals or university departments, which also may enhance the image of the company in the academic world.

There is also a feeling in companies that closer control of the studies is possible if third-party organisations are not involved. If this means higher standards, better science and better medicines, then it is to be encouraged, but if it means suppression of unwelcome findings, then it is a disservice to therapeutics and the pharmaceutical industry in general.

Clinical research programmes for the development of new drugs are extremely expensive and span long periods of time. Statistics like $150 000 000 and 10 years are by no means exceptional, so the stakes are high and maximal use of resources is essential. It is surprising, therefore, to find that many large pharmaceutical companies have only the roughest idea of the real costs of conducting a clinical trial. On questioning such a company, the payments made to investigators may be quoted, to which may be added approximate estimates of the man-weeks or -months or -years involved, which may be multiplied by some equally approximate sum of money which represents average earnings of the personnel involved. But these are not the true costs, which have to include a multiplicity of overheads and have to take into account periods of time when personnel are less than 100% occupied. Experience suggests that even in busy clinical departments underutilisation of resources may reach surprisingly high levels, partly because it is intrinsically difficult to devise work schedules that make the best use of the time available and partly because there is little pressure on company clinical research departments to provide accurate estimates of real overall costs.

In contrast to this situation, contract clinical research organisations cannot take such a relaxed attitude. Success or failure in the market-place for them depends upon costing studies accurately. Estimates that are too low will lead to financial loss and estimates that are too high will be uncompetitive and thus lose business to rival organisations.

The needs of a pharmaceutical company may be summarised under three headings: (1) completion of research programmes on schedule, (2) completion of research programmes within budget and (3) production of high-quality data that will meet the requirements of national regulatory authorities in the major countries of the world.

Completion of Programme on Schedule

Almost anyone who has worked in the pharmaceutical industry will be able to quote examples of drugs that, for one reason or another, have suffered interminable delays in their development. In some cases delays have been so prolonged that interest in the product has seriously decreased by the time it reaches the market. This is frustrating for the researchers, bad for the company's business and, if a potentially useful compound is involved, bad for the patient.

A typical example might concern a major new product for which a large clinical research programme is being conducted involving a full range of short- and long-term trials in patients meeting certain diagnostic and other clinical and demographic criteria. In one of the trials conducted early on in the programme, an investigator reports a number of cases in whom an unexpected abnormality, say, for example, changes in thyroid function, is observed. This finding is not reported in other studies being conducted at the same time, so it is dismissed as one of those inexplicable quirks that occur in clinical trials. After 2–3 years, when a significant part of the development programme has been completed, an overall review of the data is undertaken, which shows sporadic cases of abnormal thyroid function in some of the later trials. The company undergoes a panic reaction, people are blamed for not having acted earlier, recriminations abound, additional trials are planned for which people are diverted from other essential tasks, and large parts of the programme are postponed until more information is available. The system is suddenly overloaded, so endangering the successful completion of the project.

It is essential for the company to maintain the impetus right from the start of the programme. Delays inevitably lead to more delays, which can, in turn, have long-term adverse effects on the success of the drug.

Completion of Programme within Budget

The desirability of keeping a research programme within budget may seem so obvious that it hardly needs stating. Unfortunately, however, as was stated earlier, the clinical research departments of many pharmaceutical companies do not have responsive and accurate systems to estimate their real costs, particularly the costs of delays and the costs involved in the underutilisation of personnel. Working time and costs are inextricably linked, and it may well be that going outside the company in order to complete important studies in time will, in the end, save money.

Production of High-quality Data

The need for high-quality data cannot be overemphasised. It is the experience of those who have worked with national regulatory authorities that the data provided by companies in their submissions for marketing approval vary from the excellent to the deplorable. Poor-quality data are not only of little or no value, they are also time-consuming and frustrating for the regulatory authority officials to evaluate. Good-quality data are the result of successful collaboration between the sponsors and organisers of the study on the one hand and the investigators on the other. Studies conducted by pharmaceutical companies through their own medical departments are subject to just the same variability in quality as those conducted by third-party contract orga-nisations. The key to good quality lies in good study design, the selection of the best investigators and diligent monitoring. Those functions are just as accessible to contract organisations as to the companies themselves.

The USA has led the way in establishing official principles of 'Good Clinical Practice' which are the extension of already existing guidelines on

'Good Laboratory Practice'. Good Clinical Practice has proved to be considerably more difficult to apply, certainly on the international scale, than Good Laboratory Practice. This is partly due to the inherently more subjective and less scientific aspect of clinical medicine and partly due to large differences in the way in which medicine is practised from country to country. Experience suggests, at least in the UK and Europe, that pharmaceutical company medical departments have embraced the principles of Good Clinical Practice with rather less enthusiasm than their counterparts in the USA. This does not necessarily mean that the actual investigations are of any poorer quality; it just means that they lack the seal of approval that is needed in the USA.

There is no doubt that good-quality data facilitate regulatory approval and for that reason every pharmaceutical company needs the best possible data. What is possibly less obvious is that poor-quality data may actually obstruct regulatory approval. Consider again the previously quoted (apocryphal) example of the clinical trial that seemed to have revealed cases of disturbed thyroid function. If it were of poor quality (i.e. protocol violations, poor monitoring, careless reporting, etc.), then doubts will always exist concerning the interpretation of the study. The optimists will point out that it was a bad study, so the findings can be discounted, while the pessimists will claim that what has been observed is just the tip of the iceberg. Unfortunately, optimists and pessimists exist both in pharmaceutical companies and in regulatory authorities. In the former situation long delays may occur while decisions are made concerning the status of the project, and in the latter situation rejection of the submission and demands for detailed elucidation may occur.

FACILITIES OFFERED BY CONTRACT ORGANISATIONS

Clinical research contract organisations exist in many different forms, varying from large internationally orientated companies to small units employing a handful of people working on a mainly local basis. Some are independent companies or partnerships solely engaged in early phase clinical research; others are divisions of larger contract research companies involved in a wide range of toxicity and environmental safety testing. Thus, the facilities they provide vary from a restricted range of short-term clinical tests right up to and including comprehensive services covering all aspects of drug development in animals and humans.

Meeting Schedule Requirements

One of the major claims of a contract research organisation is that it can conduct studies at certain times and within certain time constraints. This is one of the most important benefits that such organisations can bring to the pharmaceutical industry; they can relieve the pressure that occurs when clinical research demands within the company become overloaded, thus threatening long development delays. It is the business of the contract organisation to provide facilities that can come to the rescue of hard-pressed companies, so permitting the overall developmental plan to proceed on schedule.

The contract organisation has a number of advantages over the pharmaceutical company in providing services on time. Anyone who has worked with a major pharmaceutical company will know that along with great size goes an immensely complex bureaucracy which is not conducive to rapid decision making.

In addition, many companies have management structures that require decision making to go through numerous different groups (medical, R & D, marketing, line management, etc.), which may have differing aims and differing motives. A secondary consequence of this organisational complexity is the development of inflexible personnel structures which, on the one hand, may be wasteful through retaining staff who are underutilised or, on the other hand, may be inadequate to meet an unexpected increase in demand.

Those who have worked in company medical departments will also know that clinical research is not the only activity that occupies their time. Many medical departments are also involved in the approval of advertising material, medical information, regulatory affairs, adverse reaction reporting, presentations at conferences and an endless succession of internal company meetings.

In contrast to this, contract organisations must be more responsive, more flexible and leaner working units. It is essential for the success of their business that they make accurate estimates of time and work involved and therefore can make accurate estimates of costs. Many such organisations are able to call upon experienced temporary personnel and part-time helpers without having to go through time-consuming bureaucratic procedures. The contract organisation is also differently motivated, in that it is dedicated to the conduct of certain specific studies to a standard that will meet all reasonable expectations and ensure business for the future. It is not concerned with the diverse responsibilities that may arise in company medical departments, and so may concentrate on timely completion of studies.

The contractual nature of such studies is of fundamental importance, in that it sets out clearly the terms under which the work is to be done. It is usual for certain standards of performance to be included in the contract, which may involve penalties if time and cost targets are not achieved. Thus, independent research organisations are highly motivated to provide accurate costings and schedules that are realistic when the nature of the study is taken into account. The study protocol may be an integral part of the contractual agreement or it may take the form of an appendix to the contract. This relationship between contract and protocol is another motivating factor in setting up a well-thought-out study.

MEETING BUDGETERY REQUIREMENTS

It has already been emphasised that independent research organisations have to make accurate estimates of costs if they are to be successful in business. In order to make accurate cost estimates, it is necessary to draw up detailed schedules covering every aspect of the proposed study, so that precise costs and requirements for personnel and materials will be known before the study starts. If the company should exceed budgetary restrictions, they would then be in a position to modify the study if that seemed appropriate. It is the experience of contract research organisations that their clients are not infrequently surprised at the high price of clinical research when it is looked at in detail. The cost implications of increasing patient numbers, extending the duration of observation, bringing in additional observation points or including laboratory or other specialist investigations are often underestimated. There is a tendency to forget that designing and setting up a clinical study may well be very time-consuming, and it is easy to neglect to take into account the hours medical advisers and clinical research associates spend in writing protocols and developing report forms.

MAKING QUALITY REQUIREMENTS

The independent research organisation works within the terms of a contractual agreement with the client company. The contract will define certain standards of performance that are to be expected. The requirements of the protocol will be complied with, the study will be conducted within specified time limits and the data will be of the quality needed to meet the regulatory or other requirements of the study. Most contract research organisations conduct all their studies in compliance with internationally accepted guidelines on Good Laboratory Practice. Compliance is monitored by a Quality Assurance Unit reporting directly to the top level of line management. There seems little doubt that the better contract research organisations maintain quality standards that are at least as high as and in many cases higher than those aimed at by the major pharmaceutical companies. High-quality data are not easily obtained from clinical trials. The varying diligence and enthusiasm of the university or hospital investigator, whose motivation may vary throughout a trial, has to be taken into consideration, as does the capricious behaviour of healthy volunteers or patients, who unaccountably fail to return or who decide, for reasons of their own, to discontinue. All the best efforts to adhere to protocol and to keep good records may be frustrated by uncontrollable outside factors which spoil the best-laid plans.

ADVANTAGES OFFERED BY CONTRACT RESEARCH ORGANISATIONS

In addition to meeting some of the needs of the pharmaceutical companies when their own medical research departments are overloaded or when particular specialist requirements occur, the independent research organisations may also provide certain advantages over studies conducted by the company itself.

Of foremost importance is the advantage of independence. The contract organisation's major aim is to conduct studies of sufficient merit to warrant further contracts from the sponsor company and to promote their capabilities and skills to other companies. It is sometimes implied that 'he who pays the piper calls the tune' and that contract organisations will provide the results their sponsors wish to see. The world being what it is, there is little doubt that such things may sometimes have happened, but it is only the most short-sighted of contract organisations that would be influenced by less than honest sponsors. The livelihood of the contract research organisation is dependent upon the quality and integrity of its work; it is far better to offend one client by refusing the bend the rules of good science and good medicine than to run the risk of being labelled as dishonest. The results of most clinical research investigations end up on the desks of assessors in national regulatory authorities, where they are subjected to detailed scrutiny and are later judged by expert committees. Studies of doubtful integrity are easily detected, so the contract research organisation is highly motivated to be seen as independent and honest.

This measure of independence does much to enhance the credibility of clinical research reports. It is difficult, and probably impossible, for even the most honest company to report findings that may be damaging to a potential new drug with the same degree of objectivity as an independent organisation that has no direct interest. There is little doubt that regulatory authorities regard research conducted by reputable contract organisations in a quite different light from that conducted by the company itself. Not only does the contract organisation enjoy enhanced credibility on acount of its independence, but also it is bound by its contractual relationship to the sponsor company to achieve certain standards of performance within defined time limits.

The contract research organisation also provides essential services to companies with limited resources of their own—in particular, the smaller pharmaceutical companies, companies requiring studies conducted in countries in which they have no resources and, in recent years, biotechnology companies.

The small- and medium-sized pharmaceutical companies are usually unable to cover the broad range of clinical research activities required for new drug development, so they become the most frequent users of outside contract services. As has been stated already, even the large companies find difficulty in making maximal use of personnel and time resources, and for the smaller company this problem is essentially insoluble. The demand for an unbroken series of clinical studies, which is the only way in which clinical research staff can be kept fully occupied, simply does not exist in a company with only a single product in development. Medically qualified personnel are the most expensive staff involved in new drug development and no company can afford to retain their services unless their skills are used to the full.

It frequently happens, during the course of drug development, that studies have to be conducted in countries other than the home base of the company concerned. A common example at the present time is the growing number of new drugs developed by Japanese companies. With few exceptions, the Japanese companies are largely unrepresented by subsidiary companies outside Japan, and since most national regulatory authorities expect new drug submissions to contain a certain proportion of clinical research conducted in their own countries, the only way forward is to make use of the contract organisations.

Another section of the industry that is increasingly making use of contract services is the rapidly growing biotechnology business. Almost without exception, biotechnology companies are purely biological and/or biochemical research organisations with virtually no resources for clinical research. This problem has been overcome either by licensing agreements with the major pharmaceutical companies or by contracting out large parts of the clinical development programme.

POTENTIAL DISADVANTAGES OF CONTRACT RESEARCH ORGANISATIONS

A major consideration for the prospective customer of a contract research unit is to assess its stability and permanence. Studies conducted for regulatory purposes are likely to be used over a period of several years, and it is important to be assured that the people who conducted the study will still be in business if and when their support is needed. In the case of the larger contract organisations this is not seriously in doubt, but for the smaller units lack of stability may be a problem. It not unfrequently happens that the registration of a new product in all the major markets of the world may span a considerable period of time, with five or more years elapsing between the first and the last licence being granted. During that time questions may be raised relating to the properties of the drug that were not apparent in the early years of marketing. It is during that time that the most critical studies on absorption, distribution, metabolism and excretion were conducted, and support from the contract organisation for the validity and integrity of those studies may be invaluable.

The most commonly raised criticism of the independent contractors is that they are more expensive than conducting the same studies in-house. The question of estimating costs has already been discussed and emphasis has been placed on the need for contract organisations to make accurate assessments.

Companies contemplating the use of a contract unit should also take into account the cost involved in delaying a development programme while resources are found in-house, which can be very considerable if several months are involved.

CONCLUSION

In conclusion, it may be stated that the contract research organisations provide services to the pharmaceutical industry which meet a wide range of needs in the early phase development of new drugs. In particular, they can provide a timely completion of major projects with independently conducted studies, giving a high level of regulatory credibility. In recent years several of the larger contract organisations have been able to provide a virtually complete new drug development programme from single-dose animal studies up to large-scale Phase III and Phase IV clinical trials. In addition, many of these contract organisations also provide regulatory writing and advisory services for the smaller companies and the newer research biotechnology groups.

10
Decision Points in Human Drug Development

Richard D. Mamelok and Jan Lessem

Section of Cardiology, Syntex Inc., 3401 Hillview Avenue, Palo Alto, CA 94303, USA

Making decisions in the development of drugs is a multifaceted and continuing process. Decisions must be made for scientific and commercial reasons in an ever-changing environment. In addition, the recent advent of molecular biology and a better understanding of cellular biochemistry are providing new perspectives on the initiation and progression of pharmacological research. The purpose of this chapter is to discuss scientific aspects of pharmacological and pharmaceutical development which go into decisions bearing on development programmes. While mention of commercial considerations will be made, these will not be covered in any depth. Furthermore, this chapter will not cover decisions to discontinue pharmacological development because of toxicological data or severe adverse reactions in people. For a detailed treatment of decisions in drug development, a monograph by Gross (1983) provides considerable information.

The classic approach to developing a therapeutic agent has been to screen a series of compounds in some model system, with some well-defined end-point as the initial measure of a drug's activity. When the animal model is chosen, both the disease to be treated and the likely indications are usually known. Promising compounds detected in the first model are further screened in other models. Concurrently a general pharmacological profile is obtained. Next a lead compound is chosen, usually on the basis of selectivity and potency. After both detailed pharmacological research and preliminary toxicology are performed, a decision as to whether to pursue research in humans is made and, if warranted, initial experiments are commenced in humans. A tolerable dose range is established, followed by preliminary trials of efficacy. Then larger studies for efficacy and safety are carried out in the heterogeneous population. Ancillary studies which confirm the mechanism of action proposed by the pharmacological studies are also carried out, as well as specially selected studies in appropriate subpopulations of patients. Each succeeding step in such a development scheme is initiated if the preceding step confirms the expected hypothesis regarding the effects of a compound—if, that is, the compound behaves similarly to a preconceived notion of how it should behave.

The most important piece of the development plan outlined above is the choice of the various models used along the way (Drews, 1983). Implicit in the choice of each model is that the model somehow serves a predictive function as to how a compound will affect a particular pathological process or disease (Davey, 1983). The choice of a model is more obvious at some times than at others, depending on our knowledge of the underlying pathological mechanisms. For example, in developing an antibiotic, initial screening will utilise the bacteria which are the ultimate 'target' in a well-defined infection. In contrast, when the ultimate target is not well identified, as in rheumatoid arthritis, a model which reflects the inflammatory process is chosen. In such a setting it is likely that the model chosen represents an epiphenomenon, not a critical step in the pathogenetic pathway. That rheumatoid arthritis is not well controlled or cured by currently available therapy reflects the lack of precision in screening models when the cause of a disease is not known and when the pathological biochemistry of a disease is not fully understood. Thus, in a drug development project the choice of animal models is crucial. The choice itself and the ultimate effectiveness of the choice are heavily dependent on the understanding of the disease process. Because a model is not a precise replication of a disease, there is no guarantee that a drug will be clinically effective, even if results from the model are encouraging. Unfortunately, a model often is chosen because it is what is available, even in the absence of any direct evidence that the model is representative of the disease for which a drug is being developed.

In *in vivo* modelling the problem in choosing a model is compounded by the variation in pharmacokinetics of a compound in different species. Differences in absorption, first-pass and subsequent metabolism, and excretion must be examined. Pharmacological activity in man may depend heavily on how closely man and the particular test animals compare in their pharmacokinetics. Unfortunately, much, if not all, of the animal pharmacology is performed prior to any testing in humans. Thus, a discrepancy between effects in people and animals can sometimes be explained by pharmacokinetic data; *a priori* predictions as to which animal will mimic most closely the pharmacokinetics of man are difficult, however (Nwangu, 1983).

Because of the inexactness of models, the decision to proceed on the basis of results of a model or series of models is made with still a fair amount of uncertainty as to the actual efficacy of the compound in man. Another dilemma presented by the choice of specific models occurs when a compound is active in a way that was not anticipated when a project was initiated. Unless the people performing the experiments are aware that the experimental results bear on the unintended, though possibly important, indication, a potential benefit will be missed. Thus, primarily out of ignorance, no decision will be made to continue developing a drug. A similar result occurs if the model used cannot even reflect the unanticipated beneficial effect.

As the molecular processes that lead to, or protect from, diseases are becoming understood, an increasing part of pharmacological research is turning towards particular molecules as targets for particular drugs. Agents designed specifically to interact with a particular receptor thought to be important in a disease process are becoming more numerous. Tissue-derived plasminogen activator, β-adrenergic blockers and H_2 blockers are some of the most successful examples. The synthesis of compounds designed to interact with a receptor, such as a specific enzyme, is forming an increasing amount of the work basic scientists perform in the pharmaceutical industry. Examples of these are inhibitors of renin and inhibitors of various protein kinases. A variation of this theme is the synthesis of endogenous molecules, or closely related analogues, with the goal to administer these in order to augment a normal biological response to a particular stimulus. Examples of such molecules are thromboxane A_2 and interleukins. In some programs, the decision process in drug development has been turned around from the classic method. The compound is now synthesised and screened for a particular biochemical effect at a specific molecular site. After this activity is confirmed, the effects of the compound in several disease settings in which the particular biochemical target was thought to be active is examined. Again the choice for models for the particular disease state is crucial, and the decision to pursue a particular model or group of models will heavily influence the direction in which the compound is developed.

The chances of success in the biochemical approach to drug development are increased in proportion to the understanding of how a particular molecule or enzymatic reaction acts in a particular disease. Thus, the decision to pursue certain biochemical targets is most likely to lead to success when the role of the biochemical target is well known. Such was the case with H_2 blockers, for example. On the other hand, the decision to pursue a compound which interacts with a biochemical target which is thought to be important, but whose exact role is unknown, is fraught with higher risk. However, the payoffs in this riskier setting, such as discovering a novel treatment or increasing the understanding of the disease *per se*, are potentially higher.

Beyond the judgement about the performance of a drug by the standards established by a model, a drug must meet other criteria to warrant a decision to proceed with further development. These decisions are based on work in basic toxicology to determine, for example, the therapeutic index, the potential for carcinogenesis and teratogenesis, and the effects on fertility. The physical properties of a drug must be assessed, to aid in pharmaceutical development. Knowledge of the pharmacokinetics and duration of action may require a decision to develop a controlled-release preparation.

When a development project starts, early input is useful from a variety of sources. Questions to be answered are: how successful is current therapy? what problems exist with current therapy? what are the new treatments being researched and what is the status of this research? Such input can help to guide the decision to pursue a project in the first place, and it is also useful in setting criteria to judge success or failure as the development plan unfolds. Exchange of ideas from basic scientists, toxicologists, clinical researchers and clinicians who have a broad view of the pertinent therapeutic field is essential in making well-considered decisions. Some general input from the marketing divisions may be helpful in making initial assessments of the size of a given market and in giving a commercial 'wish list' for the characteristics of the drug; but because of the time it takes to move a compound through development and regulatory approval, the accuracy of marketing information with respect to the ultimate commercial environment at the time of launch must be very tentative. For novel agents, as opposed to 'me too' compounds, very little information as to a compound's therapeutic utility will be available, and an accurate marketing forecast will be very difficult until the clinical effects of the drug are well described late in the development process. Thus, marketing may have some utility in presenting a general size of a market or the general frequency and duration of a disease, but it is very difficult, especially early in the development process, to make accurate forecasts.

The decision to discontinue a project in development or to modify a research plan may be influenced any time along the way by changes in the clinical or regulatory environment. These must be monitored closely during development, and the development plan must be altered accordingly. New therapeutic approaches may emerge which change a way that a particular drug will fit into a therapeutic scheme. The results of testing, especially clinical testing, that would be required to justify a 'go' decision for continued development might change. For example, the discovery that inhibitors of angiotensin-converting enzyme can improve survival in patients with severe heart failure has changed the criteria by which to measure the benefit of other drugs being tested for use in congestive heart failure. Even the current developmental plans for unapproved inhibitors of angiotensin-converting enzyme must be altered. Another example in which new information could affect the outcome of a drug development programme is in the area of hypertension. Recent evidence suggests that different antihypertensive agents affect left ventricular hypertrophy differently. This could ultimately lead to a different view of treating hypertension. Whereas the current accepted practice is to use a decrease in blood pressure as an indicator of clinical utility, it may become more important, even crucial, to examine the effects of an agent on organ damage, especially considering that there are a plethora of drugs which are effective in simply lowering blood pressure. Up until now a drop in blood pressure has been assumed to be a surrogate end-point for the beneficial effects on mortality and morbidity associated with untreated hypertension. Because of the differential effects of drugs on organs, at least in the case of ventricular hypertrophy, the use of the surrogate end-point may no longer be appropriate. At present this is a theoretical concern, but it illustrates the difficulty in planning a clinical development programme in a changing environment, especially when the time from the start of a clinical programme to a regulatory decision of approval will usually take significantly longer than half a decade.

The decision to discontinue a development project is often difficult, and it is usually made with incomplete knowledge. The likelihood of success has to be based on assumptions about the probability that, given a set of data, a desired outcome will result. The formality of this process is variable from person to person and from pharmaceutical company to pharmaceutical company. Several approaches which rely on formal decision analysis have been proposed but these have not gained universal acceptance (Balthasar *et al.*, 1978; Gittens, 1981; Boschi, 1982). It is probably a truism that the longer a project takes to find a particular drug the less likely it is that a successful result will occur in the 'near future' (Gittens, 1981). However, progress in different projects will occur at different paces, because of the nature of the drug or the disease being studied. What may appear as a reasonable development time to one investigator or to one project may appear excessive to another. That there is not a generally accepted approach to making 'go/no go' decisions testifies to the inadequacy of all approaches. Some have advocated computer-assisted modelling and analysis of the decision-making process as a method to improve the quality and strategic consistency of decisions (Wade, 1986). The uncertainty with regard to the success of a research and development project, especially prior to clinical testing, is high. The difficulty in reducing this uncertainty is a major problem for decision makers in pharmaceutical development. The analysis of methods of decision making is hampered because the payoff (either scientific or commercial) of a discontinued project, had the project been allowed to continue, will never be known. Thus, it is impossible to judge, in an absolute or purely objective way, how useful one's decision-making process is in making right and wrong decisions.

Finally, a difficult, but critical, decision in drug development consists of setting priorities within a pharmaceutical company. Clearly, therapeutic need is an important, probably the most important, criterion on which to build priorities. Therapeutic need could be greater efficacy, reduced toxicity or cheaper therapy. Therapeutic need must interact strongly with scientific and technical feasibility and with economic returns, in order to make the most effective and efficient decision (Hubbard, 1983). These, in turn, are partially determined by the perceived need, risks and benefits of a society (Keeney and Winkler, 1985; Larson *et al.*, 1985). A balance must be formed between basic science and purely applied research. As pointed out by Jolles (1983), 'fundamental science should not be emphasised to the exclusion of its practical applications; and commercial objectives (in general) are most likely to be achieved by appealing to true innovation and, therefore, to basic research'.

In summary, decision making during a drug development programme is difficult because of uncertainties with respect to the final outcome. In pharmaceutical development, these uncertainties are rarely resolved in a definitive way prior to clinical testing, since most models of disease do not fully reflect the clinical problem. Thus, decisions in early preclinical development must be made very deliberately, with careful attention to scientific issues. A wrong decision to continue a project will be extraordinarily costly with respect to money, resources and time. A wrong decision to discontinue a project could deprive patients of a new or successful treatment. The challenge to decision makers in drug development is to make a correct decision as early as possible in a setting of high uncertainty.

REFERENCES

Balthasar, H. U., Boschi, R. A. and Menke, M. M. (1978). Calling the shots in R&D. *Harvard Business Rev.*, May–June, 151–60
Boschi, R. A. A. (1982). Modelling exploratory research. *Eur. J. Operating Res.*, **10**, 250–9
Davey, D. G. (1983). The validity of animal and other laboratory models. In Gross, F. (Ed.), *Decision Making in Drug Research*. Raven Press, New York

Drews, J. (1983). Experimental models relevant for therapy. In Gross, F. (Ed.), *Decision Making in Drug Research*. Raven Press, New York

Gittins, J. C. (1981). RESPRO—an interactive procedure for planning new product chemical research. *R&D Management*, **11**, 139–48

Gross, F. (1983). *Decision Making in Drug Research*. Raven Press, New York

Hubbard, W. N. (1983). Therapeutic need as a criteria for setting priorities of projects for pharmaceutical research and development. In Gross, F. (Ed.), *Decision Making in Drug Research*. Raven Press, New York

Jolles, G. (1983). Strategic considerations in industry for setting priorities of projects in drug research. In Gross, F. (Ed.), *Decision Making in Drug Research*. Raven Press, New York

Keeney, R. L. and Winkler, R. L. (1985). Evaluating decision strategies for equity of public risks. *Operations Res.*, **33**, 955–70

Larson, L. N., Bootman, J. L. and McGhan, W. F. (1985). Demystifying cost-benefit/cost-effectiveness analyses. *Pharm. Exec.*, **5**, 64–6

Nwangwu, P. U. (1983). The process of new drug development: Current deficiencies and opportunities for improvement. In Nwangwu, P. U. (Ed.), *Concepts and Strategies in New Drug Development*. Praeger, New York

Wade, R. C. (1986). Computer-aided decisions. *Pharm. Exec.*, **6**, 58–62

11
Good Clinical Research Practice and Quality Assurance

Brian Gennery

Lilly Research Centre Ltd, Erl Wood, Windlesham, Surrey GU20 6PH, UK

INTRODUCTION

The terms 'Good Clinical Practice' and 'Good Clinical Research Practice' have entered the everyday vocabulary of the clinical researcher and imply a mystique around the subject that really does not exist. The purpose of good clinical practice is several-fold. It is to ensure, first, that persons who agree to participate in any clinical research protocol are protected from unnecessary risk as the study is conducted in accordance with a set of well-thought-out procedures; second, that the data collected from the study are of sufficiently high quality to fulfil the original purpose; third, that there is a means of auditing; finally, that the resources that have been expended on the study, human and financial, have been used to their best effect.

The principles and procedures that enshrine the conduct of good clinical practice were first set out in a number of regulations and draft regulations issued by the Food and Drug Administration (FDA) in the USA. These have been further refined in that country and now virtually all aspects of good clinical research practice have been codified.[1] Two other countries, France[2] and West Germany[3] have also incorporated these principles into their legislation and the countries of the Nordic area are currently drafting proposals to do so. In the United Kingdom the subject has been addressed by the Association of the British Pharmaceutical Industry[4] and the Commission of the European Economic Community are in the process of drafting a Guideline.

As a general principle, all elements of good clinical research practice should apply to all phases of drug development, although emphasis on some areas more than others will be dependent on the type of study under consideration.

The principles of good clinical research practice are set out in Table 11.1: all apply, in some degree or other, to studies in Phase I and Phase II of a drug development programme.

SELECTION OF INVESTIGATORS AND CENTRES

Many large pharmaceutical companies have their own clinical pharmacology facilities and do most of their early Phase I work in normal volunteer subjects

Table 11.1

Selection of investigators and centres
The protocol
Case report form (CRF) design
Ethics committees
Informed consent
Monitoring of clinical studies
Investigator agreements
Reports of volunteer studies and clinical trials
Statistics
Supplies for clinical trials
Quality assurance
Archiving

in-house. If these are not available, it is necessary to go to an institution that has the appropriate experience and facilities for carrying out such studies. Although many university departments of clinical pharmacology are able to do Phase I work and, indeed, their contribution to the programme can be invaluable, many of them do not find that early Phase I fits easily into their environment. Thus, a number of facilities have been established by commercial organisations which focus very much on Phase I and are able to offer a service that guarantees work being done within a specified time-frame. Many of these facilities are either within the structure of a major hospital or are close to one. Because their very existence depends on not only working within the agreed time-frame, but also being able to withstand the most vigorous inspection, most of them equip themselves to the very highest standards in terms of both medical technology and personnel. Whatever institution is selected, it is very much up to the sponsor to ensure that the appropriate facilities and equipment are available. Although acute catastrophic accidents are extremely rare during the first administration of a drug to man, one must plan for the worst possible eventuality.

In some special situations it is necessary to go straight to patients rather than normal volunteers, such as with antineoplastic agents, and there are oncology centres that have acquired considerable experience in doing such studies.

During recent times there has been an increasing need to study drugs in particular populations, e.g. the elderly, those with renal or hepatic dysfunction and children, in addition to looking at drug–drug interactions. These are all situations that require careful and thoughtful ethical considerations, and it is incumbent upon the sponsor to ensure that the sites he has selected for these other components of the Phase I programme have an ethical committee or institutional review board that is adequate for this purpose.

Most Phase II studies are done in hospitals or clinics that have over the years developed an interest in and expertise for this type of study. This makes the selection of centres for such work relatively simple, but one of the problems is that their very reputation means that they tend to be very popular. Thus, it may be difficult to get a study done in a reasonable timetable, especially if the compound under consideration is not a major breakthrough.

THE PROTOCOL

The protocol is central to any study. It is the road map to lead the investigator through the study plan, both in overall terms and for each individual subject. It is also the archival document that records what was planned at the outset of the study. Each company will have its own standing operating procedure for protocol development and layout. All protocols should include the following, with appropriate emphases for Phase I and Phase II studies:

Standard cover page with the title, including draft number and date of preparation, name of product (often only a laboratory number at this stage of development), nature of formulation with strengths, any comparator products (unlikely in Phase I or II), regulatory status and the names, addresses and telephone numbers of both the sponsors and the investigators.

Objectives of the study.

Rationale for the study, including the history of the development of the product and for Phase I studies a description of its intended therapeutic application.

Subject selection to include details of sex, age, and inclusion and exclusion criteria. This is of particular importance at these early stages of development, as only a limited number of animal reproduction studies may have been done.

Study design, open or blind (many Phase I studies will not be blinded), if blind, parallel or cross-over.

Drug treatment plan, which may be of special significance in Phase I to allow dosing to increase until side-effects are observed and in Phase II to allow dose ranging to take place with some degree of flexibility.

Parameters to be measured.

Follow-up procedures.

Adverse events, with special emphasis on the definitions of those events that require urgent reporting to the regulatory bodies.

Monitoring of the trial.

Conditions for modifying or terminating the study. This may be very important at this early stage, where new knowledge is being accumulated each day and rapid changes in plans may be necessary.

Statistical plan and administrative section that describes the CRF, data handling procedures and how the clinical trial material will be supplied.

Auditing procedures.

Ethics review and informed consent (any documents to be used in obtaining consent should be appended to the protocol).

Compensation or insurance arrangements.

Study flow chart.

Criteria for closing the study, including the conditions under which it may be closed prematurely.

Publication policy.

Signature page.

Some companies may attach to the protocol various other documents such as a copy of the investigator Letter of Agreement.

CASE REPORT FORM DESIGN

It should go without saying that in all studies the case report form should be designed to collect the data that have been specified in the protocol. They should be easy to use, but at the same time allow for the data to be easily transferred onto a database. Many companies have attempted to standardise their report forms to fit with their computer systems. This has considerable merit, but there are two points that should always be borne in mind. One is that the system should not drive the design of the study or the type of data that is collected, and the second is that only the data needed to answer the questions posed by the protocol should be solicited.

With some Phase I studies it may not be appropriate to put all the data onto a major corporate database, and care needs to be taken in ensuring that time and effort is not wasted in trying to create a form that will fit a particular system when it would be much simpler to handle the data by alternative means. This may also be true of many early Phase II studies.

ETHICS COMMITTEES (INSTITUTIONAL REVIEW BOARDS)

No experimental medical or surgical procedures should ever take place without some form of independent review of the plan being held. This normally takes the form of a review of the proposal by an ethics committee or institutional review board. These groups consist not only of medical and scientific personnel, but also of an adequate number of other people who can represent the non-scientific view. Indeed, in the USA the composition of these bodies is laid down in the Federal Register, and in the UK the British Medical Association has made recommendations as to their composition, although this does not carry the force of regulations.

Committees reviewing studies at the Phase I and Phase II level have a particularly difficult task as they are approving the earliest use of a compound in man and therefore will have to rely to a large extent on preclinical data. This to some degree helps to determine which institutions are suitable for doing such studies, as those who have become experienced will have an ethics committee that is comfortable with this type of study and knows what critical points to look for in the proposal.

INFORMED CONSENT

The issue of informed consent is one of the most difficult and controversial in the whole area of clinical research. No one suggests that it should not be obtained; the only issue is how.

The purpose of informed consent is to enable any outside witness to satisfy himself or herself that the agreement entered into by the subject and the investigator was done without any coercion or pressure. This protects the subject, the investigator and the institution.

There are some points on which everyone does agree—regulators, sponsors and investigators: first, that consent should be obtained; second, that the fact that it has been obtained is documented and attested to by an independent witness. Hereafter, however, views diverge. The main difference of opinion is over the issue of whether it is necessary or, indeed, appropriate to have the subject sign a document which certifies that he or she has read and understood the contents of that document; or whether it is satisfactory to have him or her sign to the effect that he or she has had the nature of the study explained and participates in it freely. The Declaration of Helsinki recommends that consent be obtained in writing, as do the ABPI Guidelines. The Food and Drug Administration require that the consent be in writing and that all the necessary elements be on the document that the subject signs. The draft Nordic Guidelines only recommend that it should be obtained, without saying how, and the French do not recommend written consent.

When one looks at the particular situation in the early phases of clinical research, there does seem to be some persuasive arguments that consent should be in writing and that the document signed should contain a summary of all the information known about the substance under study. Often the subjects in early Phase I studies will be students or even employees of the company who discovered the compound. They will, therefore, be intelligent enough and have appropriate background knowledge to understand the information in the document. (One of the arguments against complex written informed consent documents is that they cannot be understood by the persons for whom they are intended and they therefore become no more than a barrier to potential litigation.) It is particularly important to have it clearly documented in both these populations that their participation is entirely voluntary. These two points alone seem to be reason enough to have the type of consent suggested for Phase I studies.

On the other hand, in Phase II the population under study will come from the same cross-section of the community as in any other phase of clinical research, and the above arguments do not apply. While there are good reasons and a large body of opinion in favour of having a well-thought-out written informed consent document, there may be some environments in which this is not possible, and again one should rely on the protection offered in the Declaration of Helsinki and backed where appropriate by national legislation.

MONITORING OF STUDIES

The monitoring of a study can be divided into three stages: (1) those areas that need to be attended to before a study starts; (2) the monitoring needed during the course of the study; and (3) the tasks to be completed at the end of the study.

If a company has a large in-house facility, most of the monitoring will actually be done by the clinical pharmacologist conducting the study along with his team. In this case it may be that the role of the medical quality assurance group assumes an even greater responsibility than normal.

Where the study is being done in a unit outside the company, then before the study starts the monitor must satisfy himself on the following points:

(1) The unit has the ability and facilities to carry out the study. This may be of particular importance in Phases I and II, as special equipment may be needed to establish the expected pharmacological action of the test compound.

(2) A start-up meeting is held to ensure that all the participants know what is required of them in the study.

(3) There is full mutual understanding of the agreed procedures for adverse event reporting, publication plans, etc.

(4) Confirmation that ethics committee approval has been obtained and that informed consent documents and procedures will be used as agreed.

(5) The study compound will be stored in an appropriate manner, as will the randomisation code, where it exists. Also, there is understanding as to the conditions under which the code can be broken.

(6) If the statistical analysis is to be done at the centre, there are adequate resources for that.

One of the main functions of a clinical monitor is to regularly visit study sites and ensure that the study is proceeding to plan. In the case of very early studies in the life of a compound, there is a good argument to be made for the study monitor being present when the first patients go through their first visit. With a Phase I study they may well wish to be there on many more occasions, especially at the time of each major dose escalation. Their presence at this time in a Phase II study does ensure the earliest possible identification of problem areas in the protocol which can be attended to immediately and thus avoid difficulties later. Indeed, in some companies a small pilot study is always done at the start of the programme, just to ensure that such problems are picked up before too much effort has been expended.

Otherwise, the monitoring visits serve the same function as any other phase of clinical research, but will usually be done at a higher frequency.

At the end of the study the company monitor should collect all the case report forms and ensure that they are clean; account for and, where appropriate, arrange for the destruction of, unused study compound; collect randomisation codes; and arrange for the compilation of a final study report.

Other points that need to be considered in any study are the special issues of multicentre studies. Although not applying to Phase I studies (except possibly with some oncology studies), it is becoming increasingly common to do fairly large fixed-dose Phase II studies. In this case it is very important to ensure consistency in observation between centres and, if at all possible, the use of only one laboratory for the safety monitoring.

INVESTIGATOR AGREEMENTS

There are no specific differences in the nature and format of Investigator Agreements between the different phases of clinical research. The purpose of all such agreements is to set out in a simple way the obligations of the sponsor and the investigator to each other and, hence, to the study subjects.

STATISTICS AND REPORTS

A statistical plan should form part of the protocol for every study. It is not acceptable simply to state that 'the study will be analysed'. The statistical plan should give a rationale for the choice of the number of subjects to be studied, including a discussion on type 1 and type 2 calculations that have been used. It should also state the type of analysis that will be used at the conclusion of the study. In particular, there should be a clear statement as to whether there is to be an interim analysis. As Phase II studies are in large part there to determine the most appropriate dose, it is often desirable to carry out an interim analysis, as it is inappropriate to expose more than the minimum number of subjects to a higher dose than is necessary for maximum benefit.

A report should be prepared at the end of each study. This is not the same as a paper for publication or presentation, but such publications would normally be derived from the study report. Each company will have its own standard format for report writing, and the timetable within which such reports should be finished. Although the amount of detail in a particular report may vary, depending on whether or not the study is part of a registration package, it is as well to ensure that all reports do contain common elements. These include the following: introduction (in Phase I this will indicate the new nature of the compound); methods; results; discussion; conclusions; references; and appendices (e.g. curriculum vitae of each principal investigator, tabulations of data on each individual patient).

SUPPLIES FOR CLINICAL TRIALS

Often during the early development of a compound the amount of material available is limited. Also, little is known about the compound in man, and therefore drug accountability at this stage is of particular importance.

Often in Phase I only enough doses are supplied to complete the study in the number of subjects defined in the protocol.

In Phase II there may be many more doses than required, in order to accommodate the rapidly changing state of knowledge with regard to dose. Such excess may tempt an investigator to treat occasional patients outside the protocol. This is more likely if the trial is not blinded and the medication is in a therapeutic area in which there is a considerable degree of dissatisfaction. Such temptations must be vigorously withstood at this early stage of development, and drug accountability, with reconciliation of inventories, is a vital mechanism for managing this issue.

QUALITY ASSURANCE

The concept of medical or clinical quality assurance is a relatively new one, but one to which many companies are now paying a lot of attention. The idea of auditing a study from start to finish is simply a method of someone independent of the conduct of the study being able to say that what was meant to happen did in fact happen. It is not necessary (but it is helpful) to have a totally separate unit in order to carry out satisfactory audits. Audits can be done by anyone with the necessary technical knowledge, but no intellectual or personal interest in the study.

Audits on Phases I and II are of particular importance for a company, as it is on the basis of these studies that major investment decisions are made.

One of the areas that seems to give people many problems is that part of the audit which requires verification of the original patient records. In Phase I this will not normally be a problem, as the study subjects are in most cases normal volunteers and part of the informed consent process is to ask their permission for the records to be inspected and the records are only those collected during the course of the study. In Phase II, however, the study patients will be attending hospital and much of the documentation that allows them to participate in the study will be in the hospital records. In many countries these are quite properly regarded as confidential and not subject to inspection by anyone other than those having clinical care of the patient. This problem can be overcome by first making sure that this need for audit is explained to the investigator, who may not wish to participate if he or she feels that he or she cannot fulfil this requirement. Second, it must be part of the patient consent process. Third, the audit must be carried out in such a way as to preserve the integrity of patient confidentiality and maintain the value of the audit. This can be done by using the 'across the table' approach, which does not require the auditor personally to inspect the records.

ARCHIVING

Archiving all the documents that are relevant to and part of a study is the final action in closing down a study. The process does not change with the phase of clinical research.

CONCLUSIONS

The early phases of clinical research present no major difficulties in fulfilling the principles involved in Good Clinical Research Practice. The best policy is to follow the published guidelines and regulations, but to interpret them in an intelligent fashion, depending on the study that is being carried out.

REFERENCES

1. FDA guideline issued under 21 CFR 10.80
2. *Bonnes Practiques Cliniques*, issued by the Ministère des Affaires Sociales et de l'Emploi et Ministère Charge de la Sante et de la Famille, 1987
3. *Klinische Prufung von Arznelmittel*, Krankenhauspharmazia, 9 Jahrg, Nr. 3, 1988
4. *Guidelines on Good Clinical Research Practice*, issued by the Association of the British Pharmaccutical Industry

III
Ethical and Legal Considerations

12
Ethical Aspects of Research in Healthy Volunteers

Steven J. Warrington

Medical Director, Charterhouse Clinical Research Unit, Boundary House, 91–93 Charterhouse St, London EC1M 6HR, UK

INTRODUCTION

Let us begin by making a series of statements with which no reasonable person is likely to disagree:

(1) Society derives great benefit from our existing stock of medicines, many of which have been generated by research programmes which include experiments done in healthy volunteers.

(2) Present and future research programmes will yield new medicines which will be of great value to society.

(3) The development of medicines would be slower, more difficult and more expensive without the participation of healthy volunteers, but it could be done nevertheless.

(4) Delay in development of medicines is to the disadvantage of patients.

(5) The extra costs of development of drugs are borne by patients, consumers and taxpayers, not by the manufacturer.

Thus, we cannot escape the early conclusion that research in normal volunteers can yield benefits for society. If it were not so, further discussion of the ethics of such research would be pointless, since an activity which entails even an infinitesimal risk to life or health but which produces no benefits for anyone must be unethical. The real ethical difficulties arise in the consideration of how studies in volunteers should be organised and executed. Before confronting these problems, I shall consider how some general ethical principles impinge upon research in volunteers.

Ethics are a reasoned analysis of moral duty. For the purpose of this discussion, we might take our moral duties to be as follows (Beauchamp and Childress, 1983): justice—being fair; beneficence—doing good; non-maleficence—not doing harm; respect for autonomy—allowing the individual to determine what happens to him or her.

JUSTICE

The moral duty of justice requires us to be fair in our treatment of others. Thus, our treatment of volunteers should be equitable: they should be compensated adequately for inconvenience, discomfort and loss of time when participating in studies, and this is an ethical justification for the payment of research subjects. The duty to be just also clearly requires us to ensure that volunteers are properly and promptly compensated for any injury arising from their participation in a study, irrespective of the question of legal liability. Thus, justice here gives the individual rights which are additional to any to which he is entitled under the law.

The principle of fairness may also require us to study volunteers instead of, or in addition to, patients. Should not we healthy members of society share with victims of disease the burden of helping in the development of medicines from which there is no certainty that those victims will benefit?

BENEFICENCE

Beneficence requires that our actions should, when possible, benefit others. While it is clear that conducting research in healthy volunteers complies with this requirement in so far as the wider community is concerned, it might seem at first sight that we must fail in our duty to do good to the individual volunteer. In fact, the volunteer may benefit in several ways. Most obviously, she (or he, as I shall write from now onwards) gains financially. Furthermore, the experience of participation in a study may well be socially rewarding in that it involves contact with doctors, nurses, technical staff and other volunteers. And is it not pleasant sometimes to be the centre of attention, and to have one's slightest complaints taken seriously and recorded for posterity? Nor is it flippant to suggest that volunteers may regard as a benefit the opportunity to contribute to the welfare of others. In the special case of medical students, participation in a research study allows them to gain insight into the experiences of their patients—so benefiting both the student and his future patients, it is to be hoped.

Beneficence imposes upon us a most powerful ethical obligation to maintain the highest standards in the design and execution of research. A badly designed study is unethical because it must fail to yield as much useful data as a well-designed one. A badly executed project is even worse: it offends against both beneficence and non-maleficence, for not only will the yield of the experiment be less than it might have been, but also the risk of injury to the volunteers must be greater.

A final consideration is that beneficence requires us to be nice to our volunteers, just as we should be nice to our patients (Gillon, 1986). None of us can claim to be nice to all of our patients or volunteers all of the time, and it follows that we are each more or less frequently guilty of (mildly) unethical behaviour. Since we are not generally condemned because of these lapses, it follows that occasional unethical behaviour is condoned. Presumably the medical duty of beneficence is realistically regarded as an ideal to which we should aspire, rather than as a norm to which we must conform.

NON-MALEFICENCE

At first sight, observance of the duty not to harm others might appear to preclude the use of healthy volunteers in research, since no study can be entirely without risk. Indeed, if the principle of non-maleficence is accepted as absolute (*primum non nocere*—above all, do no harm), then almost all medical activities would cease. Clearly, non-maleficence must be linked with beneficence, and cannot have complete priority over it. The risk of causing harm has always to be set against the benefits to be derived, and *primum non nocere* has to be rejected as a strict instruction, although it remains a useful and pithy reminder of the dangers of medical intervention. Thus, the duty of the physician conducting research in healthy volunteers must be to minimise the risks and to maximise the benefits. If risks are to be minimised, the investigator must be highly trained, experienced and conscientious. Similarly, beneficence requires extreme competence in the investigator in order that the obligation to do good may be fulfilled.

Although non-maleficence cannot be an absolute principle, it clearly is a crucial one when the ethics of research in volunteers are considered. All are agreed that the risk of injury to volunteers in research should be kept to an extremely low level, and the safety record to date does appear to be good (Cardon *et al.*, 1976; Royle and Snell, 1986; Vere, 1988; Orme *et al.*, 1989). However, problems do arise in defining what is meant by an 'extremely low' level of risk. Should participation in a research study be as safe as crossing the road (what road? at traffic lights? on a pedestrian crossing? in rain or sunshine?) or smoking ten cigarettes (low, middle or high tar? inhaled or not?) or travelling in a passenger aircraft (how far? how many take-offs and landings?) or working in a mine or on a construction site?

Cardon *et al.* (1976) deduced that the risks of participation in non-therapeutic research were no greater than those in everyday life, as follows. Annual rates for accidental injuries that were temporarily disabling, permanently disabling and fatal were, respectively, 50, 2 and 0.6 per 1000 Americans. The corresponding figures for a population of nearly 100000 US research subjects were 0.37, 0.01 and zero per 1000. These authors reasoned that, since the average duration of a study might be about one-hundredth of a year, the risks of non-therapeutic studies were similar to those of everyday life. The only real weakness in this argument is that the incidence of adverse events in non-therapeutic research was probably underestimated: the authors used a postal questionnaire and telephone calls to investigators to quantify adverse events occurring during the previous 3 years, and this would surely lead to substantial underreporting. Furthermore, the 15% of investigators classified as 'non-responders' might well have encountered more adverse events than those who did respond.

These workers' findings, although not above criticism, are at least corroborated by surveys of volunteer studies in the UK (Royle and Snell, 1986; Orme *et al.*, 1989). A finding common to both US and UK studies was the high frequency of minor adverse symptoms occurring in relation to research studies, but Reidenberg and Lowenthal (1968) found a remarkably similar frequency of such symptoms in people who had not received either active medication or placebo.

Balancing non-maleficence against beneficence in volunteer studies is by no means the same thing as balancing risks and benefits in the treatment of patients. The crucial difference is that no volunteer research is ethically acceptable if it entails more than a tiny risk of injury, and this remains true however large the rewards to the volunteer and however great the value of the project to society in general. In contrast, extreme risks may be taken quite ethically in the therapy of a life-threatening condition—although such risks should be accepted only with the patient's knowledge and consent (in other words, with due respect for autonomy). Non-maleficence obliges us to keep risk of injury in any experiment to an extremely low level, while beneficence requires that we maximise the benefit that is derived from research.

RESPECT FOR AUTONOMY

Respect for autonomy signifies our obligation to preserve the right of the individual to determine what should or should not be done to him. In the context of our moral duties to healthy volunteers, this obligation clearly has priority over justice, beneficence and non-maleficence. We cannot, for example, ethically coerce anyone to participate in a research study on the grounds either that enormous benefits would flow from such participation or that great harm would ensue if the experiment were not done. Nor can we insist that justice requires that the subject share with others the burden of developing a drug or testing a hypothesis.

Consent

Respect for autonomy is almost tangibly expressed in the universal requirement that a person must give his consent to participate as a volunteer in a research project. The obtaining of consent is one area in which ethical obligations coincide with legal requirements (Dodds-Smith, 1985). The autonomy of the volunteer is manifestly abused if he is pressed into agreement to participate, or if he gives consent on the basis of inadequate information; if it is to be valid, consent must be both informed and freely given. We must give the subject a fair description of what will be done to him and what the risks of discomfort or injury are. The information has to be given in a form that the volunteer can understand; we fail in our ethical duties if we supply comprehensive but incomprehensible explanations. One potentially satisfactory way to inform volunteers about a study is to provide them with a detailed leaflet, the contents of which have been reviewed by both medical and non-medical assessors, and some ethical committees can provide invaluable help with such a review. Verbal explanation of a study may be ethically satisfactory but has two severe drawbacks: it is inaccessible to critical review, and it is unlikely to be as fresh after multiple repetition as it was when first propounded. Written information is, of course, valuable, but the volunteer must also have the opportunity to ask questions of the investigator.

The subject must also be of sufficient maturity and intelligence to understand the implications of the study; I shall return later to the ethical problems of non-therapeutic research in children, who by their very nature lack maturity (if not intelligence). Whereas the investigator may have little difficulty in assessing approximately the level of a volunteer's intelligence, the detection of psychopathology is a knottier problem altogether. How many physicians responsible for Phase I units would claim to be able at the prestudy examination to spot, say, a patient with treated schizophrenia? Such patients are sometimes said to appear more normal than normal people. Not only is the validity of such a patient's consent in serious doubt, but also the long-term medication of psychiatric illness may interact—perhaps fatally (Darragh *et al.*, 1985)—with the drug being studied. Invalid consent offends against the principle of respect for autonomy, and placing the volunteer at appreciable risk offends against non-maleficence to a degree which surely none would find acceptable. The investigator is therefore ethically bound to notify the volunteer's personal physician of the subject's intended participation in a study. In the UK, at least, individuals must very rarely receive treatment for chronic illness without their general practitioner's knowledge.

The validity of consent is perhaps most often questioned on the grounds that the potential subject is not adequately informed. However, we should also question whether consent is truly 'freely given'. Does the promise of a large financial reward compromise the volunteer's autonomy by inducing him to consent to procedures which he would otherwise be too afraid to want to undergo? If a teacher suggests to his student that participation in a study might be interesting and worthwhile, can the student's consent subsequently be regarded as valid? Similar reservations must be held about the use of junior staff in research projects, in both academic and industrial environments. I shall return to these questions when considering the problems of recruitment and payment of special groups of volunteers.

PAYMENT

There is no fundamental objection to the payment of volunteers; for example, in the armed forces volunteers have never been rewarded any less than conscripts. Failure to reward volunteers for their efforts would offend against justice and beneficence, whereas excessive reward must compromise the subject's autonomy. Relating the reward to the perceived risk would not in itself be ethically wrong; many readers will recall that, in the debate on the remuneration of miners, the risks to which these workers are exposed were generally accepted as a justification for paying them well. It is rather the exposure of volunteers to anything other than negligible risk which would be unacceptable, offending as it does against justice and non-maleficence.

The issue, then, is not whether volunteers should be rewarded, but how much they should be given. I find it helpful to regard participation in a study as analogous to doing part-time unskilled work—although lawyers would object to such an analogy on the grounds that volunteers lack all the legal rights (and obligations) which have been granted to employees. If we pay our volunteers at rates similar to those which apply locally to part-time unskilled workers, then the individual has, except in time or areas of high unemployment, the freedom to choose between a research study and (say) lugging carpets around a warehouse. Participation in a research study carries a risk of mild and moderate adverse symptoms, and a very small risk of severe injury—but so, too, do most unskilled jobs. For example, work on a construction site is notoriously dangerous, and even in a warehouse one might be crushed by a falling roll of carpet or transfixed by a forklift truck. Payment of volunteers at locally available rates for part-time work should help us to fulfil the moral duties of justice and respect for autonomy. Beneficence, on the other hand, might encourage us to reward the volunteers at higher rates, and such generosity may surely be ethically acceptable on occasion; the difficulty is in deciding at what point the size of the reward compromises the subject's autonomy and becomes ethically dubious. Furthermore, the analogy with part-time work is not helpful in assessing the correct level of reward for undergoing a safe but uncomfortable procedure such as swallowing an orogastric or nasogastric tube. The opinion of lay people, including lay members of ethical committees, may be a valuable guide.

One unexpected problem associated with large payments is that the very size of the payment may make the volunteer believe that the study involves a substantial risk, even when it is quite safe. Medical students at least 'expected to be rewarded for taking risks as well as for inconvenience' (Chaput de Saintonge *et al.*, 1988). As investigators, we concern ourselves mainly with what we believe to be the actual risks of the study; for the volunteers, in contrast, it is the perceived rather than the actual risk which may do the damage.

What are the moral duties of the investigator whose valuable (and ethical) research is stymied because the supply of volunteers is inadequate? If he follows the analogy with part-time work, he should simply increase the size of the reward until sufficient volunteers come forward. Is this ethical? The answer is not straightforward. I have already concluded (and you will have agreed) that the research must involve no more than a tiny risk of severe injury, and that volunteers may be rewarded for both time spent and discomfort suffered. If insufficient volunteers come forward, should the project be delayed or abandoned, or should it be more widely advertised, or should the payment be increased? What should be the attitude of the ethics committee to this problem? Abandoning a valuable project offends against beneficence; wider advertising has its own problems (see below) and increasing the payment may compromise the subject's autonomy, particularly in the case of the impoverished. The reader of this book may find it hard to believe that such a modest sum as £600 (about US $1000) could persuade anyone to submit himself to a research procedure against his inclination and better judgement, but a straw poll of students in London suggested that this might indeed be the case. The argument that the 'reluctant volunteer' is happy with his money, and that his health has not been placed at risk, is not tenable; we know, albeit from anecdotal reports, that some volunteers do regret their participation and feel guilty that they risked (as they see it) their health in return for a reward.

The resolution of these difficulties must lie in a compromise between the investigator's conflicting ethical duties. This may mean some delay in finishing the project, which may, in turn, delay or reduce the good which is achieved; somewhat wider advertising; and higher payments, which may compromise the autonomy of susceptible individuals. Ethics committees can be genuinely valuable in helping the investigator to balance these conflicting issues, although researchers often feel that the committees underestimate the value of their projects and that they function mainly as guardians of the volunteer's welfare.

Some investigators attempt to circumvent or diminish the ethical difficulties of payments to volunteers by making payment 'in kind'—that is, with goods rather than cash. This manoeuvre is clearly ludicrous (although not necessarily unethical), because goods which are desirable in the volunteers' eyes are as much of an inducement as cash; and if the goods provided are not desirable to the volunteer, he will feel cheated, and valuable research funds will have been wasted. Thus, the investigator fails miserably in his duties of justice, beneficence and non-maleficence.

Another ploy which aims to reduce the ethical difficulties of paying volunteers is not to announce the payment until the study is completed. This is not so disastrous a scheme as payment 'in kind', but nevertheless creates more ethical problems than it solves. Potential volunteers learn mainly from their peers of the existence of research units, and so are well aware of the 'going rate' for participation in studies. And if the volunteer is genuinely in ignorance of the likely payment until the very end of the study, what are we to do if he is profoundly dissatisfied with what he receives? Will not the volunteer correctly accuse us of failing in our obligations to be just, beneficent and non-maleficent (though he will probably use more blunt terminology)? 'Ah yes,' you may say, 'but we will avoid such a scene by paying our subjects so well that no one will be disgruntled'; but this, too, is ethically unsound, since payments which *everyone* would regard as generous must surely be an excessive inducement to a sizable minority.

Subjects who have to withdraw from a study for medical reasons relating to the medication or procedures are normally given payment in full, which seems fair. Should subjects be told in advance that they will be treated thus? If they are told, might they not be inclined to magnify (or even invent) adverse symptoms in order to receive their fee earlier and in return for less effort ('work')? This would lead to misleading conclusions about the drug, which might be to the detriment of the manufacturer, other volunteers and future patients. On the other hand, if the volunteer believes that he has to complete the study in order to receive full payment, he might stoically minimise and endure unpleasant symptoms—to the detriment of both himself and (possibly) future recipients of the drug. Thus, neither policy is free from offence against justice, non-maleficence and respect for autonomy. One compromise might be not to inform the subject that he will receive full payment if he has to be withdrawn, unless and until he experiences anything more than trivial adverse symptoms; this places a heavy responsibility upon the investigator to enquire energetically into any hint that the volunteer might be suffering unduly. This is evidently not entirely satisfactory, but then neither are the alternatives.

RECRUITMENT

Volunteers should be recruited by means of a general notice rather than by direct approach, which might compromise the subject's autonomy—particularly in the case of students or staff within the researcher's institution. However, I see no ethical objection to supplying, by letter or telephone call, information about forthcoming studies to individuals who have previously participated in research projects—the so-called 'volunteer panel'. General advertising for volunteers is often regarded as suspect and is, remarkably, condemned without explanation in the current Association of the British Pharmaceutical Industry 'Guidelines for Medical Experiments in Non-Patient Volunteers' (ABPI, 1988); perhaps this is a reflection of the restrictions upon doctors' freedom to advertise. In fact, there is strong ethical justification for advertising for volunteers. The duty of justice surely obliges us to distribute the opportunity to volunteer equally among those who might wish to do so, and it is hard to see how this offends against beneficence, non-maleficence or respect for autonomy. The 'targeting' of advertising at the impoverished is unethical, not because it is wrong to offer to the poor the opportunity to volunteer, but because it is wrong to deprive others of the same opportunity.

Advertisements for volunteers may reasonably mention payment, but should not give any indication of the amount. Failure to mention the fact of payment is ethically unsatisfactory, because it deprives the individual of information which is important in forming a decision about whether to volunteer. On the other hand, the size of the payment cannot be correctly interpreted by the subject unless it is accompanied by the full details of the study, and such details are unlikely to be contained in any advertisement.

SPECIAL GROUPS

Students

Students have long been used as research subjects in the study of both pharmacology and physiology. I have already alluded to the question of whether consent can be deemed to be freely given when the volunteer is a student and the investigator his teacher, but this is not the only ethical objection. The student might also feel undue pressure not to disappoint the teacher/investigator by withdrawing from the study, or might be diffident about 'giving up' in front of his classmates or friends. In class experiments, the subject might well be reluctant to divulge full medical information. The widespread use of students in studies at their own teaching hospital seems to be an example of a practice which continues mainly because it has gone on for so long that the ethical issues are not given the consideration which they deserve (Vere, 1986). An acceptable solution in the case of volunteer studies is for researchers to use students from other institutions only, although the arrangement is much less convenient for everyone.

Staff

The use by academic departments or pharmaceutical companies of their own staff as volunteers raises ethical difficulties similar to those encountered with students. The relationship between the junior and senior staff in an academic unit is not unlike that between student and teacher, but the head of department has even greater control over the destiny of his juniors than does the teacher over his students. Thus, questions must arise in relation to respect for autonomy; the validity of consent and freedom to withdraw from the study are particularly threatened.

The ethical considerations are no less troublesome if junior staff volunteer to participate in their colleagues' studies. Beneficence requires that we help our peers whenever we can do so, and justice seems to demand that the action of volunteering be reciprocated. These duties may lead to disturbing or intolerable conflict with autonomy both at the stage of consent ('He agreed to participate in my paracetamol single-dose pharmacokinetic study; am I not therefore obliged to help him similarly with his air embolism tolerance project?') and when the volunteer wishes to withdraw ('I I pull out now, this final study for his PhD thesis will not be finished before he returns to Matabeleland').

Pharmaceutical manufacturers are no doubt scrupulously careful not to exert any pressures upon employees to act as volunteers, and to recruit subjects by general notice only. Furthermore, justice might seem to demand that the employees should share the burden of testing a drug from which they might ultimately derive benefit in the form of greater success for their company. On the other hand, there must at least occasionally be a risk that the staff-volunteer's autonomy will be threatened at the stage of consent (when full medical information might not be divulged) or of withdrawal from the study. A further (perhaps purely theoretical) problem is that the status of an employee by its nature requires some surrendering of autonomy, whereas in research respect for the autonomy of the volunteer should be paramount.

The Impoverished

Justice surely requires not only that the poor should be given opportunity equally with others to act as volunteer subjects, but also that they should receive the same rewards. Furthermore, is not our duty of beneficence better satisfied by the distribution of rewards to the poor than by giving similar rewards to the rich? Unfortunately, there is at least one real ethical problem in the use of impoverished subjects in research: a level of payment which is judged appropriate by normal criteria (see section on 'Payment', above) might be an excessive inducement to the impecunious. Thus, autonomy might be compromised at the stage of obtaining consent, and non-maleficence when the subject later experiences regret or guilt. The worst possible solution to this ethical conflict would be to lower the level of payment so that only the poor would consider it worthwhile to volunteer, since they would then bear a disproportionate burden and in return would receive a reward which was less than the job demanded. The best that we can do is to set payments at a level which an ordinary person would consider to be reasonable; to inform the subjects fully, even when they are overeager to complete the formalities and start earning the money; to remain sensitive to any indication that the volunteer is having second thoughts about the wisdom of continuing; and to treat subjects generously if they do decide that participation in research is not for them.

The directing of advertising at the poor or unemployed has been condemned (ABPI, 1988) but is only objectionable on ethical grounds in so far as it implies that the well-to-do and employed are deprived of adequate information. It would be intolerably patronising to keep the poor in ignorance in order that the ethical issues might simply be 'ducked'.

Children

It is impossible to see how children could be considered as true volunteers, because of their inability to give valid consent. The parents' consent to their children's participation could not be accepted, because even a child surely has some expectation of autonomy. Could the 'volunteering' of progeny even be a form of 'child abuse by proxy'? Justice also demands that the child be rewarded for his efforts, and there are several methods of ensuring that money paid can be kept for the benefit of the child when full age is reached.

Women of Child-bearing Potential

There are no ethical problems which are peculiar to women volunteers; the issues are concerned with safety. Participation in a research study should involve no more than minimal risk, and women of child-bearing potential must be excluded from any study which entails risk to the individual or her future offspring. Because these risks are often unquantified until late in the development of the drug, most early studies are done in men. This is regrettable because it offends against the principle of justice, and may appear insulting to women who are certain that they intend never to bear any children. Unfortunately, women (and men, of course) are notorious for changing their minds as time goes by.

Elderly

Since the risk of any given study must inevitably be higher in the elderly than in the young, we should only ask the elderly to volunteer if the risk remains acceptably minute and if the project could not equally well be done in the young. Studies in the elderly may be required by the regulatory authorities, but there must be some doubt as to whether they are always needed. Much is already known about changes in drug disposition with age, and most problems of drug toxicity in the elderly in recent times could have been predicted from studies in the young. The investigator's ethical duties, then, are to ensure that the experiment is really necessary and that the risks are truly negligible. Poverty and mental incapacity may, perhaps, be more common in old age, but the ethical problems arising therefrom are not confined to the elderly.

Prisoners

Use of prisoners as 'volunteers' is now impossible in the UK, and there is little point in agonising here over the ethics of the matter. However, the issues involved are most interesting and challenging, and the reader is invited to debate them alone or with others, forearmed with the prejudices formed while reading the preceding pages.

REFERENCES

Association of the British Pharmaceutical Industry (1988). *Guidelines for Medical Experiments in Non-patient Human Volunteers*. ABPI, London
Beauchamp, T. L. and Childress, J. F. (1983). *Principles of Biomedical Ethics*, 2nd edn. Oxford University Press, Oxford, pp. 148–58
Cardon, P. V., Dommel, F. W. Jr and Trumble, R. R. (1976). Injuries to research subjects—a survey of investigators. *New Engl. J. Med.*, **295**, 650–4
Chaput de Saintonge, D. M., Crane, G. J., Rust, N. D., Karadia, S. and Whittam, L. R. (1988). Modelling determinants of expected rewards in healthy volunteers. *Pharm. Med.*, **3**, 45–54
Darragh, A., Kenny, M., Lambe, R. and Brick, I. (1985). Sudden death of a volunteer. *Lancet.*, **1**, 93–4
Dodds-Smith, I. C. (1985). The legal implications of studies in healthy volunteers. *BIRA Jl.*, **4**, 88–91
Gillon, R. (1986). Philosophical medical ethics: Doctors and patients. *Br. Med. J.*, **292**, 466–9
Orme, M., Harry, J. Routledge, P. and Hobson, S. (1989). Healthy volunteer studies in Great Britain: the results of a survey into 12 months' activity in this field. *Br. J. Clin. Pharmacol.*, **27**, 125–33
Reidenberg, M. M. and Lowenthal, D. T. (1968). Adverse nondrug reactions. *New Engl. J. Med.*, **279**, 678–9
Royle, J. M. and Snell, E. S. (1986). Medical research on normal volunteers. *Br. J. Clin. Pharmacol.*, **21**, 548–9
Vere, D. W. (1986). Ethics. In Glenny, H. and Nelmes, P. (Eds.), *Handbook of Clinical Drug Research*. Blackwell Scientific Publications, Oxford, pp. 1–32
Vere, D. W. (1988). The ethics of adverse drug reactions. *Adverse Drug Reaction Bulletin* No. 128, 480–3

13
Ethical Aspects of Research in Patients

Frank Wells

ABPI, 12 Whitehall, London SW1A 2DY, UK

INTRODUCTION

The involvement of patients in experiments is an emotive issue. Nevertheless, most members of the public are largely unaware that clinical trials are being conducted to the extent that currently exists, and know even less about how they are conducted, and of their own possible involvement. The issue of informed consent is vitally important, and not only must be fully understood by those involved in conducting clinical research, but must also inspire confidence in those who are the subjects in clinical trials.

Medical advances have always depended on the confidence of the general public in those carrying out investigations on human subjects. Such confidence will only be maintained if the public believes that such investigations are submitted to rigorous ethical scrutiny and self-discipline. Most patients trust their doctors, and will consent to any proposal, but they may not understand what is really involved, and for practical purposes the doctor carries a moral responsibility for investigations which he proposes to carry out on his patients.

It is because there are such mixed emotional reactions to the idea of being involved as a guinea-pig when ill that ethical guidance and clearance are needed; this must be carefully considered before necessary and proper clinical research can be carried out. Such care may not always appear to be given to the concerns of the community on these matters as is desirable, although the Association of the British Pharmaceutical Industry makes it quite clear in its *Guidelines on Good Clinical Research Practice*[1] that ethical clearance should always be sought and obtained from an independent ethics committee before any clinical research project is carried out.

A conference at Lugano in 1984 attempted to produce consensus statements about controlled clinical trials.[2] It was only partially successful, but many of the statements are of interest (see Table 13.1).

INFORMED CONSENT

The concept of informed consent was first discussed early in the twentieth century, in relation to surgery. Informed consent was first applied to medical

Table 13.1 The Lugano statements on controlled clinical trials (CCTs)

Obtaining informed consent is problematic because the patient	
is never truly free to decide	63%
often does not fully understand the implications of a CCT	86%
There should be no fundamental difference between the information given to a patient in order to obtain informed consent in a CCT and that given to a patient in daily practice	75%
Withholding active, safe and efficacious therapy in a CCT is acceptable provided that the omission of the active drug causes minimal and short-term discomfort and an ethics committee and the informed patient agree.	86%
Prescribers fail to see that opinion based on 'personal experience' is not good enough and that the results of CCTs are needed to make medical decisions.	95%
Clinical investigators and medical journals distort the truth by favouring CCTs with positive results instead of basing the decisions to publish on quality alone.	84%
The public must be told that	
patients often benefit from taking part in a CCT	94%
progress in medicine relies on CCTs	99%

experimentation during the Nuremberg Trials in 1947, and current standards are those set out in the Delaration of Helsinki in 1965, subsequently modified at Tokyo and Venice. Informed consent may be defined as the process whereby explicit communication of information is provided, which would be relevant to enable a patient or experimental subject to decide whether or not to have a particular treatment or to participate in a particular experiment. It has three components—informed, voluntary and competent.

Guttentag,[3] who is frequently quoted on this subject, defined informed consent to take part in a clinical trial (somewhat long-windedly, but quite accurately) as the experimenter's willing obligation to inform the experimental subject, to the best of the experimenter's knowledge, about the personal risk that the experimental subject faces in the proposed experiment, the significance of the experiment for the advancement of human knowledge and welfare, and, last but not least, the stakes involved for the experimenter himself. Or, in other words, informed consent implies that the experimenter has honestly tried to say everything that will assist the experimental subject in making the best choice of which he is capable, in agreeing or refusing to take part in the proposed experiment. That this effort should be made with unreserved sincerity is the antithesis of negligence. Current philosophical justification for informed consent, as expressed by Dyer and Bloch[4] is held to rest on the principle of autonomy—namely, that a person has basic human rights, including the right to self-determination.

Much criticism, perhaps not surprisingly, has been expressed in the media, and indeed by doctors themselves, on the ineffective way in which informed consent from those taking part in clinical research has been sought. Indeed, until 1984 the purely legal aspect of what information should be given to patients in the context of consent was left to doctors to decide. Provided that doctors acted in accordance with the practice accepted by another responsible body of medical men, they would not be held negligent in law.[5] Nevertheless, the profession has been urged for some years to confront the issue of informed consent squarely, and to examine all the implications with the aim of hammering out an acceptable working ethic for future practice.[6] Efforts to achieve this have also been made by the British Medical Association, the Royal College of Physicians, the Royal College of General Practitioners and the Association of the British Pharmaceutical Industry.

Attitudes towards informed consent differ in various countries. For example, in Italy patients have to sign a document on admission to hospital that they agree to any treatments the doctors may recommend; and in Belgium, at the hospital in Louvain, doctors are seeking to achieve agreement that anyone who comes into the hospital has by doing so given implied consent to being used as a research subject! In Canada it may now be illegal to carry out non-therapeutic research in children.

The US position is to regard patients as being 'prudent'. The prudent patient being (an adult) of sound mind, has the right to determine what is done with his or her body, and should only consent to treatment (or, it follows, experimentation) if given the opportunity of informed choice, and of evaluating the options available and the risks attendant upon each; material risks, so far as they are known, must be disclosed by the doctor.

The 'Sidaway' judgement delivered on appeal by the House of Lords in 1985 shifted the English position towards that of the Americans, in that the 'professional standard' position of doctors required modification towards allowing patients to make their own decisions about *treatments* which involved material or substantial risks or which might have disadvantages or dangers.[7]

The most common criticism from patients concerning clinical trials is that they were unaware of the fact that they were being used in experiments. The doctor must explain the reasons behind the trial, and the date of consent should be entered into the record sheets in addition to the patient signing a consent form. It is ethically essential that the doctor ensures that the patient is not subjected to any form of undue influence to secure this consent, especially when in the doctor's enthusiasm to recruit patients into a trial he may allow his clinical judgement to be impaired. It is well recognised that the proponents of any new treatment are naturally enthusiastic and commonly have an almost total and uncritical belief in their new ideas. Thus, it is easy for doctors involved in clinical trials to pursuade patients to take part, particularly if they are suffering from a disease for which conventional treatment has been unsuccessful. As a result, despite systematic or random bias, the results of treatment from uncontrolled studies carried out by enthusiasts almost always look encouraging, and a position may rapidly be reached where the doctors involved begin to think it is unethical *not* to include a patient in a clinical trial. These attitudes must be guarded against.

There are dilemmas in obtaining informed consent. One such dilemma arises where a patient is eligible for entry into a randomised clinical trial, but the doctor shrinks from revealing that consent includes the patient's agreeing to random allocation of treatment. It is not simply a matter of explaining the scientific principles behind the practice; there is also the very understandable problem of having to explain the reason for the practice—which is that the doctor does not know what is best for his patient. This causes a major shift in the doctor–patient relationship. From being solely dedicated to his individual patient's well-being, the doctor implicitly admits that the interests of other patients are also his concern and are at stake in the patient's answer. Yet such a patient may well accept this situation willingly, provided that the difference between the treatments is not too great. Suitable though randomised clinical trials may be for many treatment comparisons, if they ignore patient preference or jeopardise the doctor–patient relationship, then ethically other methods of research may be needed. However, the randomised clinical trial is now such a well-tried method of conducting clinical research that it is bound to continue. Nevertheless, it might be appropriate for patients to ask: 'Is this treatment you are suggesting to me part of a trial? If so, please inform me fully about it so that I can make up my mind whether I wish to participate or not'.

A recent editorial in the *Journal of the Royal College of General Practitioners*[14] covers the issue of informed consent. The problem of full and honest information given to the patient in terms that he can understand complicates his consent to clinical trials; Western society now concerns itself with human rights, whereas before it concerned itself with duties, and it is now felt that the patient must be given an understanding of the advantages, disadvantages and risks of any experiment, so that he may come to an autonomous decision. Thus, the physician is required to protect the patient's rights, and one of the common problems for a physician in this context is knowing whether or not the patient has understood. There are several reasons for a failure of understanding, ranging from inadequate or incomplete disclosure on the part of the doctor, through a numbing fear that prevents the intelligent patient from hearing what is being said, to a simple disability of mind. It is not surprising, therefore, that many patients still regard informed consent as 'letting the doctor do what he thinks is best'.

ETHICS COMMITTEES

It is quite clearly stated in the *Philosophy and Practice of Medical Ethics*, published by the British Medical Association, that doctors should only participate in trials which they are convinced are necessary, and in which the protocol has been given ethical clearance.[8] The topic has been aired freely over the last two decades; in 1967 the Royal College of Physicians published a report of its Committee on the Supervision of the Ethics of Clinical Investigations and Institutions, which sought to highlight the need for ethical standards to be maintained in research projects carried out in hospitals.[9] No project which was unscientific, the report stated, should be considered ethical, and evidence following the publication of this report confirmed that it had a certain impact. In 1973 details were published, again by the Royal College of Physicians, of the recommended composition and scope of ethical committees for clinical research, based on hospital districts.[10] The stated object of such ethical committees was to safeguard patients, healthy volunteers and the reputation of the profession. They were to be hospital-based, small in size and so constituted that they would not cause unreasonable hindrance to the advancement of medical knowledge. The report concluded that applications for ethical clearance for all proposed clinical research and investigations should be made through such committees, and two years later, in 1975, the Department of Health issued guidelines advising health authorities to implement these recommendations.[11]

These guidelines did not cover clinical trials undertaken in general practice, and the reason for this at the time was undoubtedly because the significance of general practitioner clinical trials was not fully appreciated. However, as 90% of medical care is provided by general practitioners in the United Kingdom and only 10% by the hospital service, it follows that the vast majority of medicines are in fact dispensed to patients who have them prescribed in general practice; thus, research which is general-practice-orientated is relevant and important. The location of multicentre Phase IV studies is bound to involve general practice, and it is considered quite essential, therefore, that the highest possible ethical standards are seen to be maintained in conducting general practitioner trials, as well as hospital trials. It is also essential that marketing exercises are not confused with clinical trials. Separate guidance exists for general practitioner trials, to which reference is made below.

To assist in the effective working of local ethical committees, the British Medical Association in 1983 recommended a revision to their constitution, to include general practitioners and a member of the lay public.[12] These proposals were considered by the national committees and the Royal Colleges representing both hospital doctors and general practitioners, and were accepted.

Apart from their altered membership, their remit was extended to cover research in all fields of medical practice. Based on Health Districts, of which there are 190 in England and Wales, the model constitution includes two hospital consultants, one junior hospital doctor, two general practioners, one community physician, one nurse and one lay member. All the practitioners on such a committee are nominated by the committees representing the various professional disciplines in the district concerned.

Although this is national policy, not every district has such an ethical committee for clinical research operating effectively; therefore, to ensure that research projects in general practice may be cleared by an appropriate ethics committee, the Royal College of General Practitioners established a central committee with a similar constitution to that recommended for local committees, originally under the chairmanship of Sir Eric Scowen, previously chairman of the UK Committee on Safety of Medicines.

Because of the importance of ethical approval, it is perhaps not surprising that even ethics committees themselves may be criticised; the lay person on such committees has a particularly important role to play, representing the interests of the patient. At an inquest held in 1982 into the death of a patient who was taking part in a clinical trial without being aware of his involvement in such a trial, the importance of seeking consent from any patient taking part in a clinical trial was highlighted.[6] Although this particular case referred to a patient who was being investigated in hospital, no fewer than 11 local ethical committees had agreed that the patients taking part in this trial should not be informed of their participation in it. None of these ethics committees had lay representation. Fortunately the situation has considerably improved in this regard over the past 6 years. Formal written consent is now virtually a requirement, and the manner in which such consent is obtained should be viewed by ethics committees as a top priority, bearing in mind the Declaration of Helsinki and other national and international codes and regulations.

There is another drawback associated with ethics committees, referred to in an article published in 1984; this relates to the possible perceived devolution of responsibility from the investigator to the ethics committee.[13] When a committee gives approval to a protocol, an investigator might feel relieved of some responsibility, and do things to patients which neither the ethics committee nor the investigator might countenance if either had sole responsibility.

An early-day motion was tabled in the House of Commons on 28 June 1988, entitled 'Medical Ethical Committees'. It reads: 'That this House notes with deep concern the revelation that Professor X was himself a member of the ethical committee at the Y Centre for Neurosurgery and Neurology which authorised him to proceed with medical operations involving the transplant of fetal tissue into the brains of sufferers from Parkinsons Disease; it believes that such a situation brings into disrepute the whole current working of such committees; and calls upon the Secretary of State [for Social Services] to introduce measures forthwith to prevent ethical committees considering applications from their own members.' This motion proceeded no further through Parliament, but it highlights a particular dilemma which should be avoided.

INTERNATIONAL RESEARCH

A series of interesting conclusions were reached at a bioethics summit conference held in Ottawa in April 1987[16] regarding the ethics of clinical research on an international basis. As national standards are established, so consideration must be given to evolving international guidelines for research involving human subjects. This will stimulate sharing of results among nations, and avoid unnecessary duplication and mutiplication of research. In order to safeguard the rights and well-being of patients and research subjects, research ethics committees need to be established in all countries where research is conducted. It is recognised that the pharmaceutical industry is a major source of medical innovation, and that the research it conducts is often carried out in a number of different countries. This makes it particularly important, ethically, that no nation should support in other countries research which does not conform to ethics review standards at least equivalent to those in force within its own country. In Phase II studies, therefore, where just a few patients are first given a novel therapy, the protocols should be subject to the highest ethical judgements that apply. Special consideration should be given to limiting the number of subjects entered into pilot studies.

ACADEMIC RESEARCH

The increasingly close links which are becoming established between university-based and industry-based research mean that academic physicians or institutions, as well as independent clinical investigators, may have financial interests in the outcome of the research; any such potential conflicts of interest should be declared in the research ethics review process.

COMPENSATION

Human research subjects should be fully informed concerning the availability—or lack of availability—of mechanisms of care and compensation to subjects who are injured as a result of their participation in research. The Association of the British Pharmaceutical Industry published in 1983 clear guidelines on the subject of compensation to patients for injury brought about by their involvement in clinical research, and pharmaceutical companies have invariably followed this guidance.[15]

COMMERCIAL CONFIDENTIALITY

In the context of industry-sponsored research, it has to be recognised that sometimes the confidentiality of commercially sensitive material may not be consistent with the requirements for ethics review. This can, therefore, create a dilemma, the resolution of which must not mean that ethical standards are lowered.

PHASE IV STUDIES IN GENERAL PRACTICE

Reference has been made to discussions which have taken place in the past between representatives of the medical profession and of the pharmaceutical industry in drawing up a Code of Practice for the Clinical Assessment of Licensed Medicinal Products in General Practice. Without this Code of Practice both the British Medical Association and the Royal College of General Practitioners might have advised doctors not to participate in clinical trials promoted by pharmaceutical companies—which would have been disastrous to the conduct of Phase IV studies in the UK. The agreement reached between all interested parties was, and continues to be, of great importance, and many clinical trials take place in the UK within the context of general practice. Nevertheless, members of the general public, and some doctors, have criticised some of the ways in which general practitioners have been involved in multicentre projects. Much of this criticism has been ill-founded, but some of it has been justified. The existence and use of this Code of Practice should minimise the chances of such criticism being made at all.

There are many and substantial reasons for conducting clinical trials; multicentre GP trials, however, are particularly valuable in deciding the merits of medicines prescribed outside hospital. The reasons are substantial, and include the facts that (a) general practice encompasses a wider, more diverse population than that found in hospital; (b) the condition of ambulant patients, particularly those at work, may be different from those in hospital; (c) the results of treatment outside hospital may differ considerably from those obtained inside hospital, where the environment is tightly controlled; (d) side-effects and other events caused by the drug under trial may appear in normal daily situations which would not appear in hospital; (e) patient compliance with treatment may be quite different away from hospital; and (f) the usefulness of some medicinal products in clinical practice may require comparison with existing products over prolonged use.

All such trials must have ethical approval, given by an independent ethics committee, and it is essential that every doctor taking part in such a trial be satisfied that appropriate ethical clearance has been given. Although it was previously considered adequate for any single independent ethics committee to give such clearance for the whole trial—while accepting the right of any doctor to seek local clearance as well—it now seems prudent to ensure that each trialist obtains ethical approval for any given trial locally, before taking part. Nevertheless, central clearance may also be given by an independent committee operating nationally, such as the ethical committee set up by the Royal College of General Practitioners, referred to earlier. Ethics committees set up by pharmaceutical companies, however reputable the company concerned, may inevitably be biased, and are consequently unacceptable.

AIDS RESEARCH

Particular problems could arise over the need to conduct research on treatment for acquired immune-deficiency syndrome (AIDS). Perry recently commented on the various ethical considerations which apply in such research.[20] He emphasised that we must be aware of: confidentiality problems; the need to do research on anything which looks hopeful; the high expectations of AIDS patients taking part; and the need to do research on HIV-infected patients who are symptomless, and the problems associated with informed consent in such subjects.

RESEARCH IN CHILDREN

Concern has arisen over the involvement of children in clinical trials; Nicholson, in his textbook on medical research with children, comments on the ability of a child to consent to research.[21] He concludes that at a developmental age of greater than 7 years there should be an attempt to obtain the child's consent and that as the child approaches the age of 14 years, so the necessity for his/her consent increases.

PAYMENT TO TRIALISTS

Doctors taking part in a clinical trial inevitably take on a greater commitment during the period of the trial than would otherwise apply for the patient concerned. This ethically justifies a fee to be paid by the company sponsoring the trial, but it is important that the fee is not seen as an inducement to participate in the trial, rather as realistic remuneration for work done, the time involved, the complexity of the assessments and the degree of expertise required.

POST-MARKETING SURVEILLANCE AND MARKET RESEARCH

The General Practitioners' Code of Practice does not cover post-marketing surveillance or marketing exercises. Post-marketing surveillance has its own guidelines, again jointly devised by the pharmaceutical industry, the Committee on Safety of Medicines, the Royal College of General Practitioners and the British Medical Association.[18] Promotional exercises, recognised for what they are, are covered by the Code of Practice for the Pharmaceutical Industry, first drawn up in 1958, and now in its 7th edition.[19]

There can be no objection to the principle of post-marketing surveillance of new medicines in general practice as a most useful method of finding out about events associated with the large-scale use of the medicine concerned. Indeed, the Licensing Authority in the UK is now effectively demanding that such surveillance take place as a condition of granting a Product Licence for certain new chemical entities. What must be resisted, and what has led to criticism of some marketing exercises, is a pseudoscientific approach which has made it appear that a purely marketing exercise is a properly controlled clinical trial. Conversely, what must also be resisted is the involvement in any way of any of the marketing personnel of a pharmaceutical company with the conduct of a clinical trial. This certainly includes multicentre GP trials, which must be wholly the responsibility of the medical department, with a named medical adviser to the company responsible personally for each trial.

CONCLUSION

Society should make the human subject an active and educated participant in which he or she contributes from a sense of basic human altruism and a desire to serve the common good, rather than as a 'subject of research', as has sometimes been the case in the past. Doctors should be (better) educated in medical ethics, as should medical students, and the general public should be made aware of the ethical commitment of doctors undertaking research.

Recent English legal history pinpoints the newly emerging issue of whether a doctor can be considered negligent because he has obtained consent on the basis of inadequate information. Judges appear to take a benign view of the integrity of the traditional medical viewpoint, but most doctors probably now agree that the patient has a right to free choice. All of this makes the decision to involve patients in clinical trials a much greater responsibility than has previously been appreciated, and confirms the importance of the ethics of all aspects of clinical research.

REFERENCES

1. Association of the British Pharmaceutical Industry (1988). *Guidelines on Good Clinical Research Practice*. ABPI, London
2. Blum, A. L. *et al.* (1987). The Lugano statements on controlled clinical trials. *Journal of International Medical Research*, **15**, 2–22
3. Guttentag, O. (1968). Ethical problems in human experimentation. In Torrey, E. F. (Ed.), *Ethical Issues in Medicine*. Little, Brown, Boston
4. Dyer, A. R. and Bloch, S. (1987). Informed consent and the psychiatric patient. *Journal of Medical Ethics*, **13**, 12–16
5. Editorial (1985). Adequately informed consent. *Journal of Medical Ethics*, **11**, 115–16
6. Peckham, M. J. (Chairman) (1983). Informed consent. *British Medical Journal*, **ii**, 1117–21
7. Anon. (1985). Sidaway v. Bethlem Royal Hospital and the Maudsley Hospital Health Authority and others (law report). *The Times*, 22 February
8. British Medical Association (1988). *Philosophy and Practice of Medical Ethics*. BMA, London, p. 75
9. Royal College of Physicians (1967). *Report on the Ethics of Clinical Investigations and Institutions*. RCP, London
10. Royal College of Physicians (1973). *Report on the Composition of Ethics Committees*. RCP, London
11. Department of Health and Social Security (1975). HSC (IS) 153
12. British Medical Association (1983). *The Handbook of Medical Ethics*. BMA, London, p. 30
13. Lewis, P. J. (1982). The drawbacks of research ethics committees. *Journal of Medical Ethics*, **8**, 61–4
14. Editorial (1987). Informed consent. *Journal of Royal College of General Practitioners*, **37**, 242–3
15. Association of the British Pharmaceutical Industry (1983). *Clinical Trials— Compensation for Medicine-induced Injury*. ABPI, London
16. Report on Bioethics Summit Conference (1987). Towards an international ethic for research involving human subjects. *IME Bulletin Supplement 6*, May

17. Association of the British Pharmaceutical Industry (1988). *Code of Practice for the Clinical Assessment of Licensed Medicinal Products in General Practice*. ABPI, London
18. Anon. (1988). Guidelines for the conduct of postmarketing surveillance studies. *British Medical Journal*, **i**, 399–400
19. Association of the British Pharmaceutical Industry (1988). *Code of Practice for the Pharmaceutical Industry*. ABPI, London
20. Perry, S. W. (1988). Ethical considerations in AIDS research. *IME Bulletin*, March, 2–3
21. Nicholson, R. H. (Ed.) (1986). Review of medical research and children. In *Medical Research with Children: Ethics, Law and Practice*. Oxford University Press, Oxford

14
Legal Liabilities in Clinical Trials

Ian C. Dodds-Smith

McKenna & Co., Inveresk House, 1 Aldwych, London WC2R 0HF, UK

INTRODUCTION

There is a voluminous literature on legal issues in clinical research and, more particularly, the relationship between law and ethics. Medicine is international but the law often varies from country to country. This chapter must, therefore, inevitably be less than comprehensive and the approach will essentially be to indicate how the main issues are addressed by English law, making comparisons with other jurisdictions only where these are particularly striking or relevant to the likely development of English and European Community law.

DEFINITION

There is no universally accepted definition of clinical trials. In this chapter the term will be used in the widest sense as meaning the scientific study of drugs in man. It therefore encompasses several different types of study falling within clinical pharmacology, ranging from those involving therapy in circumstances where there is no accepted mode of treatment but where the aim is to help the particular patient and at the same time advance medical science, to those involving non-patient volunteers where no prospect of personal benefit arises. It will be seen that the very different nature of the volunteers carries with it important legal consequences. Non-patient volunteers are often referred to as healthy volunteers but this is a misleading expression, as any group of people will include the normal percentage in any population who suffer from allergies and other minor illnesses and abnormalities. However, the expression is widely used and will be used in this chapter to describe a person who has no significant illness relevant to a proposed study and agrees to participate other than with a view to personal medical benefit. Volunteers enrolling with a view to treatment will be termed 'patient volunteers' and the term 'clinical research' will be used to denote both fields of research.

LAW AND ETHICS

The medical profession has traditionally had to conduct clinical research against the background of a society that desires and applauds new drug treatments for disease but at the same time has a deeply suspicious view of the use of human beings in medical experimentation. The appalling examples of prisoners used for experimentation during World War II did little to allay that suspicion but at least provoked the first serious set of international ethical guidelines on a subject where both the law and medical ethics was notoriously vague.[1] For once, the law has an excuse for being vague. Legal rules tend to reflect the decisions within society as to what is ethically right and proper, and, therefore, until the medical profession and society at large has established the ethical framework within which medical research should be conducted, the law is bound to be hamstrung.

The ethics of many aspects of medical research remain controversial and the law on the subject is unsatisfactory. Indeed, the main feature of the law is its very limited intervention in the form of specific legal rules. Even where the courts have explored the legal requirements of a particular aspect of research—such as consent—the decisions of the judges have often been conflicting. Even as late as the 1950s there was some doubt as to the legality of certain research, with Regan noting that although it was the duty of a physician to ensure that his practices reflected changing knowledge, it was also his duty 'to refrain from experiments'.[2]

If this statement were to be taken at face value, clinical trials could not take place, for the randomised controlled clinical trial is the very essence of an 'experiment'. However, there is now no doubt that most controlled clinical trials are both ethical and legal. Legislatures the world over have formally accepted that only experimentation in patients produces reliable information and helps to protect the public at large from ineffective and unsafe medicines. Results from increasingly sophisticated trials of this nature are now a legal requirement for the registration of new medicinal products throughout the western world.

In contrast, the same legislatures have been slow to establish detailed rules relating to the manner in which clinical research is to be performed. Thus, the European Directives[3] relating to marketing authorisations and the Medicines Act legislation in the UK applicable to dealings in medicinal products[4] require applicants for licences to produce clinical trial data, and most member states require some type of approval before commencing trials and the reporting of adverse events encountered. However, such legislation does not normally provide detailed guidance on matters such as trial design and patient consent.

Furthermore, in the UK (and six other member states of the Community) the supply of drugs for healthy volunteer studies remains wholly unregulated by statute. A committee set up in the UK after the thalidomide catastrophe in the 1960s to recommend what legislation was required relating to the safety and efficacy of drugs declared that 'responsibility for the experimental laboratory testing of new drugs before they are used in clinical trials should remain with the individual pharmaceutical manufacturer'.[5] Records of debates in Parliament at that time reflect the fact that the primary concern was to ensure that new drugs were not put on the market before possible harmful side-effects had been evaluated rather than to protect the rights of either patients or healthy volunteers. The unwritten assumption was that the medical profession could be relied upon to look after the former and the latter were well able to look after themselves.

Since that time such an assumption has increasingly been questioned in the UK. The requirement since 1967 that all clinical research conducted in institutions within the National Health Service should be referred by the investigator for vetting by an independent ethics committee,[6a] and the fact that such a practice is now also standard in respect of research conducted in private institutions and companies, has only partly alleviated public concern. In October 1989, the Department of Health in the UK began consultation on revised guidance to research ethics committees in the face of 'widespread uncertainty about requirements and a great variance in operational procedures'. Reports continue to appear of patients enrolled in clinical trials without being fully aware of this fact, and there is widespread criticism within and outside the medical profession of the increasing commercialisation of healthy volunteer studies. Emotive headlines such as 'Students are cancer drug guinea-pigs' and 'Tests go on at drug death clinic'[7] not only typify the approach of a media keen to sensationalise any issue concerning drugs, but also underline more general misgivings about the notion that self-regulation by the pharmaceutical industry and the professions offers adequate safeguards to volunteers in the absence of clear ethical or legal rules in conformity with which clinical research will be conducted.

To date, the pressure for change in the UK has been limited by the fact that, despite the ethical and legal confusion, very few people are injured in clinical research.[8] Care in selection of subjects and the high level of monitoring of subjects have led to a dearth of cases to test the legal waters. However, faced with a more litigious society, today even the medical profession is becoming increasingly troubled by the legal uncertainties that periodically envelop them and recognise that a more formal framework would provide benefits in terms of their own legal protection. However, all legislatures face a dilemma. They recognise the need for some statutory intervention to protect both the volunteer and the investigator, but the difficulty of developing rules that are practical to apply in a field as disparate as clinical research, but not so restrictive as to encourage over-defensive medicine, has so far been difficult to resolve. For the present, in the UK at least, fears about defensive medicine appear dominant and a Bill entitled 'Unethical Experiments' failed to get a second reading in Parliament when introduced in 1977.

But the position in the UK is not exceptional—the majority of member states of the Community have taken no initiative to control the performance of clinical research by statute. The German Drug Law of 1976[9] contains some provisions specific to this issue and the Republic of Ireland has embraced more detailed statutory control through the Control of Clinical Trials Act 1987,[10] but only after several requirements of the draft Bill were watered down in the face of major opposition from the medical profession and pharmaceutical industry. Moreover, although the focus for many legal initiatives relating to the marketing of pharmaceuticals has switched to Europe, attempts to fill the vacuum from that quarter have suffered from the inevitable problem of getting agreement on what is, or is not, ethically acceptable within a Community where medical and social traditions are markedly different. In France, for instance, a clause in the French Constitution which declares illegal the use of one's body for profit for a long time hindered the use of healthy volunteers in research. Despite a new law passed in December 1988,[11] directed at the protection of volunteers for biomedical research, there is still in France strong opposition to such studies in some parts of the medical profession.[12]

The most comprehensive initiative in this area has been the Report of July 1987 from the EEC/CPMP Working Party on Efficacy of Drugs, which drafted a 'Recommended Basis' for the 'Conduct of Clinical Trials of Medicinal Products' within the Community.[13] The CPMP guidelines—described by one member of the Working Party[14] as 'a modest start towards common regulation in this field'—are based upon international codes of practice and seek to provide a common basis for clinical evaluation of new chemical entities, in order to promote the development of safe products at lowest possible risks. The Guidelines cover all phases of clinical trials and make recommendations for everything, from the qualifications of investigators, design of protocols and ethics committee approval, to issues of consent and liability for injury to subjects. The European Parliament recently adopted a resolution on the harmonisation of medico-ethical questions in the EEC proposing a European Code of Ethics that will emphasise the rights of patients, and therefore the harmonisation of practice in relation to ethical issues is undoubtedly now part of the political agenda. The CPMP is preparing an extension of its 1987 guidelines through a recommendation on Good Clinical Practice for trials on medicinal products in the Community which seeks to harmonise this whole area of activity.[15] It is a formidable task.

LEGAL REGULATION UNDER GENERAL PRINCIPLES OF LAW

Codes of Practice ranging from international initiatives such as the Nuremberg Code and Declaration of Helsinki[16] to the many guidelines from national institutions, industrial associations and professional bodies provide rules which reflect (albeit inconsistently) the three fundamental ethical principles—namely the requirement of respect for persons, the requirement to minimise the risk of harm and the requirement to treat persons fairly. For persons seeking to establish that certain behaviour was, or was not, contrary to general principles of law, guidelines based on these principles may have evidential value through indicating prevailing standards of medical practice. In Germany and the Republic of Ireland the statutory provisions clearly draw heavily on such guidelines.

In the UK, as in many other countries, none of these principles are yet mirrored in comprehensive and clearly defined legal requirements relating to research. Nevertheless, principles of judgement made law—'common law'—

such as the duty to avoid causing injury through lack of care, have general application and in a wider sense regulate all the activities of those initiating or conducting clinical research, from the selection of volunteers and the organisation and execution of the study to the counselling of volunteers and their rights (if any) to compensation in the event of injury. Overall, however, English law has not noticeably impeded the carrying out of research, except perhaps in a few areas where the lack of clear judicial authority (e.g. in relation to the capacity of children or the mentally incapacitated to give consent) has had an inhibiting effect. Equally, little guidance can be found from the decisions of the courts of other countries, as few cases relating specifically to planned medical research have come to trial anywhere in the world. This absence of authority means that any description of the legal obligations of the parties to research must normally be extrapolated from general principles of law such as negligence and trespass to person. These principles are, broadly speaking, common to all parts of Europe, although their basis (common law or code) and their detailed application vary.

THE LEGAL OBLIGATIONS OF THE MANUFACTURER

In Relation to the Investigator

The legal relationship between the sponsoring company (invariably the manufacturer of the drug under study) and the investigator will be governed primarily by the terms of the contract they enter into. In most cases of research in healthy volunteers or patient volunteers it is desirable that there be a written contract between the sponsor and the investigator; this is the case whether the latter be an individual physician contracting to perform the research or a contract research establishment. The express terms of the contract may be supplemented by conditions implied by operation of law. Thus, under English law, in any contract for services there are implied terms relating to the exercise of reasonable care and skill and the need to complete the work in a reasonable time.[17] Furthermore, statutory provisions may limit the extent to which liability on the happening of certain events may be excluded by either party.[18]

Deciding what legal obligations are to be accepted by each party and thereafter translated into specific terms of the agreement are essentially commercial matters, and while some guidance[19] on issues to consider has been issued by the Association of the British Pharmaceutical Industry (ABPI), a standard form of agreement has not been developed for member companies. In practice, letters agreements are common. These usually define at the very least the protocol to be followed, the information to be made available in relation to the compound to be studied, the time limit for the study, the fee for carrying out the work, the reporting procedure for adverse events, confidentiality and publication of results, intellectual property rights and liability for injury to subjects. None of these matters give rise to particular difficulties, except perhaps the question of liability for injury to volunteers and indemnities, which are considered later in this chapter.

In Relation to the Research Subject

Under English law, the sponsor will typically not be in a contractual relationship with the research subject, although ethical guidelines relating to compensation for injury may require a contractually binding undertaking on this question to be given by the sponsor to a healthy volunteer. However, independent of contract, the sponsor has long been exposed to liability for negligence and more recently in strict liability. A similar legal remedy in negligence exists in each of the member states of the European Community, although the burden of proof in relation to establishing it varies and the strict liability provisions are not uniform throughout the Community.

Negligence

The sponsoring manufacturer under English law owes the research subject an obligation to exercise reasonable skill and care, and any careless act or omission that leads to injury may expose the sponsor to liability to pay compensation.[20] Such an act or omission could in theory arise in a number of ways touching upon the supply of the test compound.

He will be exposed if a defect (such as contamination) arises in the course of the process of manufacturing the drug. Such cases are very rare, as quality control standards are very high in the industry. More likely is the possibility of some harmful propensity of the drug, implicit in its design, going undetected prior to administration to humans. This will always be a major concern for a manufacturer, but the manufacturer's exposure to liability is, in fact, limited. His duty in this regard is to carry out reasonable preclinical research with a view to establishing that it is safe to proceed from administration to animals to administration to humans. When assessing later whether the manufacturer exercised the standard of care required, the courts will judge the likelihood of harm—and therefore his decision to proceed—by reference to the state of scientific knowledge at the time—the 'state of the art' as it is commonly known. The state of the art would essentially comprise prevailing knowledge of both animal and human toxicology as gleaned from both the international literature on the compound in question (or the class of compounds of which it is a member) and the preclinical research conducted by the manufacturer. Any preliminary clinical data already obtained by the company or an associated company may also be relevant.

A research subject who is injured and brings a claim for compensation will need to establish that the manufacturer had insufficient evidence to justify introducing the drug into humans or that he should have established the harmful propensity of the drug by virtue of the observations which were made—or should have been made—in the course of the preclinical work or from the published literature. Failure to follow authoritative guidelines relating to the testing results to be available before administration to humans may be used as evidence of negligence, although each case will turn on its particular facts. Such an inquiry is rarely simple, and the outcome in terms of liability may ultimately depend upon who carries the burden of proof. Under English law the burden is upon the injured research subject. The obligation to take proper steps to discover any harmful characteristic of the drug is an exacting one, but the manufacturer will not automatically be liable if he fails to isolate that harmful characteristic, provided that he exercised reasonable care. He is not liable for unforeseeable effects, as by definition no amount of care can guard against injuries arising from the unforeseeable.

More straightforwardly, the manufacturer may be vulnerable if he has failed to supply adequate information on the preclinical testing of the drug to the investigator so that the investigator can satisfy himself that it is safe to proceed and rule out subjects who may be particularly at risk from the drug in question. Dukes and Swartz[21] have emphasised the degree to which 'investigators' carrying out studies for the pharmaceutical industry are reliant upon the planning and expertise of the sponsor's own medical department. For this reason they prefer the use of the expression 'clinician in charge' as indicating their more limited role in practice. The manufacturer undoubtedly has a crucial obligation to apprise the investigator of the research that has been done with the drug under trial and explain the results (and also to provide information in relation to knowledge acquired later), but equally this does not remove entirely the responsibility of the investigator in law to make an independent judgement and indeed it is he who must be prepared to discuss fully the perceived risks and benefits (if any) with the ethics committee.

The manufacturer is not likely, as a matter of English law, to be found legally liable for injuries arising solely through the negligence of his investigator, where that person is not his employee. The manufacturer who delegates responsibility for carrying out the study to an outside investigator or contract research company must exercise reasonable care in the choice of his investigator. However, provided that he makes reasonable inquiries to establish the competence and experience of that person and the adequacy of the facilities for conducting the research, he should not be liable for his investigator's negligence in the performance of any procedure contemplated by the protocol.[22] Arguments to the contrary based upon the concept of non-delegable duties where hazardous operations are involved have been canvassed but find little support in English law.

Strict Liability

The legal exposure of the manufacturer might have been expected to change as a result of the imposition of strict liability upon 'producers' under domestic legislation implementing the EEC Directive of 1985 on Liability for Defective Products.[23] In fact, this is not the case, and indeed doubt has been expressed as to whether the supply of research products is covered by the new law at all.

In the UK the Directive is implemented by the Consumer Protection Act 1987,[24] and at the consultation stage the Department of Trade suggested that strict liability only applied to freely marketed products because research products were not 'put into circulation' in the normal sense of this phrase.[25] Early drafts of the Consumer Protection Bill actually provided a defence to producers if a product found to be defective was put into circulation solely for the purpose of a test to be conducted with or upon it. In the event, the matter was clearly reconsidered, as such an exemption did not appear in the Act itself.

Therefore, most commentators agree that the Directive is applicable to research products, but the application of the particular form of strict liability it introduces will probably have very limited impact for research. The new law impacts primarily on 'producers' and the manufacturer of a medicinal product is a 'producer' under the Act. However, a product is treated as defective only if its safety is not such as persons generally are entitled to expect, having regard to all the circumstances, including the manner in which, and the purposes for which, the product has been marketed and any instructions or warnings given in relation to it. It would appear to follow that the very status of research products would mean that any volunteer, aware that he was participating in research, would have difficulty in getting over the first hurdle, namely establishing that he was entitled to expect the product to be safe. In the case of processing defects such as contamination, this may not be a problem, but even if on the facts of a particular case a product's defective nature is established, the producer may still be able to avoid liability by proving that the development risk defence (otherwise known as 'the state of the art defence') applies. Under the Directive, member states are allowed to grant the producer this defence in their implementing legislation if they so wish, and where incorporated in the implementing legislation, it protects the producer if: 'the state of scientific and technical knowledge at the time when he put the product into circulation was not such as to enable the existence of the defect to be discovered'.[26]

So far most members of the Community have incorporated the defence, but interpretation of the defence has also been the subject of much controversy. Even while the Directive was under negotiation, somewhat different attitudes were adopted by member states. In the UK, after much discussion in Parliament, the Act was passed with the defence applying where: 'the state of scientific and technical knowledge at the relevant time [essentially the time of supply of the product to another] was not such that a producer of products of the same description as the product in question might be expected to have discovered the defect if it had existed in his products while they were under his control'.[27]

On the face of it, therefore, discoverability in its purest sense—without regard to the practicability of discovery—is not made the test but rather whether a producer could be expected by reference *inter alia* to prevailing industry standards, to have discovered the defect. This notion, while arguably more consistent with the Directive's practical objective of balancing the need for better consumer protection against the need not to stifle innovation, varies little from the traditional negligence standard and indirectly allows the question of the economic feasibility of discovering the defective nature of the product to be considered.

This is particularly relevant to clinical research, given that preclinical testing tends to focus upon a limited number of experiments, in a limited number of laboratory species, using a limited number of animals in the treatment and control groups. Primate testing, while technically feasible and often more likely to reveal potential hazards in man, is still not routinely performed and ethical pressures are increasingly operating somewhat differently in that area. If the harmful characteristics of a drug could have been established in one particular species used in animal experiments but not habitually used, any maufacturer faced with the allegation that a harmful characteristic of the drug would have been revealed by a sufficiently large study in that species would hardly be able to say that the defect was not discoverable in a technical sense.

This controversy is yet to be settled and will not be resolved finally until the issue is argued before the European Court. Attempts by consumer associations to make the European Commission bring proceedings under the Treaty of Rome, challenging HM Government's interpretation, finally bore fruit in December 1988, when the Commission announced that proceedings would be commenced against the UK and Italy for failing to implement the defence correctly. Pending the decision in those proceedings, it is reasonable to draw the conclusion that strict liability in the UK barely changes the legal obligations of the pharmaceutical manufacturer in relation to research, except that the manufacturer has the burden of establishing non-discoverability rather than the injured volunteer. In other member states denying the defence, or adopting the narrow interpretation of the defence, the change might turn out to be quite significant.

Criminal Liability

Setting aside criminal sanctions under any regulatory requirements providing for notification or approval of clinical research proposals, suppliers in the UK of certain products for clinical trials must, so it seems, also satisfy the 'general safety requirement' imposed on all goods intended for private use or consumption under Section 10 of the Consumer Protection Act 1987.[28] Licensed medicinal products are specifically excluded from the provisions of this part of the Act but not unlicensed medicinal products. To satisfy the law, the goods must be 'reasonably safe having regard to all the circumstances'. Under the legislation, an investigator may also be treated as a supplier when administering a drug to volunteers. However, it would seem that if the risk has been reduced to a minimum and all regulatory requirements have been met, compliance with the 'safety requirement' will also have been met. The European Commission has recently proposed a 'Product Safety Directive' aimed at prohibiting the supply of any product which presents an 'unacceptable risk', and harmonising safety controls. There is considerable opposition in some member states to this initiative which would give the Commission power to take steps against products thought to be hazardous.

THE LEGAL OBLIGATIONS OF THE INVESTIGATOR

In the absence of a contractual relationship between investigator and volunteer, which is only likely to arise under English law where a patient is treated privately or in the case of arrangements for healthy volunteer research, the investigator's obligations are primarily determined by the law of negligence—the duty to exercise reasonable care. The standard of care required of a physician is in this respect the same as would apply in relation to conventional treatment, although in practice the investigator arguably has a stricter responsibility to supervise the actions of other health professionals assisting him. In non-experimental contexts the duty has been well defined in a series of recent decisions,[29] and if the investigator acts in accordance with the professional norm and adopts the practice that a body of opinion skilled in his field would have adopted in similar circumstances, he is most unlikely to be found negligent. There is inevitably, therefore, a wide band between what is the prevailing consensus on any given issue and what is indefensible in law.

All research involves risks and the exercise of reasonable care in practice obliges the investigator to make a careful judgement that these are proportionate to the possible benefits. Where no benefit for the individual is envisaged because he is a healthy volunteer, the risks must be kept to the minimum independent of any issue of consent. The same principle applies where Phase I research is conducted in patient volunteers but the administration is not related to the condition being treated, except that the investigator must also be alert to the issue of drug interactions between the trial compound and the patient's own treatment drug. In the case of therapeutic research where the patient is being treated with a new drug because established treatments have failed to provide an acceptable level of efficacy or produced unacceptable side-effects for the patient, the prospect of benefit enables the investigator reasonably to advise the patient to embrace the somewhat greater risks. It is of interest that in the light of the more complicated balancing exercise to be conducted in research, German law requires[30] that a physician must have at least 2 years' experience in clinical research of drugs before he may conduct a study as principal investigator. The fact of approval by an ethics committee may assist the investigator if his conduct is challenged. The extent to which, in each case, the investigator must advise the volunteer of the nature and seriousness of those risks that cannot be excluded raises the wider issues of consent described in detail below.

Depending upon the manner and circumstances of recruitment of healthy volunteers, including, perhaps, whether payment is made in return for participation, a contractual relationship may arise between the investigator and the volunteer. Today it is common to see consent forms extended into documents that in truth amount to written contracts under which each party expressly accepts certain obligations. Obligations concerning confidentiality, compensation, etc., may be accepted by the investigator and obligations to disclose details of existing or recent medication and report promptly any deterioration of health during participation may be accepted by the volunteer. Breach of such obligations by one party may in theory give rise to a claim for damages by the other party, although in practice breach of the volunteer's obligations is at most likely to prejudice his right to full payment or, on grounds of contributory fault, his position under compensation arrangements. Independent of these express terms, where an investigator contracts with a volunteer, English law will also imply a warranty on the part of the investigator that reasonable care and skill will be exercised in relation to the study. This obligation is broadly comparable with that which arises under the law of negligence, independent of a contract.

The introduction of strict liability for product defects should not have major repercussions for the investigator, for, as explained above, strict liability will impact primarily on the manufacturer. However, if investigators prepare their own research products, they will be strictly liable for defects in them on the same basis as manufacturers. Furthermore, the liability of a producer is imposed upon any person supplying a defective product, if he is unable within a reasonable time to inform the injured person of the identity of the actual producer/importer into the Community or, at the very least, the person who supplied him with the product.[31] Given the discrete nature of clinical research, investigators should not be troubled by issues of identification and their liability will continue to rest firmly in negligence.

In practice, this means that the investigator will only be vulnerable to claims for compensation if he has negligently failed to consider carefully the preclinical and other information supplied by the sponsor and therefore has allowed an unsafe proposal to go forward or if he has not passed material information to the volunteer, or if he has failed to screen out volunteers unsuitable for participation in the light of the advised contraindications of the drug, or has failed to perform ancillary procedures carefully or supervise the study and response of subjects adequately. In this regard, it must be noted that if a patient is improperly removed from treatment that is required, the injury may arise out of the absence of the existing treatment following randomisation to placebo or an ineffective new drug under trial. Patient selection and monitoring is, therefore, vital.

Consent

The legal effect of consent under English law is embodied in the maxim *volenti non fit injuria*, meaning 'to one who is willing no harm is done'. In law this has been reframed as the proposition that one who expressly, or by implication, consents to the commission of a wrong against him (or an act that would have been wrongful apart from the consent) cannot thereafter claim damages for any harm suffered. However, the nature of the defence has been confused by the fact that it may arise in two distinct circumstances. The first of these is where the patient consents to an invasion of this physical integrity that would otherwise be actionable as a trespass to person. The second is where, having consented to that medical intervention, he also agrees to assume the risk of a specific injury to which he is exposed by the study in circumstances where, if inadequate information about that risk had been provided, the investigator would have been exposed to a claim in negligence for failure to take proper care in counselling the volunteer.

Consent and Trespass to Person

Through the concept of trespass to person, the English common law reflects the fundamental ethical principle that we should respect each other's physical integrity. An act which intentionally leads to some physical contact amounts, in the absence of consent, to a battery.[32] However, the law does allow a person to consent to the use of a reasonable degree of force on his person and so no wrong is committed where consent is freely given. Therefore, it has long been understood that if a doctor touches or examines a person in his care or adopts any invasive procedure, provided that he has obtained consent the patient cannot thereafter claim compensation for any resulting injury on the grounds of trespass to person. The exceptions to obtaining consent, such as acting out of 'necessity' to preserve life, are most unlikely to arise in clinical research.

Consent may be expressed or inferred from conduct. Accordingly, a volunteer offering himself for participation in a research study and proffering his arm for an injection required by the protocol to the study will almost certainly be found to have consented to the physical contact involved. To operate as a defence, the consent must be real in the sense that the volunteer must be informed in broad terms of the nature and general purpose of the study and the consent must not be procured by fraud or misrepresentation.[33] In 1970 the ABPI noted in its *Guidelines* relating to research in healthy volunteers[34] that a volunteer suffering an ill-effect, which he believed should have been made the subject of a warning, might be expected to put forward a claim at law based on the combined allegation of trespass to person and negligence. One advantage of a claim in trespass is that damage need not be proved to have resulted from the wrongful act. In contrast, liability in negligence depends upon the claimant showing not only a breach of the duty of care, but also that the injury complained of is causally related to the breach of duty.

However, it is doubtful whether claims based on trespass will now feature greatly in the context of research. First, the Court of Appeal in England recently suggested[35] that to succeed in trespass the plaintiff must prove that the physical contact not only was deliberate, but also was made with an element of hostility. On this basis, actions for battery against physicians would normally be completely untenable, but the meaning of 'hostility' is somewhat unclear in this context and subsequent decisions have followed the traditional distinction, which recognises deemed consent only in respect of physical contact falling within the reasonable and generally acceptable band of conduct which may occur in the ordinary course of daily life but requires express consent for contact falling outside the ordinary course. For the present, therefore, it would perhaps be unwise to treat trespass to person as a dead letter in the field of clinical research on this basis alone. Indeed, in a recent case the need for any element of malice or hostility was suggested to be wrong in law.[36]

However, the English courts have also made it tolerably clear that failure to disclose the risks of the procedure does not vitiate consent that is real in all other respects.[37] Such failure will not, therefore, expose the investigator to an action in damages for trespass to person, although it may provide grounds for an action in negligence based on failure to disclose material information. This is a more significant reason why a claim in trespass is now unlikely in practice unless it can be argued that any sort of consent was lacking.

Consent in Children and the Mentally Handicapped

Having regard to the matters to be explained to volunteers, there arises the issue of competence to understand that explanation. The law in relation to consent competency—the legal capacity to give consent—is very unclear, as regards both children and those suffering from mental disability. The Nuremberg Code does not expressly cover either group, but the Declaration of Helsinki states in relation to non-therapeutic research that, where the subject is 'legally incompetent', the consent 'of the legal guardian' should be procured.[38] As the ethical and legal legitimacy of research which offers no direct benefit to the individual is based firmly on obtaining valid consent, the implication is obvious—essential research is less likely to be performed, to the longer-term disadvantage of these classes of person. Indeed, the phrase 'therapeutic orphans' has been coined in relation to children. The key to this issue is, therefore, ultimately the validity of proxy consent.

In relation to children, following a recent decision of the highest appeal court in England, the position appears to be that in relation to clinical research as part of treatment, a child over 16 may validly consent to treatment without regard to the wishes of his parents. Below that age, a minor's capacity to consent depends upon his having sufficient understanding to make a reasonably informed decision and is not to be determined by reference to any judicially fixed age limit.[39] Where he does not have such understanding, the parents have a legal right to give consent on his behalf. Nevertheless, most ethical guidelines advise that even if an investigator believes that a child is capable of giving valid consent, the approval of a parent or guardian should still be obtained.

There is no direct authority on the issue of consent in relation to non-therapeutic research, but the general principle that one should focus upon the particular child's capacity to make a rational decision would seem to apply. In the case of children unable to give a valid consent themselves, the more difficult question arises as to whether a parent can properly consent in law to a child being subjected to a procedure which carries no prospect of direct personal benefit but only risk. There is no authority on this point. Some commentators have argued that the duty of a parent to act in the best interests of a child can equally be termed an obligation not to do anything clearly against the interests of the child.[40] As Dworkin[41] has argued, this would allow consideration of wider issues than direct medical benefit, including social responsibility, and on this basis, provided that approval of an ethics committee has been obtained for a study (which will only be forthcoming if it involves minimal risk and considerable benefit to children as a group), it is unlikely that English courts would declare ineffective a fully informed parental consent. This would appear to be ethically sound, but in practical terms the uncertainty that hinders research will only be resolved by a clear decision of the courts. In this regard, the reluctance of physicians to adopt the above approach has undoubtedly been fuelled in the past by the statements from the Medical Research Council to the effect that a strict view of the law would prohibit proxy consents by parents in respect of non-therapeutic research.[42] This view was later underwritten by a Department of Health circular,[43] despite the fact that no authorities could be cited to support the MRC's statement, and it appeared to be based on one legal opinion only. The question may, in any event, be somewhat academic where drugs are involved, as most bodies—including recently the Medicines Commission in the UK[44]— have recommended that no approach should be made to recruit children as healthy volunteers in studies of medicinal products. The Department of Health's draft guidance of October 1989 still adopts a cautious approach, saying that parents responsible for allowing a child to be subjected to any risk (unless *de minimis*), without the prospect of benefit for that child, could be said to be acting illegally.[6b]

The position in relation to clinical research into mental illness, using the mentally handicapped as subjects, is equally unclear. The traditional legal analysis was that the law protects the physical integrity of all persons, and therefore any intervention may only take place when, in a lucid moment, the mentally handicapped subject can give consent. On this basis, in relation to an adult not subject to any lucid moment, it was said that the proxy consent of a relative would not suffice and the physician could not proceed.[45] Indeed, even where the subject is a child, doubt over the legal position of those concerned with care in a recent case was sufficient to prompt an application to make a child a ward of court so that the court could be asked to approve sterilisation, applying the traditional test of what was in the best interests of the child.[46]

Likewise, in a recent case involving a mentally handicapped adult, where wardship is not an option, the physicians involved in the patient's care refused to terminate pregnancy and sterilise the patient without the protection of the court. The mother therefore applied for a declaration that the intervention envisaged did not constitute trespass to the person. The declaration was granted on the basis that the only consideration was what was in the best interests of the patient and consistent with good medical practice. That decision has been upheld by the highest appeal court which found that a doctor could lawfully treat an adult incapable of consenting provided it was in the patient's best interests. However, although not strictly necessary, it was suggested good practice in the case of sterilisation to involve the courts.[47]

Such an approach might be invoked in relation to clinical research, for the recent case law is support for the principle that if the treating physician believes that there is the prospect of benefit if the patient participates in a trial of a new treatment for his mental illness, and in this sense it is good medical practice to enrol him in the study, an extended principle of necessity will protect the investigator from legal sanction. In all cases, however, it would still obviously be important on ethical grounds to obtain the approval of the responsible relative and ethics committee approval before proceeding.

However, these cases do not suggest that the doctor can dispense with consent in the case of non-therapeutic research. Indeed, the decisions of the appeal courts suggest the contrary, but in any event there is a general consensus that testing of medicinal products can never be justified in mentally handicapped subjects who could not expect personal benefit. The UK Department of Health's draft guidance of October 1989 appears to exclude research on mentally disordered people unless their mental state still allows 'freely given' consent.[6b]

The recent legislation in the Republic of Ireland has seemingly ruled out proxy consents except in relation to the participation of patients in research for their direct therapeutic benefit.[48] Likewise, in the UK the Medicines Commission has advised that the recruitment of healthy volunteers unable personally to give a valid consent should not take place in relation to studies involving medicinal products.[49]

Consent and Negligence

One element of the general duty of care owed by the investigator to the patient or healthy volunteer is the duty to disclose and counsel the volunteer in relation to any material risks to his health and well-being that might result from participation in the study. The duty flows from the ethical requirement that one should respect the autonomy of others, i.e. the right of self-determination. The investigator must in law provide sufficient information to give meaning to that right.[50] In English law, where a person volunteering for research is warned of the nature and extent of a specific risk—and freely and voluntarily agrees to run that risk knowing that if he is injured because the risk materialises, he will have no legal right of redress—he has assumed the risk himself and his consent to do so acts as a defence to any claim in negligence based upon the existence of the risk.

However, the assumption of a specific risk prior to participating does not imply acceptance of the consequences of any unrelated failure by the investigator to take reasonable care in supervising the research or in treating him should he suffer an adverse reaction. Furthermore, any attempt by the investigator, in a consent form or otherwise, to exclude or restrict his liability generally for death or bodily injury resulting from the investigator's negligence will in English law be void.[51]

The Doctrine of Informed Consent

From these principles, it is often suggested that for the investigator to avoid an action in negligence all the possible risks must have been fully explained and understood, i.e. fully 'informed consent' must be obtained. However, a series of recent cases show that this proposition is not correct as a matter of English law. All of these cases dealt with consent in the context of treatment but in the absence of any cases concerned with research they are a proper starting point. Indeed, there is little reason to argue that the principles ought to be different purely because in research personal benefit is more speculative (or indeed entirely lacking). However, this is a much discussed area of law where from the outset policy decisions appear to have distorted the logical progression from ethical principle to legal decision.

In England, as the author of the previous chapter has remarked, the traditional view in relation to medical treatment has been that the issue of information on risks is a matter of clinical judgement and not of legal doctrine. Early cases suggested that the physician must decide what risks were material and should be communicated to the patient. At its most extreme this approach was used to justify misrepresenting the facts to the patient.[52] In contrast, in many jurisdictions in the USA there has been a trend towards a general rule of law—based in part on the proposition that a fiduciary relationship exists between physician and patient—requiring full disclosure, so that all risks must be disclosed which *the patient* might consider material to the decision as to whether to accept treatment or not.[53] The physician is invited to presume that he is dealing with a rational person and disclose all relevant risks, even if he believes that the risks are remote. In this regard, the right to know is treated as taking precedence over the need to know. The notable exception to this rule is where the physician has good reason to believe that proper disclosure will be detrimental to the physical or mental well-being of the patient, in which case it is the 'therapeutic privilege' of the physician to limit his counselling accordingly. The rule has come to be called the 'doctrine of informed consent'.

In recent cases in England[54] patients injured during conventional therapy have invited the courts to adopt the North American approach but the courts have declined to do so. It has been unequivocally stated that there is no difference between the standard of care required in giving advice on risks and that required in diagnosis and treatment. The primary obligation to disclose risks with a view to allowing the patient to make a rational choice has been re-emphasised, but the obligation has been limited to making such disclosure as is reasonable in the light of all the circumstances, so that the physician will normally have discharged his duty if he acts in accordance with practice accepted as proper by a body of physicians skilled in the relevant field. In cases where the question is whether the reasonable physician should have disclosed a particular risk, the courts will hear expert evidence before determining whether it should have been disclosed. This falls some way short of the North American approach, although the courts have warned the medical profession to be on its guard against being overpaternalistic and 'playing at God', specifically declaring that the court has an inherent right to intervene and declare that a risk must be disclosed, even if evidence of medical practice to the contrary is shown to exist. As an illustration of this it has been suggested that no court would sanction the failure of a physician to disclose a 10% chance of serious harm.[55]

Thus, both in North America and in England, while the legal criterion for disclosure is the materiality of the risk, the determination in law of what risks are material, and should therefore be disclosed, varies. Whereas in some jurisdictions of North America a risk is treated as material where a reasonable person in the patient's position would be likely to attach significance to it when deciding whether or not to accept the medical intervention, the English courts have only wavered slightly from a standard under which materiality is judged by reference to the professional norm in any given case.

Disclosure of Risks and Research

In the USA the central features of the 'doctrine of informed consent' have been reproduced in FDA requirements for all clinical research.[56] Investigators must state the immediate purpose of the research and the significance of the data to be generated, and must explain the procedures envisaged, how often they will be carried out and the overall length of time each will take. In addition, a full description of any 'reasonably forseeable risks or discomfort' to the subject is required and the subject must also be told specifically of the possibility of 'unforseeable risks'. Such a standard of disclosure, requiring notification of what is 'reasonably forseeable', is perhaps more onerous than the Nuremburg standard of disclosing what is 'reasonably to be expected' or the Declaration of Helsinki requirement that subjects should be 'adequately informed'. Certainly, what is in theory foreseeable might still not be expected. Indeed, some researchers have drawn attention to the potential risk of overdisclosure and confusion as the essential features of the study's safety profile become blurred by a sea of detail and ill-defined possibilities.

The present approach of English law to disclosure of risks has been widely criticised as being out of line with the aspirations of modern society, which is more informed and questioning on matters relating to health. Inevitably, it has been suggested that a different test for judging materiality might apply outside the field of conventional treatment. However, it is difficult to see that this would be consistent with the overall approach of the English courts and above all the apparent concern of the judges to avoid defensive medicine—a concern that is all too obvious in their decisions. There is no logical basis for adopting an entirely different approach to patients simply because one form of treatment happens to take place in an experimental context, although one would expect the application of a 'reasonable physician' test to materiality to focus more closely on the possible risks and particularly the risk of the unknown. For the time being, there is certainly no case law relating to the therapeutic research that would support the approach of the Canadian courts that 'there can be no exceptions to the ordinary requirements of disclosure in the case of research as there may well be in ordinary medical practice'.[57]

Although it is tempting to try to place research using healthy volunteers in an entirely different category, logically there is, again, no compelling reason why a different test should be applied. However, in non-therapeutic research, whichever standard is applied to judge materiality, the outcome should be the same. When dealing with healthy volunteers, there is no question of disclosure not being in the best interests of the subject on the grounds that it might dissuade him from accepting appropriate treatment. Accordingly, the reasonable physician will surely decide what is material by reference to what the 'reasonable person' in the position of the healthy volunteer would want to know and, moreover, would attempt to learn whether the subject might indeed wish to know more. It is unlikely that the courts, no longer affected by the dangers of promoting defensive medicine, would find that any reasonable physician could properly adopt a practice that did not involve warning of all foreseeable risks, including a suspicion of risk where the outcome would be serious if the risk materialised. In short, because the volunteer is not being treated for illness, any foreseeable risk must be material when it is set against the absence of any prospect of compensating personal benefit.

This is not to say that the physician must teach volunteers the essence of clinical pharmacology, but he must ensure that the volunteer knows enough to make a rational decision. Even with healthy volunteers, irrelevant information which may distort the picture may justifiably be ignored. Equally, any request by the subject to limit the amount of information he is given must be taken into account, because real respect for autonomy dictates that it should—although failure to request information that the reasonable person would seek should raise a question mark in the investigator's mind as to the suitability of the volunteer for participation in the study. It is, therefore, difficult to justify anything less than comprehensive disclosure with healthy volunteers, and whether the courts choose to explain the result as arising from the application of a 'reasonable physician' or 'reasonable healthy volunteer' standard of materiality is of little practical significance.

Some indication that a consistent approach will be adopted by the English courts arises from two recent cases, the first[58] where the duty to inform was considered in the context of advice about the risks of failure associated with female sterilisation. The judge at first instance suggested that a distinction could be made between advice in the therapeutic and 'non-therapeutic' context, by which he meant where the 'patient' was psychologically and medically normal, so that in the context of female sterilisation the duty of disclosure need not be determined exclusively by reference to the practice of competent professionals. The Appeal Court overruled the decision. Likewise, in a case concerning a warning of the risks of the long-term contraceptive Depo-Provera to a perfectly healthy patient, a similar professional standard was applied to disclosure.[59]

This is not to say that the approach of English law is to be preferred. Indeed, there is evidence that the medical profession itself has taken the warnings about paternalism to heart and in guidelines developed for ethics committees or professional codes of practice is developing an approach more consistent with the North American doctrine than that espoused by the English courts. The CPMP guidelines of 1987[60] recommend informing patients and healthy volunteers 'verbally, and if possible also in writing' about 'the possible risks and discomforts involved'. Significantly, the first direct legislative intervention in the Community—the Control of Clinical Trials Act in the Republic of Ireland—has enshrined an approach to clinical research of all types that would appear to involve full disclosure. The 'person conducting the clinical trial' is obliged by Section 9 to ensure that the subject is made aware of, *inter alia*, 'the risks and any discomfort involved in, and the possible side-effects of, the trial'. It may be argued that this leaves open the definition of 'risks' but, on the face of it, the intention appears to be that the obligation is unqualified. The Irish Department of Health guidelines on the Act go further and recommend that the consent form itself include 'details of any forseeable risks which may arise'. Furthermore, under the Irish legislation, after the explanation of the objectives, risks and other features of the trial, the subject must be allowed a period of 6 days within which to consider whether to participate, and except with the agreement of the Minister of Health the trial cannot begin in the interim.

Whatever the present state of English law—and it suggested that the approach adopted is only likely to be altered by legislation—if clinical research and, in particular, research in healthy volunteers is to be accepted by society as a whole, those supervising it must be seen to have made careful disclosure of all relevant information. This is one area where the ethical and legal requirements should certainly coincide. Properly informed consent has been described as 'an obstacle to research',[61] but the trend of professional ethical guidelines is towards more comprehensive counselling on risks and alternative treatments, and it will become less easy for physicians seeking to justify non-disclosure to find expert evidence to support their case.

Randomisation and Placebo Controls

Studies that are methodologically unsound are incapable of providing valid data and thereby lose their ethical underpinning. The randomised controlled clinical trial conducted under 'blind conditions' has been developed as the optimal design for experimental purposes. However, the physician responsible for the patients, though partly in search of new knowledge, must also not lose sight of the fact that he has an overriding duty in law to act reasonably and in the best interests of the patient. On this basis, it is difficult to see how he can advise a patient to enter a study unless it appears to him that the patient's health will not be prejudiced by his being part of either the case or control group. After taking account of the risks attending the treatment, and the benefits of the current treatment options, participation of his patients must hold out the chance of 'saving lives, re-establishing health or alleviating suffering', to use the Helsinki phraseology.

Where the design of the trial involves two therapeutic groups, problems in practice are seldom of great medico-legal significance, although the fact of randomisation is so fundamental to the trial method that ethically and legally it should, except where 'therapeutic privilege' is involved, be disclosed to the patient as part of the consent procedure. It has been persuasively argued, and would seem correct, that since the patient's assumption is that the physician will choose what he considers is the best treatment for the patient, any failure to explain the facts of randomisation may involve the physician in 'straying outside the terms of his patient's consent'. The fact that many patients are not aware that they have been enrolled in a trial has given rise to considerable adverse publicity in the UK, to the detriment of the research community.[62]

Where the control group is intended to receive a placebo, the medico-legal difficulties may be greater. It has been suggested by some that placebo controls are always unethical.[63] However, placebo groups are often considered essential, especially where the end-point of treatment is difficult to assess and observer bias is a potential problem. Feinstein sums it up as follows: 'If the question is worth asking, if its answer requires the use of placebo, and if the answer is worth getting, then the plan to use a placebo is justified.'[64] He argues strongly that the ethical question boils down to one of consent. Patients must be informed of the plan and they are then free to refuse to participate. Certainly, the more commonly held view is that placebo controls are acceptable ethically and legally, notably where there is no alternative to the treatment under trial (or serious doubt as to efficacy of that treatment) or when the effect of adding a new treatment to an established one is under study. Such a position is adopted by the Medical Research Council in the UK. As a matter of English law, it is suggested that provided that a patient is made fully aware of the possibility and risks to health of being randomised to placebo, and the risks are minimal, it is doubtful that the courts would rule that the patient's consent was invalid or that the investigator was negligent.

The view that the problem is essentially one of consent is supported by the new Irish legislation, which requires that any subject asked for consent must be made aware, where appropriate, of the possibility of receiving a placebo.[65] The CPMP guidelines[66] make a similar recommendation. There has always been a degree of discomfort about placebo trials, but, as Gilbert has pointed out,[67] an absolute requirement for fully informed consent in all randomised controlled clinical trials may have a significant effect on trials comparing transparently different types of treatment (e.g. surgery versus drug therapy) where patients are likely to have marked personal preferences, but will have a limited effect on the viability of drug trials which compare active treatment with placebo or new drugs with standard drugs.

Consent Forms

Under German law the consent of a patient volunteering to participate in trials of unlicensed drugs must be in writing or, if made orally, must be independently witnessed.[68] The requirement for written consent (with certain exceptions) also applies in the Republic of Ireland. However, few other states have laws directly regulating consent. All that is required under English law for consent to be effective is an actual statement from which it is reasonable to deduce that a volunteer has freely given his consent. An effective consent may be given orally, although as a matter of evidence it is desirable for it to be witnessed by someone other than the investigator himself. The UK Department of Health has proposed witnessed consent and suggests that such consent need only be recorded in the patient's case notes.[6b]

However, it is the case that most ethical guidelines advise that the consent and the nature of the information disclosed as the basis for that consent should be recorded in writing. The CPMP guidelines adopt this approach. Where consent forms are employed, and Dukes and Swartz have suggested that this is less frequent in countries where there is 'no tradition of patient litigation', it is sometimes recommended, particularly in relation to healthy volunteers, that the investigator confirm in writing on the same form that he has advised the volunteer of the relevant features of the study. Increasingly, investigators cross-reference this statement to a volunteer information sheet, which contains written confirmation of the nature, purpose and risks of the research.

However, a signed consent form is not decisive evidence that the consent was validly obtained or that proper care was exercised in counselling the subject. Consent issues essentially focus upon the volunteer's state of mind in deciding whether to participate and the true nature of the counselling received, rather than upon a signature on a document. Indeed, it is right that a volunteer should be able to withdraw consent at any time; no volunteer should feel contractually bound by having signed a consent form. This right is, in fact, enshrined in the new Irish legislation. There is, however, a presumption under English law that the document has been read before signature and, at the very least, the preparation of consent forms directs the minds of those performing the research to the various ethical considerations, and provides a record that an attempt has been made to address them.

THE LIABILITY OF OTHER PARTIES TO RESEARCH

There are, of course, other parties to most research whose lack of care can cause injury. The hospital or other establishment in which the research takes place has a legal obligation to ensure, as with conventional therapy, that their facilities and the medical products and equipment made available for research are in proper order and are sterile and safe for normal use. However, the potential liability of hospitals and health authorities does not raise issues specific to clinical research. Equally, it must also be remembered that the volunteer, too, has certain obligations, breach of which in law may have implications—principally by reducing or extinguishing the volunteer's ability to claim compensation for any injury suffered by virtue of his own contributory negligence. The position of ethics committee and regulatory authorities requires special mention.

Ethics Committees

In 1964 the Declaration of Helsinki clearly established the need for all research protocols to be considered by an independent committee for guidance and, implicitly, approval. Ethics committee approval has now, in practice, become a necessary step in the performance of most research in Europe, although submission to ethics committees is not legally required in most member states of the Community. Furthermore, in the absence of statutory intervention, progress in formalising the status of ethics committees has been slow.

In the UK the Royal College of Physicians recommended in 1967 that all research projects performed in medical institutions should be approved by an independent group of doctors, and in 1973 the College made further recommendations concerning the composition and functions of such committees. In a circular in 1975[69] the Department of Health endorsed the College's proposals and required that they be implemented by health authorities. However, it was not until 1984 that the College issued detailed guidelines on the constitution and functions of ethics committees, but the practices of ethics committees remain far from uniform.[70]

The sole reference to ethics committees in the Medicines Act legislation appears in an Order relating to notification of clinical trial proposals.[71] This Order requires any refusal by an ethics committee to sanction a trial to be reported by the sponsor to the Licensing Authority. More recently, the Medicines Commission was called upon to advise the Minister of Health on whether healthy volunteer studies should be brought under statutory control. While reporting that there is 'inadequate reason on the basis of presently available information to recommend this course of action', the Commission made various proposals[72] for a better system of self-regulation and notably recommended that 'the role and constitution of ethics committees should be codified and elaborated by those concerned' and that the Department of Health should communicate guidance after consultation with interested bodies. In October 1989 the Department of Health began consultation on guidelines which will supersede the 1975 circular.[6b] It relates to all research concerning patients or healthy volunteers or fertilization *in vitro* or fetal material and provides detailed guidance on the constitution of ethics committees and their functions and procedures. In some respects the guidance conflicts with that provided by the Royal College of Physicians, whose own ethics committee's guidelines are under revision at the same time as the College prepares new detailed guidelines for research in patients. Clear and consistent guidance still seems some way off.

In contrast, in the USA Food and Drug Administration regulations[73] define the constitution and purpose of 'Institutional Review Boards' to which all clinical investigations requiring the consent of the FDA must be submitted for approval, and in the Republic of Ireland the Control of Clinical Trials Act now requires all clinical research to be submitted to an Ethics Committee, whose constitution is subject to review by the Minister of Health. The approval of a study by the Committee must be reported to the Minister, and the Act also lays down the ethical issues to be considered by the Committee.[74] New legislation in France[75] will in due course require research to be submitted to ethics committees.

In the UK, even without the existence of legislation to focus attention upon their role, ethics committees, and particularly the lay members, have become more concerned about their own legal position in the face of an increasingly litigious environment. As a matter of English law, 10 years ago few would have doubted that a body which, *inter alia*, held itself out as there to protect the interests and health of research volunteers did not owe a duty of care in law to those volunteers, breach of which could make the members vulnerable to claims for compensation on the grounds of negligence. The trend in English law has in recent years[76] been away from making bodies carrying out public functions liable in negligence, but on balance it is suggested that an ethics committee does owe volunteers a duty of care as a matter of private law. The claim would have to be made against the individual members for failure to exercise reasonable care in approving the trial, as committees are informal bodies and have no legal personality in their own right. This theoretical risk has certainly led some ethics committees to seek and obtain full indemnities from the authority appointing them in respect of any claim that might be advanced by an injured volunteer.

Regulatory Authorities

Where a government regulatory authority reviews a proposal for research and consents to its performance, it may be exposed to claims if its review can be said to have been performed negligently. Under English law, although there is no direct authority on this matter, the Licensing Authority and the Committee on Safety of Medicines have been sued in relation to the approval of drugs for marketing,[77] and the principle ought to be the same. However, as mentioned above in relation to the status of ethics committees, recent decisions of the appeal courts in other areas of activity have raised question marks as to whether a public body, such as the Licensing Authority or its expert advisory committees, owe private law obligations to individuals who might be affected by their actions. The issue remains uncertain, but even if a right of action does exist, the likelihood of such an action succeeding is comparatively small. The Licensing Authority would no doubt argue that in acting on the advice of its expert committee it was acting reasonably. In turn, the expert committee might reasonably be expected to defend a claim on the basis that the decision of a distinguished body of medical experts by definition could not be challenged as inconsistent with the opinion or practice of a reasonable body of professional opinion. As regards clinical trial exemptions, it would be particularly difficult to show negligence, as neither the Licensing Authority nor its expert committees are in a position to consider the preclinical data fully and the system of negative clearance rests on the certification of the company's medical advisor or of the consultant engaged by the company.

COMPENSATION FOR INJURY

In Germany legislation relating to clinical trials provides for compulsory insurance, which must respond in relation to injury caused by participation.[78] In Sweden injury arising in clinical trials should be compensated under the pharmaceutical insurance-based scheme (although there has not been a case so far). Equally, in the Republic of Ireland by law the person conducting the research must satisfy the ethics committee that adequate funds are available to provide compensation for any injury resulting from the trial, independent of negligence.[79] But in the UK and indeed most member states, where a patient volunteer is injured in the course of research, his right in law to compensation will be determined solely by application of the principles of negligence and strict liability described above. It follows from what has been said about the nature of these remedies that the fact of even a serious injury occurring in research does not automatically imply a right to compensation.

As a matter of English law the volunteer will be hard pressed to establish a right to compensation in negligence provided that the investigator ensured that the volunteer consented to participate in the study, and in all other respects both the manufacturer of the drug and the investigator exercised reasonable care in the planning and performance of the study. The nature of research is that injury can arise however much care is taken by the participants and in all cases negligence will not be easy to prove for a private individual operating outside his field of knowledge with the burden of proof lying firmly with him. In terms of strict liability, whatever interpretation of the 'state of the art defence' is adopted, certain 'development risks' will remain with the volunteer.

There has been considerable criticism in the UK of the fact that such risks should be left with individuals seemingly less able to bear the burden of the unexpected than the manufacturer or the institution under whose auspices the research is conducted. Once a product has completed its main research phase and is freely marketed, the arguments for leaving some risk with the consumer are more finely balanced, but a fundamental ethical principle of research is the requirement for fairness and this translates into the need to ensure that the burden and benefits of research are properly shared. The argument to compensate those injured in research through no fault of their own is therefore formidable, although interestingly the Declaration of Helsinki does not raise the issue. In the UK both the Medical Research Council and the Department of Health have represented[80] that they would consider making ex gratia payments in appropriate cases. However, the Royal Commission on compensation for personal injury (Pearson) commented:[81] 'We think that it is wrong that a person who exposes himself to some medical risk in the interests of the community, should have to rely on ex gratia compensation in the event of injury. We recommend that any volunteer for medical research . . . who suffers severe damage as a result should have a cause of action on the basis of strict liability, against the authority to whom he has consented to make himself available.' Even with the increasing tendency of some healthy volunteers to treat participation in research as merely another form of 'work', where it is questionable whether the desire to serve society is uppermost in their minds, the greater commercialisation of such research arguably makes the case for compensation even stronger.

However, not all groups that have looked at this question felt able to support the idea of a strict liability remedy in law—a remedy that the Pearson Commission appeared to believe should be against the investigator's employer or perhaps the sponsor of the research. A group convened by the Ciba Foundation came out against the concept of claimants still having to seek redress through the courts against a named defendant, at least in relation to injuries other than those arising from processing or labelling defects.[82] In their view the objective of providing volunteers 'with the sure knowledge that they would receive a quick and just response to their quest for compensation' required the introduction of a 'no fault compensation scheme' operating outside the system and financed jointly by those promoting and involved in research on an insurance-orientated basis.

Contrary to the intentions of the Pearson Commission, strict liability as established by the EEC Directive does not provide volunteers with a much improved prospect of compensation, especially in those jurisdictions such as the UK, where a 'development risk defence' has been made available to the producer. However, the ethical imperative has long been recognised by the Association of the British Pharmaceutical Industry, first in 1970 in relation to healthy volunteers from its own staff[83] and later all healthy volunteers[84] and clinical trial patients.[85] Through separate contractual or quasi-contractual arrangements with volunteers the right to compensation is based solely on proof of a causal connection between the administration of the drug and the injury complained of. A study-based approach of this type avoids some of the significant problems of funding and administering a national 'no-fault scheme' of the type envisaged by the Ciba Working Group.

In the case of healthy volunteers the present ABPI guidelines to member companies recommend that a specific contractually binding undertaking is given to volunteers to compensate them (or their dependants) in the event of 'any significant deterioration in health or well-being' caused by 'participation' in the study, with compensation calculated by reference to the level of damages that would be awarded by the English courts for similar injuries had legal liability in negligence been established. The undertaking goes on to provide that any dispute as to the application of the compensation provisions is to be referred to an arbitrator. The guidelines provide that this undertaking should not seek to exclude compensation where there is an issue as to whether the negligence of the investigator may have caused the injury. The overriding consideration is to provide for the volunteer and it is suggested that the sponsoring company merely preserves its rights of recourse against third parties so that indemnity in respect of, or contribution towards, compensation paid to a volunteer can be recovered from third parties where they have been negligent. In England such a right of recourse will normally arise by operation of law but separate indemnities can be sought as appropriate and are freely given by the major commercial contract research companies. Most important-ly, the guidelines do not preclude a volunteer from pursuing a claim in negligence or strict liability if he so desires. The Medicines Commission has recommended[86] not only that companies should give an undertaking to provide compensation, but also that they should 'provide evidence of their ability to fulfil it'. The Department of Health has recently endorsed that suggestion.[6b]

In the case of patient volunteers, somewhat different arrangements apply to research sponsored by members of the ABPI. Some patients entering clinical trials suffer from minor disorders but others from life-threatening diseases where discussion of compensation arrangements in the event of injury may well cause unnecessary alarm and not be in their best interests. For these reasons many doctors are reluctant to expose their patients to elaborate consent forms or the separate paperwork required to establish a binding contractual obligation to compensate. Instead, member companies are asked to give an 'undertaking' to the investigator, to compensate for injuries caused by the 'medicine under trial' which, while not legally binding, is unquestion-ably binding as a matter of commercial reality. Clearly, in the event of injury an ethics committee would monitor the fact that the undertaking was honoured and a company that did not might find sponsoring future research very much more difficult for it, not to mention the adverse media comment that the failure would generate. The undertaking to pay compensation under the guidelines ends with the trial, so that patients continued on the trial drug thereafter are not covered.[87]

In practice, therefore, interests are protected in industry-sponsored research, although some commentators have drawn attention to the narrower basis for paying compensation to patient volunteers as compared with healthy volunteers and, in particular, the fact that the wider expression of injury arising 'through participation' is not used and payment may be excluded where negligence of the investigator may have caused the injury. The fact that compensation is denied where the drug has failed to produce the desired effect—as might happen in an oral contraceptive trial—has also been criticised.[88] Certainly, compensation for injury only due to the 'medicine under trial' would exclude injury not due to the drug but to a medical intervention directly contemplated by the protocol. However, the infinite variety of clinical trials presents difficulties when drafting simple guidelines and in appropriate cases experience shows that companies are prepared to vary them to accommodate particular concerns.

The arrangements made by industry have yet to be followed by government and academic interests initiating research, whose volunteers still must rely, at best, upon vague representations about ex gratia payments. This double standard has been criticised by the Royal College of Physicians,[89] which in relation to healthy volunteer studies has recommended that the concept of contractual undertakings developed by industry be extended in principle to universities and other institutions performing research. Ethics committees are advised by the Royal College to check carefully to see that arrangements have been made for compensating volunteers where the study is sponsored by industry but the College appears to accept that the funding of academic research (or rather the lack of it) makes this impracticable for the moment in relation to research not industry sponsored. The Medicines Commission has now advised that government should formally indicate 'that sympathetic and comparable consideration' would be given to healthy volunteers injured in studies performed by publicly funded bodies.[90] The October 1989 Draft Guidelines from the Department of Health[6b] state that an injured volunteer would be 'entitled to enter a claim for ex gratia payment', but add that 'Each case would of course have to be considered on its merits'. The guidelines do state that ethics committees should ensure that volunteers are made aware of the compensation arrangements. One can speculate whether the absence of a formal arrangement—now so commonly available—should be treated as a material fact to be disclosed by the investigator to the volunteer. One can envisage some volunteers, after sustaining injury, arguing that had they known compensation was not available they would not have volunteered. Certainly, DHHS regulations in the USA state that non-availability of such compensation must be disclosed on the basis that it is a reasonable presumption for a volunteer to make that in the event of injury he will be provided for.[91] Surprisingly, however, special compensation arrangements do not appear to be a common feature of research in the USA.

PROOF OF CAUSATION

Whether claims in respect of injury are made in negligence or strict liability or pursuant to a special contractual arrangement or under a centrally funded no-fault scheme, the common feature of all of these approaches is that the claimant must prove causation. In English law causation is a matter to be determined by the court as a reasonable inference to draw from admissable evidence and must be established on the balance of probability. Although tribunals of the type envisaged by the supporters of 'no-fault' schemes might well be encouraged in practice to set aside the strict rules of evidence applied by courts in assessing what is reliable evidence of the facts alleged (this appears to be the case with the Swedish schemes), the burden of proving causation inevitably still rests with the claimant.The burden will sometimes be difficult to discharge, particularly in clinical trials where deterioration in health may simply reflect the progression of the underlying disease or the effect of a concomitant therapy. The Ciba Working Party concluded, in relation to healthy volunteer studies, that because injuries during research are rare the problems of establishing causation are unlikely to be substantial, it being ' . . . reasonable to assume that any deterioration in health which occurs within a short time of the experiment, in the absence of any other evident explanation, is attributable to the experiment and should be compensated'. In contrast, as regards clinical research with patients, the Working Party recognised that 'detailed consideration of the probability of a causal relationship between therapy and event would . . . be unavoidable particularly when larger scale and prolonged studies are carried out'.[92]

Difficult cases will arise but in practice, where corporate sponsors are involved, because of the commercial setting within which the injury has arisen, the pressure will be to give the benefit of the doubt to the volunteer. This was apparent in the case of a student who died after the administration of midazolam in a healthy volunteer study sponsored by Roche Products, where a payment was made despite the fact that there was little scientific evidence to suggest that the compound could have caused the aplastic anaemia from which the volunteer died. Likewise, in its evidence to the Pearson Commission the MRC noted that it had recommended an ex gratia payment in a case where a volunteer taking part in a trial of live attenuated influenza vaccine developed a neurological lesion shortly after administration, despite the fact that such a lesion had not previously been reported in association with vaccination.

INDEMNITIES FOR INVESTIGATORS AND OTHERS CONNECTED WITH RESEARCH

The concern of ethics committees that they might be drawn into litigation if a volunteer is injured in clinical research has been mirrored in the UK by the concern of investigators and also the health authorities in whose hospitals research takes place to see that they are adequately protected from claims. In part the concern of the investigators has been heightened by discussions as to whether medical protection societies, faced with an increasing number of claims and the need to demand much higher premiums, will automatically continue to defend and indemnify their members in respect of activities that arguably fall outside their normal professional duties. Acting as investigators for the pharmaceutical industry not only might be viewed as more commercially motivated, but also is widely thought to increase the physician's potential exposure to claims. The protection societies in the UK have denied that they have any present intention of changing the basis upon which members' benefits are granted; acting as an investigator (unless as an employee of a pharmaceutical company) is treated as part of professional practice. However, the fact that the right to be indemnified is discretionary (membership does not amount to an insurance contract in the strict sense) has encouraged physicians to investigate whether further protection can be gained from those requesting their services as investigators.

As a result, it is now standard practice for an investigator to request a person who has instituted and sponsored the research to provide an indemnity for his benefit and that of his co-workers against any liability and expenses that the investigator may suffer as a result of claims in respect of personal injury made by volunteers involved in the study. As the majority of clinical research is today sponsored by the pharmaceutical industry, it is the individual company that is asked for such an indemnity. Typically, this will be drafted only to extend to injury which was not caused by the negligence of the investigator or the failure of the investigator to adhere to the protocol to a material extent. In the event that a claim is made, but is unsuccessful, the investigator not covered by a protection society can reasonably anticipate a significant loss in terms of irrecoverability of legal fees and other expenses, and the principal advantage of an indemnity of this type is that such costs will be paid for him. A corollary of the indemnity however, is that the sponsor will make the indemnity conditional upon his receiving proper notice of any claim or circumstances likely to give rise to a claim, coupled with a right to take over the defence of the claim in the name of the investigator. Such provisions often concern investigators but are normal commercial practice in relation to indemnities which otherwise expose the person granting them to significant exposure, as there is no obligation in English law to mitigate loss in such circumstances and all costs and expenses arising from the event to which the indemnity relates are prima facie recoverable.

Occasionally, as the price for agreeing to act as an investigator, some investigators will ask that the indemnity cover them against the consequences of their own negligence. The rationale of this appears to be that the opportunity for negligence only arises because the investigator is assisting the company and because of the limited practicability of the investigator obtaining separate professional indemnity insurance. The ABPI has advised that such indemnities should normally not be given, no doubt partly on the basis that the giving of the indemnity by the sponsoring company is too easy to characterise as an encouragement to the investigator to exercise less care than he might otherwise do. It seems very doubtful that this concern is valid, but when the relationship between physicians and the industry is so frequently the subject of criticism, it is entirely understandable.

More recently, certain health authorities have taken the initiative in seeking to establish a standard form of indemnity for all studies which will cover not only investigators but also the health authority against loss arising other than as a result of their own negligence. Some health authorities request evidence of security for such an indemnity in the form of a parent company guarantee. These would seem to be matters of a commercial nature which must be negotiated in the light of particular circumstances. Of concern, however, is the fact that it is understood that some ethics committees have been asked to make approval of protocols conditional on the provision of such indemnities. This arguably requires the ethics committees to participate in commercial arrangements which fall outside their proper remit. Such an approach is in marked contrast to the lack of initiative taken by health authorities to ensure that unequivocal commitments to pay compensation may be made to volunteers who may be injured in studies that are not initiated by industry interests.

REFERENCES

1. *The Nuremberg Code; Trials of War Criminals before the Nuremberg Tribunals* (1949). No. 10, Vol. 2, pp. 181–2, Washington D.C., US Government Printing Office
2. Regan, L. J. (1956). *Doctor and Patient and the Law*, 3rd edn, Mosby
3. 65/65/EEC (as amended), OJ No. 22, 09.02.65, p. 369
4. Medicines Act (1968). Chapter 67, HMSO, London
5. See English and Scottish Standing Medical Advisory Committee and Hansard, 15 February 1968, at p. 1608
6a. See HM(68)33 and Supervision of the Ethics of Clinical Research Investigations and Fetal Research, HSC (IS) 153, Department of Health, 1975
6b. Draft Guidelines for Local Research Ethics Committees. Department of Health, October, 1989
7. *Nature*, **307**, 09.02.84, and *Daily Telegraph*, 31.05.84
8. Orme, M. *et al.* (1989). Healthy volunteer studies in Great Britain. *Br. J. Clin. Pharm.*, **27**, 125–33; and Spiers, C. J. and Griffin, J. P. (1983). A survey of the first year of the operation of the new procedure affecting the conduct of clinical trials in the UK. *Br. J. Clin. Pharm.*, **15**, 649–55
9. Federal German Pharmaceutical Law, dated 24.08.76, BGBle.1.1976, p. 2445; see Sections 40–42
10. Control of Clinical Trials Act, Number 28 of 1987. The Stationery Office, Dublin
11. French law on the protection of persons undergoing biochemical research, No. 88-1138-1988, Dec 20th
12. Arpaillange, *et al.* (1985). Proposal for ethical standards in therapeutic trials, *Br. Med. J.*, **291**, 887
13. EEC/CPMP. Working Party on Efficiency of Drugs, July 3, 1987, III/411/87/EN-Rev
14. Hvidberg, E. F. (1988). Presentation to Interscience Conference on Conduct of Clinical Trials, Copenhagen
15. *Good Clinical Practice for Trials or Medicinal Products in the European Community*. European Commission, III/3976/88-EN Rev 1, 17.02.89
16. World Medical Association. Declaration of Helsinki: Recommendations Guiding Medical Doctors in Biomedical Research Involving Human Subjects. Adopted 1964 and revised in Tokyo (1975) and Venice (1983)
17. Supply of Goods and Services Act (1982). Chapter 29, HMSO, London
18. The Unfair Contract Terms Act (1977). Chapter 50, HMSO, London

19. Association of British Pharmaceutical Industry, Circular 87/89
20. For an explanation of the general principles see Donoghue v. Stevenson (1932), A.C. 562 H.L.; and Vacwell Engineering Co Ltd v BDH Chemicals Ltd (1971), 1QB 88
21. Dukes, M. N. G. and Swartz, B. (1988). *Responsibility for Drug-induced Injury*, Elsevier, p. 299
22. Cynat Products Ltd v. Landbuild (Investment & Property) Ltd (1984), 3 All ER 513
23. Directive 85/374/EEC, OJ No. L 210/29
24. Consumer Protection Act (1987). Chapter 43, HMSO, London
25. Implementation of the E.C. Directive on Product Liability. An Explanatory and Consultative Note, Department of Trade, Nov. 1985, at ¶56, p. 14
26. Directive 85/374/EEC, Supra at 23, Article 7(e)
27. Consumer Protection Act, Supra at 24, Section 4(1)(e)
28. Consumer Protection Act, Supra at 24, Section 10(7)(e)
29. Sidaway v. Bethlem Royal Hospital Governors (1985), AC 871, applying Bolam v. Friern Hospital Management Committee (1957), 2 All ER 118
30. Federal German Pharmaceutical Law, Supra at 9, Section 40(1.4)
31. Consumer Protection Act, Supra at 24, Section 3(3)
32. Collins v. Wilcock (1984), 1 W.L.R. 1172
33. Freeman v. Home Office (No. 2) (1984), QB 524
34. The Report of the Committee to Investigate Medical Experiments on Staff Volunteers (1970). Association of the British Pharmaceutical Industry, ¶3.3. (Updated as Guidelines for Medical Experiments on Non-patient Volunteers, 1984)
35. Wilson v. Pringle (1987), QB 237, 253
36. Re F. (1989) 2 WLR 1025
37. Freeman v. Home Office (No. 2), Supra at 33
38. Declaration of Helsinki, Supra at 16, see Section I(ii)
39. Family Law Reform Act (1969), S.8(1), Chapter 36; and Gillick v. West Norfolk and Wisbech Area Health Authority and the Department of Health (1985), 2 All ER 402
40. Kennedy, I. *The Patient on the Clapham Omnibus*, MLR, Vol. 47, 454
41. Dworkin, G. (1978). *Arch. Dis. Child.*, **53**, 443
42. Report of the Medical Research Council of 1962–63 entitled *Responsibility in Investigations on Human Subjects*, Cmnd 2382, HMSO, London
43. HSC (15) 153, Department of Health, Supra at 6
44. *Medicines Commission Advice to Health Ministers on Healthy Volunteer Studies* (1987), HMSO, London
45. See Report of the Medical Research Council, Supra at 42 and TvT 1988 Fam. 62
46. In Re B. (a minor) (wardship: sterilisation) 1988, AC199
47. In Re F., Supra at 36
48. Control of Clinical Trials Act (1987), Supra at 10, see S.9(7)
49. Medicines Commission, Supra at 44
50. Sidaway, Supra at 29
51. Unfair Contract Terms Act (1977), Chapter 50, Supra at 18
52. Hatcher v. Black (1954) *The Times*, July 2nd
53. Canterbury v. Spence (1972), 464. F 2d 772; and Reibl v. Hughes (1981), 114 DLR (3d)1
54. Sidaway, Supra at 29; Gold v. Haringey Health Authority (1987), 2 All ER at 888; Blyth v. Bloomsbury Health Authority (1987), *The Times*, Feb 11, CA
55. Sidaway, Supra at 29
56. Food and Drug Administration Rules and Regulations Part 56 (1981). *Federal Reporter*, **46** (17), Jan 27th

57. Halsuska v. University of Saskatchewan *et al.*, 1965, 52 WWR 616
58. Gold v. Haringey Health Authority, Supra at 54
59. Blyth v. Bloomsbury Health Authority, Supra at 54
60. EEC/CPMP Working Party Guidelines, Supra at 13
61. Fost, N. (1979). Sounding board. Consent as a barrier to research. *New Engl. J. Med.*, **300**, 1272–3
62. See, for instance, *The Observer*, Editorial of 09.10.88
63. For a general discussion see Vere, D. (1981). Editorial, *J. Roy. Soc. Med.*, **74**, Feb; and Report of Cancer Research Campaign Working Party (1983). *Br. Med. J.*, **286**, April 2nd
64. Feinstein, A. R. (1980). *Eur. J. Clin. Pharm.*, **17**, 1–4
65. Control of Clinical Trials Act, Supra at 10, see S9(4)(d)
66. EEC/CPMP Working Party Guidelines, Supra at 10
67. Gilbert, J. (1988). Letter, *I.M.E. Bulletin*, Oct, p. 10
68. Sections 40(2) and 41(6) Federal German Pharmaceutical Law, Supra at 9
69. HSC (15) I53, Supra at 6
70. *Guidelines on the Practice of Ethics Committees in Medical Research* (1984). Royal College of Physicians, London
71. The Medicines (Exemption from Licences) (Clinical Trials) Order SI 1981, No. 164
72. Medicines Commission, Supra at 44
73. FDA Rules, Supra at 56
74. S8(4) Control of Clinical Trials Act, Supra at 10. In contrast, in Denmark until March 1989, trials could begin before ethics committees had completed their review, which often took place after trials were completed! (See *Scrip*, No. 1389, 24.02.89)
75. Title III of new French law, Supra at 11
76. See for instance Peabody Donation Fund v. Sir Lindsay Parkinson & Co Ltd (1985), AC 210, and Rowling v. Takaro Properties Ltd (1988) AC 473
77. See for instance the Opren (benoxaprofen) litigation settled before trial—Davies v. Eli Lilly and Others (1988), unreported
78. S.40(3) Federal German Pharmaceutical Law, Supra at 9
79. S10 Control of Clinical Trials Act, Supra at 10
80. See ¶1339 of Royal Commission on Civil Liability and Compensation for Personal Injury, March, 1978, Cmnd 7054, HMSO, London; and letter (unpublished) of October, 1973 from Chief Medical Officers of Department of Health to President of Royal College of Physicians, London
81. Royal Commission, Supra at 80
82. *Medical Research: Civil Liability and Compensation for Personal Injury* (1980). The Ciba Foundation
83. ABPI Report, Supra at 42
84. ABPI Guidelines for Medical Experiments in Non-patient Human Volunteers (1988). March
85. ABPI Guidelines (1983). Clinical Trials—Compensation for Medicine-induced Injury, August
86. Medicines Commission, Supra at 44
87. *Legal Liability and the Supply of Investigational Drugs* (1986). ABPI Circular No. 494/86
88. Diamond, A. L. and Laurence, D. R. (1983). *Br. Med. J.*, Sept 3rd, p. 676
89. Research on Healthy Volunteers (1986). A Report of the Royal College of Physicians, London
90. Medicines Commissions, Supra at 44, see ¶6.16
91. FDA Rules, Supra at 56, S.50.25(a)(b)
92. Ciba Foundation, Supra pp. 9 and 11

IV
Measuring Drug Activity in Man

15
The Assessment of Tolerance and Side-effects in Non-patient Volunteers

Derrick Jackson

Biosciences Research Centre, Beecham Pharmaceuticals Research Division, Yew Tree Bottom Rd, Epsom, Surrey KT18 5XQ, UK

INTRODUCTION

Tolerance studies in non-patient volunteers help to bridge the gap between animal and patient studies and reduce exposure to ineffective therapy during the early evaluation of a new drug in man. The management of patients is improved by the information gained on the nature of side- and toxic effects and the dose level at which they occur.

Volunteer studies also provide an opportunity to acquire preliminary information on the kinetics of new drugs and knowledge of their metabolism. Such studies should be a feature of all early volunteer studies, since not only do they help to validate the preclinical toxicology and choice of species for subsequent longer-term investigations, but also they may highlight differences between the handling of a drug in man and the species used to demonstrate its therapeutic potential. Even with similar metabolism the dose at which the desired therapeutic effect is produced may produce side-effects only seen at much higher doses in animals. This often occurs with central nervous system effects—for example, sedation.

Various factors need to be considered in the conduct and design of tolerance studies, and these are considered below.

PRECLINICAL TOXICOLOGY

A number of guidelines have been published by the Association of the British Pharmaceutical Industry (ABPI), WHO, etc., which describe preclinical toxicology testing, and these should be taken as a minimum and additional investigations considered, depending on the nature and actions of the experimental compound concerned. An important feature is the need to look for possible unwanted cardiovascular effects, and acute studies in the

195

anaesthetised dog are an important feature of almost all preclinical toxicity testing.

Preclinical toxicity testing is designed to demonstrate and characterise the toxicity of a new compound in animals and does not always predict its safety for the initial studies in man. There must be a clear distinction between the non-toxic effect level and doses at which effects predicted from the animal pharmacology can occur, since the latter are the inevitable consequence of giving multiples of the assumed human therapeutic dose. Experience dictates that the initial human dose should be one-fiftieth of the animal dose producing the desired pharmacological effect in the most sensitive animal species, or one-tenth of the minimum dose which produces toxi effects in animals, if this is less. The initial test dose should be administered to two or three volunteers, this and subsequent doses being adjusted for body weight, the dose increases determined by the response of these volunteers together with the data from the preclinical toxicology and pharmacological investigations.

Choice of Pharmaceutical Preparation

The pharmaceutical formulation should be as simple as possible so as to avoid variations in absorption. Ideally these initial studies should be with the compound in aqueous solution, but if this is impossible, a good pharmaceutical opinion must be obtained. At some time in a new compound's progression, tolerance studies should be conducted with the formulation intended for use in the clinical trials, but where possible the initial studies should be with the compound alone.

Qualification and Training of Physicians Conducting the Study

The physician with responsibility for the study must have adequate experience—preferably at least 2 years, full-time, including extensive experience of cardiovascular and CNS techniques in new drug investigations in non-patient volunteers. In particular, he or she should have access to, and an intimate knowledge of, resuscitation equipment, i.e. defibrillators, ECG monitors, laryngoscopes, airways, cardiac pacers and appropriate drugs for i.v. and intratracheal administration. The protocol should list the standard equipment together with the emergency drugs available plus details of any extra equipment and drugs thought necessary, depending on the compound concerned and its postulated pharmacological action in humans. An appropriate antidote should also be available. All medical and nursing staff should have regular resuscitation practice sessions and examination of their abilities by an independent physician.

Training manikins (Simons, 1986) which enable a proper assessment to be made of an operator's technique together with simulation of possible problems, e.g. cardiac arrhythmias, are extremely useful. The resuscitation trolley should at all times be in the ward with the volunteers, since it is known that recovery from cardiac arrest is dependent on the time between arrest and the start of treatment. In the case of volunteers the objective should be to ensure that treatment is always started within 45 s, since studies have shown that if resuscitation is delayed for more than 4 min and defibrillation for 8 min, then, in patients, the survival rate is only 43% (Eisenburg *et al.*, 1979). Obviously, the sooner resuscitation is started the less chance of brain damage or death, and for non-patient volunteer studies a 100% survival rate must be the objective.

Properly trained medical and nursing staff must therefore be in close proximity to the volunteers for the duration of the study and for at least three times the plasma half-life, when this is known. If not, then observations must be for at least 24 h after the last dose. After the study the volunteers must have access to an emergency system whereby they can have direct contact with the study director, e.g. via a telephone call system.

CLINICAL AND LABORATORY SAFETY TESTS

Drugs can affect clinical laboratory tests, whether by direct chemical interference or by their pharmacological action (Elking and Kabat, 1968; Sher, 1982), and so the opinion of an experienced clinical chemist on the potential of a new drug to interfere with such tests should always be obtained. All volunteers should have a full clinical examination and full haematology and clinical chemistry profiles before being considered for investigation. Experience suggests that the 'normal' range of any parameter in volunteers should be determined for that particular laboratory, since what is normal for the average hospital patient may not be so for young healthy volunteers. One particular difficulty is with the white blood count (WBC), especially when the parameter is examined at frequent intervals. The WBC is often low in healthy young males, and additionally exercise, stress and adrenaline release can affect its value (French and MacFarlane, 1970). All volunteers should have a chest X-ray before entering a volunteer panel, to exclude those cardiac conditions, albeit rare, which may have been missed by clinical examination. Other essential prestudy tests are for hepatitis, for undisclosed drug therapy, including drugs of abuse (e.g. by use of the TOXI-LA Drug Screening 7 System) and for alcohol if the volunteers are not known to the investigator.

Other sets of investigations have been demonstrated by experience to be useful additions to the prestudy screen. A pretreatment endocrine screen allows a proper investigation of endocrine function should this be proved necessary by subsequent events. Endocrine disorders are relatively common, and although many will be detected by the common screens described above, some may not. Changes in thyroid function can profoundly affect drug kinetics (O'Connor and Freely, 1987) and it is reasonable to assume on the available evidence that minor clinically undetected changes of other endocrine functions may do likewise. Equally, the drug being investigated may affect endocrine function itself. Individuals with a history of unexplained rash should routinely be excluded from tolerance studies unless the protocol calls for their inclusion. Violent exercise can also produce anomalies in clinical chemistry, particularly creatine phosphokinase and WBC estimations. All studies should be conducted according to the principles laid down in the Declaration of Helsinki (1964), as amended at Tokyo (1975) and Venice (1983). The Royal College of Physicians of London published guidelines in 1984 for the composition of ethics committees, which are particularly suitable for studies in non-patient volunteers. One useful addition to the College's recommendation is to ensure that one or more of the members of the committee have special skills in the art of communication so as to ensure that the information given to volunteers, which should always be included in the protocol, really does allow them to give proper informed consent. The protocol author often has too much special knowledge of the drug under investigation and the associated sciences properly to appreciate the difficulties of the unknowledgeable volunteer.

Use of Female Volunteers

The use of both males and females in prepatient tolerance studies is important, since both in animals and in man there may be differences in the susceptibility of the two sexes to a particular drug. The use of females taking oral contraceptives is open to criticism and should be avoided until proper interaction studies have been conducted, since oestrogen and progestogens can interfere with the absorption of some drugs. Females should have a pregnancy test and a test for the recent occurrence of ovulation prior to the clinical investigation and at appropriate intervals during the study. Teratogenicity testing is no guarantee of safety (Larson *et al.*, 1982). If the female volunteers are not well known to the investigators, then, ideally, only single-dose studies should be undertaken, to ensure that no differences exist between the sexes in the kinetics of the drug or sensitivity to the pharmacological and other effects.

Design of Studies

In general, four major types of tolerance studies should be conducted in non-patient volunteers. First, single-dose studies up to the maximum dose where signs indicative of possible toxicity occur or the level at which side-effects are shown to be unacceptable for patient studies. The upper limit will also be determined to some extent by the findings in preclinical toxicology. The second study should investigate the tolerance of the drug at the dose and duration of therapy proposed for the initial patient studies. If not covered by this investigation, a third tolerance study should be undertaken with those drugs destined for long-term use, of at least 3 weeks' duration. The fourth group of studies consists of special investigations to determine more fully by special tests the effects on specific symptoms, such investigations being determined by the animal experiments and the human tolerance studies. The use of 'step-up' designs, i.e. gradually increasing each sequential dose in any one volunteer, to provide information on the maximum tolerated dose in man should be avoided, since they provide no information on the tolerance of a standard repeat dose and also no information on the tolerance of any particular single dose unless the times between doses are sufficiently great to ensure that there are no residual effects from any previous administration. One of the repeat-dose studies should be with the formulation intended for clinical study.

Diet can either impair or enhance the absorption of drugs (Vessell, 1984) and so affect their tolerance. In initial studies the compound should be administered in the fasting state. The duration of the fast should be 8–10 h and not more than 12 h since the level of albumin-bound free fatty acids rises after 12 h (Reidenberg, 1977), which will affect the free level of some albumin-bound drugs. Some foods, e.g. fat, may enhance a particular drug's absorption, so, although it is possible to conduct the early clinical studies in hospital patients based on tolerance studies conducted in fasting individuals only, it is important to determine the effect of food (e.g. low fat, high fat, liquid means, solid meals) on absorption before the drug is administered to relatively poorly supervised outpatients. If it is decided to conduct tolerance studies with drug administration with food, then the precise timing in relation to food intake should be clearly stated, since differences in the rate and amount of drug absorption can occur if the drug is administered with the first mouthful of food, with the meal or more than 30 min after food.

Posture can also affect drug absorption, presumably by changes in the rate of gastric emptying (Rainbird *et al.*, 1987), but specific protocol instructions on posture are probably best avoided except during those investigations which include an assessment of pharmacokinetics. Multiple-dose studies with limitation on the posture to be adopted during the period of drug absorption from the gastrointestinal tract are difficult to control adequately and could be misleading, as such control contrasts sharply with the situation in therapeutic practice. However, in comparative studies there should be uniformity between the groups, and similarly it is good practice to ensure that the amount of exercise undertaken is similar for all study participants.

Informed consent invariably involves telling the volunteer what side-effects and toxicity may occur and thus inevitably suggesting that these effects are probable—hence the need for the inclusion of a placebo and a comparative drug at some stage in the prepatient investigations. Most tolerance studies give a good indication of the nature and severity of possible adverse events, but little knowledge of the incidence of clinical practice. The classical example is antibiotics, where the incidence of gastrointestinal effects can be up to ten times higher in volunteers than in patients. In the initial single-dose and early multiple-dose studies the volunteer should be asked a simple question (e.g. have you noticed any symptoms since your last examination?) and then each volunteer should be asked in the same order whether they have experienced specific symptoms, this list being determined by the pharmacology and toxicology of the drug under investigation. The use of trick questions at this stage of the investigations is best avoided. An attempt should be made to assess the severity of any symptoms by the use of visual analogue scales.

The following sequence of tolerance studies is suggested for a new drug suitable for administration to new patient volunteers.

(1) Single-dose studies, one dose per volunteer up to at least twice the dose intended for multiple-dose studies or the maximum tolerated dose, whichever is the lesser dose.

(2) Multiple-dose study employing the proposed therapeutic regimen in a small number of volunteers.

(3) Multiple-dose placebo-controlled study employing at least the maximum dose intended for patients. If these investigations are conducted at more than one centre, differences are often apparent in the incidence of particular side-effects between centres, even in placebo-controlled studies, suggesting that tolerance studies are at best a qualitative assessment. If the volunteers are all recruited from one institution, then it is instructive to compare the incidence of side-effects on both active and placebo therapy by laboratory or office, and it will be noted on some occasions that one particular complaint is found in one group of people working together, irrespective of therapy. The most 'infectious' side-effects are gastrointestinal, demonstrating the need for large numbers of volunteers in tolerance studies with drugs producing such symptoms.

(4) It may be necessary in some instances also to include a multiple-dose study using a multiple of the proposed maximum therapeutic dose, provided that the animal toxicity and early tolerance studies permit such an investigation. Such studies are extremely useful in helping to assess the tolerance of new drugs in patients with a clinical condition where it is difficult to determine the contribution of a new drug, if any, to the pattern of side-effects observed—for example, the assessment of antiemetics in patients receiving anticancer chemotherapy.

The methodology described so far will provide details of the symptoms and signs resulting from the pharmacological action of the drug, i.e. side-effects and/or direct drug toxicity. It is unlikely that any of the other types of adverse events will become manifest, in view of the volunteer selection procedures and the numbers involved. Special investigations are almost invariably required, either as components of the tolerance study itself or as separate studies, the type and nature of which are determined by the pharmacology of the compound and the nature of the toxicity observed in the preclinical studies or any subsequent investigation, including the initial non-patient volunteer studies.

Other chapters in this book describe in detail the specialist investigations employed in patient and non-patient volunteer studies, but the following investigations should be included in evaluation of all new compounds.

Cardiovascular Screen

All the initial single-dose studies should include a continuous recording of heart rate and ECG with frequent determination of blood pressure, and this continuous monitoring should continue throughout the intial multiple-dose studies, with trained staff available to note any untoward events.

A good practice is to have a continuous display with recording of lead II for at least twice the anticipated beta half-life of the drug with 12 lead ECGs before treatment, at C_{max}, if known, and 2 h and 24 h later. The 12 lead ECG tracing should be followed by high-speed ECGs for measurement of conduction intervals. Ambulatory monitoring for up to 24 h per day, depending on the drug, is an essential part of multiple-dose studies. However, such intensive monitoring can cause problems in interpretation, since food ingestion can produce small falls in blood pressure and increases in heart rate. Minor changes in the T wave with even inversion in some subjects have also been described (Fagan *et al.*, 1986). Any real or suspect changes in the early volunteer studies or any suggestion from the preclinical toxicology of a cardiac effect should lead to more detailed investigations, to include assessment of cardiac output and myocardial contractility, e.g. by the use of echo cardiography, Doppler systolic time intervals and impedance cardiography.

Central Nervous System

The assessment of drugs designed to affect the central nervous system will of course include detailed studies of pharmacology and effects on psychomotor performance. A wide range of tests is needed for such an assessment. However, all drugs, including those with primarily a non-central action, may affect the CNS and produce drowsiness and impaired performance resulting in potential hazards when operating machinery or car driving and also affect decision making. Therefore, all new drugs should be tested for effects on the CNS at some stage of their evaluation—if possible, when the therapeutic dose has been established. For examples of such tests see Bond and Lader (1974); Nicholson (1978); Peet *et al.* (1981); Lewis *et al.* (1985); Francis *et al.* (1986); Mattilla *et al.* (1986) and McClelland *et al.* (1987).

Intravenous Studies

The general plan is the same as for oral studies, with the following considerations.

Whenever possible, the intravenous solution should be isotonic. Vasovagal attacks during intravenous effusion, with pulse rates as low as 20 beats per minute, are liable to occur even with mildly irritant solutions. A good plan is to start with a dose one-fiftieth of that which produces the full pharmacological effect in experimental animals, provided that this dose is less than one-tenth of that which produces toxic effects in the preclinical toxicity studies. The duration of the infusion should be 20 min and this period can gradually be reduced by steps to 10 min, then 5 min, then 2 min, provided that this progression takes place at one particular dose level. As a general rule, no drug dose, other than anaesthetic agents, should be given intravenously in less than 2 min. All doses should be given on a unit/weight basis. A satisfactory plan is to double the dose for the first four increments and then limit any increment to 50% of the preceding dose. Safety is of paramount importance, and any sign of intolerance should lead to, first, a repeat, if ethical, in more volunteers of that dose, and if this is satisfactory, then progression with much smaller dose increments.

The assessment of safety, particularly on the cardiovascular system, is equally important. A scheme devised by Dr J. Upward is a good guideline for such investigations, and is set out below.

(A) Compounds with no effect on the ECG or circulation of animals at doses 2 × those which produce the desired pharmacological effect.

Electrocardiographic monitoring
(1) Oscilloscope display of lead 2 (during infusion and for at least one hour after the end of the infusion, depending on the presumed half-life of the drug.
(2) 12 lead electrocardiogram (pre-treatment, immediately after infusion and at 2 and 24 hours post infusion).
(3) High speed electrocardiogram (50 or 100 mm/sec), recorded immediately after the 12 lead recording; for measurement of PR interval, QRS duration and QT interval.
(4) Ambulatory electrocardiographic monitoring (recording started before infusion and continued for 8 hours post infusion).

If significant changes are produced, then proceed as in (B).

Monitoring of circulation
Blood pressure and pulse rate—measured before infusion, immediately after infusion and at intervals for 8 h.
(B) Compounds which produce effects on the ECG or circulation of animals at dose 2 × those which produce the desired pharmacological effect.

Electrocardiographic monitoring
(1) Oscilloscope display of lead II, during infusion and for at least 1 h after the end of the infusion. Electrocardiographic monitoring continued until the PR interval, QRS duration and QT interval (the latter corrected for heart rate) have returned to the normal range.
(2) 12 lead electrocardiogram (as for Section A).
(3) High-speed electrocardiogram (recorded as in Section A, but additional recordings will be taken at 2 h intervals until the PR interval, QRS duration and QTc lie within the normal range).
(4) Ambulatory electrocardiographic monitoring (recording starting before infusion and continued for 24 h post-infusion; subjects remain under supervision until the end of the recording or until the electrocardiogram has returned to normal; whichever is later).

Monitoring of circulation
Blood pressure and pulse rate—measured before infusion immediately after infusion and then at 1–2 h intervals over the next 24 h, or at greater intervals, e.g. 6 h, if all readings have been normal for at least 4 h.

Following the single-dose studies, a full tolerance study should be performed to mimic the maximum dose and usual duration of therapy expected in therapeutic practice.

Intramuscular Formulations

Many intramuscular preparations are special formulations of an intravenous product and, apart from the intravenous clinical programme and intramuscular pharmacokinetic studies, little or no additional work is necessary. It is our practice to give the preparation in therapeutic doses up to steady state, and this is usually enough to determine tolerance. Lignocaine is added to the preparation for the initial investigations. Where no intravenous data are available, tolerance studies of the same duration as that proposed for therapeutic use are advised.

Topical Products

Skin Preparation

The majority of topical products will have been subject to systemic toxicological assessment, and it remains to establish topical tolerance by an assessment of the product's dermal irritancy and sensitisation potential (Gollhauser and Kligman, 1985). An example of the clinical pharmacology assessment of a topical product is given in Jackson *et al.* (1985) and Wuite *et al.* (1985). Whenever possible, it is desirable to use objective methods of laser Doppler flowmetry for the assessment of irritancy (Nilsson *et al.*, 1982). Any constituent of a topical preparation which penetrates the skin poorly may be negative in such tests but, when applied therapeutically to non-intact skin, be sufficiently well absorbed into the skin to stimulate a sensitisation response. This possibility can be lessened by the use of concentrations many times in excess of that proposed for therapeutic use plus an experiment in 20+ volunteers with total body application of the test substance under a plastic body suit.

Intranasal Preparations

As for topical products, plus a full therapeutic course at the maximum dose in comparison with the vehicle used for the drug in an adequate number of volunteers, such a number to be estimated on the basis of pilot trials involving at least 12, and preferably 24, subjects. If there is any possibility of the drug reaching the pulmonary system, then the precautions recommended for intravenous products should be taken.

Intravaginal and Sublingual Preparations

As for topical products, plus a full therapeutic course at the maximum dose in comparison with placebo, plus a standard preparation in suitable patient volunteers.

Eye and Ear Preparations

As for topical products, plus a full therapeutic course at the maximum proposed therapeutic concentration. In both these situations experience shows that animal studies can be misleading, particularly with eye preparations. Subjects must be examined daily by slit lamp fluorescent staining of the cornea, measurements of visual acuity, ophthalmoscopy and regular measurements made of intraocular pressure. A good strategy is as follows:

(1) Tests on skin for irritation and sensitisation.
(2) Single conjunctival applications in 12 subjects.
(3) Three conjunctival applications in 12 subjects.
(4) The full proposed therapeutic regimen, with placebo comparison, the numbers of subjects involved being decided in consultation with a statistician.

LIMITATION OF TOLERANCE STUDIES

Provided that the handling of the drug in man is similar to that in the animals used to demonstrate its therapeutic potential and toxicity characteristics, then tolerance studies are a good qualitative indication of the likely side-effect pattern of a compound and its potential toxicity for man. In particular, they give a good indication, when properly conducted and assessed, of a suitable starting dose for patient studies. Quantitative assessments of side-effects and other adverse reactions based on tolerance studies in non-patient volunteers are best avoided, in view of the frequently observed differences between healthy adults and patients.

REFERENCES

Bond, A. and Lader, M. (1974). The use of analogue scales in rating subjective feelings. *Br. J. Med. Psychol.*, **47**, 211–18
Eisenberg, M. S., Bergner, L. and Hallstrom, A. (1979). Cardiac resuscitation in the community; importance of rapid provision and implementation for programme planning. *J. Am. Med. Ass.*, **241**, 1905–7
Elking, M. P. and Kabat, H. F. (1968). Drug induced modifications of laboratory test values. *Am. J. Hosp. Pharm.*, **25**, 485–519
Fagan, T. C., Sawyer, P. R., Gourley, L. A., Lee, J. T. and Gaffney, T. E. (1986). Postprandial alterations in haemodynamics and blood pressure in normal subjects. *Am. J. Cardiol.*, **58**, 636–641
Francis, G. R., McClelland, G. R. and Pettitt, K. E. E. (1986). Measurement of body sway using ultrasound. *Br. J. Clin. Pharm.*, **21**, 123P
French, J. E. and Macfarlane, R. G. (1970). The reactions of the blood to injury. No. 2 Cellular reactions. In Florey, H. W. (Ed.), *General Pathology*, 4th edn. Lloyd-Luke, London, pp. 246–7
Gollhausen, R. and Kligman, A. M. (1985). Human assay for identifying substances which induce non-allergic contact urticaria: the NICU test. *Contact Dermatitis*, **13**, 98–106

Jackson, D., Tasker, T. C. G., Sutherland, R., Mellows, G. and Cooper, D. L. (1985). Clinical pharmacology of Bactroban: pharmacokinetics, tolerance and efficacy studies. In Dobson, R. L., Leyden, J. J., Noble, W. C. and Price, J. D. (Eds.), *Bactroban. Excerpta Medica Current Clinical Practice Series 16*, Amsterdam, pp. 54–67

Larson, S. K., Elwin, C. E., Gabrielsson, J., Paalzow, L. and Wachtmeister, C. A. (1982). Do teratogenicity tests serve their objectives? *Lancet*, **ii**, 439

Lewis, R. V., Jackson, P. R. and Ramsay, L. E. (1985). Side effects of β-blockers assess using visual analogue scales. *Eur. J. Clin. Pharm.*, **28** (Suppl), 93–6

McClelland, G. R., Loudon, J. M. and Raptopoulos, P. (1987). Paroxetine and oxazepam: effects on psychomotor performance. *Br. J. Clin. Pharm.*, **23**, 117P

Mattila, M. J., Mattila, M. and Konno, K. (1986). Acute and subacute actions on human performance and interactions with diazepam of temelastine (SK&F 93944) and diphenhydramine. *Eur. J. Clin. Pharm.*, **31**, 291–8

Nicholson, A. N. (1978). Visual analogue scales and drug effects in man. *Br. J. Clin. Pharm.*, **6**, 3–4

Nilsson, G. E. and Wahlberg, J. E. (1982). Assessment of skin irritancy in man by laser Doppler flowmetry. *Contact Dermatitis*, **8**, 401–6

O'Connor, P. and Feeley, J. (1987). Clinical pharmacokinetics and endocrine disorders, therapeutic implications. *Clin. Pharmacokinet.*, **13**, 345–64.

Peet, M., Ellis, S. and Yates, R. A. (1981). The effect of level of depression on the use of visual analogue scales by normal volunteers. *Br. J. Clin Pharm.*, **12**, 171–8

Rainbird, A. L., Pickworth, M. J. W., Lightowler, C., Mitchell, M. and Wingate, D. L. (1987). Effect of posture and cold stress on impedance measurements of gastric emptying. *Pharm. Med.*, **2**, 35–42

Reidenberg, M. M. (1977). Obesity and fasting—effects on drug metabolism and drug action in man. *Clin. Pharm. Ther.*, **22**, 729–34

Sher, P. P. (1982). Drug interferences with clinical laboratory tests. *Drugs*, **24**, 24–63

Simons, R. S. (1986). Training manikins. In Evans, T. R. (Ed.), *ABC of Resuscitation*. British Medical Journal, London, pp. 35–9

Vessell, E. S. (1984). Complex effects of diet on drug disposition. *Clin. Pharm. Ther.*, **36**, 285–96

Wuite, J., Davies, B. I., Go, M. J., Lambers, J. C., Jackson, D., Mellows, G. and Tasker, T. C. G. (1985). Pseudomanic acid, a new antibiotic for topical therapy. *J. Am. Acad. Derm.*, **12**, 1026–31

16
Design of First-administration Studies in Healthy Man

Colin Broom

SKF Research Ltd, The Frythe, Welwyn, Herts AL6 9AR, UK

INTRODUCTION

The progression of a drug from animal to human studies probably represents the single most important step in drug development. However, the design of the initial human evaluation study is associated with a great deal of uncertainty. Although there are a number of general reviews of Phase I studies (Vaidya and Vaidya, 1981; Burley and Glynne, 1985; Rogers and Spector, 1986), there is a lack of guidance regarding the initial human evaluation; consequently, practice varies considerably between investigators. It is the aim of this chapter to review the important decisions to be made after completion of satisfactory preclinical work and the relative advantages and disadvantages of different study designs, all of which allow the dose of a drug to be escalated from a low to a high level with safety as a primary concern.

MEASUREMENT OF BIOLOGICAL EFFECT

When the drug to be studied is unlikely to have a measurable biological effect in healthy man, the investigator will be limited to making a preliminary assessment of the pharmacokinetics and the tolerability of the drug. However, the majority of drugs have a biological effect, even in healthy man, and it is desirable to monitor such effects, even during the initial study. The advantages of doing this are that, first, the study will have a biologically based end-point rather than a toxicological one; second, the data generated will allow early evaluation to proceed more efficiently by allowing the investigator to obtain data over a relevant dose range; and third, it may provide valuable early information that may require the drug development strategy to be reappraised. The potential disadvantage is that the measurement of biological effect could compromise the safety of volunteers, and this factor should be carefully considered for each study. However, the development of non-invasive methodology and the established safety of many standard procedures for measuring the biological effect of drugs now mean that extensive evaluation is often possible. It may be argued that knowledge of the onset of biological effect will enhance the safety of a study by making the investigator aware that an active dose level has been reached and subsequent dosing increments may need to be reduced.

In all study designs the monitoring of tolerability in terms of effects on heart rate, blood pressure, ECG, laboratory measurements and symptoms should be performed as outlined in the preceding chapter. Investigators should be experienced in the conduct of first-administration studies and familiar with the relevant technique being used to evaluate the biological effect of the drug. Additionally, the healthy volunteers taking part in the study should have been made familiar with the conduct of clinical pharmacology studies, ideally by previous participation in volunteer studies, and should have no doubts about the competence of the investigator and his staff.

CHOICE OF DOSE

Ideally, doses to be administered should be calculated on a dose per unit body weight or a dose per square metre of body surface area basis. Limitations due to the pharmaceutical preparation may make this impossible, in which case this loss of flexibility will need to be addressed in the study design. The starting dose in first-administration studies should be determined from data on the pharmacological profile of the drug in animals. It is generally taken to be around one-fiftieth of the pharmacologically effective dose in the most sensitive animal species studied. This general rule has evolved rather than being part of any formal guideline, and has been widely discussed (Dollery and Davis, 1970; Pitts, 1974; Vaidya and Vaidya, 1981).

The top dose to be used may also be based on animal pharmacology, particularly if the drug to be studied is relatively non-toxic in animal studies. The maximum dose permissible should otherwise be a fraction between one-tenth and one-fifth of the 'no effect' dose in toxicological studies (i.e. a fraction of the dose producing no toxicological effect in the animal species studied). For drugs likely to have a low therapeutic index this level of safety may not be possible; therefore, each drug will need to be judged on an individual basis. Obviously the top dose actually administered will be dictated by the findings in the study.

The choice of dosing increments in the escalating dose regimen will be chosen depending on the dose–response relationships in animal studies. These may predict how steep the dose–response curve is likely to be in man and in what dose range the biological effect is likely to be seen. In general, doses are no more than doubled, at least until the predicted biologically effective dose range is reached. Dosing increments are often limited to no more than 50% in the predicted biologically effective dose range, where relatively large absolute increases in dose occur. However, the dosing increments need to be determined in part by the findings during the study. The study design needs to allow flexibility of dosing so that lower or intermediate doses are permissible if necessary. There are alternative schemes for dosing increments, such as the modified Fibonacci search scheme

(Hansen, 1970; Carter *et al.*, 1977), which is particularly favoured in the study of cytotoxic agents in patients. Using this scheme, dosing increments are based on the initial starting dose (× mg per square metre of body surface area) and increased in the order ×, 2×, 3.3×, 5×, 7×, 9×, 12× and 16×. First-administration studies in cancer represent a specialised area of early studies (Von Hoff *et al.*, 1984). If the same group of subjects are to be studied during the dose escalation, each individual subject should receive no more than four single doses of drug, even though there may be adequate animal data to support further dosing.

ROUTES OF ADMINISTRATION AND FORMULATION

The chemical and pharmaceutical properties of the drug to be studied, together with its proposed therapeutic uses, will dictate what drug formulations are available. Some investigators advocate using the intravenous route for the first administration of a drug, since slow infusions (i.e. at least 15 min duration) can be turned off at the earliest suggestion of the occurrence of adverse effects. This is clearly so for drugs likely to exert pharmacological or toxicological effects rapidly, but the advantage of this route is no longer present when there is a lag time to effect, longer than the duration of the infusion. An additional important advantage is that there is less variability in systemic exposure, both within and between subjects, than is obtained following oral administration, when rate and extent of absorption may vary enormously. Thus, a further variable is taken away during the process of dose escalation. In practice, most drugs are developed primarily for oral administration and the majority of initial studies will, therefore, be by this route. As a generalisation, less variability in absorption is likely with solutions or simple suspensions of drug and the onset of effect is often quicker. Solutions allow drug dose to be based on body weight or proportional to body surface area. This individualisation of dose is clearly not possible when pharmaceutical problems dictate a solid dosage form. Additionally, some dose-escalating designs make individualisation of doses less of a limitation, particularly those using a within-subject escalating regimen (see below). The oral dosing form for use in subsequent clinical studies is almost invariably tablets or capsules, and therefore there are merits in studying these in the first study if development time is to be reduced.

Most other routes of administration follow similar principles to that of the oral formulation, and once a dose is given, it is difficult to get back!

STUDY DESIGNS

A dose range and the route of administration with a suitable formulation of the investigative drug having been chosen, the next major decision is regarding the dose-escalating design to be adopted. There is no definite right or wrong study design; however, the data generated in preclinical studies need to be carefully evaluated and decisions made regarding the most suitable design for the drug being studied.

A few generalizations can be made. One is that the study should ideally be single-blind rather than open. If the study is double-blind, prompt access to the randomisation code should be available to the investigator. Thus, the use of a placebo treatment is to be recommended (or rarely a comparator drug) in the first study. However, a number of theoretical and practical problems are caused by the use of a placebo treatment, which will be discussed for each design.

SPECIFIC DESIGNS

Simple Rising Dose Designs

This design (Table 16.1) is commonly used for first-administration studies. The groups are studied sequentially at suitable intervals. Group size needs to be relatively large, i.e. at least four subjects on active treatment, in order to obtain some degree of confidence before going on to study a subsequent group at a higher dose level. One problem with this design is that of between-subject variability. For instance, a member of a group studied may be more sensitive to the drug than any member of a preceding group. He or she will receive a dose twice as large as the preceding group and consequently may suffer an adverse event related to excess pharmacological effect or toxicological effect of a drug. Placebo-treated subjects need to be incorporated into each group to make the study subject blind; thus, the numbers of subjects studied will need to be large, i.e. about 48 subjects required for the example in Table 16.1. An advantage of the design is that the study can be completed expeditiously.

There are a number of variations on the above simple rising dose design which allow groups to be studied on more than one occasion; an example is given in Table 16.2.

Table 16.1 Simple rising dose design

	Dose							
	×	2×	4×	8×	16×	32×	48×	72×
Group 1	+							
Group 2		+						
Group 3			+					
Group 4				+				
Group 5					+			
Group 6						+		
Group 7							+	
Group 8								+

Table 16.2 Combined between + within-subject dose escalation

	Dose							
	×	2×	4×	8×	16×	32×	48×	72×
Group 1	+		+		+		+	
Group 2		+		+		+		+

This is an attractive design in terms of reduced subject numbers; however, it is complicated by incorporating a placebo treatment. If a different subject within each group is given placebo on each occasion (so that every subject is studied once on placebo), significant safety concerns arise, since subjects given placebo will always receive a dose at least four times as great as their preceding dose and twice as great as the maximum dose given to preceding subjects. An alternative is to continue to treat the same subjects with placebo throughout the study but the measurement of biological effect without comparative placebo data for each subject is difficult. Once again the group sizes will need to be relatively large.

Within-subject Rising Dose Design

One of the main problems associated with first-administration studies is the difference in response between subjects with regard to the pharmacological effects (and toxicity) of the investigational drug. This problem can be overcome to a certain extent by studying increasing doses within each subject (Table 16.3). This is feasible in healthy volunteers, since their physiological state is constant, and does not change with time. This is not always true in patients. The use of a single dose of placebo can also be incorporated in a randomised order for each subject within a group, so that, in the example given, subjects would be studied four times on active drug in the order indicated, with a single, additional placebo treatment somewhere within that order. This design allows within-subject dose–response relationships to be determined, relative to a placebo response. The second group is subsequently studied at a dose higher than that of the first group, with further dose escalation. The large increase in dose between subjects is a potential safety problem but can be overcome by overlapping the dose levels studied within each group, as depicted in Table 16.4.

One or more dose levels may be overlapped between the sequentially studied groups. This design has a number of significant attractions when a measurable biological effect is being studied. The number of subjects required is often smaller, e.g. each group may be no more than about four subjects and all of these subjects can receive a placebo in a randomised order, i.e. four active doses and one placebo. Greater numbers of subjects will be studied within the relevant dose range—for instance, 8–48× in the example. Second, the safety inherent in the design arises from the fact that only within-subject escalation of dose takes place. Between-subject variability is allowed for by the overlapping design, such that the dose studied in each new group is either less or no greater than that studied in a preceding group.

Table 16.3   Within-subject dose escalation

	Dose							
	×	2×	4×	8×	16×	32×	48×	72×
Group 1	+	+	+	+				
Group 2					+	+	+	+

Table 16.4   Within-subject, rising dose design, with overlap of consecutive groups

	Dose							
	×	2×	4×	8×	16×	32×	48×	72×
Group 1	+	+	+	+				
Group 2				+	+	+	+	
Group 3					+	+	+	+

Dose–response relationships within subjects can be determined and the variability in response between subjects can also be addressed. Further groups can be added to elaborate on the relevant part of a dose–response relationship, if required, and to allow further intermediate doses to be studied, if necessary. The data will also allow a preliminary pharmacokinetic evaluation of within-subject dose proportionality in addition to the between-subject variability.

One of the disadvantages of such a design is the time taken to study the effect of a drug, since even for drugs with rapid elimination the time between consecutive doses within each subject should be at least 48 h, to allow post-study-day safety evaluation. When the elimination of a drug is likely to be long or where the biological effect is likely to persist for some time, e.g. irreversible H^+/K^+ ATPase inhibitors, the duration between consecutive study days may need to be 1 week or more. Also, potential carry-over effects need to be borne in mind.

The presentation of biological data from such a study will not be as straightforward as using more simple designs, owing to the different numbers of subjects studied at each dose level. However, it is possible to present data very elegantly by analysing data statistically by an appropriate modelling procedure.

Other Designs

A limited number of other designs are possible, depending on the type of drug being studied. One such design is the stepwise increase in infusion rates within a subject on the same study day (Figure 16.1). Clearly this type of design is only possible with safety when the elimination of an intravenous drug (or drug rapidly and consistently absorbed by another route) is short and time to biological effect shows little or no lag phase. This information will be indicated from animal studies but may not necessarily apply in man. Any

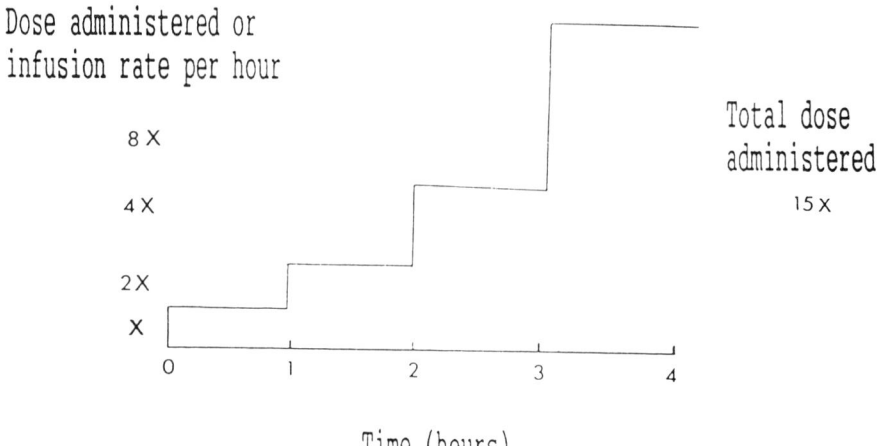

Figure 16.1 Stepwise increase in drug infusion rates

subsequent toxicological effect, e.g. haematological effect or effect on liver enzymes, will not be evident early enough to prevent relatively high doses from being administered. Also, there is no information on the effect of a single larger infusion that has not been preceded by smaller doses. In situations where tolerance to biological or adverse effects occurs rapidly, the investigator can be misled into believing that the tolerability is better than it really is. Thus, there are significant disadvantages to this approach. The only advantage is that escalation of dosing is rapid.

CONCLUSION

There is no ideal design for a first-administration study in man. The choice of design must be based on the pharmacodynamics and pharmacokinetics expected in man. All designs must have safety as their primary concern, particularly when a drug's biological effect is also to be measured. A well-designed first-administration study will allow a dose–response relationship to be identified and will provide preliminary pharmacokinetic data. The more definitive, more rigorously controlled studies of pharmacodynamics and pharmacokinetics in volunteers and patients may subsequently be performed with earlier knowledge of the appropriate dose range.

REFERENCES

Burley, D. M. and Glynne, A. (1985). In Burley, D. M. and Binns, T. B. (Eds.), *Pharmaceutical Medicine Clinical Trials*. Edward Arnold, London, pp. 70–109

Carter, S. K., Selawry, O. and Slavik, M. (1977). Methods of development of new anti cancer drugs. Clinical trials in cancer chemotherapy. *Cancer*, **40**, 544–57

Dollery, C. T. and Davies, D. S. (1970). The conduct of initial studies in man. *Br. Med. Bull.*, **26**, 233–6

Hansen, H. H. (1970). Clinical experience with 1-(2-chloroethyl)3-cyclohexyl-1-nitrosourea (CCNU NSC 79037). *Proc. Am. Ass. Cancer Res.*, **11**, 43

Pitts, N. E. (1974). In MacMahon, F. (Ed.), *Principles and Techniques of Human Research and Therapeutics*, Volume II: *Drug-induced Clinical Toxicity*. Futura, New York, pp. 19–35

Rogers, H. J. and Spector, R. G. (1986). In Glenny, G. and Nelmer, P. (Eds.), *Handbook of Clinical Drug Research. Phase I Studies*. Blackwell Scientific, Oxford, pp. 33–58

Vaidya, A. B. and Vaidya, R. A. (1981). Initial human trials with an investigational new drug. *J. Postgrad. Med.*, **27**, 197–213

Von Hoff, D. D., Kuhn, J. and Clark, G. M. (1984). In Buyse, M. E., Staquet, M. J. and Sylvester, R. J. (Eds.), *Cancer Clinical Trials Methods and Practice; Design and Conduct of Phase I Trials*. Oxford University Press, Oxford, pp. 210–20

17
The Detection and Assessment of Adverse Reactions in Early Phase Patient Trials

Jan N. Lessem and Richard D. Mamelok

Section of Cardiology, Syntex Inc., 3401 Hillview Avenue, Palo Alto, CA 94303, USA

INTRODUCTION

Great difficulties exist in detecting and assessing adverse reactions in clinical trials. These difficulties are even more pronounced in early Phase I and Phase II trials, since knowledge about the chemical entity under evaluation may be scarce and only a few subjects and patients participate in these early trials. An adverse drug reaction has to be defined prior to initiating any trial; the WHO definition of an adverse drug reaction is any response to a drug 'which is noxious and unintended and which occurs at doses used in man for prophylaxis, diagnosis or therapy'. This definition takes into account therapeutic failures.

If the mode of action of a particular drug is known, it may be possible to predict some side-effects. Other adverse reactions are totally unexpected. Another factor, especially in early clinical trials with the drug, is determining causality. Does a certain drug cause a specific reaction (Karch and Lasagna, 1975)? In early controlled or open clinical trials these reactions may appear to be very sporadic, and the observer does not have the benefit of large multicentre and well-controlled trials to aid him in his judgement. It is still important to try to solve the causality issue, since a very severe reaction could or should lead to an appreciation of the risk–benefit ratio early in development, and thus lead to an informed judgement as to whether the development of a certain drug should continue or not. In our discussion of early clinical trials we shall focus on how to detect serious side-effects, but it is equally important to recognise the minor ones, which may be of more daily irritation to the patient than the odd or unusual event. Even for these minor events, it is indeed important to establish, if at all possible, causality. Sometimes these minor events can be expected from the pharmacology, e.g. a headache may be expected as a finding when a vasodilator is given. However, the question as to whether the incidence of such an adverse event is high or low relative to other vasodilators can only be answered appropriately by large long-term trials, and thus is beyond the scope of this chapter.

The goal of Phase I studies is usually to define the highest dose tolerated by a volunteer population. This goal may sometimes be impossible to achieve, if the tested entity does not produce any adverse reactions causing termination, or pharmacological unwanted effects such as, for example, an extreme slowing of the AV-conduction time. However, it is possible that in some Phase I studies adverse reactions will occur that will be dose-increase-limiting, and these may again range from severe pharmacological effects to subjective symptoms.

If the tested entity is a so-called 'me-too' agent, it is possible that knowledge about the adverse reaction profile occurring with the original first-generation agent may guide the physician in the search for the adverse reactions associated with the agent being tested. When the second-generation angiotensin-converting enzyme inhibitors were developed, the search for rashes, proteinuria, taste disturbances and neutropenia was carried out vigorously, and all possible tests used to ensure a better side-effect profile. However, cough, which is a rather frequent occurrence with all ACE inhibitors, was overlooked, until large postmarketing studies were carried out. For the third generation cough was then originally searched for.

Guidance as to which side-effects to expect may be obtained from animal toxicology studies. These, although often short-term in duration, prior to starting Phase I, may indicate a specific target organ or organ system where toxic reactions occur. It may then be critical to include an evaluation of this organ system in the early studies. If one were to develop a drug that was found to affect the bone marrow, it would of course be vital to include laboratory tests that were directed at detecting deficiencies in bone marrow function. Similarly, if one knew that the stomach was a toxic target organ, it might be important to include gastroscopy already in Phase I studies.

METHODOLOGY

In early Phase I and Phase II clinical trials certain instruments should be employed in order to detect all adverse reactions and to make an informed judgement as to their causes.

Among these instruments are checklists and questionnaires. Patients or healthy subjects can be given checklists of some common events known to occur with the class of drug being tested, and asked to check occurring symptoms. The clinical investigator can use checklists for recording adverse events. If checklists are used, it is important not only that checkboxes for expected adverse events be available, but also that additional space be available to the individual to utilise when an unexpected adverse event occurs. This space could be used by the subject to describe the event in detail. Huskisson *et al.* (1977) found that the use of a checklist encourages the reporting of solicited adverse events, but suppresses the true frequency of unsolicited events. Therefore, if checklists are to be used early in drug development, extreme caution in interpreting the results is advisable. Questionnaires ask the user to answer a standard set of questions, usually defined on the basis of the known pharmacology of the drug. The reproducibility and validity of questionnaires in soliciting adverse drug reactions may impact the understanding of causality, as Hutchinson (1986) discusses. They may also introduce both observer and user biases and objectivity may be lost because of subjective evaluations, mainly on the part of the investigator. One other valid point of criticism against these methods is that subjectivity, which may be the most important lead, will be forfeited in the search for objectivity and completeness.

The design of early clinical trials can be important in detecting advance events and in assessing their importance. All trials, whether they are exploring aspects of the pharmacokinetics or of the pharmacodynamics of a drug, should be controlled studies. There may be more patients or subjects receiving the new chemical entity compared with placebo, but there should always be a placebo control in this early stage. Such a design at least gives the observer an opportunity, albeit small, to put into perspective a certain adverse reaction. When early trials are placebo-controlled, statements about causality and prevalence can be somewhat more definite, at least when several trials are looked at in the aggregate.

Placebo-controlled studies may also allow for estimating a dose response for a particular reaction. The advantage of early trials is detecting drug-induced adverse events. Subjects or patients participating should not be allowed to take any concomitant medications. An adverse event occurring under these circumstances will be easier to attribute to the introduction of the experimental drug, and not confounded by drug interactions or by the effects of another agent. Karch and Lasagna (1975) pointed out the difficulties in interpreting adverse reactions arising from drug interactions. If an adverse reaction is thought to have occurred, and was thought to be due to the drug described, a rechallenge can be helpful in distinguishing an effect of the drug from a chance occurrence.

It is also important early in clinical development to try to establish whether a particular complaint is a drug reaction, part of the disease progression or an event which occurs with significant frequency in normal adults in the absence of any drug treatment.

Placebo-controlled studies are also favoured in this context. Examples of events which occur frequently in the normal population are complaints such as headache, sleep disturbances, nausea and fatigue. Events which could be disease progression are illustrated by an increase in angina pectoris in patients with coronary artery disease. Complaints are often serious, and therefore it behoves the clinical monitor to try to separate these different categories.

Detection and recognition of drug-induced adverse events may have a very profound effect on a development programme. The detection of such a serious adverse event may actually be the crucial decision point in a go/no go decision chain of drug development. Early identification of serious untoward events may save a corporation vast sums of money in development costs, compared with discovering these events during the postmarketing surveillance. An example of the latter is the ophthalmological side-effects of practolol and the thalidomide catastrophe.

Despite the perceived advantage of controls in early clinical trials, it is rare for a Phase I study, owing to its small size, to yield enough information on a non-serious adverse effect to definitely assign causality. However, the suggestion of causality must be entertained seriously by the observers. The close observation of subjects in early clinical trials is extremely valuable, because the monitor is able to gain first-hand knowledge of adverse events. This supervision is usually only possible in Phase I and in early Phase II, owing to the small number of subjects. However, if the study remains open-labelled and uncontrolled, the validity of any assessment of adverse reactions, be they serious or not, is open to question. When designing early studies, in order to evaluate safety, it is important and useful if the demography of subjects is not too restricted, so that events which are more frequent in a particular subset of patients or subjects might be suspected early in development, although confirmation of such a predilection will require a large safety trial. However, the earlier in a development programme this is considered, the better the long-term and multicentre programme will be designed.

To more definitively determine causality of an adverse event, several methods have been developed. The most reliable is the rechallenge, as described by Karch and Lasagna (1975). By definition, a specific adverse event is described as drug-related if it disappears on stopping the drug and reappears in the same form on reintroduction. This technique is more readily employed for rare events in very early clinical trials, where the participating number of patients, or subjects, is small, and therefore renders such a rechallenge manageable. It is advisable to perform a rechallenge under strict medical supervision, so that one can treat any further side-effects that may arise from the rechallenge. At times the adverse event may be so serious that the attempt to induce it is too risky, since the patient or subject will rarely gain a personal advantage from the experience.

So far very little has been said about the usage of specific laboratory tests. It is self-evident that all clinical trials include history and physical examination, both at screening for enrolment and at preset times during the duration of the study. The physical examination should be thorough and the case report form be detailed enough to capture all clinical information obtained. If drug therapy is aimed at a specific organ, the physical examination of that organ and its related function become particularly important, not only to detect adverse reactions, but also to obtain efficacy information. Other laboratory parameters used to obtain early information should include ECG and a broad biochemical screen. It is possible that a certain adverse reaction may be detected by these methods at an earlier stage than by clinical symptomatology, either objectively or subjectively. AV-block I with certain antiarrhythmic drugs is a good example of such a reaction, where the ECG will be more helpful than the clinical examination. Leakage of microproteins through the kidney membranes is another such example, where sophisticated laboratory methods are more useful than clinical examination. Depending on the pharmacological activity of the test agent, a specifically designed laboratory protocol may be used, already in Phase I, and certainly in Phase II studies.

The assessment of adverse reactions in early clinical studies must also take into account whether a certain reaction was present prior to the subject or patient entering the study. Here it is important to evaluate whether a change of status has occurred during treatment, and whether this change should be attributed to the test agent or possibly an underlying disease. Is, for example, increased angina in a subject treated with a dihydropyridine an expression of progression of disease or an adverse reaction caused by vasodilatation? Another very common example is headache, which even during short studies may change in severity. If such is the case, it is very important for the investigator to try to assess whether the severity changes were due to pharmacological actions of the test agent or not. In this assessment he/she may be guided by the questionnaire method discussed above.

DISCUSSION

Most of the published literature on adverse drug reactions has addressed causality, and has defined different algorithms to try to reach objective decision points. Kramer *et al.* (1979 provided such an algorithm, which takes into account previous general experience with the drug, alternative aetiological candidates, timing of events, drug concentrations and evidence of overdose, and rechallenge. All these factors are important and will be useful, but only a few of them will be helpful in very early clinical development, since some are not known until a large number of patients have been exposed to the experimental drug. Therefore, the production of a probability score may not be as important as a particularly objective assessment of the subjective symptoms in combination with widespread knowledge of the pharmacological properties of a drug or a class of drugs. This was pointed out by Naranjo *et al.* (1981), who demonstrated the relative lack of interobserver variation when a questionnaire included at least one question which asked for an evaluation of an adverse event within the context of the known pharmacology of the drug. Such a question was thus assigned a weight different from that assigned to less directed questions. Such a process was considered to introduce biases but it remains unclear how it affects the conclusions.

The pharmacological properties of a test agent may also cause its more serious adverse reactions. An example of this is the first-dose blood-pressure-lowering effect of the ACE inhibitors. These adverse events may also be dose-related—namely the higher the dose is pushed to achieve maximum pharmacological effect, the more dangerous this effect may be as an adverse event. This may and probably should lead to development of new drugs that maintain the pharmacological benefits without turning them into adverse events. The development of a renin inhibitor may be such an example, where more specific enzyme blockage may lead to higher tolerability. This, however, has to be proven to be the case. Similar examples could be found within groups of drugs used in other therapeutic areas—for example, antiplatelet drugs, antineoplastic drugs.

Phase IV studies with large patient populations have also been used to describe adverse reactions to drugs. Several methods, such as spontaneous reporting (Rossi *et al.*, 1983), formal postmarketing surveillance (Inman, 1981) and record linkage (Pere *et al.*, 1987), have been described to better characterise an individual event. However, as is evident from previous discussions, these techniques do not lend themselves to application in the early Phase I or Phase II trials. The only method which it may be possible to use in Phase II clinical pharmacology studies is record linkage. It is possible to link adverse reactions, as single events, to events recorded in hospital records and in clinical follow-up of the patient's condition. An example of where record linkage may be useful is neutropenia or agranulocytosis. Hospital charts may provide a good record to follow these patients on a clinical basis. The number of white blood cells prior to and after introduction, as well as after withdrawal of the experimental drug, could be determined.

A methodology described by Venulet *et al.* (1986), utilising in-house monitoring, does not easily lend itself to early detection of adverse events, since only a large experience can give definitive information. However, the data collected should start early in clinical testing.

It is imperative that clinical monitors closely follow the results of early trials, as was described in the previous section. By doing that, their awareness of events will be raised and they will more readily detect serious events.

In early clinical trials the pharmacological knowledge becomes important as well as a mind open to analysing unexpected adverse events. Knowledge about previous drugs in a certain class may direct the search for certain side-effects in a preconceived way. There exists a danger that other new equally serious or important adverse reactions are overlooked in the early development phases. Rechallenge is probably our best method of assessing the causality of an event in our early clinical trials, but it cannot always be attempted.

REFERENCES

Huskisson, E. C. and Wojtulewski, J. A. (1977). Measurements of side effects of drugs. *Br. Med. J.*, ii, 698–9

Hutchinson, T. A. (1986). Standardized assessment methods for adverse drug reactions: a review of previous approaches and their problems. *Drug Inf. J.*, **20**, 439–44

Inman, W. H. (1981). Postmarketing surveillance of adverse drug reactions in general practice. *Br. Med. J.*, **282**, 1131–2

Karch, F. E. and Lasagna, L. (1975). Adverse drug reactions. *J. Am. Med. Ass.*, **234**, 1236–71

Kramer, S. M., Leuenthal, J. M., Hutchinson, T. A. and Feinstein, A. R. (1979). An algorithm for the operational assessment of adverse drug reactions. *J. Am. Med. Ass.*, **272**, 623–32

Naranjo, C. A., Busto, V., Sellers, E. M., Sandor, P., Ruiz, I., Roberts, E. A., Janecek, E., Domecq, C. and Greenblatt, D. J. (1981). A method for estimating the probability of adverse drug reactions. *Clin. Pharm. Ther.*, **30**, 239–45

Pere, J. C., Begaud, B., Haramburu, F. and Albin, H. (1987). Less croisements de fichiers une technique intéressante en pharmacovigilance. *Therapie*, **72**, 59–62

Rossi, A. C., Knapp, D. E., Anello, C., O'Neill, R. T., Graham, C. F., Mendelis, P. S. and Stanley, S. R. (1983). Discovery of adverse drug reactions: a comparison of selected Phase IV studies with spontaneous reporting methods. *J. Am. Med. Ass.*, **279**, 2226–8

Venulet, J. Ciucci, A. G. and Berneber, G. C. (1986). Updating of a method for causality assessment of adverse drug reactions. *Int. J. Clin. Pharmacol. Ther. Toxicol.*, **24**, 559–68

18
The Assessment of Pharmacodynamic Effects

J. D. Harry

Head, Clinical Pharmacology Unit, ICI Pharmaceuticals, Mereside, Alderley Edge, Cheshire, UK

INTRODUCTION

Important objectives of the early studies in man, and particularly of volunteer studies, of a putative compound include the generation of data to allow decisions to be made about the further development of the compound. This further development will include studies in patients with the disease for which the compound is targeted with the aim of producing a useful therapeutic agent. The data from early studies in man (Phase I and early Phase II studies) consist of aspects of the pharmacodynamic properties of the compound (what the compound does to man), pharmacokinetic properties (what the body does to the compound) and safety and tolerance. If these aspects of the data generated in early studies suggest that the compound should proceed in development, then early studies should, where possible, provide data on what end-points might be useful in patient studies, what dose and what dosing regimen is sensible to start in patients, and what side-effects should be looked for. Ideally, both pharmacokinetic and pharmacodynamic studies are important in producing data of the kind required for later work. However, in selecting dose and dosing regimens, in particular, pharmacodynamic assessments are especially important. Unfortunately, measurements of pharmacodynamic parameters are not always easy and may require sophisticated and expensive equipment. Considerations of this kind may help to explain the emphasis of the past years on developing pharmacokinetic data rather than dynamic data for new compounds in early studies. This is not to decry the value of pharmacokinetic data in drug development in general. Certainly, the metabolism of a compound in man is useful to know early in development, to put into context the toxicological studies performed in animals; however, it is very unusual for a compound to be removed from 'development' if it is producing anticipated pharmacodynamic effects in man, and no side-effects and yet is metabolised differently in man compared with the animals used in toxicological evaluation. Such situations might require further toxicology of the compound in another animal species which does produce similar matabolism to man, or further toxicology to be performed with the major metabolites seen in man but not present in the species used for toxicology studies (Parke,

1987). These answers would be required to satisfy some regulatory authorities. Further, it must be accepted that it is not always possible to measure pharmacodynamic effects with all compounds, e.g. antibiotics, where the essential measurement for 'efficacy' in volunteer studies will be the concentrations of a drug in the blood which will be known from *in vitro* studies to be effective against the bacteria concerned. Therefore, it is clear that pharmacokinetic and pharmacodynamic assessments are important in the early phases of developing a new compound, the relative importance of each depending upon the compound under consideration.

However, in the main, where pharmacodynamic assessments can be made in early studies they should be made, ideally together with kinetic assessments. This chapter deals with pharmacodynamic assessments in early development (particularly in volunteer studies), highlighting their value in making decisions about compounds at this stage of development, but at the same time adding a word of caution that the assessments have to be performed correctly to obtain reliable evidence.

VALUE OF PHARMACODYNAMIC ASSESSMENTS TO EARLY DRUG DEVELOPMENT

Pharmacology in Man

During the preclinical development of a putative compound, the animal pharmacology is clearly delineated. Such pharmacology is presumed to be a relevant model of the eventual clinical usefulness of the compound, e.g. an antiulcer agent which should produce its efficacy by reducing acid secretion from the stomach would be expected to show such pharmacology in animals, with evidence to support how it reduces acid secretion. Therefore, these pharmacological effects seen in animals, being possible models of the disease status, should be identified in man as soon as possible. Only when they are seen in man can evidence be gained that the compound is likely to have therapeutic activity.

The demonstration of pharmacological properties in man can be achieved in many ways. In many cases the pharmacology seen in animals can be measured in man with the same tests. Thus, a compound which is a β-adrenoceptor blocking agent in animals would be expected in man to reduce the heart rate response to exercise or to antagonise the effects of a full β-adrenoceptor agonist (Harry, 1977). In other instances the investigations in man may be indirect assessments which are related to the pharmacology seen in animals. An example of this may be the *ex vivo* test of a thromboxane antagonist, where the compound can be given to man and blood taken from the subject and tested against *in vitro* platelet aggregation induced by a thromboxane agonist (Patscheke *et al.*, 1986). An estimate of a biochemical end-point may also be considered to demonstrate that a compound has pharmacological activity in man. As an example, diuretic agents shown in animal studies to alter excretion of Na^+ and K^+ in the urine can be shown to produce the same effect in normal volunteers after a single dose (Baba *et al.*, 1968). Thus, the demonstration in man that a putative compound has the same pharmacology as in animals can be achieved in several ways.

In early drug development, if a compound should be expected to produce pharmacodynamic effects, then these should be sought in appropriate studies. If no such effects are seen in properly designed studies using sensitive and validated test models, then questions must be asked before progressing to further studies. There may be several reasons for the lack of effect, some of which are listed below:

(1) The lack of effects might be related to not achieving a blood level sufficient to produce the pharmacodynamic effects. Higher doses than expected may therefore be required to demonstrate the expected effects. Pharmacokinetic investigations may be needed to identify whether factors such as absorption, metabolism or the blood–brain barrier are responsible for the lack of effect.

(2) The pharmacological test may not be sensitive enough to allow the pharmacodynamic effect to be seen. The 'sensitivity' of the method should have been estimated before testing a new compound. This can be achieved with the use of compounds known to produce changes in a subject which can be detected by the method. Such a study will produce confidence in the methodology, as well as data on the size of effect expected (e.g. Harry *et al.*, 1988).

(3) The compound may not produce the same pharmacology in man as in animal models.

If the expected pharmacodynamic effects can be measured with a compound, then clearly the next stages of development can proceed. A greater difficulty, however, is what to do if no pharmacodynamic effects are seen and should be expected. The answers may be obvious, e.g. there may be lack of absorption of the compound, or a massive 'first pass effect', leaving no active drug in the circulation. In these instances development may be terminated. However, if the reasons are not obvious, further investigations should be performed in patients with the disease for which the compound is targeted. It is possible that the pharmacology of the compound may not be related to its therapeutic effect, e.g. the antihypertensive effect of β-adrenoceptor blocking agents, and so therapeutic efficacy may be missed. If results in one or two such studies are negative, i.e. no therapeutic effects, then development should be abandoned. If no pharmacodynamic effects are seen (when looked for) in early volunteer studies, then limited patient exposure should be investigated. Further work in other areas, e.g. toxicology, should await these results.

Dose to Produce Pharmacodynamic Effects

If pharmacodynamic effects are seen in normal volunteers which are related to the expected therapeutic action of the compound, then a clear estimate of the dose to give to patients for efficacy studies can be obtained. This is particularly applicable to the H_2 antagonist group of drugs which are used to suppress acid secretion. The therapeutic effects of the H_2 antagonists are dependent upon their ability to suppress acid secretion. If the range of doses is known to prevent secretion (e.g. stimulated by pentagastrin, histamine or food), then these doses would be the ones to determine whether acid secretion is prevented in patients with peptic ulcers (e.g. Brogden *et al.*, 1978). If patients behave differently compared with volunteers, then adjustment of dose will be required. However, the important point is to decide at which dose to commence patient studies, and this should be similar to that which produces the pharmacological effects seen in animal studies and reproduced in man.

Duration of Action of the Pharmacodynamic Effect

Assessments of the pharmacodynamic effects in normal volunteers not only allows the unit dose around which to proceed into studies in patients to be determined, but can also give some indication of the dosing regimen to be followed. This can be estimated by measuring the duration of the pharmacodynamic effect following a single dose in normal volunteers. To illustrate this point, Visacor (ICI; a selective β_1-adrenoceptor partial agonist) has been shown to produce blockade of β_1-adrenoceptors following single oral doses of 10–400 mg (Harry *et al.*, 1984; Pringle *et al.*, 1986) at various time points after dosing, but of these doses only the 200 mg dose was effective for over 24 h after a single dose. Thus, Visacor should be able to produce effective blockade of β_1-adrenoceptors in man for over 24 h when administered once daily. The antianginal (and possibly the antihypertensive) effects of β-adrenoceptor blocking agents are related to the ability of these compounds to produce blockade of β-adrenoceptors. Therefore, pharmacodynamic results in normal volunteers predict that Visacor should be an effective antianginal agent at a dose of 200 mg once daily. Studies in patients with angina pectoris have confirmed this (Berkenboom *et al.*, 1987).

By estimating the duration of action of pharmacodynamic effects of a compound, especially where this may be a model of the therapeutic effect, the unit dose to produce the dosing regimen required can be ascertained. Thus, by using a range of doses, the dose producing an approximately 8 h duration of pharmacodynamic effect will allow dosing three times per day; 12 h, twice per day; and 24 h, once per day. In practice, it is not possible to have a range of doses to allow such a range of durations, because of various factors, e.g. absorption may be saturated at doses required for longer duration, transit through the gut will not allow sufficient time at an absorption area and larger degrees of absorption may be associated with higher blood levels and resultant side-effects. However, the introduction of slow-release formulations can overcome some of these problems. Such formulations can be tested for extended duration of action with pharmacodynamic effects, as shown for the long-acting preparation of the β-adrenoceptor blocking agent propranolol (McAinsh *et al.*, 1978).

Ideally, to determine a unit dose for a given dosing regimen, both pharmacokinetic and pharmacodynamic data are required. By measuring the elimination half-life $(T_{\frac{1}{2}})$ of a compound from the blood and assessing the minimum blood level to produce the desired pharmacological effect, a dose can be accurately estimated to give the desired duration of effect (Figure 18.1).

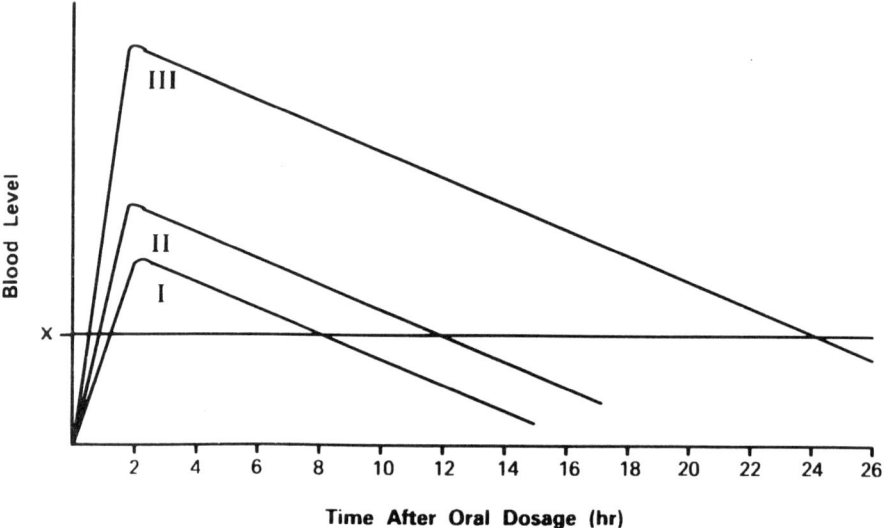

Figure 18.1 Relationship between blood levels and time after oral dosing with 3 doses (I, II, III) of a putative new compound. X = Minimum blood levels to produce desired pharmacological effect. Dose I would allow tid dosing. Dose II would allow bid dosing. Dose III would allow once daily dosing

Determination of Possible Side-effects of Putative Compounds

The animal pharmacology of a putative compound may show effects in biological systems other than that system in which the chemical should be effective, e.g. a β-adrenoceptor blocking agent, which should affect essentially the cardiovascular system, may be shown to affect some tests of central nervous function. These effects in the central nervous system may be investigated in man during the early studies. Thus, by performing pharmacodynamic tests of CNS function, e.g. single or complex reaction times, tests of mood with visual analogue scales and EEG effects (either waking or sleeping), a β-adrenoceptor blocking agent could be 'screened' for possible CNS effects (e.g. Salem and McDevitt, 1984). If effects are seen, the relevance to the clinical therapeutic effects may be positive or negative, but at least possible central nervous system side-effects should be investigated more fully during later clinical studies.

FACTORS TO BE CONSIDERED IN PERFORMING PHARMACODYNAMIC ASSESSMENTS IN MAN

As alluded to earlier in this chapter, it is vitally important that pharmacodynamic assessments of putative drugs in man during the early assessment period be properly performed. No decisions on the future progress of a compound in the development process can be properly made unless the results of studies can be relied upon. Consequently, as with any other clinical trials or investigations, design of studies is crucial. It is not intended to discuss aspects of study design exhaustively in this chapter, but certain basic philosophies need to be mentioned when considering the assessment of pharmacodynamic effects of drugs in man.

Design of the Study

Important in any study involving man, and in particular when assessing pharmacodynamic responses to new compounds, is the problem of variability within human subjects. This problem can be considered either troublesome or fascinating, but needs to be considered carefully in designing studies of drug effects. Variability in responses to compounds can be caused by such factors as age, body size, disease states, etc. In many instances subjects may show a profound placebo effect, in particular if the end-effect being estimated involves subjective rather than objective criteria. Thus, design of studies to assess pharmacodynamic effects has to try to minimise variability. The design will always depend upon the questions posed in any particular study, but, in general, all studies should be placebo-controlled and randomised. 'Blindness' of the study will depend upon the assessments being estimated. Inclusion and exclusion criteria can reduce variability inherent with age, body weight, etc. 'Within-volunteer' studies can further help to reduce variability and reduce the number of volunteers required in early studies.

Reliability of Methodology for Assessing Pharmacodynamic Responses

Methods used to measure the pharmacodynamic effects of compounds need to relate to the assessments and be reliable and reproducible. Invariably, where initial studies in volunteers are concerned, the methods used will be 'non-invasive'. Reproducibility of the method must be established, possibly both when used by a single observer (intraobserver variability) or by several observers (interobserver variability), before any study with a new compound is performed. The method should be tested with established drugs to prove that it is measuring the assessment it should be measuring and to estimate its sensitivity to any changes induced by these drugs, so that the kind of change looked for from a new compound can be expected to be seen. To illustrate the above, a validation of a new portable infrared device for measuring the pupil diameter in man has been carried out. To show that the method was measuring the pupil size, a study was performed comparing known mydriatic and miotic compounds with placebo on pupil size after instilling the compounds into the eyes of normal volunteers. The results gave the expected answer (Figure 18.2: Millson *et al.*, 1988b). Some estimate of within-observer variability was obtained and the method was then used to determine whether a new anti-5HT$_2$ agent affected the pupil (Millson *et al.*, 1988a).

Resting Pupil Diameter
(Mean ±95% Confidence Limits)

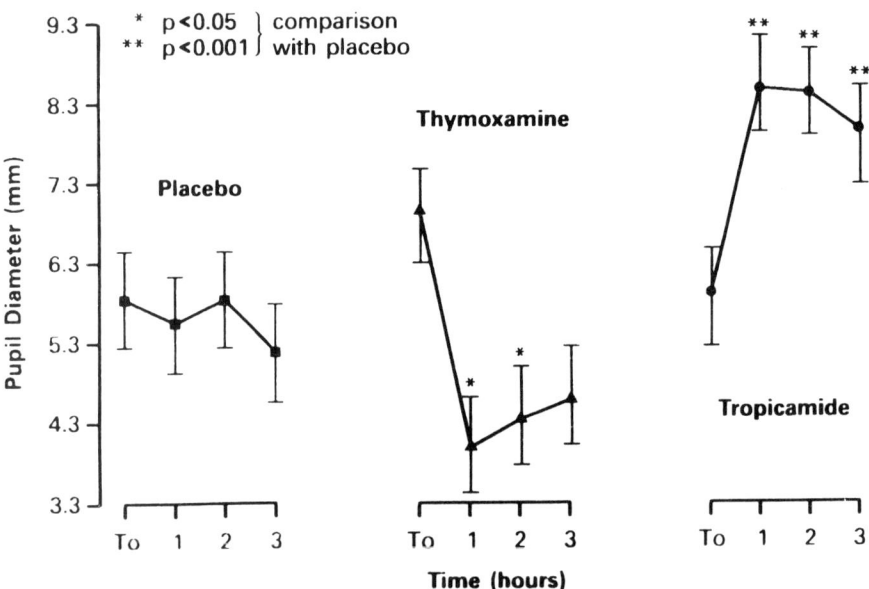

Figure 18.2 Mean (±95% CL) of resting pupil diameter before (T_0) and 1, 2 and 3 h after instillation into the eye of placebo, thymoxamine and tropicamide *$p < 0.05$, **$p < 0.001$, comparing postdose values after thymoxamine and tropicamide with those after placebo

Statistical Power of the Studies

It is important in studies to determine the pharmacodynamic effect of a new compound that the numbers of subjects in a study are sufficient to detect the type of changes which might occur. It is important not to make decisions about the action of a compound if Type II errors, in particular, cannot be eliminated (i.e. finding no differences from placebo when one exists). When pharmacodynamic investigations with a new compound begin, it may not be possible to assess the numbers of subjects required in a study to allow a reasonable value for β (probability of finding no difference when one exists). Thus, to answer a specific question of activity over placebo, two or three studies may be required. The first one uses small numbers (say 4–6) of subjects to obtain an estimate of effect, so that a second or third study can then be designed with adequate power to determine whether an effect is present or not.

CONCLUSIONS

Pharmacodynamic assessments in early studies of a compound in man (especially volunteer studies) can provide vital evidence to aid future investigations in patients. The dose and dosing regimen obtained from volunteer studies in which the pharmacological effects are seen should be the ones around which to commence early patient studies. Evidence may be collected to direct specific questions in patient studies to find early possible side-effects of a new compound. In general, pharmacodynamic and pharmacokinetic assessments should be made together in early studies, to obtain most information for future studies. However, studies to measure pharmacodynamic effects in man must be properly designed, using validated techniques, to prevent wrong conclusions being drawn.

REFERENCES

Baba, W. I., Lant, A. F., Smith, A. J., Townsend, M. M. and Wilson, G. A. (1968). Pharmacological effects in animals and normal human subjects of the diuretic amiloride hydrochloride (MK-870). *Clin. Pharm. Ther.*, **9**, 318–27

Berkenboom, G. M., Ibrahim, T., Abramounicz, M. and Degre, S. G. (1987). Comparison of the immediate effects of two beta-blocking drugs; non-selective and cardioselective with modest ISA in exercise induced angina. *Cardiology*, **74**, 43–8

Brogden, R. N., Heal, R. C., Speight, T. M. and Avery, C. S. (1978). Cimetidine: A review of its pharmacological properties and therapeutic efficacy in peptic ulcer disease. *Drugs*, **15**, 93–131

Harry, J. D. (1977). The demonstration of atenolol as a beta-adrenoceptor blocking drug in man. *Postgrad. Med. J.*, **53** (Suppl. 3), 65–9

Harry, J. D., Millson, D. S. and Morton, P. B. (1988). Use of Doppler echocardiography to determine the cardiac effects of dobutamine in volunteers. *Pharm. Med.*, **3**, 173–83

Harry, J. D., Norris, S. C., Young, J., Wardleworth, A., Corlett, C. and Morton, P. (1984). The demonstration of ICI 141,292 as a β-adrenoceptor blocking agent in man. *Br. J. Clin. Pharm.*, **18**, 291P

McAinsh, J., Baber, N. S., Smith, R. and Young, J. (1978). Pharmacokinetic and pharmacodynamic studies with long acting propranolol. *Br. J. Clin. Pharm.*, **6**, 115–21

Millson, D. S., Harry, J. D., Howarth, S. J. and Wilkinson, D. (1988a). Effects of a 5-HT$_2$ antagonist (ICI 169,369) on human pupillary responses. *Br. J. Clin. Pharm.* (in press)

Millson, D. S., Harry, J. D. and Wilkinson, D. (1988b). Measurement of pupillary responses to miotic and mydriatic drugs in human volunteers using a portable infrared pupillometer. *Br. J. Clin. Pharm.*, **26**, 200P

Parke, D. V. (1987). Metabolism and toxicokinetic studies in the safety evaluation of drugs and other chemicals. In Berford, D. J., Bridges, J. W. and Gibson, G. C. (Eds.), *Drug Metabolism—From Molecules to Man*. Taylor and Francis, London, pp. 477–92

Patscheke, H., Staiger, C., Neigebauer, G., Kaufmann, B., Strein, K., Endele, R. and Stegmecer, K. (1986). The pharmacokinetic and pharmacodynamic profiles of the thromboxane A-2 receptor blocker BM13.177. *Clin. Pharm. Ther.*, **39**, 145–50

Pringle, T. H., O'Connor, P. C., McNeill, A. J., Finch, M. B., Riddell, J. G. and Shanks, R. G. (1986). Effects of ICI 141,292 on exercise tachycardia and isoprenaline induced β-adrenoceptor responses in man. *Br. J. Clin. Pharm.*, **21**, 249–58

Salem, S. A. M. and McDevitt, D. G. (1984). Central effects of single oral doses of propranolol in man. *Br. J. Clin. Pharm.*, **17**, 31–6

19

The Assessment of Pharmacokinetics

Stephen Toon

Medeval Ltd, University of Manchester, Manchester M15 4SH, UK

INTRODUCTION

Pharmacokinetic assessment of new drug entities forms a pivotal part of any pharmaceutical development programme. Although primarily providing data to support toxicological and efficacy studies, carefully designed and executed pharmacokinetic studies in early drug development can greatly enhance decision-making processes involved in formulation development, as well as providing indications of potential problems that may arise later in the clinical assessment of the new drug entity.

To some individuals, Phase I pharmacokinetic studies are synonymous with the assessment of bioavailability. Undoubtedly, bioavailability testing forms an important component of Phase I pharmacokinetic assessment, but one must remember that for the optimum design and execution of a bioavailability study, the pharmacokinetic characteristics of the drug in question must be known.

As one might envisage, increasing scientific awareness ultimately influences the expectations of regulatory authorities as they relate to data filed in support of New Drug Applications (NDAs), and in turn the design and objectives of Phase I pharmacokinetic studies. The importance of considering the pharmacokinetics of the individual enantiomers of chiral drug substances intended for clinical administration as the racemate is already being highlighted in regulatory documentation. Consequently, it is essential that the design and interpretation of Phase I pharmacokinetic studies involving chiral drugs be based on an understanding of the potential influences of stereochemistry.

The assessment of bioavailability is thus an established and integral part of any Phase I pharmacokinetic programme, but to what extent stereochemical aspects of the pharmacokinetics of chiral drug substances should be investigated in early drug development is still a highly debatable issue. Therefore, this chapter intends to focus on these two areas of investigation: one established practice and one causing increasing concern to the regulatory agencies.

THE ASSESSMENT OF BIOAVAILABILITY

The current definition of bioavailability is one relating to both the extent and rate of drug absorption and delivery to the systemic circulation. Previous definitions had solely emphasised the extent of absorption by expressing bioavailability as that fraction of the administered dose of drug reaching the systemic circulation intact. For certain drugs, however, the rate of entry into the systemic circulation has been shown to influence the ensuing pharmacological response.

Assessment of bioavailability is a key element in the pharmacokinetic characterisation of any new drug entity, but particularly for drugs with a narrow therapeutic index, a high clearance, or variable or poor absorption. The bioavailability of a drug has important implications with respect to the proposed route of administration, formulation design and the protocol by which preclinical toxicology studies are undertaken.

The extent of absorption is much more readily quantified than the absorption rate and is usually equated with the fraction of the administered dose that reaches the systemic circulation as unchanged drug (F). Most bioavailability assessments require pharmacokinetic characterisation of the drug on two separate occasions, with the extent of absorption being quantified by comparison of either the area under the plasma drug concentration–time curve (AUC) or the amount of drug excreted into the urine unchanged (A_e) associated with the two administrations, one of which is regarded as the reference dose and the other as the test dose. Quantification of the absolute bioavailability is achieved by the administration of the drug of interest intravenously (reference dose) and orally (test dose; a solution, suspension or solid dosage form), characteristically according to a randomised two-way crossover design. The extent of absorption is then calculated as the ratio between either AUC or A_e following oral administration and that following intravenous administration. Direct comparison of these independent administrations, sometimes separated by a period of several weeks, is undertaken with an assumption of constancy of various pharmacokinetic parameters between treatments. Comparisons of AUC assume that the total clearance is constant between doses. When urinary excretion measurements are utilised, it is assumed that the ratio between renal and non-renal clearance is constant. It is often difficult to ascertain whether such assumptions are always valid.

There have been several mathematical approaches proposed which are designed to take into account the intrasubject variability encountered in bioavailability assessment. Kwan and Till (1973) reported a method of assessing the extent of absorption based upon estimation of the changes in clearance which occur between treatments. A knowledge of the relative magnitude of the pathways of elimination of the drug in question enables the appropriate correction to be made in the assessment of bioavailability. For instance, for a drug that is predominantly eliminated via the renal route, one might assume that intrasubject variations in renal clearance (Cl_R) may be a major determinant in any observed variability in F and that non-renal clearance (Cl_{NR}), the minor route of elimination, may be regarded as constant between treatments. The equation derived for this situation by

Kwan and Till is shown below:

$$F_{\text{p.o.}} = \left(\text{Cl}_{\text{R,p.o.}} - \text{Cl}_{\text{R,i.v.}} + \frac{D_{\text{i.v.}}}{\text{AUC}_{\text{i.v.}}} \right) \frac{\text{AUC}_{\text{p.o.}}}{D_{\text{p.o.}}}$$

where the suffixes 'i.v.' and 'p.o.' refer to the intravenous and oral (or extravascular) routes, respectively, and D is the dose of drug given. Comparison of this equation with the standard equation used to calculate F,

$$F_{\text{p.o.}} = \frac{D_{\text{i.v.}} \, \text{AUC}_{\text{p.o.}}}{D_{\text{p.o.}} \, \text{AUC}_{\text{i.v.}}}$$

indicates that $\text{Cl}_{\text{R,p.o.}} - \text{Cl}_{\text{R,i.v.}}$ is the correction factor compensating for the variability in renal clearance. A similar approach could be applied for drugs eliminated primarily via non-renal pathways. Toon *et al.* (1989) examined differing mathematical approaches to the assessment of the absolute bioavailability of clonidine delivered transdermally. In this instance little difference was observed between the methods utilised to calculate F, indicating that the renal and non-renal routes of clonidine elimination were equally variable. Other mathematical approaches aimed at compensation for intrasubject variability observed both between and within the phases of a study designed to assess the extent of absorption have been discussed in detail by Cutler (1981).

Stable isotope methodology has been used as an experimental approach to overcome the problems of intrasubject and intersubject pharmacokinetic variability which may compromise statistical analysis and interpretation of bioavailability data. Assessment of bioavailability using stable isotopes involves the simultaneous administration of the test dose of drug and the reference dose (the intravenous dose, if absolute bioavailability is being assessed). The drug contained in one of the doses is labelled (enriched) with one or more stable isotopes (i.e. ^2H, ^{13}C, ^{15}N). Chemically, therefore, the drug originating from the two routes of administration may be distinguished by a difference in molecular mass. This mass difference may be detected by use of mass spectrometry; for instance, operating the mass spectrometer in the selected ion monitoring mode, one can quantify unlabelled drug delivered by one route at mass m and drug labelled with ^{13}C delivered by the other route at $m + 1$. Coupled with gas chromatography, mass spectrometry (GC-MS) provides a highly specific and sensitive analytical technique. Intraindividual variability, as encountered on administering drug to an individual on two discrete occasions, is for all intents and purposes eliminated with this experimental approach; at least within subject, error is constant for both forms of the drug. The reliability of the comparison between the two doses of drug is, therefore, greatly enhanced by their simultaneous administration. Statistical statements relating to the comparison are also strengthened, with the same levels of significance and power being achieved with fewer volunteers (Heck *et al.*, 1979). More practical aspects of bioavailability design are also benefited by the stable isotope approach. In essence, both phases of a conventionally designed study are undertaken simultaneously, thereby reducing the duration of the study by half. Similarly, as both labelled and unlabelled drug can be quantified in the same sample, the number of assays required to facilitate an assessment of bioavailability is also halved.

However, the utilisation of stable isotope-labelled drug in the assessment of bioavailability is not without problems. The major assumption underlying the simultaneous administration of a labelled and non-isotopically-labelled drug is that the body cannot distinguish between the two species. This need not be the case, especially when dealing with molecules labelled with deuterium (Blake *et al.*, 1975). Molecular isotope effects may result in differential pharmacokinetics and/or toxicity (Baillie, 1981) between the labelled and unlabelled species, making comparisons between the two species invalid. Although positioning of the label in a metabolically inert position on the drug molecule may avoid the influence of isotope effects, prestudy investigations into the potential manifestation of such phenomena are obligatory, especially when employing deuterated homologues. Furthermore, simultaneous administration of two clinically relevant doses of drug could lead to undesirable toxicity or pharmacokinetic non-linearity should any dose dependency exist. Availability, either synthetic or commercial, of the labelled drug is also a major determinant in the undertaking of bioavailability assessment using stable isotope techniques.

Assessment of the extent of absorption almost invariably relies upon an estimation of the area under the plasma drug concentration–time curve (AUC). Following single-dose administration, comparison between the test and reference formulations is made with values of AUC estimated between time zero and infinity. Practically, AUC estimation is split into two parts: that which may be determined empirically ($AUC_{(0,t)}$) and that which is calculated via extrapolation from the last experimental data point to infinity ($AUC_{(t,\infty)}$).

The most commonly adopted approach of estimating $AUC_{(0,t)}$ is the linear trapezoidal method (Gibaldi and Perrier, 1982). The underlying assumption of this method is that two consecutive concentration–time points are related linearly. Therefore, any deviation from this linear approximation may result in an error in area estimation. Chiou (1978) and Yeh and Kwan (1978) have investigated the errors associated with area estimation by the trapezoidal method. For a function which declines monoexponentially it has been shown that the log-trapezoidal method provides a better estimate of area. Here the underlying assumption is that two consecutive concentration–time points are related through an exponential function, which, for declining *in vivo* drug concentrations, is not unreasonable. However, for ascending concentration–time data, as observed during drug absorption, it has been shown that application of the log-trapezoidal method produces very large errors in area estimation. The ideal combination of approaches, therefore, seems to be to adopt the linear-trapezoidal method up to the peak concentration and the log-trapezoidal method thereafter.

Estimation of the residual area between the last experimental data point and infinity is normally estimated by the equation

$$AUC_{(t,\infty)} = \frac{C_t}{k}$$

where C_t is the plasma drug concentration at time t and k is the elimination rate constant. The accuracy of estimation of $\text{AUC}_{(t,\infty)}$ is therefore dependent upon the quality of the estimate of C_t and k. Utilisation of the experimentally determined value for C_t assumes that there is no error in its estimation. In reality this is unlikely to be the case. A more appropriate approach, therefore, is to utilise a predicted value for C_t ($\hat{C}_t$) obtained from the model describing the parent data set, as in this situation precision in the estimation of $\hat{C}_t$ is determined by the quality of the entire data set (i.e. several data points as opposed to one). In many instances the terminal slope of a plasma drug concentration–time profile following extravascular administration reflects elimination, and the rate constant associated with the slope is the elimination rate constant k. The situation may arise, however, where absorption of the drug is sufficiently slow for it to become the rate-limiting step in the overall absorption–disposition process, so that the terminal slope primarily reflects absorption and not elimination ('flip–flop'). Under these circumstances the calculation of $\text{AUC}_{(t,\infty)}$ poses a dilemma. Figure 19.1 shows two plasma theophylline concentration–time profiles relating to single oral doses of theophylline, one a solution and the other a controlled release (CR) formulation, but both administered to the same volunteer on separate occasions. We know that the terminal rate constant associated with the

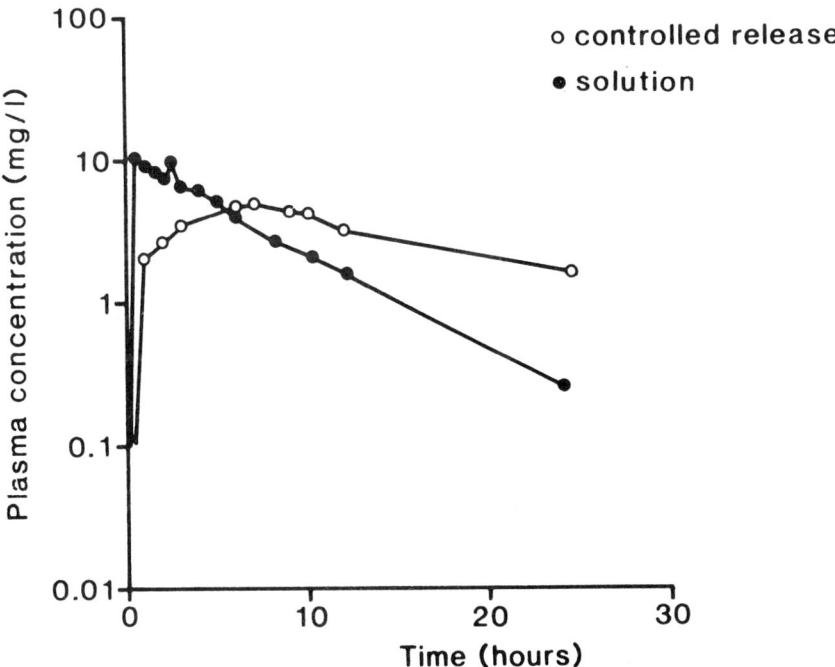

Figure 19.1 Plasma theophylline concentration–time profiles following the oral administration of 400 mg of theophylline either in solution or as a controlled release formulation to a healthy non-smoking male volunteer

solution solely reflects elimination and so, even graphically, it is apparent that the terminal slope of the controlled release formulation is primarily reflecting absorption. The dilemma is in deciding which rate constant to use in estimating $AUC_{(t,\infty)}$ for the controlled release formulation. If the terminal rate constant from the CR profile is used, then we are saying that theophylline absorption will continue to be the rate-limiting process between time t and infinity. Obviously this cannot be the case, as at some point in time absorption will be complete and elimination of theophylline will predominate; thus, the utilisation of the CR terminal rate constant as opposed to k ($k > k_{CR}$) will lead to an overestimation of $AUC_{(t,\infty)}$.

Should we, therefore, be using k, obtained from the solution, to assess $AUC_{(t,\infty)}$ for the controlled release product? Examination of the CR profile indicates that theophylline absorption is still occurring over the later points, and thus calculation of $AUC_{(t,\infty)}$ for CR product using the elimination rate constant could potentially result in an underestimation of the extrapolated area. This dilemma has to be solved empirically, and not theoretically. The contribution of any extrapolated area to the total AUC should ideally be less than 10%. The objective of any study design is, therefore, to maximise $AUC_{(0,t)}$ and minimise $AUC_{(t,\infty)}$. This is accomplished by extending the blood sampling time over a time period equivalent to approximately 3–4 times the terminal half-life of the drug. By reducing the contribution of the extrapolated area to the total AUC, selection of the appropriate rate constant by which $AUC_{(t,\infty)}$ is estimated is less critical. For certain drugs, however, notably those drugs with long half-lives or those which undergo enterohepatic recycling, following the terminal phase over 3–4 half-life equivalents may pose logistical problems. The problems associated with the assessment of the extent of absorption of such drugs have been discussed by Shepard *et al.* (1985a, b).

Assessment of the extent of absorption based on comparison of AUCs arising from two individual dosage administrations assumes that there is pharmacokinetic linearity between the two treatments. Plasma concentration–time profiles relating to the administration of identical doses of drug but by different routes may exhibit large differences in their respective plasma concentration ranges; for instance, when assessing the absolute bioavailability of a controlled release product (i.v. bolus versus oral dose). Any concentration dependence of the pharmacokinetics of the drug may therefore lead to a non-linear relationship between the two modes of administration. Concentration-dependent plasma protein binding could potentially result in non-linearity between the two formulations used in the assessment of absolute bioavailability of a solid oral dosage form made with reference to an i.v. bolus dose due to marked differences in the range of drug concentration produced by the two routes of administration. Ideally, therefore, the reference formulation (i.v.) should produce plasma concentrations of similar magnitude to those produced by the formulation under test. For assessment of absolute bioavailability, this can be achieved by the intravenous dose being delivered as a constant rate infusion. By careful selection of the infusion rate and duration of infusion, the plasma profile relating to the i.v. dose of drug can be made to match that relating to the oral dose, thereby avoiding complications of concentration-dependent pharmacokinetics. The use of drug administration by intravenous infusion to investigate non-linearities in bioavailability assessment has been demonstrated for theophylline by Steinijans *et al.* (1987). This approach obviously depends on a knowledge of the formulation-dependent plasma drug concentration–time profile of the drug which is being assessed; indeed, a knowledge of the bioavailability of the substance prior to the assessment of this parameter would be ideal! For the assessment of comparative bioavailability where there is no i.v. formulation, it is unlikely that the input profile of the drug from the reference formulation, normally a solution, can be controlled, and thus alternative approaches to correcting for non-linearity are required. The calculation of bioavailability based on AUC ratios cannot be used when the pharmacokinetics of the drug are non-linear. Under such circumstances, bioavailability may be obtained from modelling of the blood level data, but this approach may be quite complex (Metzler and Tong, 1981).

Verapamil is a chiral channel-blocking agent used in the treatment of cardiovascular disease, and is clinically administered as a racemic mixture (50:50 mixture of the (+)- and (−)-verapamil enantiomers), even though it is acknowledged that the (−)-enantiomer is the more pharmacologically active species. Although the bioavailability of (±)-verapamil for the two volunteers depicted in Table 19.1 is identical, the stereochemical composition of the plasma verapamil concentrations in these two individuals differs markedly (as shown by the ratio of AUC for the two enantiomers). As the pharmacological activity of the two enantiomers differs markedly, the ensuing pharmacological response from an identically available dose of (±)-verapamil could potentially be quite different. Data such as these have resulted in suggestions that, for drugs producing a quantifiable pharmacological effect, bioavailability may be more relevantly (from a clinical viewpoint) quantified by comparison of the pharmacological response produced by the reference and test doses of drug (Smolen, 1982). Under these circumstances bioavailability assessment is based on the fraction of the administered dose of drug reaching the systemic circulation intact or as pharmacologically active species (active metabolite or active enantiomer). An alternative approach proposed by Rowland (1986) has suggested that under such conditions bioavailability may be more appropriately quantified by comparison of the doses required to produce the same pharmacological response.

The importance of quantifying the rate of absorption in any assessment of bioavailability is being acknowledged increasingly. Pharmaceutical formula-

Table 19.1 Bioavailability of verapamil in two healthy male volunteers following the oral administration of 160 mg of pseudoracemic verapamil (based on data from Vogelgesang *et al.*, 1984)

Subject	Bioavailability (F%)	$\dfrac{AUC\,(+)}{AUC\,(-)}$
1	39	6.54
2	38	3.26

tion development has tended to emphasise the importance of controlled rate of drug input in the optimisation of bioavailability. Clinically, however, a constant or zero-order rate of drug input may not always be desirable. Quantification of the rate of drug absorption may be achieved most simply by determination of the maximum plasma drug concentration (C_{max}) and the time taken to reach C_{max} (t_{max}). More rigorous mathematical approaches to the *in vivo* assessment of absorption rate have been reviewed by Cutler (1981).

Therapeutically, the rate of drug input, certainly as it relates to bioavailability, has generally been considered to be of little importance. Nifedipine was originally marketed as a rapid release capsule formulation, but was later formulated as a controlled release tablet. Although the extent of nifedipine absorption from the two formulations was identical, differences in the pharmacological profile of the drug were observed. Both formulations were shown to produce the desired antihypertensive effects, but the tablet was found to produce a much lower increase in heart-rate than the capsule formulation. The difference in pharmacological profile was attributed to the difference in the input rate of nifedipine between the two formulations, a hypothesis later substantiated by comparison of i.v. bolus and i.v. infusion data (Kleinbloesem *et al.*, 1984; Kleinbloesem, 1985). From the studies with nifedipine it is apparent that the rate of drug absorption may be as important a determinant of efficacy as the extent of absorption.

STEREOCHEMICAL PHARMACOKINETICS

At the turn of the century it was reported by Cushny (1904) that the individual optical enantiomers of hyoscyamine isolated from *Atropa belladonna* had marked differences in anticholinergic activity. Since that time, there have been many reports detailing differences in the pharmacological activity profiles of the individual enantiomers of chiral drug substances (Smith, 1974; Ariens *et al.*, 1983); however, the potential for stereoselective differences in enantiomeric disposition was seldom acknowledged until relatively recently.

Surveys of prescription drugs have shown that an appreciable number are chiral and administered as racemates (50:50 mixture of the individual enantiomers). Mason (1984) showed that, of the 398 synthetic chiral pharmaceuticals appearing in the 1980 edition of the US Pharmacopeial Dictionary of drug names, 82% were administered as their racemate. A Scandinavian survey showed that, of 666 drugs listed in a Swedish physicians' desk reference, 174 were marketed as racemic mixtures (Simonyi, 1984). It is clear that optically active drug substances are not infrequently prescribed, but in doing so a mixture of two or more chemical species of, more often than not, unknown pharmacokinetic and pharmacodynamic characteristics is blindly administered.

Much criticism has been levelled at the lack of 'stereospecific awareness' within the pharmacokinetic and clinical pharmacology literature (Ariens, 1984; Testa, 1988), with the inference that the failure to acknowledge the importance of stereochemistry results in scientifically meaningless data.

With respect to drug development, the counterargument could be that if it is intended to market the drug as the racemate and all the toxicological and clinical studies have been satisfactorily undertaken with respect to registration of the drug in this form, then stereochemistry is unimportant. This is a naïve attitude and one that is becoming less acceptable to regulatory bodies.

The failure to acknowledge the importance of stereochemistry in the pharmacokinetic assessment of new drug entities has undoubtedly been in part due to methodological difficulties in undertaking stereochemical analysis of such drugs in biological fluids.

Many early attempts at investigating underlying stereochemical changes in pharmacokinetics of the individual enantiomers of chiral drug substances involved the administration, on separate occasions, of the individual enantiomers, with subsequent quantification using conventional analytical methodology (O'Reilly, 1980; White *et al.*, 1980). The underlying assumption of this approach is that the pharmacokinetics and pharmacodynamics of the individual separated enantiomers are totally independent and additive; this is not always the case. George *et al.* (1972) reported that the elimination half-life of (*R*)-propranolol was shorter when given alone than when administered as a component of the racemate. The basis of this observation resides in the differences in the pharmacological properties of the individual propranolol enantiomers. (*S*)-Propranolol, unlike its optical antipode, produces a reduction in hepatic blood flow to which, as a drug of high extraction ratio, the clearance of propranolol, and its individual enantiomers, is proportional. The decrease in hepatic blood flow produced by (*S*)-propranolol consequently results in a decrease in the clearance of the (*R*)-enantiomer, which in turn, in the absence of any alteration in distribution, manifests as a prolongation in the elimination half-life of this species. The pharmacokinetics of the individual enantiomers when administered as a racemic mixture cannot, therefore, necessarily be predicted from data obtained from administration of the individual enantiomers in isolation.

An approach to the investigation of stereochemical pharmacokinetics that is particularly suited to Phase I investigative studies involves the utilisation of stable isotope methodology—in particular, the use of pseudoracemates (Baillie, 1981). A pseudoracemic mixture is an artificially produced racemic mixture of the individual enantiomers of a chiral drug substance in which one of the enantiomers has been enriched synthetically with a staple isotope label, with the mass difference of the individual enantiomers being detected by selected ion monitoring (SIM) mass spectrometry. A major benefit of assessing enantiomeric pharmacokinetics using pseudoracemates is that the stereochemical origins of identifiable metabolites can immediately be assessed and quantified, because, as with parent drug, the enantiomers of the metabolites also exhibit a mass difference. The application of stable isotope methodology has been used with much success in the quantification of the metabolic fate of (*R*,*S*)-warfarin and (*R*,*S*)-phenoprocoumon (Toon *et al.*, 1985, 1986). As with all investigations involving stable isotopes, suitable controls must be undertaken to eliminate the potential influence of isotope effects and analytical quantification must account for the natural abundance of the isotope in question (Bush and Trager, 1981).

The most commonly reported approach to the quantification of the pharmacokinetics of the individual enantiomers of a chiral drug substance following administration of the racemate involves some form of chromatographic separation of the individual enantiomers, with or without prior derivatisation. Advancing developments with chiral columns (both GC and HPLC) and the increasing commercial availability of optically pure derivatising reagents mean that chromatographic separation of enantiomers is becoming increasingly tenable (Souter, 1985).

Although there are as yet no regulatory requirements relating to the pharmacokinetic assessment of the individual enantiomers of a drug to be administered clinically as the racemate, a failure to acknowledge the importance of stereochemistry can seriously compromise the interpretation of any pharmacokinetic observations.

Figure 19.2 shows the single-dose plasma concentration–time profiles of (R,S)-warfarin in two young healthy male volunteers in the absence and in the presence of chronic sulphinpyrazone administration. In both cases sulphinpyrazone was shown to potentiate the hypoprothrombinaemic response produced by the anticoagulant. While consistent with the changes in the plasma concentrations of (R,S)-warfarin in subject 1 (i.e. increase in concentration and increase in response), the observed changes in warfarin pharmacokinetics in subject 2 on the surface completely contradict the pharmacological observations. Examination of the underlying pharmacokinetics of the individual warfarin enantiomers was found to resolve the problem (Toon *et al.*, 1986). (S)-warfarin is approximately five times more potent an anticoagu-

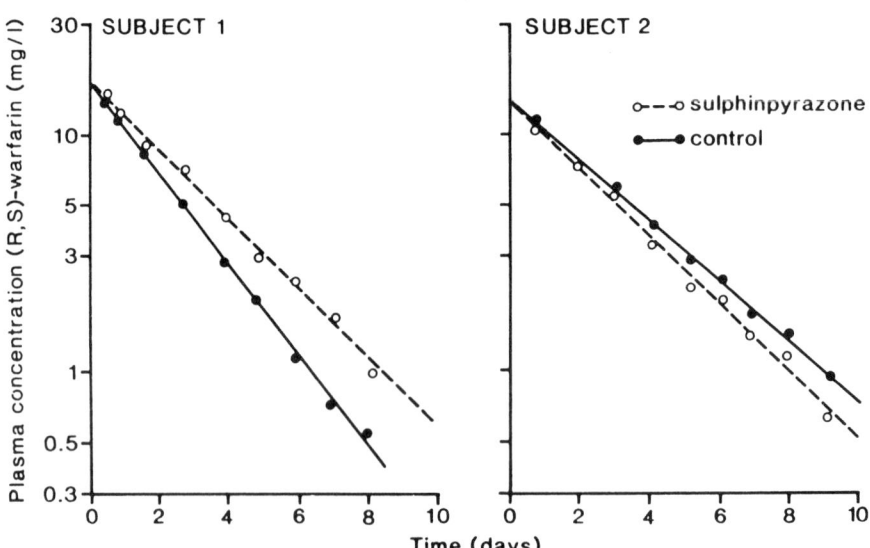

Figure 19.2 Plasma (R,S)-warfarin concentration–time profiles in two volunteers following the oral administration of racemic warfarin (1.5 mg/kg body weight) in the absence and in the presence of concomitant sulphinpyrazone administration

lant than its optical antipode, and while the apparent clearance of (*R*)-warfarin was found to increase in the presence of sulphinpyrazone, resulting in a decrease in the plasma concentration of this species, the apparent clearance of the more pharmacologically active (*S*)-enantiomer simultaneously decreased, resulting in higher plasma concentrations of this species and, consequently, an increase in pharmacological response. Thus, the net effect of the opposing changes in the individual enantiomers determines the magnitude and direction of the change in racemic warfarin concentrations.

Discrepancies between pharmacological response and drug concentration may often be the first indication in the drug development programme of underlying stereochemical complexities.

Stereoselective first-pass elimination has been reported for several chiral drug substances of high extraction ratio (Von Bahr *et al.*, 1982; Lennard *et al.*, 1983). Interpretation of pharmacokinetic data relating to such drugs can easily be confounded by a failure to acknowledge this phenomenon. Stereoselective inhibition of the first-pass elimination of (*R*)-metoprolol, the least pharmacologically active enantiomer, provided the apparent discrepancy between the relatively large increase in the AUC of (*R*,*S*)-metoprolol observed in the presence of chronic cimetidine and the lack of change in pharmacological response over that observed in the absence of H_2-antagonist (Toon *et al.*, 1988).

The non-steroidal anti-inflammatory agents (NSAIDs) are a very widely prescribed class of drugs. Within this therapeutic class the arylpropionic acids have been shown to exhibit a particular stereochemical peculiarity. Administered clinically as the racemate, it has been shown for many of the arylpropionic acids that the less active (*R*)-enantiomer is converted *in vivo* to its more pharmacologically active optical antipode (Hutt and Caldwell, 1983). The (*R*)-to-(*S*) interconversion (the (*S*)-enantiomer is not converted to the (*R*)-form) appears peculiar to this class of compounds, but is a phenomenon to be borne in mind when developing new chemical entities which contain centres of asymmetry.

The basis of any observed difference in the pharmacokinetics of the enantiomers of a chiral drug substance is often assumed to be metabolic in origin. This need not necessarily be the case. Just as the hepatic clearance of highly extracted drugs is rate-limited by hepatic blood flow, the hepatic clearance of poorly extracted drugs is rate-limited by the degree of binding of the drug to plasma proteins. The total clearance (Cl) of a lowly extracted drug may be described by the equation:

$$Cl = Cl_{int} \cdot f_u$$

where Cl_{int} is the intrinsic clearance, an index of metabolic processes, and f_u is the fraction of drug not bound to plasma proteins. It is apparent therefore that any differences in the plasma protein binding (changes in f_u) of the individual enantiomers of a poorly cleared chiral drug substance would manifest as an observed stereoselectivity in the total clearance of enantiomers, even though there may be no difference between the enantiomers at a metabolic level (as quantified by Cl_{int}). The importance of this interrelationship has been discussed by Toon and Trager (1984).

Stereoselectivity in plasma protein binding could also potentially manifest as a difference between the renal clearance of the individual enantiomer of a chiral drug that is excreted renally by glomerular filtration, as only unbound drug is filtered. Stereoselectivity in renal elimination has been reported for quinine and quinidine (Notterman *et al.*, 1986) and also for the enantiomers of the β-blocking agent pindolol (Hsyu and Giacomini, 1985). Stereoselective differences in plasma protein binding were not, however, implicated in either of these reports, and thus stereochemical factors appear to be influencing renal elimination at a more fundamental level.

In summary, therefore, it is essential to recognise the importance of underlying stereochemical factors when interpreting pharmacokinetic observations relating to chiral drug substances. Further, there is no reason why any *in vivo* process should not exhibit stereoselectivity towards the individual enantiomers of a chiral drug substance, and this should be borne in mind in the early development of such compounds.

REFERENCES

Ariens, E. J. (1984). Stereochemistry, a basis for sophisticated nonsense in pharmacokinetics and clinical pharmacology. *Eur. J. Clin. Pharm.*, **26**, 663–8

Ariens, E. J., Soudijn, W. and Timmermans, P. B. (Eds.) (1983). *Stereochemistry and Biological Activity of Drugs*. Blackwell Scientific Publications, London

Baillie, T. A. (1981). The use of stable isotopes in pharmacological research. *Pharm. Rev.*, **33**, 81–132

Blake, M. I., Crespi, H. L. and Katz, J. J. (1975). Studies with deuterated drugs. *J. Pharm. Sci.*, **64**, 367–91

Bush, E. D. and Trager, W. F. (1981). Analysis of linear approaches to quantitative stable isotope methodology in mass spectrometry. *Biomed. Mass Spectrom.*, **8**, 211–18

Chiou, W. (1978). Critical evaluation of potential error in pharmacokinetic studies of using the linear trapezoidal rule method for the calculation of the area under the plasma level–time curve. *J. Pharmacokin. Biopharm.*, **6**, 539–46

Cushny, A. R. (1904). Atropine and the hyoscyamines—a study of the action of optical isomers. *J. Physiol.*, **30**, 176–94

Cutler, D. (1981). Assessment of rate and extent of drug absorption. *Pharm. Ther.*, **14**, 123–60

George, C. F., Fenyvesi, T., Conolly, M. E. and Dollery, C. T. (1972). Pharmacokinetics of dextro-, laevo- and racemic propranolol in man. *Eur. J. Clin. Pharm.*, **4**, 74–6

Gibaldi, M. and Perrier, D. (1982). *Pharmacokinetics*, 2nd edn. Marcel Dekker, New York

Heck, H. d'A., Buttrill, S. E., Flynn, N. W., Dyer, R. L. Anbar, M., Cairns, T., Dighe, S. and Cabana, B. E. (1979). Bioavailability of imipramine tablets relative to stable isotope labelled internal standard: increasing the power of bioavailability tests. *J. Pharmacokin. Biopharm.*, **7**, 233–48

Hsyu, P. H. and Giacomini, K. M. (1985). Stereoselective renal clearance of pindolol in humans. *J. Clin. Invest.*, **76**, 1720–6

Hutt, A. J. and Caldwell, J. (1983). The metabolic inversion of 2-amylpropionic acids.

A novel route with pharmacological consequences. *J. Pharm. Pharmacol.*, **35**, 693–704

Kleinbloesem, C. H. (1985). Nifedipine: Clinical pharmacokinetics and haemodynamic effects. PhD Thesis. University of Leiden, The Netherlands

Kleinbloesem, C. H., van Brummelen, P., van de Linde, J. A., Voogol, P. J. and Breimer, D. D. (1984). Nifedipine: Kinetics and dynamics in healthy subjects. *Clin. Pharm. Ther.*, **35**, 742–9

Kwan, K. and Till, A. (1973). Novel method for bioavailability assessment. *J. Pharm. Sci.*, **62**, 1494–7

Lennard, M. S., Tucker, G. T., Silas, J. H., Freestone, S., Ramsey, L. E. and Woods, H. F. (1983). Differential stereoselective metabolism of metoprolol in extensive and poor debrisoquine metabolisers. *Clin. Pharm. Ther.*, **34**, 732–7

Mason, S. (1984). The left hand of nature. *New Scientist*, No. 1393, 10–14

Metzler, C. M. and Tong, D. D. M. (1981). Computational problems of compartment models with Michaelis–Menten-type elimination. *J. Pharm. Sci.*, **70**, 733–7

Notterman, D. A., Drayer, D. E., Metakis, L. and Reidenberg, M. M. (1986). Stereoselective renal tubular secretion of quinidine and quinine. *Clin. Pharm. Ther.*, **40**, 511–17

O'Reilly, R. A. (1980). Stereoselective interaction of trimethoprim-sulfamethoxazole with the separated enantiomorphs of racemic warfarin in man. *New Engl. J. Med.*, **302**, 33–5

Rowland, M. (1986). Can bioavailability assessments be made from pharmacodynamic data? In Proceedings of *Bioavailability Update: Industrial and Legal Aspects*. Conference organised by Swedish Academy of Pharmaceutical Sciences, Gothenberg, Sweden

Shepard, T. A., Reuning, R. H. and Aarons, L. (1985a). Interpretation of area under the curve measurements for drugs subject to enterohepatic cycling. *J. Pharm. Sci.*, **74**, 227–8

Shepard, T. A., Reuning, R. H. and Aarons, L. (1985b). Estimation of area under the curve for drugs subject to enterohepatic cycling. *J. Pharmacokin. Biopharm.*, **13**, 589–608

Simonyi, M. (1984). On chiral drug action. In *Medicinal Research Reviews*. John Wiley, New York, pp. 359–413

Smith, D. F. (Ed.) (1984). *CRC Handbook of Stereoisomers: Drugs in Psychopharmacology*. CRC Press Inc, Boca Raton, Florida

Smolen, V. (1982). In Bozler, G. and van Rossum, J. M. (Eds.), *Pharmacokinetics During Drug Development: Data Analysis and Evaluation Techniques*. Gustav Fischer Verlag, Stuttgart, pp. 242–98

Souter, R. W. (1985). *Chromatographic Separations of Stereoisomers*. CRC Press, Boca Raton, Florida

Steinijans, V. W., Schulz, H.-U., Böhm, A. and Beier, W. (1987). Absolute bioavailability of theophylline from a sustained-release formulation using different intravenous reference infusions. *Eur. J. Clin. Pharm.*, **33**, 523–6

Testa, B. (1988). Substrate and product stereoselectivity in mono-oxygenase-mediated drug activation and inactivation. *Biochem. Pharm.*, **37**, 85–92

Toon, S., Davidson, E. M., Garstang, F. M., Batra, H., Bowes, R. J. and Rowland, M. (1988). The racemic metoprolol H_2-antagonist interaction. *Clin. Pharm. Ther.*, **43**, 283–9

Toon, S., Heimark, L. D., Trager, W. F. and O'Reilly, R. A. (1985). Metabolic fate of phenprocoumon in humans. *J. Pharm. Sci.*, **10**, 1037–40

Toon, S., Hopkins, K. J., Aarons, L. and Rowland, M. (1989). Rate and extent of absorption of clonidine from a transdermal therapeutic system. *J. Pharm. Pharmacol*, **41**, 17–21

Toon, S., Low, L. K., Gibaldi, M., Trager, W. F., O'Reilly, R. A., Motley, C. H. and Goulart, D. A. (1986). The warfarin–sulfinpyrazone interaction: stereochemical considerations. *Clin. Pharm. Ther.*, **39**, 15–24

Toon, S. and Trager, W. F. (1984). Pharmacokinetic implications of stereoselective changes in plasma-protein binding: Warfarin–sulfinpyrazone. *J. Pharm. Sci.*, **73**, 1671–3

Vogelgesang, B., Echizen, H., Schmidt, E. and Eichelbaum, M. (1984). Stereoselective first-pass metabolism of highly cleared drugs. Studies of the bioavailability of L- and D-verapamil examined with a stable isotope technique. *Br. J. Clin. Pharm.*, **18**, 733–40

Von Bahr, C., Hermansson, J. and Tawara, K. (1982). Plasma levels of (+)- and (−)-propranolol and 4-hydroxypropranolol after administration of (±)-propranolol in man. *Br. J. Clin. Pharm.*, **14**, 79–82

White, P. F., Ham, J., Way, W. L. and Trevor, A. J. (1980). Pharmacology of ketamine isomers in surgical patients. *Anesthesiology*, **52**, 231–9

Yeh, K. and Kwan, K. (1978). A comparison of numerical integrating algorithms by trapezoidal, lagrange and spline approximation. *J. Pharmacokin. Biopharm.*, **6**, 79–98

20
Radiolabelled Metabolism Studies in Man

J. McEwen*† and Ian H. Stevenson†

*Drug Development (Scotland) Ltd, Ninewells Hospital and Medical School, Dundee DD1 9SY, UK
†Dept of Pharmacology and Clinical Pharmacology, Ninewells Hospital and Medical School, Dundee DD1 9SY, UK

INTRODUCTION

Over recent decades a revolution in analytical methodology has led to a better understanding of the processes of drug absorption, distribution, metabolism and elimination, allowing pharmacokinetics to emerge as a distinct discipline. The justification for an increased interest in pharmacokinetics is presumably based upon the premise that a drug will be used more appropriately when its behaviour in the body is better understood: a drug's action must be related in some way to its presence in the body. Sophisticated pharmacokinetic modelling may, in addition, provide some clue to the penetration of drugs into receptor sites outside the plasma compartment.

The purpose of this chapter is to discuss the value of one particular category of pharmacokinetic study in man, using radiolabelled drug, concentrating on practical features of planning and study design.

OBJECTIVES OF LABELLED STUDIES

At some stage in a typical development programme, it is usual to perform special isotope studies in man. Nearly all such 'metabolism' studies involve beta-emitting isotopes, either ^{14}C or ^{3}H or, less frequently, ^{35}S. Although standard 'cold' analytical techniques, including the use of stable (non-radioactive) isotopes, can also give some useful metabolic information, the measurement of radioactivity in biological samples (usually after some form of chromatographic separation) is the only sure way of following the patterns of hitherto unknown metabolites in plasma, urine or faeces. In addition, radiolabelled methods remain the only practicable means of measuring overall balance of administered and excreted medication, offering a degree of precision which is usually unobtainable by other methods. This helps to ensure that there is no residual unexcreted portion with the potential for long-term cumulation with multiple dosage.

The use of radiolabelled drugs in such studies should be regarded essentially as a preliminary step to the full characterisation of the fate and routes of metabolism of a drug by more specific means, such as gas–liquid or high-performance liquid chromatography procedures (both of which require pure samples of individual metabolites to be available). The ultimate identification procedure is, of course, mass spectrometry or its derivative technique, mass fragmentography, often preceded by GLC or HPLC separation. Martin and Reid (1981) have reviewed some of the techniques of isolation and identification of drug metabolites. Relatively few purely radiolabelled pharmacokinetic studies are now published and the technique is to an extent becoming a tool of the pharmaceutical industry in the early characterisation of drug disposition in man. Two examples of published work from industry involving radiolabelled methods are given by Rising *et al.* (1977) and Chamberlain *et al.* (1980).

A further reason for characterising the patterns and pathways of drug metabolism in man is to compare these data with preclinical work in laboratory animals, helping to interpret interspecies differences in a compound's pharmacological and toxicological profile, and justifying the choice of preclinical species for long-term toxicity studies.

PHARMACOKINETICS AND RADIOACTIVITY

Radioactivity has the advantage of ease of detection; however, it should always be remembered that plasma or urinary levels of activity are non-specific and only follow those fractions of the parent molecule which happen to be labelled. This lack of specificity means that levels of total radioactivity cannot be used in pharmacokinetic calculations or modelling as if they represented drug levels. Thus, care should be taken in using labelled intravenous–oral crossover studies to predict drug bioavailability. Using total radioactivity, all that will be measured in such circumstances is the bioavailability of radioactivity. Intravenous and oral studies with radiolabelled drug can still give very useful information about the routes and rates of metabolism of drug by the two routes, which can be particularly relevant when a drug is subject to extensive 'first-pass' presystemic elimination. Investigations with radiolabelled propranolol in man, for example, were able to demonstrate that the active metabolite, 4-hydroxy propranolol, appeared in the circulation after oral dosage to a much greater extent than after intravenous dosage (Coltart and Shand, 1970). Suitable chromatographic isolation of parent compound can sometimes be very helpful in circumstances where analytical problems are so great that a radioactive study proves the only practicable means of obtaining any clinical pharmacokinetic data. Although levels of total radioactivity do not necessarily represent drug concentration, the plasma profile of isotope can sometimes be used in multiple-dosage extrapolations to predict the possible accumulation of any form of drug-related material. Johns *et al.* (1964) describe an unusual radiolabelled study in man, in which the presence of tissue-bound methotrexate was demonstrated by release of radioactivity following administration of subsequent doses of unlabelled parent compound and analogues several weeks after the original administration of radiolabelled methotrexate.

BACKGROUND DATA REQUIRED

Before a dose of radiolabelled drug can be given to man, considerable planning is needed. A special radiolabelled synthesis has to be commissioned; it is important to place the label appropriately, avoiding side-chains which are easily cleaved, since one would then be following the fate of the side-chain and not the main structure. In very complicated molecules where metabolism can result in two or more significant fragments, consideration should be given to more than one labelled synthesis, and more than one labelled study, so that the progress of different parts of the molecule can be followed. It may, alternatively, be possible in such circumstances to use both ^{14}C and ^{3}H to follow two portions of the molecule at the same time.

Given a suitably labelled supply of drug, with appropriate checks on chemical purity of the radioactive molecule, a series of investigations in at least two species of laboratory animals are then required. The purpose of these studies is to ensure an adequate recovery of radioactivity, to develop appropriate separation and identification procedures for candidate metabolites, and to measure the time-course of tissue distribution of radioactivity in order to calculate the estimated whole-body and tissue radioactivity exposure in man. It is an advantage if whole-body autoradiography can also be performed in at least one laboratory species (not an albino) to give a qualitative picture of the distribution of drug throughout the body. An overview of the techniques of whole-body autoradiography is given by Franklin and Ross (1989).

These preclinical data then allow a decision to be made as to whether a radiolabelled study is justified in man. In the UK all experiments involving radioactivity have to be approved by the Administration of Radioactive Substances Advisory Committee (ARSAC), who have published guidelines on the investigative use of radioactivity in man (Department of Health and Social Security, 1988). A general guideline is that studies should fall within a Category I WHO radiation exposure, which is within the range of variation in natural background radioactivity (Table 20.1). It is usually possible to achieve

Table 20.1 WHO classification of radioactive exposure

	Dose limits (μSv)	
Exposure category	*Total body*	*Single organ*
I	<500	<2500
II	500–5000	2500–25 000
III	5000–50 000	25 000–250 000
IV	>50 000	>250 000

this with 1850 kBq (50 μCi) of ^{14}C or 3700 kBq (100 μCi) of ^{3}H, suitably diluted with non-labelled drug, to achieve an appropriate chemical dose.

STUDY DESIGN

Drug Formulation

Although most early pharmacokinetic studies in man are performed using gelatin capsules, an oral solution may prove the most convenient formulation for the rather specialised case of radiolabelled metabolic studies. A specially manufactured batch of radiolabelled capsules will be more wasteful of the limited quantity of labelled drug: in addition, dose-to-dose variation in content of radioactivity between individual capsules means that the calculation of administered label will be less precise, since the administered capsule cannot itself be sampled. Using an aliquot of the actual dosage solution, the dose of administered radioactivity can be precisely calculated, against which recovered activity can be accurately compared.

As in the case of any other clinical investigation, it is important to involve a pharmacist in the development of the dose formulation, especially if there are any uncertainties regarding stability. Appropriate analytical certificates of drug content and purity should be prepared, in addition to quality control of radiochemical purity.

Dosage

Although radiolabelled metabolism studies are usually performed as early as possible in the clinical development programme, it is advisable to wait at least until clinical investigations give a reasonable idea of the effective dose in man. The routes and rate of drug metabolism can vary with dosage, so an investigation which uses too low a chemical dose may prove misleading.

Selection of Subjects

Radiolabelled studies usually involve relatively small numbers of subjects—between 3 and 12. Partly to avoid any use of radioactivity in undiagnosed early pregnancy, and partly because this type of investigation is performed before full teratogenicity studies have been carried out, females are not usually considered to be suitable subjects. In order further to reduce any risk of cumulative radiation exposure in any given subject, it is preferable to select older rather than younger males as volunteer subjects—avoiding individuals younger than, say, 30 years old. In order to evaluate the significance of any variability between subjects, consideration should be given to prior metabolic typing to define hydroxylator or acetylator status.

As is the case in any pharmacokinetic investigation, it is important to standardise dosage conditions with respect to administration of food, posture, mobility, other medication, alcohol intake, etc.

Sampling Procedures

Quite a number of sequential blood samples can be taken by direct venepuncture in the course of a metabolic study, but there is a limit to the endurance of even the most robust patient or subject, especially if technique is less than perfect. Although the insertion of an indwelling cannula is sometimes a little more uncomfortable than direct venepuncture, it is generally preferred to multiple venepunctures and in most circumstances can remain patent for up to 36 h without difficulty. Cannulae can be either a rigid indwelling needle of the 'butterfly' type, which should be placed well away from both wrist and elbow, to avoid the need for temporary splinting, or the flexible plastic variety (e.g. 'Angiocath'), which can be placed in the generally more visible veins in the antecubital fossa, and which allow a much fuller range of movement. Cannulae need to be treated with care, however, and patients or subjects should remain under supervision while they are in use. They need to be regularly flushed with sterile saline; the addition of a small amount of heparin (e.g. 5 units/ml) can help to keep the lumen patent, although saline alone can be adequate for short periods if heparin could cause problems (for example, altering the protein binding of a highly bound drug or influencing platelet aggregation). The varieties of cannulae with an 'intermittent' multipuncture seal are cleaner and neater than those which need a three-way tap.

When a large number of blood samples are being processed together, separation of plasma or serum after centrifugation can be speeded up by the use of plastic separation aids (Sarstedt), which squeeze plasma or serum from the centrifuge tube. These devices are much quicker than Pasteur pipettes and also have the advantage of maximising the recovery of supernatant.

Attempts to collect saliva often result in a bottle of froth; flow can be stimulated by biting on a suitably inert substance, such as a small square of Teflon, placed between the molar teeth. Salivary drug levels can often give a good kinetic profile, usually in equilibrium with unbound circulating concentrations, and it may be useful to establish any relationship between plasma or serum and salivary concentrations in a metabolic study, since salivary collections may be helpful in later clinical studies in which blood sampling is undesirable or impracticable—for example, in children. After oral dosage with a solution, it is, of course, necessary to make sure that residual dosage solution has been rinsed away before collecting salivary samples.

Urine samples are best collected into preweighed containers so that the volume of urine can be measured by weight, assuming that 1 ml weighs 1 g. This method of measuring volume is much more convenient and more hygienically acceptable than the use of graduated cylinders, and in fact provides greater accuracy, even if no correction is made for specific gravity. Although in other types of pharmacokinetic study there is usually no need to keep more than a small 30 ml aliquot of urine from each collection, complete urine collections are usually saved over at least 5 days in metabolic studies: the structure of labelled metabolites in urine is more likely to be characterised if the total amount excreted can be concentrated by techniques such as freeze-drying.

Enthusiastic designers of pharmacokinetic studies should remember that some people have considerable difficulty in micturating on demand, especially at very frequent intervals: if 1 h collections are needed, then adequate hydration will be needed to ensure an adequate flow.

Faecal samples are almost invariably collected in radiolabelled metabolic balance studies, again over at least 5 days. If a subject becomes constipated during such a study, or if the rate of production of faeces appears slow, it may be useful to specify a minimum number of stool samples, say six, and prolong the collection period appropriately. Because faecal samples cannot usually be collected over a precisely timed interval like urine, it is better to collect them in numbered order as they are produced, keeping a careful record of date and time of collection. It is worth the effort to make the collection procedure as acceptable and convenient as possible. One technique is to collect faecal samples directly into stout plastic bags which have been placed inside airtight containers of suitable dimensions. Once delivered to the laboratory, the plastic bag can be transferred to a suitable apparatus (Seward Ltd) for homogenisation by external flat paddles after addition of water (in proportion to the weight of the specimen), without the need to transfer faeces to another container. Alternatively, faecal collections can be made directly into airtight Thurger–Bolle plastic collection pots which are compatible with the high-shear type of homogenisation apparatus (Silverson Machines Ltd).

Expired air is occasionally collected in a labelled balance study, if it is possible that the label could be cleaved from the molecule and eliminated as radioactive carbon dioxide: however, it should be possible to design a labelled molecule in which this will not occur. There is no need to sample expired air continuously in claustrophobic hoods in these circumstances, since regular collections can be taken at selected intervals by breathing through a suitable mouthpiece into a scintillation vial containing a trapping medium for carbon dioxide together with an indicator such as phenolphthalein, up to the point at which the indicator changes colour. This allows the ^{14}C content of a known mass of carbon dioxide to be measured, and if the levels are plotted out against time, the area under the curve gives a good estimate of the amount of radiolabel eliminated by this route.

Liquid Scintillation Counting

The conventional method of measuring beta-radiation is liquid scintillation counting. For maximum efficiency, the biological sample has to be solubilised in the scintillation fluid. In addition, coloured samples are frequently bleached to avoid loss of counting efficiency as a result of colour quenching: however, this process can itself cause problems through chemical quenching. Although biological samples such as plasma and urine can often be added directly to scintillation vials without too much loss of efficiency, aliquots of whole blood or faeces cannot be handled in this way, and are usually combusted on filter paper in a special oxidising apparatus which collects the products of combustion as radiolabelled carbon dioxide and/or water. Especially towards the end of a set of study samples, when radioactivity approaches background levels, the counting process can be quite a lengthy procedure—for example, 100 minutes per vial—so it is not usually feasible to expect rapid feedback of results in order to decide whether to extend the collection period. It is usually better to plan to collect samples for rather longer than the minimum predicted period: if a complete balance is subsequently attained, and counts are low, unwanted extra samples can be discarded. It is an expensive and tedious business to repeat an investigation when the final calculations show that collections were prematurely terminated.

ETHICS: RADIATION SAFETY

Radioactivity is an emotive subject in which careful assessment of relative risk–benefit ratios is rarely presented with any degree of objectivity. A recent symposium published by the Royal College of Physicians of Edinburgh on the medical implications of the use of nuclear technology included a presentation by Fry (1989): Table 20.2 is abstracted from this paper. Radiation exposure within WHO Category I from a typical metabolic study (Table 20.1)

Table 20.2 Average annual dose of radiation in the UK

Source	Dose (μSv)
Natural radiation (ground level)	2200
Weapons fallout	5
Chernobyl accident	<1
Medical procedures[a]	300
Occupational exposure[b]	1100
Miscellaneous[c]	10

[a] Average of toal population.
[b] Average of exposed workers.
[c] TV sets, watches, air travel.

compares favourably with exposure to natural and man-made sources. It can, indeed, be argued that in early metabolic studies it is more important to consider the ethical and safety implications of the chemical burden of a new investigative drug than those of administered radioactivity. It remains important, however, that all aspects of investigative studies in man, including the use of radioactivity, be carefully and objectively reviewed by an independent ethics committee; volunteers should be fully informed of the nature and potential risks of any project.

REFERENCES

Chamberlain, J., Coombs, J. D., Dell, D., Fromson, J. M., Ings, R. M. J., Macdonald, C. M. and McEwen, J. (1980). Metabolism of cefotaxime in animals and man. *J. Antimicrob. Chemother.*, **6** (suppl. A), 69–78

Coltart, D. G. and Shand, D. G. (1970). Plasma propranolol levels in the quantitative assessment of beta-adrenergic blockade in man. *Br. Med. J.*, **iii**, 731–4

Department of Health and Social Security (1988). *Notes for Guidance on the Administration of Radioactive Substances to Persons for Purposes of Diagnosis, Treatment or Research.* London

Franklin, E. R. and Ross, D. A. (1989). Whole body autoradiography. In Illing H. P. A. (Ed.), *Xenobiotic Metabolism and Disposition: the Design of Studies on Novel Compounds.* CRC Press, Boca Raton, Florida, pp. 41–66

Fry, F. A. (1989). Radioactivity in the environment: sources and relative contributions to public exposure. *Proc. R. Coll. Phys. Edin.*, **19**, 163–70

Johns, D. G., Hollingsworth, J. W., Cashmore, A. R., Plenderleith, I. H. and Bertino, J. R. (1964). Methotrexate displacement in man. *J. Clin. Invest.*, **43**, 621–9

Martin, L. E. and Reid, E. (1981). Isolation of drug metabolites. In Bridges, J. W. and Chasseaud, L. F. (Eds.), *Progress in Drug Metabolism*, Vol. 6. John Wiley, Chichester, pp. 197–248

Rising, T. J., Fromson, J. M., McEwen, J. and Johnson, P. (1977). Absorption studies with the anti-diarrhoeal agent ethacridine lactate in laboratory animals and man. *Arzneimittel Forschung*, **27**, 872–8

V
Assessment of Drug Effects on the Cardiovascular System

21
Non-invasive Measurement of Cardiovascular Response

J. D. Harry

Head, Clinical Pharmacology Unit, ICI Pharmaceuticals, Mereside, Alderley Edge, Cheshire, UK

INTRODUCTION

The title of this chapter is wide-ranging and to cover all aspects implicit in the title would require a book of its own. Consequently, this chapter needs to be restrictive—in particular, when it comes to interpreting the words 'cardiovascular response'. Just one area of the cardiovascular system will be considered, namely cardiac function (i.e. assessments of the heart function). Response will be restricted to the effects of drugs on this cardiovascular parameter at rest and during the stress of exercise. Further, the term 'non-invasive technique', while clearly understood by research workers, particularly those involved with assessing the effects of drugs on cardiac function, does lack a clear definition, which is needed when writing a chapter such as this. A working definition could be: non-invasive techniques, when applied to studies involving measurements of cardiac function (invariably left ventricular function), are those which do not employ methods of direct entry into the circulation such as occurs when measuring cardiovascular parameters from cardiac catheterisation. Such techniques, therefore, will be made from the 'surface' of the body and will not involve the breaking of the skin (other than perhaps to inject a marker into the circulation for subsequent non-invasive measurements, e.g. as radionuclide methods for assessing cardiac output).

A number of non-invasive techniques are now available to assess the effects of drugs on cardiac function. In this chapter, particular emphasis will be directed to those methods which are applicable to early development (Phase I and early Phase II) studies of the effects of new drugs affecting the cardiovascular system. Thus, it is really inappropriate to consider in this chapter such techniques as thallium scanning to detect areas of underperfusion in the myocardium or the assessments of left ventricular volumes using radionuclide techniques. These non-invasive techniques are more useful for longer-term studies of drugs in patients.

GENERAL CONSIDERATIONS ABOUT NON-INVASIVE TECHNIQUES

Non-invasive assessments of cardiovascular functions are attractive when assessing whether a new untested chemical entity affects the activity of the heart. Little discomfort is experienced by the subject and repeated measurements can be made over a period of time after dosing. However, care does need to be exercised when using non-invasive techniques that the measurement being made does faithfully reflect the change in the cardiovascular parameters that the compound is producing. Therefore, certain critical criteria about the measurements should be considered as obligatory before the method can be accepted to allow interpretation of the measurements as sufficiently meaningful to permit decisions about the effects of untested compounds. Some of these criteria are considered below.

Validation

Like any technique for measuring biological activity, non-invasive techniques for assessing cardiac function need to be validated. The validation may take various forms, but for non-invasive techniques the measurements should correlate well with the same parameters being assessed by direct invasive measurements (if this is possible). Thus, the measurement of cardiac output by the non-invasive pulsed Doppler ultrasound methods has been compared in the same patients against measuring cardiac output by the invasive thermodilution of Fick techniques (e.g. Loepky *et al.*, 1984; Rose, 1984). Most of these types of validation have been performed with the subjects at rest, and under these conditions reasonable correlations have been achieved. Very few investigations have been performed under conditions of stress, when the correlation may or may not still exist. This has been attempted for Doppler techniques, comparing with the thermodilution techniques in the same subjects, when the correlation seemed to remain when the heart was stimulated by dobutamine (Bojanowski *et al.*, 1987). One other factor to consider when non-invasive techniques are compared with invasive assessments, e.g. of cardiac output, is that the accuracy of the invasive procedure is taken as standard. Invasive assessments of cardiac output are themselves imperfect (Schuster *et al.*, 1984). However, despite these problems a non-invasive assessment of cardiac function should show some relationship to invasive assessments (at rest and under stress), to be of use in determining the effects of drugs on the heart.

Sensitivity of the Technique

To be useful to determine the effects of drugs affecting cardiac function, non-invasive techniques need to be sensitive enough to detect these changes, invariably in small groups of subjects. As an example, this has been shown to be the case for assessing the inotropic activity of dobutamine with the non-invasive technique of systolic time-intervals. Thus, Harry *et al.* (1988b) showed that doses of intravenous dobutamine (1, 2, 4 μg kg^{-1} min^{-1}) produced changes in measurements of systolic time-intervals, suggesting that a positive inotropic effect has occurred. These same doses produce changes in cardiac output when measured with invasive techniques (Jewitt *et al.*, 1974). Thus, systolic time intervals can be considered sensitive enough to detect the action of an inotropic agent such as dobutamine affecting the heart (provided that the drug has no other effect on the circulation; see later). With the Doppler techniques for assessing blood flow in the aorta, changes of greater than 13–15% induced by a compound would be required before it can be accepted that the effect is drug-induced (Gardin *et al.*, 1964; Harry *et al.*, 1988b).

Reproducibility of the Technique

The particular advantage of non-invasive over invasive assessments of cardiac function is that serial observations can be made over time, allowing the short- and long-term affect of therapeutic interventions to be assessed. The applicability of such methods to longitudinal studies does depend upon the reproducibility of the measurements. Reproducibility studies over the short (3 h) and long term (months) have been performed with systolic time intervals as an assessment of inotropic state of the heart (Kupari, 1983). The results showed that the reproducibility of the method was high over the 3 h time-period (subjects resting supine) and remained good over longer periods of time, provided that diurnal variation was taken into account. Thus, systolic time-intervals as a measure of inotropic state of the ventricle should be amenable to showing changes induced by an intervention. A similar assessment of short- and long-term reproducibility has been performed for Doppler measurements of cardiac output by Robson *et al.* (1988) and for M-mode echocardiography by Otterstad *et al.* (1987), both with similar results. Thus, before any non-invasive technique can be used to study drug intervention, reproducibility of the measurement (under the same conditions, usually resting) over the time-course of any particular study needs to be established.

'Robustness' of the Technique

Most non-invasive assessments of cardiac function currently available can assess the effects of a drug when the subject is at rest. However, few of the methods become applicable when the heart is stimulated, as, for example, with exercise. One such method is the assessment of cardiac output with the non-invasive technique of impedance cardiography. This system shows a good correlation between measurements of resting cardiac output compared with the invasive method of dye dilution (Gabriel *et al.*, 1976). Attempts have been made to assess its use in exercise by several workers, e.g. Teo *et al.* (1985). Even then, examination of the methods in this paper shows that measurements were not made while the subjects were exercising but immediately after they stopped cycling on a bicycle ergometer. While the measurements under these circumstances are clearly not 'resting' values, they are not the measurements at that given level of exercise and they are being made when changes in the cardiovascular system from exercise to non-exercise are maximal. Despite this limitation, a good correlation was obtained between two sets of exercise in 4 healthy males separated by at least 1 week. Attempts have been made in our laboratory to use the impedance cardio-graph while subjects are still exercising upright on a bicycle ergometer. The results (on 6 healthy male volunteers) are encouraging and show that the system will measure cardiac output with the subjects exercising and that the results were reproducible (Figure 21.1). Doppler echocardiography has also been reported to be capable of assessing cardiac output while the subjects were exercising (e.g. Daley *et al.*, 1985; Innes *et al.*, 1988), but experiences wth Doppler techniques in our laboratory were disappointing with bicycle exercise.

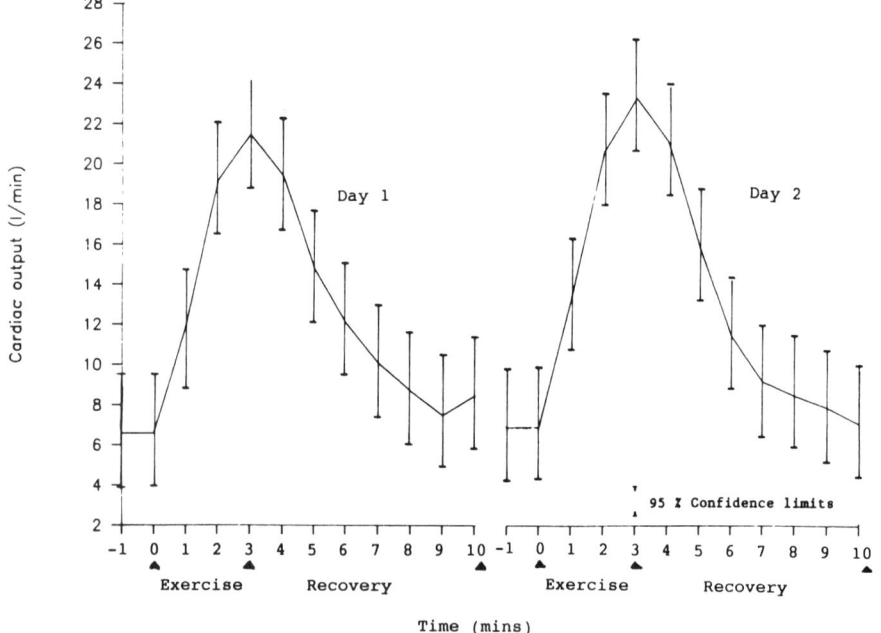

Figure 21.1 Cardiac output measured with an impedance cardiograph before, while exercising and while recovering from exercise (using a bicycle ergometer) from a group of 6 normal subjects recorded on different days (1 and 2) with the same level of exercise on each day. Day 1, day 2 at least 1 week apart

INTERPRETATION OF MEASUREMENTS OBTAINED WITH NON-INVASIVE TECHNIQUES

The interpretation of measurements of cardiac function, whether obtained by invasive or non-invasive techniques, but more especially with the latter, has to be carried out with care. Changes induced in the inotropic state of the heart by a drug or other intervention may be secondary and consequent upon changes in some other part of the circulation rather than by stimulation of the heart itself. The use of systolic time-intervals to assess non-invasive changes in cardiac function induced by drugs helps to illustrate this point. Thus, it is well known that if a change in heart rate occurs as a result of giving the drug, then changes will occur in the measurements of systolic time-intervals, which are not due to stimulation of the myocardium but due to the increase in heart rate. Thus, special formulae exist to correct for the changes in heart rate when systolic time-intervals are used (e.g. Weissler *et al.*, 1968). Similarly, changes in preload (venous pressure and venous return) and after-load (arterial blood pressure) are all known to effect inotropic states of the heart (e.g. Furnival *et al.*, 1970). Yet no such formulae exist when systolic time-intervals are used to assess drug-induced changes in the inotropic state of the heart, if changes in preload or after-load occur. In fact, it may be inappropriate to use such a measurement of inotropic activity of the heart, if it is known that blood pressure also changes with the intervention, unless attempts can be made to keep those changes in blood pressure to a minimum. It is probable that all non-invasive assessments of cardiac function suffer from the problems that changes in the measurements may be a primary effect on the heart and/or secondary to changes in other parts of the circulation. The above does not invalidate the description of the effects of drugs affecting the cardiovascular system. It does, however, make an analysis of the mechanism of action of the drug difficult. So, if a new isotropic compound is tested in early Phase I studies using non-invasive techniques, any effect that the compound produces can be faithfully recorded. If only one of the parameters changes, e.g. increase in cardiac contractility, and the animal pharmacology of the compound is such that it is an agent only stimulating the myocardium, then the mechanism of action is obvious. If, however, heart rate, blood pressure or other cardiovascular parameters change (and these are not always being measured), then the mechanism of action of the drug in man can only be established if the effects of the changes on the inotropic state are corrected for.

NON-INVASIVE METHODS AVAILABLE TO STUDY EFFECTS OF DRUGS ON THE CARDIOVASCULAR SYSTEM IN EARLY DEVELOPMENT STUDIES

Two types of questions with respect to the cardiovascular system are asked of new compounds when they are being investigated in the early trials in normal volunteer subjects: first, if the compound is a cardiovascular agent, then specific studies of its effect on the heart or peripheral circulation may be required; second, if the compound is other than a cardiovascular compound, then all that may be required is to determine any general effects that the compound may have on the circulation. In either case the use of non-invasive techniques is a major advantage, although, clearly, less sophisticated tests would be applicable in the latter situation than in the former. Thus, the type of non-invasive method to be used will depend very much on the question being asked of the compound under evaluation. Some of the techniques are easier and cheaper to set up than others, but in all cases care has to be exercised that personnel using the technique are fully familiar with it and are convinced that the method does have the capability of assessing the measurements being made, using most of the criteria considered above.

Heart Rate and Blood Pressure

Invariably, in all assessments of drugs on the cardiovascular system, measurements are made of heart rate and blood pressure. These two measurements form the basis of 'screening' the effects of compounds in man for cardiovascular activity and for safety reasons. It is not intended to discuss these methods of measurements to any major extent. Heart rate can be measured accurately and reproducibly from ECGs, and the whole system can now be computerised, so that objective records can be easily produced. Blood pressure can be measured non-invasively with standard sphygmomanometry and cuff systems. However, these systems are subjective, and new non-invasive automated machines are available to measure blood pressures. These machines do need validating, and while reasonable correlations do exist for resting supine and standing systolic and diastolic blood pressure, they cannot be used in exercise and should be considered unreliable when major changes in blood pressure are induced—for example, with isoprenaline (Arnold and McDevitt, 1985). Methods of measuring blood pressure have been reviewed (e.g. Raftery, 1978). If more sophisticated estimates of the effects of drugs on heart rate or blood pressure are required, then non-invasive 24 h ambulatory techniques are available which give valuable information on the effects of drugs on these parameters with the subjects during their normal daily lives (e.g. Stott *et al.*, 1980).

Cardiac Function

'Cardiac function' here refers essentially to left ventricular function. Therefore, the non-invasive methods considered are those which will assess inotropic state of the heart and cardiac output, both related to left ventricular activity. The following describes some of the more commonly used assessments.

Systolic Time-intervals

Systolic time-intervals are derived from a simultaneous recording of the ECG (usually lead II), the phonocardiogram and the indirect recording of the cardiac pulse from an air-filled system (Weissler *et al.*, 1969). A typical record is shown in Figure 21.2. The measurements made are left ventricular ejection time (LVET—measured from the onset of the rapid upstart of the carotid

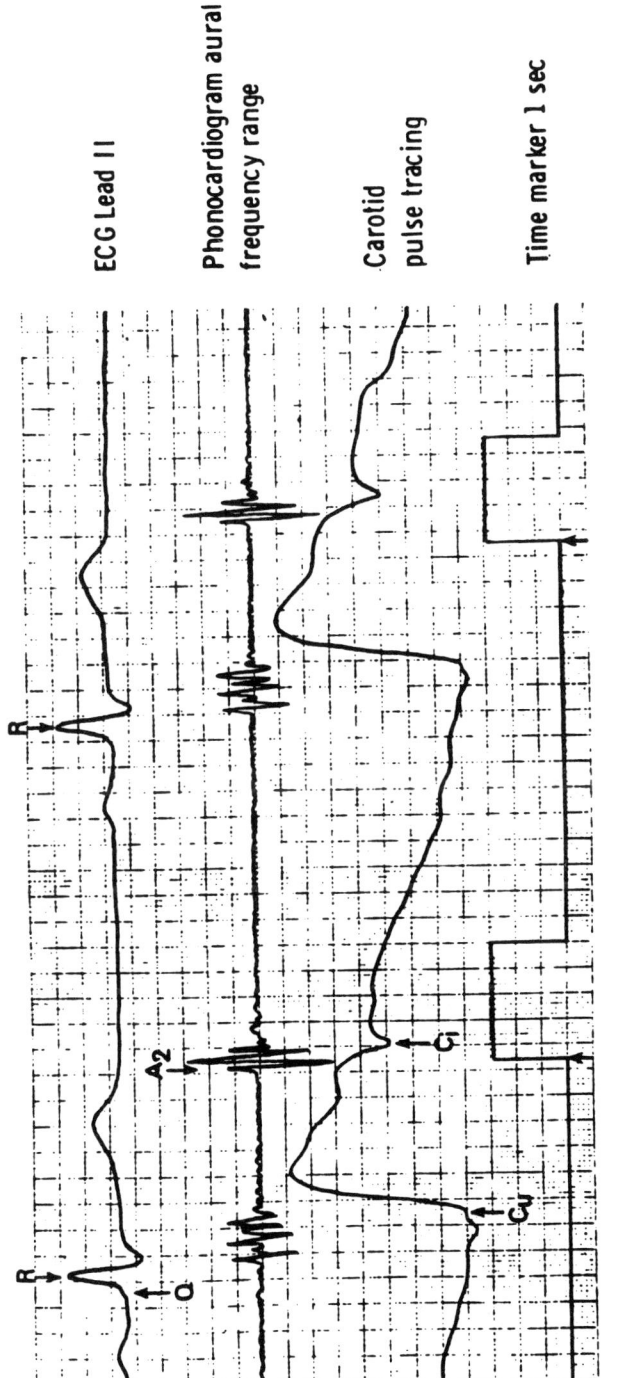

ECG Lead II

Phonocardiogram aural frequency range

Carotid pulse tracing

Time marker 1 sec

Q = onset of Q wave
R = peak of R wave
A_2 = beginning of the aortic component of second heart sound
C_u = carotid pulse wave upstroke
C_i = carotid pulse wave incisura

Figure 21.2 Simultaneous recordings of the ECG phonocardiogram and carotid pulse tracing from which the systolic time intervals can be measured

pulse to the incisura); electromechanical systole (QA_2—measured from the peak of the q-wave in the ECG to first deflection of the aortic component component of the 2nd heart sound); and pre-ejection period (PEP—which is derived from $LVET - QA_2$). The methods and techniques of making the measurements of systolic time-intervals are reviewed by Lewis *et al.* (1977)—an article which also includes data on validation and reproducibility of the method. Under conditions where no changes in heart rate, preload or after-load (blood pressure) occur as a result of an intervention, reductions in these values represent a positive inotropic change in the heart and increases represent a negative inotropic change (e.g. review by Gibson, 1975). Because changes in heart rate are known to affect these systolic time-intervals, regression equations relating each measurement to heart rate have been established and are used to correct the measurements for heart rate (Weissler *et al.*, 1968). These equations of Weissler have been used by many laboratories to correct the measurements of the intervals, but it has been argued that each laboratory should create its own equations for its own subjects rather than use those generalised by Weissler, who developed his equation on his own normal subjects (Kelman *et al.*, 1981).

Systolic time-intervals have proved useful to studies in our laboratory when trying to determine whether Xamoterol (ICI 118,557), a β_1-selective partial agonist, produced a positive inotropic effect in normal volunteers following the first administration in man. Reductions in the indices occurred and were considered relevant because there were no changes in heart rate or blood pressure; thus, Xamoterol had produced the inotropic effect (Marlow *et al.*, 1980). Further, dobutamine produced changes in systolic time-intervals consistent with a positive inotropic action and was used to determine at which dose a β_2-selective adrenoceptor blocking agent effected this predominant β_1-effect (Harry *et al.*, 1988b).

Echocardiography

Echocardiography utilises ultrasonic signals reflected from cardiac structures, thus allowing continuous recordings of the motion of these cardiac structures. Several adaptations have been developed, of which the two most important are M-mode echocardiography and two-dimensional echocardiography. Both of these systems can give information non-invasively about the function of the heart, particularly the left ventricle, but the M-mode system is probably best for considering the effects of drugs on cardiac performance. The principles and techniques of M-mode echocardiography are described elsewhere (e.g. Feigenbaum, 1976). Direct measurements that can be made are thickness of interventricular septum and left ventricular posterior wall, with the distance between the endocardial surfaces of the septum and the posterior wall representing the volume of the left ventricle. It is from the volumes of the ventricle in systole and diastole that stroke volume can be estimated and from changes in thickness of the ventricular wall that inotropic state can be assessed (various parameters have been derived from this latter assessment—Popp, 1982). Validation of the method with invasive techniques to measure stroke volume shows reasonable correlation (Kronik *et al.*, 1979), but reproducibility requires great experience on the part of the user because of the problems of standardisation of the transducer position (Popp *et al.*, 1975). Positive inotropic effects of compounds can be assessed with M-mode echocardiography, e.g. with dobutamine or milrinone, but, as with other assessments of left ventricular function, special tests need to be performed to ascertain whether the effects are on the heart or secondary to other changes in circulation (Borow *et al.*, 1986).

Doppler or Echo-Doppler Cardiography

Doppler techniques can be used to measure the velocity of blood elements (particularly red blood cells) in any large vessel (for details of techniques and instrumentation, see Baker *et al.*, 1977). If these measurements are made in the aorta just above the aorta valve (from a probe positioned in the suprasternal notch), assessments of aortic ejection velocity can be made. Integrals of this velocity signal in systole correspond to stroke volume (Calocousis *et al.*, 1977).

Other parameters which can be measured from the Doppler shift recordings are peak flow velocity, ejection time and acceleration time. All of these measurements will be affected by changes in ventricular function. Cardiac output can be measured by multiplying the systolic velocity integral by the cross-sectional area of the aorta and the heart rate. The cross-sectional area of the aorta is assessed by the use of M-mode echocardiography. Newer Doppler techniques are being developed which assess stroke volume without the need to measure the cross-sectional area of the root of the aorta (e.g. 'Quantascope'—Silke *et al.*, 1987). However, for the assessment of the effects of drugs in volunteer studies to determine whether a new compound affects ventricular function, it should not be necessary to measure cardiac output but just the Doppler markers of ventricular function, as was shown by Harry *et al.* (1988a) for dobutamine. Good correlations exist, at rest, between assessments of cardiac output made from Doppler recordings and invasive techniques (Rose *et al.*, 1984; Innes *et al.*, 1987). However, the technique is not very good on exercise, although some authors suggest that it might be (Daley *et al.*, 1985). Reproducibility of results is good (e.g. Gardin *et al.*, 1984; Harry *et al.*, 1988a), but to achieve this reproducibility training and continuous use by the user are required.

Impedance Cardiography

Impedance cardiography involves the creation of an electrical field in the chest by the passage of a small current across it. As the blood is ejected from the ventricles, its movement within the electrical field creates changes in the transthoracic impedance. These changes in electrical impedance can be monitored electrically, to yield a measurement of stroke volume. Details of the system can be found in review articles, e.g. Mohapatra (1981). There appears to be a reasonable correlation between cardiac output assessed by cardiac impedance methods and cardiac output assessed by conventional invasive techniques (e.g. Gabriel *et al.*, 1976; Teo *et al.*, 1985). The method can be used during exercise. Reproducibility is good (Teo *et al.*, 1985), with an acceptable sensitivity of the same order as that of the dilution estimates of cardiac output.

CO_2 Rebreathing Techniques

The standard Fick principle to measure cardiac output requires estimates of either oxygen (O_2) or carbon dioxide (CO_2) in the mixed venous blood and the arterial blood, so that the differences between the two (O_2 or CO_2) can be measured, from which cardiac output can be calculated if O_2 consumption or CO_2 creation over a period of time is known. Indirect methods of assessing arteriolar and mixed venous CO_2 have now been developed, using rebreathing techniques which have been made possible by the advent of rapid infrared CO_2 analysers (capnometers). Mixed venous CO_2 is estimated by a 'plateau' or equilibrium method (Collier, 1956) and arterial CO_2 by making estimations of end-tidal CO_2. The details of the operations and methods used are reviewed by, for example, Ceretelli *et al.* (1966). With the Collier equilibrium technique good correlation exists between the CO_2 rebreathing method and invasive direct Fick or dye dilution methods when assessing resting and exercising cardiac output (e.g. Franciosa *et al.*, 1976; Reybrouck *et al.*, 1978). Hinderliter *et al.* (1986) found the method to be less sensitive than Doppler echocardiography to detect changes in cardiac output induced by propranolol or cuff inflation of the limbs.

CONCLUSIONS

Various non-invasive methods are now available to assess the effects of drugs in man on cardiac function. However, each of the methods does require sophisticated technology and computer-assisted modules to make the handling of results reasonable; indeed the Doppler techniques do require spectral analysis of the waveform, which is hardly possible without computer analysis. This makes the equipment for each technique expensive. However, each of the methods outlined does allow description of the effects of drugs in early development on cardiac function in volunteers and patients, all methods at rest and a few on exercise. Whichever system is used within any one laboratory, the persons making the assessments must be trained in the technique and then validate, assess reproducibility, etc., in their own setting before meaningful results with new chemical entities can be achieved upon which to base decisions about the effect of the compound on the heart.

REFERENCES

Arnold, J. M. O. and McDevitt, D. G. (1984). Indirect blood pressure measurement during intravenous isoprenoline infusions. *Br. J. Clin. Pharm.*, **19**, 114–16

Baker, D. W., Rubenstein, S. A. and Lord, G. S. (1977). Pulsed doppler echocardiography: principles and applications. *Am. J. Med.*, **63**, 69–80

Bojanowski, L. M., Timmis, A. D., Najm, Y. C. and Gosling, R. G. (1987). Pulsed doppler ultrasound compared with thermodilution for monitoring cardiac output responses to changing left ventricular function. *Cardiovasc. Res.*, **21**, 260–8

Borow, K., Neumann, A. and Lang, R. M. (1986). Milrinone versus dobutamine: contribution of altered myocardial mechanics and augmented inotropic state to improved left ventricular performance. *Circulation*, **73** Suppl. III), 153–60

Calocousis, J. S., Huntsman, L. L. and Curreri, P. W. (1977). Estimation of stroke volume changes by ultrasonic doppler. *Circulation*, **56**, 914–17

Ceretelli, P., Cruz, J. C., Farhi, L. E. and Rahn, K. (1966). Determination of mixed venous O_2 and CO_2 tension and cardiac output by a rebreathing method. *Resp. Physiol.*, **1**, 258–64

Collier, C. (1956). Determination of mixed venous CO_2 tension by rebreathing. *J. Appl. Physiol.*, **9**, 25–9

Daley, P. J., Sagar, K. B. and Wann, L. S. (1985). Doppler echocardiographic measurement of flow velocity in the ascending aorta during supine and upright exercise. *Br. Heart J.*, **54**, 562–7

Feigenbaum, H. (1976). *Echocardiography*, 2nd edn. Lea and Febiger, Philadelphia

Franciosa, J. A., Ragan, D. O. and Rubenstone, S. J. (1976). Validation of the CO_2 rebreathing method for measuring cardiac output in patients with hypertension or heart failure. *J. Lab. Clin. Med.*, **88**, 672–82

Furnival, C. M., Linden, R. J. and Snow, H. M. (1970). Inotropic changes in the left ventricle: the effect of changes in heart rate, aortic pressure and end-diastolic pressure. *J. Physiol.*, **211**, 359–87

Gabriel, S., Atternberg, J. H., Oro, L. and Ekeland, L. G. (1976). Measurement of cardiac output by impedance cardiography in patients with myocardial infarction. Comparative evaluation of impedance and dye dilution methods. *Scand. J. Clin. Lab. Invest.*, **36**, 29–34

Gardin, J. M., Dabestani, A., Martin, K., Allfine, A., Russell, D. and Henry, W. G. (1984). Reproducibility of Doppler aortic flow measurements: studies on intraobserver, interobserver and day to day variability in normal subjects. *Am. J. Cardiol.*, **54**, 1092–8

Gibson, D. G. (1975). Assessment of left ventricular function in man by non-invasive techniques. *Mod. Trends Cardiol.*, **3**, 247–79

Harry, J. D., Millson, D. S. and Morton, P. B. (1988a). Use of Doppler echocardiography to determine the cardiac effects of dobutamine in volunteers. *Pharm. Med.*, **3**, 173–83

Harry, J. D., Norris, S. C., Percival, G. C. and Young, J. (1988b). The dose in humans at which ICI 118,557 (a selective β_2-adrenoceptor blocking agent) demonstrates blockade of β_1-adrenoceptors. *Clin. Pharm. Ther.*, **43**, 492–8

Hinderliter, A. L., Fitzpatrick, M. A., Schork, N. and Julius, S. (1987). Research utility of non-invasive methods for measurement of cardiac output. *Clin. Pharm. Ther.*, **41**, 419–25

Innes, J. A., Mills, C. J. and Noble, M. I. M. (1987). Validation of beat by beat pulsed doppler measurements of ascending aortic blood velocity in man. *Cardiovasc. Res.*, **21**, 72–80

Innes, J. A., Simon, T. D., Murphy, K. and Guz, A. (1988). The effects of exercise and subject age on pulsed Doppler measurements of left ventricular ejection in normal man. *Q. Jl. Exp. Physiol.*, **73**, 323–41

Jewitt, D., Mitchall, A., Birkhead, J. and Dollery, C. (1974). Clinical cardiovascular pharmacology of dobutamine, a selective inotropic catecholamine. *Lancet*, **2**, 363–7

Kelman, A. W., Sumner, D. J. and Whiting, B. (1981). Systolic time intervals versus heart rate regression equations using atropine in reproducibility studies. *Br. J. Clin. Pharm.*, **12**, 15–20

Kronik, G., Slany, J. and Mosslacher, H. (1979). Comparative value of eight M-mode echocardiographic formulas for determining left ventricular stroke volume. *Circulation*, **60**, 1308–16

Kupari, M. (1983). Reproducibility of the systolic time intervals: effect of the temporal range of measurements. *Cardiovasc. Res.*, **17**, 339–43

Lewis, R. P., Rittgers, S. E., Forester, W. F. and Boudoulas, H. (1977). A critical review of the systolic time intervals. *Circulation*, **56**, 146–8

Loepky, J. A., Hockenga, D. E., Green, E. R. and Luft, N. C. (1984). Comparison of non-invasive pulsed doppler and Fick measurements of stroke volume in cardiac patients. *Am. Heart J.*, **107**, 339–40

Marlow, H. F., Harry, J. D. and Shield, A. G. (1980). Duration of action of single intravenous doses of ICI 118587, a cardiac β stimulant. *1st World Congress on Clinical Pharmacology, London*. Abstract No. 0772

Mohapatra, S. N. (1981). *Non-invasive Cardiovascular Monitoring by Electrical Impedance Technique*. Pitman Medical, London, pp. 33–69

Otterstad, J. E., Hurlen, M., Michelsen, S. I. and Krutsen, K. M. (1987). Reproducibility of serial M-mode and doppler echocardiographic recordings of left ventricular dimensions and function: a comparison with traditional measurements of heart rate and blood pressure in apparently healthy men. *J. Cardiovasc. Ultrason.*, **6**, 285–95

Popp, R. L. (1982). M-mode echocardiographic assessment of left ventricular function. *Am. J. Cardiol.*, **49**, 1312–18

Popp, R. L., Fally, K., Brown, O. R. and Harrison, D. C. (1975). Effect of transducer placement on echocardiographic measurement of left ventricular dimensions. *Am. J. Cardiol.*, **34**, 537–40

Raftery, E. B. (1978). The methodology of blood pressure recording. *Br. J. Clin. Pharm.*, **6**, 193–202

Reybrouck, T., Amery, A., Billet, L., Fagard, R. and Stijus, H. (1978). Comparison of cardiac output determined by a carbon dioxide rebreathing and direct Fick method at rest and during exercise. *Clin. Sci. Molec. Med.*, **55**, 445–52

Robson, S. C., Boys, R. J. and Hunter, S. (1988). Doppler echocardiographic estimation of cardiac output: analysis of temporal variability. *Eur. Heart J.*, **9**, 313–18

Rose, J. S., Nanna, N., Rahintoola, S. H., Elkayam, U., McKay, C. and Chadraratna, P. A. W. (1984). Accuracy of determination of changes in cardiac output by transcutaneous continuous wave doppler computer. *J. Am. Coll. Cardiol.*, **54**, 1099–102

Schuster, A. J. and Nanda, N. V. (1984). Doppler echocardiographic measurement of cardiac output: comparison with a non-golden standard. *Am. J. Cardiol.*, **53**, 257–9

Silke, B., Evan, J. M., Verma, S. P., Sharma, S. K. and Taylor, S. H. (1988). A new echodoppler ultrasound method of cardiac output determination. *Br. J. Clin. Pharm.*, **25**, 147P

Stott, F. D., Raftery, E. B. and Goulding, L. (Eds.) (1980). *Isam 1979—Proceedings of the Third International Symposium on Ambulatory Monitoring*. Academic Press, London

Teo, K. K., Hetherington, M. D., Hoennel, R. G., Greenwood, V., Rossall, R. E. and Kappagoda, T. (1985). Cardiac output measured by impedance cardiography during maximal exercise tests. *Cardiovasc. Res.*, **19**, 737–43

Weissler, A. M., Harris, W. S. and Schoenfeld, C. D. (1968). Systolic time intervals in heart failure in man. *Circulation*, **37**, 149–59

Weissler, A. M., Harris, W. S. and Schoenfeld, C. D. (1969). Bedside techniques for the evaluation of ventricular function in man. *Am. J. Cardiol.*, **23**, 577–83

22
Anti-anginal Drugs

Edmond Roland

Rhône-Poulenc Santé, 20 Avenue Raymond Aron, 92165 Antony Cedex, France

INTRODUCTION

Considerable advances have been made over the past few years in the understanding of the mechanisms responsible for precipitation or exacerbating anginal pain (Maseri, 1983, 1987; Epstein *et al.*, 1988). These advances have modified the therapeutic approach to the syndrome and it seems important to review them before presenting the methods for evaluation of anti-anginal drugs.

PATHOPHYSIOLOGY OF CORONARY AND MYOCARDIAL FUNCTION IN ANGINA PECTORIS: CRITICAL ASPECTS FOR DRUGS EVALUATION

Under physiological conditions, a close correlation is observed between the increase in myocardial oxygen consumption and coronary blood flow over a wide range (Schaper *et al.*, 1985). Coronary flow is regulated by oxygen demand (momentary oxygen consumption) and by oxygen delivery. The main factors which determine myocardial oxygen consumption ($M\dot{V}_{O_2}$) are those using most of the available energy: heart rate, contractility and wall tension (Figure 22.1). In wall tension, it is mainly pressure development and left ventricular volume. In contractility, it is the velocity of fibre shortening. Unlike the situation in skeletal muscle, oxygen extraction by the myocardium is almost at a maximum level at rest: this results in a wide and constant arteriovenous oxygen difference between coronary arteries and coronary sinus in man. The normal coronary system consists of large epicardial vessels, which normally function as passive conduits and offer little intrinsic resistance to flow (Epstein *et al.*, 1985; Schaper *et al.*, 1985). The intramyocardial arterioles, on the other hand, alter their intrinsic tone in response to the demands of the myocardium for oxygen. Because of their small diameter and well-developed media, they have the capacity to alter profoundly resistance to flow (Epstein *et al.*, 1985; Schaper *et al.*, 1985). The intramyocardial arteriole resistance. Through the autoregulatory system provided by these arterioles, myocardial oxygen delivery and myocardial oxygen consumption are closely linked: when MV_{O_2} increases the resistance vessels dilate and thereby permit myocardial flow to increase in proportion to the increased

265

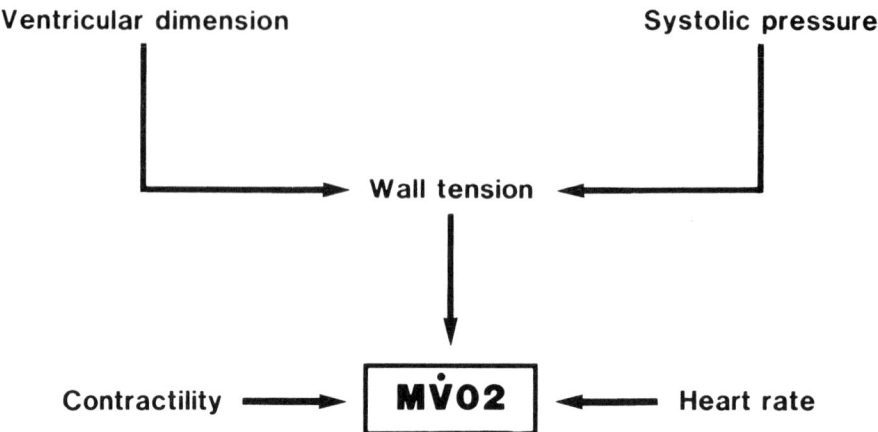

Figure 22.1   Determinants of myocardial oxygen consumption ($M\dot{V}_{O_2}$)

oxygen demands (Epstein *et al.*, 1985). Ischaemia is induced when the capacity of oxygen delivery cannot meet oxygen demand any longer, owing to increasing proximal resistance in the coronary system. This situation is provoked by either excessive increase in $M\dot{V}_{O_2}$ beyond a certain threshold or a primary critical reduction in the coronary lumen (Figure 22.2).

When a large epicardial vessel is narrowed by a fixed atherosclerotic lesion, its conductance function is compromised and it now offers considerable resistance to flow. If no other alteration occurs, the increased resistance leads to a decrease in flow and thereby causes ischaemia. However, ischaemia-induced metabolic derangements activate autoregulatory mechanisms, resulting in arteriolar dilatation and decrease in arteriolar resistance (Schaper *et al.*, 1985). Because epicardial artery resistance and arteriolar resistance are in series, total coronary vascular resistance returns towards normal (Epstein *et al.*, 1985). Further increases in large-vessel obstruction cause progressive arteriolar dilatation, and resting flow will remain normal until the vasodilator reserve of the arterioles is exceeded. Although this compensatory mechanism may prevent the appearance of ischaemia under resting conditions, it is not adequate to prevent ischaemia when large increments in flow are required, as with exercise. During exercise, once the vasodilator reserve of the arterioles is exhausted, flow can no longer increase as a result of further decreases in resistance. When this maximal flow threshold is exceeded, myocardial ischaemia and angina appear.

Although the concept of fixed obstruction provides a ready explanation for the onset of angina with exercise when $M\dot{V}_{O_2}$ increases considerably, it cannot explain the onset of angina occurring at rest without obvious increase in $M\dot{V}_{O_2}$ or why anginal threshold should vary markedly during different times of the day or of the week or during different seasons of the year, as it so frequently does in patients with angina (Crea *et al.*, 1986; Maseri, 1987). The finding that dynamic increases in either large- or small-vessel coronary resistance can also precipitate ischaemia or reduce the threshold of $M\dot{V}_{O_2}$ at which it occurs has

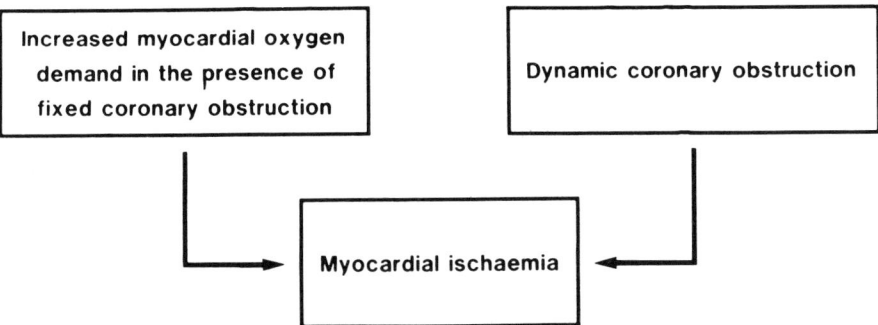

Figure 22.2 Mechanism of transient myocardial ischaemia

important implications for the therapy of angina pectoris (Epstein *et al.*, 1985). This dynamic coronary obstruction may occur within or outside a stenotic segment. The product of systolic pressure and heart rate (double product) at angina onset is a reflection of the maximal rate at which the obstructed coronary artery is capable of delivering oxygen. By examining the effect of anti-anginal agents on the double product, as indirect index of myocardial oxygen demand, two types of pharmacological interventions could be considered. If an intervention improves exercise capacity, but the double product at angina is no higher than control levels, it implies that the intervention causes the beneficial effect by decreasing oxygen demand at any level of external stress (Figure 22.3) and this type of pharmacological action

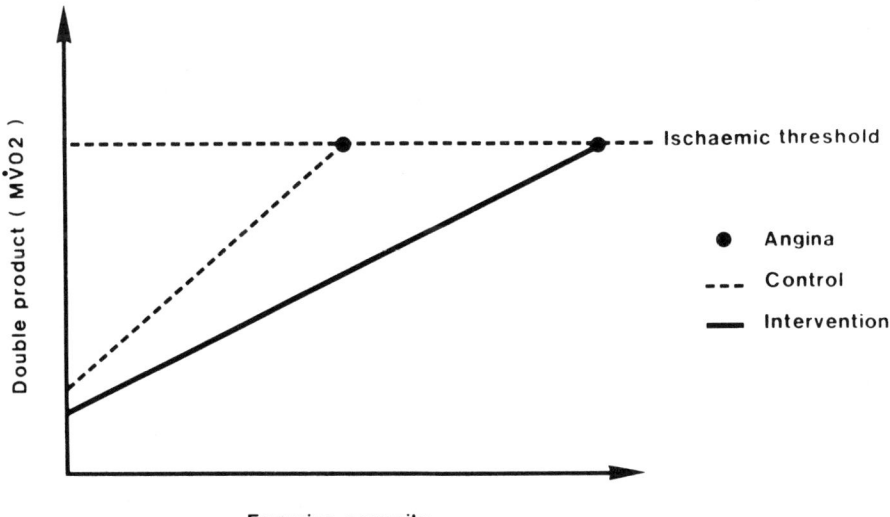

Figure 22.3 Pharmacological intervention that improves exercise capacity by reducing myocardial oxygen consumption ($M\dot{V}_{O_2}$). Exercise capacity improves but angina occurs at same or lower level of $M\dot{V}_{O_2}$ and coronary flow reserve remains constant

would be more effective against fixed coronary obstruction. If exercise capacity is improved and double product at angina increases, the implication is that the myocardium can attain a higher workload before ischaemia occurs, most probably because myocardial flow has increased (Figure 22.4) and such intervention is designed more against dynamic coronary obstruction. Of course, a single anti-anginal agent can combine both types of response.

The onset of myocardial ischaemia is followed by left ventricular dysfunction, electrocardiographic changes and angina, in that order. In the presence of ischaemia, the absence of angina does not signify the absence of ventricular dysfunction (Schaper *et al.*, 1985). The first haemodynamic changes observed during exercise-induced ischaemia are the slowing of isovolumic relaxation and contraction. This is followed by an abnormal increase in end-diastolic pressure due to the loss of contraction and increased wall stiffness in the ischaemic left ventricular wall segment. Of special importance is the relation between diastolic pressure and volume, i.e. diastolic compliance during ischaemia. Several studies have clearly shown that during ischaemia the immediate haemodynamic alterations may result primarily from a change in left ventricular diastolic compliance rather than left ventricular systolic pressure (Schaper *et al.*, 1985). Thus, the increase in left ventricular end-diastolic pressure is a very early sign of ischaemia. In addition, it has been shown that abnormalities of the level of the small coronary arteries (endocardial layers) can contribute to precipitation of myocardial ischaemia, either by dynamically increasing coronary resistance in response to vasoconstrictor influences profound enough to cause ischaemia at rest or by restricting vasodilator reserve and thus the potential to augment flow, which would

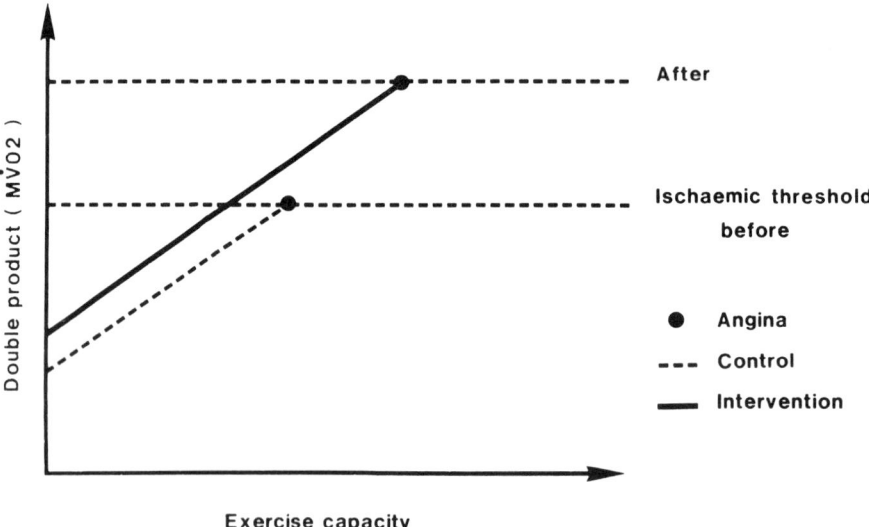

Figure 22.4 Pharmacological intervention that improves exercise capacity by increasing coronary flow. Exercise capacity improves with a higher ischaemic threshold and an improved coronary flow reserve

predispose to the development of ischaemia during interventions that in-crease myocardial oxygen requirements (Maseri, 1987). Although the abnor-mal coronary vasodilator reserve can be ascribed to vasoconstrictor influences modulating the tone of small coronary arteries, it is also possible that the inadequate vasodilator reserve could be due to abnormal myocardial com-pressive forces, i.e. increased left ventricular diastolic pressure might increase myocardial wall tension during diastole and thereby interfere with coronary flow (Schaper *et al.*, 1985; Klocke *et al.*,1987). This fact emphasises the complex relationship between left ventricular function and coronary flow, particularly in the endocardial layers (Klocke *et al.*, 1987).

In summary, pharmacodynamic effects which reduce myocardial oxygen consumption are: (1) a decrease in preload (left ventricular diastolic press-ure), (2) a decrease in heart rate, (3) a decrease in contractility, (4) a decrease in afterload through a decrease in arterial impedance. Pharmacodynamic effects aiming at reducing the dynamic coronary obstruction are: (1) spas-molytic action on coronary arteries and (2) reduction of preload through a decrease in diastolic pressure.

METHODS FOR EARLY EVALUATION OF ANTI-ANGINAL DRUGS

By definition, angina pectoris is a clinical symptom which implies acute transient myocardial ischaemia. The goal of therapy will be to alleviate ischaemia pain through a reduction of the imbalance between oxygen supply and consumption. This chapter is mainly devoted to the evaluation of drugs for exertional angina. Methods for early evaluation of anti-anginal agents can be divided into two categories: (1) measurements which give the pharmacody-namic profile in man and indirect evidence for efficacy; (2) methods which determine direct evidence of drug efficacy.

Pharmacodynamic Profile in Man

From the pathophysiology of angina pectoris, it is obvious that it is important to consider the mode of action in man of a potential anti-anginal drug, which may predict its clinical efficacy (Kraupp, 1985). However, such studies, in general, do not provide direct evidence for anti-anginal efficacy of the drug. Many anti-anginal agents act, at least in part, by causing dilatation of the peripheral vessels (Kraupp, 1985). Therefore, when animal studies indicate that the experimental drug has vasoactive effects at concentrations at all comparable with the therapeutic level, initial studies in man should include an assessment of the effects of the compound on resistance in arteries and veins. While the symptoms of angina pectoris and their relief by anti-anginal agents can be assessed only with reference to the sufferer, a full understanding of the mechanisms of action of anti-anginal drugs requires objective assessment of their circulatory effects, including those on the peripheral circulation. Such drugs can relieve anginal pain through reducing myocardial oxygen consumption by either cardiac or extracardiac effects (Kraupp, 1985). The cardiac effects may include contractility, heart rate, coronary flow and left ventricular function. The extracardiac effects involve the peripheral circulation by reducing preload or afterload. Preload is reduced when venous capacity rises as a result of venous dilatation and, hence, venous return and cardiac filling are decreased. In fact, reduction of preload and afterload is also a possible means of treating heart failure, so that the same vasodilator drug may be of benefit in both angina and heart failure. This convergence of interests strengthens the case for adequate assessment of the peripheral actions of anti-anginal drugs and the major role played by haemodynamic studies at this stage.

Haemodynamic Studies

Right and Left Catheterisation Protocol

The purpose of such study is to gain information on the effects of the anti-anginal agent on basic haemodynamic parameters, and more precisely on cardiac loading condition. The adequate population would be at the beginning patients undergoing routine right or left catheterisation for chest pain and with normal left ventricular function or patients who need a close monitoring of their haemodynamic state—for example, after an acute myocardial infarction with signs of heart failure.

Right heart catheterisation   With the technique of flow-directed right heart catheterisation, the effects of anti-anginal medication on cardiac output and left ventricular filling pressure can readily be quantified and even monitored at the bedside throughout the medical intervention. Pressures measured by flotation catheters must be referred to an appropriate zero point (related to the level of the tricuspid valve, which is usually located in the supine position at the upper border of two-thirds of the tranversal diameter of the thorax, measured from the table surface). Different types of catheter are available, ranging from the 4F end-hole latex system for single pressure recordings to the 7F double-lumen flotation catheter (Swan–Ganz type) used for double-chamber diameter pressure recordings and evaluation of cardiac output by thermodilution. With careful maintenance of the zero reference point and exact calibration, pressure may be recorded with an accuracy of ± 2 mmHg under clinical conditions. Left ventricular end-diastolic pressure is reflected by the pulmonary end-diastolic pressure in wedge position (PWP), if both mitral stenosis and pulmonary hypertension are absent. Thus, PWP is a good assessment of cardiac preload and the normal value is less than 12 mmHg.

Thermodilution is the most common technique for the determination of cardiac output because of its convenience. Ice-cold water is injected into the right atrium and the change in temperature is detected by a thermistor located 4 cm from the catheter tip, which is positioned in the main stem of the pulmonary artery. The blood need not be withdrawn, in contrast with other indicator techniques, i.e. indocyanine green. The procedure is easily carried out at the bedside by one person. The thermodilution technique meets the assumptions of Fick's law of diffusion if homogeneous temperature mixing is present. Portable computer devices providing rapid data display are commonly used for uniform sampling and calculation of the transient changes in blood temperature. To improve precision, repeated (at least three consecutive) measurements of the same conditions are advisable and the mean value should be taken.

Left heart catheterisation is only acceptable if patients have an indication for coronary angiography. Left heart catheterisation from the right femoral sheath may be performed with a variety of catheters. Manometer-tipped catheters, with which the transducer is placed in the cardiac chamber, are usually used to achieve the most accurate recording of pressures. The principal advantage of left heart catheterisation is the facility to assess left ventricular contractility or performance through measurements of left ventricular pressures, stroke volume and ventricular volume.

Pressure measurements The accuracy of the assessment of cardiac performance can be increased by adding a measurement of left ventricular end-diastolic pressure to that of stroke volume. Thus, when the ventricular end-diastolic pressure is elevated and the stroke index is reduced, myocardial contractility is probably impaired. Since changes in the maximum rate of rise of ventricular pressure (peak dp/dt) are known to be highly sensitive to acute changes in contractility, measurement of ventricular dp/dt may be employed along with filling pressure in the assessment of contractility. High-fidelity catheter-tip micromanometers should be employed to obtain a reliable assessment of peak dp/dt. Peak dp/dt is largely independent of afterload and appears to be more markedly affected by changes in contractility than by preload. However, the latter influence cannot be disregarded.

Quantitative angiography Measurements of the volumes of cardiac chambers can be made utilising cineangiograms with contrast material injected into the left ventricle. The hyperosmolarity produced by the contrast agent increases blood volume, which begins to raise preload and heart rate within 30 s of the injection, an effect which may persist for as long as 2 h. Therefore, when multiple observations in a comparable state are desired, it is essential to monitor the haemodynamics, to ensure that they have returned to control levels, before the angiogram is repeated. Selective injection of contrast material is essential to obtain the image of the opacified left ventricular cavity in either monoplane or biplane views. The ejection fraction (EF) is derived from planimetric measurements with the assumption that the ventricle is ellipsoidal in shape. The definition of the ejection fraction is:

$$\text{EF } (\%) = \frac{\text{end-diastolic volume} - \text{end-systolic volume}}{\text{end-diastolic volume}} \times 100$$

In addition to the measurement of the global ejection fraction of the left ventricle, the ventriculogram can also assess regional ejection fraction to detect segmental wall motion abnormalities (Nienaber and Bleifeld, 1985).

The wall motion may be normal or may show decreased inward movement (hypokinesis) or absent movement (akinesis). The presence of a hypokinetic or akinetic segment on the resting ventriculogram may not necessarily indicate fibrous scarring after infarction, but can also be caused by severe underperfusion of still-viable myocardium. The regional wall motion can be readily improved after acute reduction of preload by vasodilating drugs. Pharmacologically induced venous pooling has beneficial effects on both myocardial oxygen supply and demand, especially when ventricular diastolic pressures are elevated. Moreover, when coronary vessels are narrowed by atherosclerotic lesions or by spasm, relaxation of normal or increased smooth muscle tone at the site of the stenosis by a vasodilating agent may increase native and collateral flow (Klocke *et al.*, 1987), enabling critically underperfused territories to re-establish contractile function (Nienaber and Bleifeld, 1985). Depressed regional left ventricular ejection fraction due to regional ischaemia will normalise if the oxygen supply/demand ratio is normalised by any pharmacological intervention.

Quantitative Coronary Angiography

Quantitative measurement of stenosis severity could become a useful tool in the evaluation of vasoactive drugs (Nienaber and Bleifeld, 1985; Reiber *et al.*, 1985; Demer *et al.*, 1988). Adequate geometric analysis by quantitative coronary arteriography includes dimensions of percentage narrowing, absolute diameter and length combined into fluid dynamic equations to provide a single integrated measure of severity, i.e. flow reserve (Demer *et al.*, 1988). This anatomic–geometric method has been validated experimentally, completely automated and tested for routine clinical use (Reiber *et al.*, 1985). Both the area of stenosis and the cross-sectional area of a normal segment can dilate with infusion of vasodilators. In the presence of coronary stenosis involving primarily a single vessel, downstream flow may be maintained through collateral channels arising from neighbouring relatively normal coronary arteries (Klocke *et al.*, 1987). Thus, in the presence of coronary obstruction localised to a territory with collateral development, vasoactive agents may increase collateral flow through vasodilation of collateral vessels or by relaxation of normal smooth muscle tone at the site of the stenosis.

There are four different mechanisms for altered severity of coronary artery stenosis during changing vasomotor states of the distal vascular bed: (1) arterial smooth muscle relaxation and vasodilatation of the stenotic segment; (2) vasodilatation of the coronary artery adjacent to the stenotic segment; (3) the appearance of fully developed turbulence in the stenotic segment; and (4) narrowing of the stenotic segment due to decreasing intraluminal pressure caused by arteriolar vasodilatation and decreasing distending pressure.

When performing pharmacological interventions during coronary angiography, two different approaches may be used: either repeated angiography in the same single view without altering the X-ray setting, or use of multiple angiographic views (Reiber *et al.*, 1985). In the first case, if the coronary segment is non-axisymmetric, induced vasodilatation may accentuate asymmetry of the lumen by preferentially relaxing the non-atherosclerotic part of the arterial wall. Consequently, the use of a single angiographic view will be misleading (Reiber *et al.*, 1985). Thus, the effects of vasodilators are better quantified if multiple projections are obtained. This will increase the accuracy of diameter measurements and will better reflect the true luminal cross-sectional area.

The attempt to visualise the vasodilating action of drugs with anti-anginal potency by quantitative evaluation of coronary arteriograms is often difficult, since relief of angina depends on several mechanisms.

Atrial Pacing

Left ventricular catheterisation and left ventricular angiography provide further functional information if performed under stress, such as atrial pacing.

Rapid atrial pacing has been used in the catheterisation laboratory as a controlled and reproducible method of producing myocardial ischaemia in patients with coronary artery disease. In this condition, pacing has been shown to induce angina-like chest pain, electrocardiographic S–T segment depression, myocardial lactate production, increases in left ventricular filling pressure, decreases in left ventricular ejection fraction and segmental wall motion abnormalities (Markham *et al.*, 1983). Usually the right atrial pacing test is performed 30 min after the completion of coronary arteriography; using the percutaneous femoral approach, a bipolar flared pacing catheter is placed within the right atrium. When a satisfactory pacing threshold has been achieved, the pacing rate is increased by increments of 10 or 20 beats/min rapidly until angina or atrioventricular block occurs. If atrioventricular block develops at a rate that is less than 85% of the age-predicted maximal heart rate, 1 mg atropine is administered intravenously. Pacing is initiated at a rate of 80 beats/min. At each pacing rate, the presence, intensity and character of chest discomfort are recorded. Pacing is discontinued either when typical chest symptoms with significant ECG changes have developed or when a pacing rate has been achieved that is at least 85% of the age-predicted maximal rate. Three-channel ECG monitoring is continued during pacing and a 12-lead electrocardiogram is obtained before, during each pacing level, immediately after cessation of pacing and until chest pain and ECG changes resolve. The usual ECG criteria for myocardial ischaemia are 1 mm or more of horizontal or downsloping segment depression from 0.08 s or longer beyond the J point, in any lead using the PR segment as the baseline. The changes must be observed on at least three consecutive beats with a steady baseline. Haemodynamic measurements are performed at baseline, peak pacing rate and 30 s after abrupt termination of pacing.

Although atrial pacing seems to be a very simple method to produce myocardial ischaemia, the electrocardiographic, metabolic and haemodynamic alterations that may accompany pacing-induced ischaemia are specific but relatively insensitive markers of ischaemia (Markham *et al.*, 1983). Chest pain during atrial pacing is a non-specific occurrence, appearing with similar frequency in normal subjects and patients with coronary artery disease and pacing-induced ischaemia. Post-pacing ECG S–T segment depression >0.1 mV occurs in slightly more than half of those with pacing-induced ischaemia but it also occurs on occasion in normal subjects (Markham *et al.*, 1983). Both peak-pacing myocardial lactate production and postpacing elevation of left ventricular end-diastolic pressure are highly specific but relatively insensitive reflectors of pacing-induced ischaemia. This relative insensitivity might improve if atrial pacing were performed more rapidly (>140 beats/min) or for a longer period of time (>4 min).

Assessment of Coronary Blood Flow

Following the discovery that the coronary sinus could safely be catheterised in man, a variety of techniques have been developed using coronary sinus intubation and sampling (Marcus *et al.*, 1987).

Continuous thermodilution   Coronary sinus thermodilution is an inexpensive, widely available technique for the measurement of coronary flow and is the most frequently applied approach to studying coronary flow in patients. This technique needs a preformed triple-function Webster catheter. Cold saline or dextrose is infused continuously down the catheter into the coronary sinus at a high flow rate of 35–55 ml/min, to ensure adequate mixing. The resistance of the infused saline and the saline–blood mixture is recorded by two thermistors, from which sinus flow is calculated. There are several advantages to this technique. It requires only right heart catheterisation to cannulate the coronary sinus and is therefore remarkably safe. The method can be repeated on several occasions during cardiac catheterisation and is ideal for drug studies on myocardial metabolism, as coronary sinus samples can be obtained at constant heart rates by use of the pacing facilities of the catheter and the lumen of the catheter. The equipment is cheap compared with the cost of radioisotope methods, but X-ray screening is required. Despite these attractive features, the method has severe limitations. Phasic coronary flood or rapid changes in mean flow cannot be assessed, because the time constant of the technique is slow. Perfusion in specific transmural layers cannot be estimated, and regional left ventricular flow measurements are confined to crude separation of anterior vein flow (left ventricular anterior wall and septum) and perfusion to a large but indeterminate area of the left ventricle (distal coronary sinus). Convincing validation studies, coronary sinus thermodilution employed under clinically relevant conditions versus an accepted standard, have never been presented (Marcus *et al.*, 1987). In spite of its limitations, the technique of continuous thermodilution remains one of the fundamental methods available for the study of the effects of drugs on coronary flow with facilities for simultaneous study of myocardial metabolism and oxygen consumption.

Gas clearance methods   Several non-radioactive gases (nitrous oxide, hydrogen, helium, argon) and radioactive ^{133}Xe have been used in such studies (Marcus *et al.*, 1987). This approach requires obtaining simultaneous arterial and coronary sinus blood for measurements of gas concentration during the saturation or desaturation phase of gas administration. All the limitations of thermodilution methods are equally applicable to gas clearance methods. Several test curves are necessary to construct reliable arterial and coronary sinus curves with heterogeneous flow. Overall, the method takes time and is not the most suitable for studies of changes of flow following drug intervention.

Electromagnetic flow probes and Doppler techniques have been used mainly to assess flow in vein bypass grafts and rarely to measure flow in native coronary vessels (Marcus *et al.*, 1987). Although the intraoperative Doppler technique is useful for research applications, the clinical applicability is minimal because the measurement can only be obtained during open heart surgery. Recently, a small 3F Doppler catheter has been developed which can measure flow in major coronary vessels. However, because the Doppler catheters require intracoronary cannulation, there will always be some risk associated with this approach, which does not seem attractive for drug evaluation.

Positron-emission tomography could in theory be used for precise non-invasive measurement of regional myocardial perfusion. In practice, this goal has yet not been achieved, because the radionuclides available for positron-emission tomography are not ideal and many imaging artefacts continue to plague this method (Marcus *et al.*, 1987). On the horizon, a new generation of techniques, magnetic resonance imaging, ultrafast computed tomography and contrast echocardiography, may permit precise measurement of perfusion in different layers of the left ventricle without cardiac catheterisation (Demer *et al.*, 1988). Although very promising, these new techniques should be carefully validated before using them for drug development.

Radionuclide Methods

Radionuclide methods for testing anti-anginal drugs should be used at rest and when myocardial ischaemia occurs, i.e. under exercise. Two types of information could be gathered with radionuclide methods: myocardial perfusion and myocardial function.

Radionuclide Procedures for Myocardial Perfusion

^{201}Tl is the most widely used perfusion imaging agent because of its advantageous biological and physical properties, which are superior to those of older agents. Its relatively low-energy photons allow the application of high-resolution collimators and the physical half-life of 73 h provides a long shelf-life for practical clinical imaging. Following an intravenous injection, ^{201}Tl accumulates in the myocardium very rapidly and myocardial concentration is proportional to flow. The initial extraction fraction is 85–88%. Because of this high extraction efficiency during the first pass, thallium concentration in the blood is low, approximately 10% of the initial concentration 2 min after injection and less than 1% after 2 h (Adam *et al.*, 1985). In clinical use, 1.5–2 mCi of ^{201}Tl is injected intravenously with the patient at rest or while exercising. The exercise images are of better quality because of a higher myocardial concentration of thallium (a result of inward coronary blood flow) and lower background activity. In exercise studies, the patient should continue to exercise an additional 1 min after thallium injection, to ensure the distribution of ^{201}Tl at peak exercise. Images are obtained in multiple projections. The presence of a perfusion defect on the initial image may represent either ischaemia or scar or both. The distinction can be made by comparing the initial images with delayed images obtained 4 h after injection. The persistence of a defect in the delayed images denotes a fixed defect (Adam *et al.*, 1985). The advantages of ^{201}Tl over exercise ECG are higher sensitivity (80–90%) and specificity (85–95%) and ability to localize the disease vessels and to assess the viability of the myocardium (Kaul *et al.*, 1988). However, the sensitivity and specificity of exercise thallium image depend, to a certain extent, on the observer's interpretative ability and experience. The variability of observers in interpretation as to the presence or absence of a defect is 10–15%, and even higher variations are noted when the anatomical location of the defect is examined (Iskandrian *et al.*, 1985). Thallium scintigraphy is difficult to use for evaluating anti-anginal drugs, mainly because on acute test (control and drug intervention study in one session) is not feasible. After the control examination, a relatively long time has to elapse until radioactivity can be applied again. Repositioning of the patient and gamma camera is necessary, which affects reproducibility. More important, the patient has to be exposed to another dose of radiation. In addition, quantification is difficult.

Assessment of Left Ventricular Performance with Radionuclide Angiography

The approach of nuclear cardiology is based on the assumption that cyclic motion of each myocardial region can be described as a set of time-dependent count rates, forming a representative time–activity curve, which corresponds to the time–volume curve of the respective region. This can be attained by a gating procedure which produces a set of heart images describing one heart cycle. After radiolabelling the blood pool (with 20 mC 99^{m}Tc), the myocardial count rate depends on the volume changes of the heart. This technique involves external imaging of the cardiac blood pool with an external imaging device, such as a probe or gamma scintillation camera. The simplest procedure is to show the scans in rapid sequence, so that the heart motion becomes visible. Two methods of radionuclide analysis of left ventricular function have been utilised. In the first method, the transit of a bolus of radionuclide material as it passes through the central circulation is observed (first-pass technique). In the second method, the left ventricle is visualised using radioactive substances that circulate in the blood in a steady state. This equilibrium technique requires gating of multiple RR intervals to produce a summed, composite cardiac cycle (gated blood-pool technique). The latter is preferred for pharmacological intervention, since after one injection serial studies of EF and volume can be performed for several hours. Regional wall motion abnormalities can be detected immediately. This is of special interest for drug administration, because after injection of 99 ^{m}Tc-labelled erythrocytes, the heart motion can be observed for about 5–7 h. Thus, improvement of regional wall motion after administration of anti-anginal drugs can be closely monitored (Nestico *et al.*, 1985).

Rest and exercise radionuclide angiography is a useful technique to study the cardiac adaptation during exercise in patients with coronary artery disease. Most patients with coronary artery disease have an abnormal ejection fraction (EF) response to exercise (Adam *et al.*, 1985). Radionuclide angiography permits evaluation of the regional and global systolic function and the pressure–volume relationship during both systole and diastole. Reproducibility and variability in these measurements should be considered. In good laboratories, the inter- and intraindividual variability is less than 5%, but each laboratory should establish its own reproducibility results (Nestico *et al.*, 1985). A more important point, however, is the reproducibility of results when measurements are separated by days or weeks. Sequential studies in normal individuals and patients with coronary artery disease have shown up to 10% differences in EF, especially in subjects with normal resting EF. While such variation may reflect technical limitations, it could also be due to variation in sympathetic tone (Nestico *et al.*, 1985). Similar variations in EF have been observed when contrast angiography is used instead of radionuclide angiography. In addition, the drug-induced changes in EF may depend on baseline EF and the presence or absence of myocardial ischaemia. The latter is especially important in interpreting changes in exercise EF.

Non-invasive methods, such as echocardiography and systolic time-intervals, are not mentioned here, since they are discussed in another chapter of the book.

Direct Evidence of Efficacy: Exercise Tests

Exercise testing is an established method for detecting coronary artery disease, evaluating the severity of disease and prognosis (Detrano and Froelicher, 1988). In addition, exercise tolerance testing is considered the primary method for establishing prophylactic antianginal efficacy (WHO, 1984).

Exercise Test Modalities

Two types of exercise tests can be used: isometric or dynamic. Isometric exercise, defined as constant muscular contraction without movement (i.e. handgrip), imposes a disproportionate pressure load on the left ventricle relative to the body's ability to supply oxygen. Dynamic exercise, defined as rhythmic muscular activity resulting in movement, initiates a more appropriate increase in cardiac output and oxygen exchange (Froelicher, 1984). Since a delivered workload can be accurately calibrated and the physiological response easily measured, dynamic exercise is preferred for clinical testing. Using progressive workloads of dynamic exercise, patients with coronary disease can be protected from rapidly increasing myocardial oxygen demand. A maximal exercise test brings an individual to a level of intensity where fatigue or symptoms prohibit further exercise or when maximal oxygen consumption (V_{O_2} max) is achieved and no further increase in heart rate occurs. Estimates of predicted maximal heart rate may be used as a guide for test termination, but these estimates should not be used as predetermined termination points in maximal testing.

When measurement of maximal exercise capacity is intended, possibilities include the treadmill and the upright bicycle ergometer. Cycle ergometer tests provide for stable ECG and blood pressure recording. Intravascular catheters may be kept in place, expired air may be collected easily, and both echdocardiographic and scintigraphic observations may be made. Their main disadvantages are that individuals who are not accustomed to cycling will often be unable to reach maximal heart rates owing to leg fatigue, and results depend upon complete subject co-operation in order to maintain a constant work rate in following a specific protocol.

Treadmill testing permits the highest oxygen consumption rate of any common exercise device. Both speed and elevation can be varied over a wide range of exercise intensities with excellent reproducibility (American Heart Association, 1972; Froelicher, 1984). External control of the work rate is attained with a minimum of subject co-operation. It may be more difficult to obtain exact recording of the blood pressure and ECG at near-maximal workloads. In addition, treadmill exercise is not suitable for studies requiring a relatively immobile thorax, such as those involving indwelling vascular catheters or sensitive precordial detectors such as echocardiographs or scintillation cameras.

Test Protocols

For each subject an appropriate cardiovascular history and examination should be performed prior to the exercise test. The subject should be tested either after an overnight fast or no earlier than 2 h after a light meal. Patients should abstain from tobacco, alcohol and caffeine for at least 3 h prior to testing. The subject should be informed of the indications for the test, the details of its procedure and the potential hazards of testing, and should then provide written informed consent. A 12-lead conventional resting electrocardiogram must be recorded and examined for possible contraindications (Table 22.1) and the interpretation should be recorded prior to exercise. A number of different treadmill and cycle ergometer protocols are widely used (Table 22.2) (American Heart Association, 1972; Froelicher, 1984; American College of Sports Medicine, 1986). Cycle ergometer protocols use an increased external work of 25–30 W per stage. The duration of each stage should be 2–3 min.

Table 22.1   Contraindications to exercise testing

(1)	Recent acute myocardial infarction (less than 3 months)
(2)	Unstable angina pectoris
(3)	Severe aortic stenosis
(4)	Uncontrolled cardiac dysrhythmia
(5)	Acute myocarditis or pericarditis
(6)	Severe hypertension
(7)	Congestive heart failure
(8)	Intracardiac conduction block greater than first-degree
(9)	Suspected or known dissecting aneurysm
(10)	Thrombophlebitis or pulmonary embolus
(11)	Acute systemic illness

Table 22.2

	Stage	Speed (mile/h)	Elevation (%-grade)	Duration (min)
Bruce test:	1	1.7	10.0	3
	2	2.5	12.0	3
	3	3.4	14.0	3
	4	4.2	16.0	3
	5	5.0	18.0	3
	6	5.5	20.0	3
	7	6.0	22.0	3
Naughton test:	1	2.0	0.0	3
	2	2.0	3.5	3
	3	2.0	7.0	3
	4	2.0	10.5	3
	5	2.0	14.0	3
	6	2.0	17.5	3
	7	2.0	21.0	3

ECG tracing should be continuously displayed on a scope and then recorded on paper at least once per exercise stage and at each minute post-exercise. Blood pressure should be measured before exercise, at least once during each exercise stage and every 2 min post-exercise until stable. Exercise is continued by the subject until termination points are reached (Table 22.3). In the post-exercise period a complete 12-lead ECG should be recorded immediately and at 2 and 4 min post-exercise in addition to any other leads. Post-exercise observation should continue for 6 min or until all

Table 22.3 Indications for stopping an exercise test

(1) Angina-like pain that is progressive during exercise (stop at 3+ level or earlier on a scale of from 1+ to 4+)
(2) Excessive degree (≥ 0.4 mV) of ischaemic type of ST-segment depression or elevation
(3) Ventricular tachycardia, multifocal premature ventricular contractions or frequent (>30%) premature ventricular contractions aggravated or precipitated by exercise
(4) Ectopic supraventricular tachycardia
(5) Exercise-induced intracardiac block
(6) Signs of severe peripheral circulatory insufficiency: pallor, confusion, ataxia, diminished pulse
(7) Any significant drop (10 mmHg) of systolic blood pressure or failure of the systolic blood pressure to rise with an increase in exercise load
(8) Excessive blood pressure rise: systolic greater than 250 mmHg, diastolic greater than 120 mmHg
(9) Unexplained inappropriate bradycardia
(10) Excessive fatigue or dyspnoea
(11) Failure of monitoring system
(12) Subject requests to stop

exercise-induced abnormalities have disappeared. Exercise testing should be supervised by a physician trained in the procedure, and the exercise laboratory should be equipped and organised for patient safety measures.

Interpretation of Exercise Test

When interpreting the exercise test, it is important to consider each of its facets separately. A test should not be called abnormal (positive) or normal (negative); rather, the interpretation should specify which responses were abnormal or normal and each should be given a weighted value. There are other parameters besides the ECG that should be monitored, including patient appearance, blood pressure, heart rate response, symptoms and functional capacity. Criteria for stopping a test are listed in Table 22.3. Some criteria constitute an abnormal response to exercise testing. These abnormal responses may or may not be a result of ischaemia.

Evaluation of ECG Data

Many different lead systems have been used for exercise testing (Froelicher, 1984; Detrano and Froelicher, 1988). This situation has complicated making comparisons of the ST-segment response to exercise. Bipolar lead systems (CM5 Naughton test, CB5 Bruce test or Wilson leads V_2 and V_5) have been used for reasons of convenience. Since the question of how many leads need to be recorded during an exercise test has not been resolved, it seems advisable to record as many as are economically and practically possible. In patients with a normal resting ECG, a V_5 or similar bipolar lead along the long axis of the heart may be adequate. In patients with ECG evidence of myocardial damage, additional leads are needed. As a minimal approach, it is advisable to record three leads—a V_5 type lead, an anterior V_2 type lead and an inferior lead such as a VF—but a 12-lead system should usually be preferred (Mason–Likar system). The normal ST-segment vector response to tachycardia and to exercise is a shift to the right and upward. The most common manifestation of exercise-induced myocardial ischaemia is ST-segment depression. The standard criterion for this type of abnormal response is horizontal or downsloping ST-segment depression of 0.1 mV (1 mm) or more for 80 ms. It provides the optimum sensitivity and specificity (Froelicher, 1984; Detrano and Froelicher, 1988). The probability and severity of coronary artery disease are directly related to the amount of J-junction depression and are inversely related to the slope of the ST-segment. Because of these related factors, computer measurements such as the ST index and the ST integral, which take into account both slope and depression, should prove to be superior to classic criteria (Froelicher, 1984). Table 22.4 lists some of the conditions that can possibly result in false-positive responses. Digitalis, and psychotropic drugs such as tricyclic agents and other antidepressant drugs, can cause exercise-induced repolarisation abnormalities, especially in women. Anaemia, electrolyte abnormalities, meals and even glucose ingestion can alter the ST-segment and T-wave in the resting ECG and can potentially cause a false-positive response. To avoid this

Table 22.4 Conditions that can cause a false-positive exercise test

Drug administration (digitalis, psychotropic drugs)
Left ventricular hypertrophy
Bundle branch block
Wolff–Parkinson–White syndrome
Electrolyte abnormalities
Anaemia
Pericardial disorders
Mitral valve prolapse syndrome
Valvular heart disease

problem, all ECG studies should be performed after at least a 2–3 h fast. This requirement is also important because of the haemodynamic stress put on the cardiovascular systems by eating. After a meal functional capacity is decreased and the ischaemic threshold may vary. Left bundle branch block, left ventricular hypertrophy and WPW syndrome may induce ST-depression without coronary artery disease. Exercise electrocardiographic responses in men correspond more closely than in women with the presence or absence of coronary artery disease (Froelicher, 1984).

Development of ST-segment criteria other than exactly one or two divisions of the chart paper and problems with exercise artefact distortion of the electrocardiogram have set the stage for computer enhancement of ECG evaluation (Froelicher, 1984). By computerised averaging of ECG complexes, artefacts are reduced. Recognition algorithms identify the points on the ECG to be measured. This analysis made by computer has the capacity of much greater precision than is possible by visual measurement of conventional ECG. This is particularly crucial for some criteria such as determination of time to 1 mm ST-segment depression. Several computer systems have been developed and commercial adaptations are available.

Heart Rate and Blood Pressure

The normal blood pressure response to exercise is a progressive rise in systolic pressure with little change in the diastolic pressure. In most exercise protocols, the systolic blood pressure rises about 8–10 mmHg per stage. A pathological fall in blood pressure during exercise is encountered occasionally, and although an insensitive sign, it is claimed to be highly specific for severe coronary artery disease (Froelicher, 1984). The heart rate increases progressively with each increase in exercise intensity. The heart rate–systolic blood pressure product rises progressively during exercise testing, and its peak value serves to characterise the cardiovascular performance. Normal individuals usually develop a peak rate–pressure product of 20–35 mmHg $\times$ beats/min $\times$ 10^{-3}. In contrast, most patients with overt ischaemic heart disease will not be able to generate rate–pressure products exceeding 25 mmHg $\times$ beats/min $\times$ 10^{-3}. However, there is sufficient overlap in individual cases to prevent this product from being a useful single criterion of disease.

Maximal Work Capacity

Maximal work capacity is the most important measurement that can be gained from an exercise test. On a treadmill exercise protocol calling for increments of about 12 ml O_2 per kg body weight per minute per 3 min stage, the exercise endurance of adult men is about 11.5 min and that of women 7.6 min (Froelicher, 1984; American College of Sports, 1986). With the bicycle ergometer, the average maximal aerobic exercise capacity of men is about 1200 kpm/min and for women about 800 kp/m min. In spite of the wide normal variability of work capacity, the measurement of exercise protocol endurance has great value in the evaluation of patients with chest pain.

Effort Angina

Although various kinds of chest discomfort are encountered during exercise testing, the finding of symptoms characteristic of anginal pain improves the sensitivity of exercise ECG (Detrano and Froelicher, 1988). It has been reported that, whereas ST-segment changes alone detect 65% of patients with significant coronary disease, when characteristic pain was also considered a positive finding, the detection rate rose to 85%.

Criteria for Detection of an Anti-anginal Effect

The main objective criteria of efficacy are the changes in maximum work attained at the time of onset of anginal pain and/or ST-segment depression (i.e. 1 mm ST-segment depression). The time of onset of anginal pain is clearly one of the most important, since it is this that the drug is intended to prevent or alleviate (WHO, 1984). Changes in heart rate, systolic pressure, dyspnoea or tiredness, disturbances of rhythm or conduction which can be attributed to myocardial ischaemia should be recorded, but cannot be regarded as criteria for an anti-anginal effect.

Safety

The risk of exercise testing is approximately one death per 10000 tests in large, varied populations (Detrano and Froelicher, 1988). The more common risk can be detected by careful, attentive search for contraindications prior to testing (Table 22.1).

METHODOLOGICAL ISSUES IN THE EARLY EVALUATION OF ANTI-ANGINAL DRUGS

The objective of this early phase will be to identify whether with single or repeated doses there is indeed a beneficial effect in the prevention of angina and to obtain some information on the effective dosage, duration of effect and any frequent or severe adverse effects.

Patient Selection

For pharmacodynamic studies, patient selection is rather straightforward and consists mainly of subjects who have an indication for haemodynamic evaluation.

More careful attention should be paid to patients recruited in efficacy trials, i.e. exercise protocols. Those patients should be suffering from stable angina of effort which should be well characterised from the patients' history. The main task is to recruit only patients with true ischaemic heart disease. Therefore, ischaemic heart disease should be diagnosed using an acceptable objective criterion: documented past history of myocardial infarction; significant stenosis (>50%) of at least one major coronary artery on the coronary angiogram; positive symptom-limited exercise test (pain + significant ST-segment depression); positive thallium stress test. Patient condition should be stable, i.e. over a period of at least 1 month there should have been no clear deterioration or improvement. The resting electrocardiogram should be such as not to interfere with the interpretation of ST-segment changes during angina. For this reason it is advisable to recruit only male patients in early pilot trials.

Suitable study subjects should be identified by their response to exercise test. The major, and for practical reasons the only, acceptable efficacy criterion is the occurrence of anginal pain during exercise. An anti-anginal agent cannot be considered anti-anginal unless it increases the amount of exercise that a patient can perform prior to the development of angina after drug administration (WHO, 1984).

In order to be able to demonstrate an improvement in exercise capacity, selected patients should have neither too severe a form of angina nor too mild a degree of coronary artery disease. In this respect, the best population is patients who experience chest pain within 3–7 min of beginning exercise with the Bruce protocol. In addition, for purposes of being able to detect efficacy using small sample size, the reproducibility of the anginal pain in relationship to exercise becomes an important consideration. It has been reported that exercise capacity has a variability of 10–15% in good laboratories (Khurmi *et al.*, 1986; Detrano and Froelicher, 1988). Thus, prior to randomisation, the reproducibility of exercise tolerance should be evaluated and the decision to randomise patients should incorporate one additional criterion: a reproducible exercise test within the range of 15%. In contrast to a reasonably rigorous means of identifying patients with stable angina pectoris suitable for randomisation for early efficacy trials, a patient population with vasospastic angina, unstable angina or silent myocardial ischaemia is more difficult to deal with. Owing to the high variability and often critical condition of those patients, it is not recommended to focus early trials on this specific population when rough information on drug efficacy, dose–response relationship and duration of effect is not yet available. Therefore, evaluation of anti-anginal drugs in this specific setting is beyond the scope of this chapter.

In summary, the logic of the selection scheme for early efficacy trials with exercise protocols is to: select patients who have stable angina due to myocardial ischaemia; demonstrate that such patients have a positive symptom-limited exercise test and that spontaneous variation of exercise capacity is less than 15%.

Protocol Design

Treating angina is particularly challenging, because the patient's symptoms are subjective and highly prone to amelioration through a placebo effect (Benson and McCallie, 1979; Parisi *et al.*, 1982). This placebo effect may cause a 30–80% reduction in angina frequency. Even objective improvement as assessed by exercise test has been reported with an increase in exercise performance of 14–49% (Boissel *et al.*, 1986). Therefore, the most unambiguous means of demonstrating efficacy at this early stage is to use a placebo control. However, such placebo-controlled trials are not always easy to implement in symptomatic patients with coronary artery disease (Khurmi *et al.*, 1986). This difficulty could be overcome by careful selection of patients and rather short duration of treatment, from 2 days to 2 weeks. It has been shown that assignment to placebo group is not associated with increased adverse experience in short-term trials (Glasser *et al.*, 1988) or even in a long-term protocol (Boissel *et al.*, 1986).

Haemodynamic studies are usually open and performed after a single administration of the drug. However, appropriate design with use of blinding or adequate control strengthens such studies, especially pacing protocols.

For exercise efficacy protocols, a run-in period is essential. After carefully supervised withdrawal of prior anti-anginal drug therapy, the patient may be started on a single-blinded placebo run-in period of 1 week which allows: (1) assessment of exercise capacity and variability, (2) accustoming of the patient to the experimental procedure.

After randomisation, parallel designs are easiest to interpret. Cross-over studies with appropriate attention to randomisation of treatment sequence and to sufficiently long time-intervals could be used. This type of protocol is better suited to single administration of various doses of a short-acting drug. Single-dose or short-term efficacy studies should be performed with patients receiving no other anti-anginal agents except sublingual nitroglycerin for relief of anginal pain. For parallel design protocol using a placebo-controlled group, it is usual to recruit 20–30 patients per group.

The exercise tests should be performed under well-defined conditions as regards the time of the day, the period which has elapsed following administration of the drug or placebo, and the timing with respect to meals. Exercise tolerance tests should be carried out, if possible, between 9.00 and 11.00 hours in the fasting state or at least 2 h after a light breakfast. With frequent exercise testing, carried out on the same day or on successive days, a training effect may be observed. This fact emphasises the need for adequate randomisation and for a control group.

The main efficacy criteria are changes in exercise performance, and have been discussed earlier. Demonstration that an anti-anginal drug is active means that it is both anti-anginal and anti-ischaemic (WHO, 1984). This latter fact implies that the agent will delay the time to 1 mm ST-segment depression or for a given workload ST-segment depression will be reduced as compared with control state. Diary studies with counts of anginal attack rate or nitroglycerin consumption may provide supportive evidence of efficacy. However, such measurements cannot be the major data upon which a decision will rest at this early stage.

The time–effect relationship of single and multiple doses of drug is necessary to assess. This duration-of-effect evaluation should be performed with serial exercise tolerance tests. Such designs are usually flexible and do not raise safety issues. Every attempt should be made to study the relationship between blood concentrations and measures of efficacy. This can be performed during the dose–effect, time–effect studies. The correlation or lack of correlation between blood levels and effect or time-course of blood concentrations and time-course of effect should be considered a necessary description of the clinical pharmacology of the anti-anginal agent.

CONCLUSION

This early evaluation of anti-anginal drugs would need to focus upon:

(1) Defining the pharmacodynamic profile in man with haemodynamic studies which provide necessary insights into the mechanism of drug action. However, such studies, in general, do not provide primary evidence of anti-anginal or anti-ischaemic efficacy of the drug.
(2) Demonstrating the efficacy of the new anti-anginal agent when used alone with exercise tolerance protocols, performed on a homogeneous group of patients with stable angina.

REFERENCES

Adam, W. E. and Stauch, M. (1985). Radionuclide methods. In Abshagen, U. (Ed.), *Clinical Pharmacology of Antianginal Drugs*. Springer-Verlag, Berlin, pp. 213–37
American College of Sports Medicine (1986). *Guidelines for Exercise Testing and Prescription*. Lea and Febiger, Philadelphia
American Heart Association. The Committee on Exercise (1972). *Exercise Testing and Training of Apparently Healthy Individuals: A Handbook for Physicians*. American Heart Association, Dallas
Benson, H. and McCallie, D. P. (1979). Angina pectoris and the placebo effect. *New Engl. J. Med.*, **300**, 1424–9
Boissel, J. P., Philippon, A. M., Gauthier, E., Schbath, J., Destors, J. M. and the B.I.S. Research Group (1986). Time course of long-term placebo therapy effects in angina pectoris. *Eur. Heart J.*, **7**, 1030–6
Crea, F., Margonato, A., Kaski, J. C., Roohiguey-Plaza, L., Meran, D. O., Davies, G., Chierchia, S. and Maseri, A. (1986). Variability of results during repeat exercise stress testing in patients with stable angina pectoris: role of dynamic coronary flow reserve. *Am. Heart J.*, **112**, 249–54

Demer, L., Gould, K. L. and Kirkuide, R. (1988). Assessing stenosis severity: coronary flow reserve, collateral function, quantitative coronary arteriography, positron imaging and digital substraction angiography. A review and analysis. *Prog. Cardiovasc. Dis.*, **30**, 307–22

Detrano, R. and Froelicher, V. F. (1988). Exercise testing: uses and limitations considering recent studies. *Prog. Cardiovasc. Dis.*, **31**, 173–204

Epstein, S. E., Cannon, R. O., Watson, R. M., Leon, M. B., Bonow, R. O. and Rosing, D. R. (1985). Dynamic coronary obstruction as a cause of angina pectoris: implications regarding therapy. *Am. J. Cardiol.*, **55**, 61B–68B

Epstein, S. E., Quyyumi, A. A. and Bonow, R. O. (1988). Myocardial ischaemia—silent or symptomatic. *New Engl. J. Med.*, **318**, 1038–43

Froelicher, V. F. (1984). *Exercise Testing and Training.* Year Book Medical Publishers, Chicago, pp. 1–23, 38–74

Glasser, S. P., Clark, P. I., Lipicky, R. J. and Yusuf, S. (1988). What is the risk of exposing patients with chronic stable exertional angina to placebo in controlled trials of new drugs? *Circulation*, **78** (Suppl. II), II-99 (abstract)

Iskandrian, A. S. and Hakki, A. M. (1985). Thallium-201 myocardial scintigraphy. *Am. Heart J.*, **109**, 113–28

Kaul, S., Finkelstein, D. M., Homma, S., Leavitt, M., Okada, R. D. and Boucher, C. A. (1988). Superiority of quantitative exercise thallium-201 variables in determining long-term prognosis in ambulatory patients with chest pain: a comparison with cardiac catheterization. *J. Am. Coll. Cardiol.*, **12**, 25–34

Khurmi, N. S., Bowles, M. J., Kohli, R. S. and Raftery, E. B. (1986). Does placebo improve indexes of effort-induced myocardial ischemia? An objective study in 150 patients with chronic stable angina pectoris. *Am. J. Cardiol.*, **57**, 907–11

Klocke, F. J., Ellis, A. K. and Canty, J. M. (1987). Interpretation of changes in coronary flow that accompany pharmacologic interventions. *Circulation*, **75** (Suppl. V), V34–V38

Kraupp, O. (1985). Pharmacodynamic principles of action of antianginal drugs. In Abshagen, U. (Ed.), *Clinical Pharmacology of Antianginal Drugs.* Springer-Verlag, Berlin, pp. 97–115

Marcus, M. L., Wilson, R. F. and White, C. W. (1987). Methods of measurement of myocardial blood flow in patients: a critical review. *Circulation*, **76**, 245–53

Markham, R. V., Winniford, M. D., Firth, B. G., Nicod, P., Dehmen, G. J., Lewis, S. E. and Hillis, L. D. (1983). Symptomatic, electrocardiographic, metabolic, and hemodynamic alterations during pacing-induced myocardial ischemia. *Am. J. Cardiol.*, **51**, 1589–94

Maseri, A. (1983). The changing face of angina pectoris: practical implications. *Lancet*, **1**, 746–9

Maseri, A. (1987). Role of coronary artery spasm in symptomatic and silent myocardial ischemia. *J. Am. Coll. Cardiol.*, **9**, 249–62

Nestico, P. F., Hakki, A. H. and Iskadrian, A. S. (1985). Effects of cardiac medications on ventricular performance: emphasis on evaluation with radionuclide angiography. *Am. Heart J.*, **109**, 1070–84

Nienaber, C. and Bleifeld, W. (1985). Assessment of coronary artery disease and myocardial ischemia by invasive methods. In Abshagen, U. (Ed.), *Clinical Pharmacology of Antianginal Drugs.* Springer-Verlag, Berlin, pp. 239–84

Parisi, A. F., Strauss, W. E., McIntyre, K. M. and Sasahara, A. A. (1982). Considerations in evaluating new antianginal drugs. *Circulation*, **65** (Suppl. I), I38–I42

Reiber, J. H. C., Serruys, P. W., Kooijman, C. J., Wijns, W., Slager, C. J., Gerbrands, J. J., Schnurbiers, J. C. H., Den Boer, A. and Hugenholtz, P. G. (1985). Assessment of short, medium and long term variations in arterial dimensions from computer-assisted qualification of coronary cineangiograms. *Circulation*, **71**, 280–8

Schaper, W., Schaper, J. and Hoffmeister, H. M. (1985). Pathophysiology of coronary circulation and of acute coronary insufficiency. In Abshagen, U. (Ed.), *Clinical Pharmacology of Antianginal Drugs*. Springer-Verlag, Berlin, pp. 47–96

WHO (1984). *Guidelines for the Clinical Investigation of Antianginal Drugs*. Geneva

23
Anti-arrhythmic Agents

Pran K. Marrott

Director, Cardiovas Medicine, Berlex Laboratories Inc., 300 Fairfield Road, Wayne, NJ 07470–7358, USA

INTRODUCTION

Before its evaluation in man, the investigational drug will have been studied in suitable animal models in order to determine its pharmacology, pharmacokinetics and antiarrhythmic properties. The drug's antiarrhythmic action will have been classified (Vaughn Williams, 1984) and effective doses will have been determined. Acute and subacute animal toxicology (13 weeks) in two species will have been undertaken and the drug will have been shown to be free of significant toxic effects. Assay methodology for parent drug and active metabolites (if possible) will have been determined and validated, and pharmacokinetics of the drug in animal species will have been examined.

METHODOLOGIES

Appropriate methodologies are available for assessing in man the effect of the drug on cardiac arrhythmias, left ventricular (LV) performance, cardiac conduction, ventricular repolarisation and arrhythmia aggravation.

Assessment of the Drug's Effect on Arrhythmias

Continuous Long-term Electrocardiographic Monitoring

The evaluation of the effect of the investigational drug on ventricular ectopic (VPC) frequency is undertaken with the help of continuous long-term (24–48 h) electrocardiographic (ECG) monitoring (Holter tape recordings). Evaluation is made difficult by day-to-day and hour-to-hour variability in the frequency of VPCs, but various statistical principles have defined lower limits of VPC reduction for determining drug efficacy (Morganroth *et al.*, 1978; Winkle, 1978; Michelson and Morganroth, 1980; Sami *et al.*, 1980; Shapiro *et al.*, 1982). For multicentre studies, Holter tape evaluation is best undertaken by a central agency so that consistency of analysis can be guaranteed. Quality control is important, to ensure adequacy of recording instruments, quality of the tape, and accuracy and repeatability of the analysis method. Accuracy and repeatability of evaluation can be ensured by the introduction of gold standard tapes where the arrhythmia frequency has been previously verified (Morganroth, 1981). All Holter recordings are made for two successive 24 h periods, but if this is not possible, then baseline observations only are undertaken for two consecutive 24 h periods, whereas the remaining observations may be undertaken for 24 h periods. When 24 h observations are made, reduction in total VPC counts of $\geq 80\%$ ($\geq 90\%$ suppression of couplets and runs) is necessary to show that drug effect has occurred. For 48 h recordings, $\geq 70\%$ reduction of total VPC count ($\geq 90\%$ suppression of runs and couplets) is necessary to show that drug effect has occurred. The tapes (cassettes or reel-to-reel) used by the central agency should be compatible with the analysing system used by the investigator. This is necessary, as rapid analysis of the Holter tape may be required, in certain instances, to determine whether or not to continue medication. Correct electrode placement and the use of good-quality electrodes will avoid disappointment resulting from blank tapes. ECG recordings obtained for less than 18 h out of 24 h should be discarded. Evaluation of Holter tape data should be individualised for each patient and not pooled for all patients, since the between-patient variability is very large.

Transtelephonic Cardiac Rhythm Monitoring

Transtelephonic cardiac rhythm monitoring (TTM) is accomplished by the use of a portable ECG modulator to transmit the cardiac rhythm (ECG strip) of patients by telephone to a central agency where it is recorded and instantly analysed. The report of analysis is communicated urgently by telephone, or by mail (as necessary), to the patient's physician. The equipment consists of three components: an ECG transmitter that converts cardiac electrical activity to acoustic waves; a telephone wire; and an ECG receiver that transforms the message received into electrical signals. Several different types of ECG transmitters are available. These transmit ECG information from a single lead for from 30 s to 3 min. Modifications of this basic system include multiple leads and memory, allowing ECG storage when a telephone is not immediately available. Several studies have used TTM to examine the response to investigational drug therapy in patients with cardiac rhythm disorders (Bucknall *et al.*, 1984; Anderson *et al.*, 1988; Henthorn *et al.*, 1988).

Craig Pratt *et al.* (1987) have shown that the use of TTM for following up patients with chronic symptoms associated with cardiac rhythm disorders is complementary to Holter tape evaluation and successfully maintains monitoring of patients receiving anti-arrhythmic therapy. TTM should be used during the follow-up of patients with ventricular tachycardia (VT), to monitor both efficacy and safety (absence of proarrhythmia) of the drug under investigation. In patients with supraventricular tachycardia (SVT), TTM can be more reliably linked to efficacy if patients selected for the drug studies are those who are known to have clearly defined symptoms in association with their tachycardia.

Exercise Testing

Circulating catecholamines affect myocardial electrophysiological properties and influence the mechanisms that cause arrhythmias. Exercise augments sympathetic tone and is an important tool for the exposure of arrhythmia as well as for the evaluation of antiarrhythmic agents (Podrid *et al.*, 1987). Therefore, in addition to long-term ECG monitoring, exercise tests should be undertaken to assess the effect of the investigational drug on ventricular arrhythmias occurring during exercise. In the case of drugs with Class II (beta-receptor blocking) properties, the beta-receptor blocking effect of the drug, based on reduction of exercise-induced tachycardia, will also be determined.

Symptom-limited treadmill exercise tests using a modified Bruce protocol are appropriate. The exercise tests are analysed for heart rate, systolic and diastolic blood pressure, double product at peak exercise and total exercise duration. VPC frequency and complexity, and the number of runs, both before and following drug therapy, are evaluated by visual inspection and quantification of all beats from a compressed single-channel ECG that should include the upright exercise time and 10 min of supine rest, after exercise.

Programmed Electrical Stimulation Studies

Studies involving programmed electrical stimulation (PES) of the heart have been used to assess the effect of the investigational anti-arrhythmic drug on the induction of monomorphic sustained VT in patients with VT or those resuscitated from ventricular fibrillation (VF). Premature ventricular stimuli (1–3) are introduced during right ventricular (RV) pacing at 2–3 pacing cycle lengths from the RV apex and outflow tract. Monomorphic sustained VT can be induced by this technique in up to 84% patients with previously documented VT and serves as a useful objective parameter against which the response to an anti-arrhythmic drug may be assessed (Horowitz *et al.*, 1982). Non-sustained or polymorphic VT and VF are not considered to be suitable end-points of PES, since they may occur as a non-specific response to aggressive stimulation (Brugada *et al.*, 1983; Mann *et al.*, 1983; Buxton *et al.*, 1984). On the other hand, the specificity for PES induction of sustained monomorphic VT is almost 100% (Vandepol *et al.*, 1980; Livelli *et al.*, 1982; Brugada *et al.*, 1983; Schoenfeld *et al.*, 1984). Patients in whom the drug prevents induction and partial responders can be followed up in the long term to assess long-term efficacy and safety. Invasive tests such as the above do carry some risks, but these risks are low when studies are performed by experienced physicians. Baseline electrophysiological studies should be undertaken after washout of previous anti-arrhythmic drugs for at least five drug half-lives. Patients in whom sustained monomorphic VT is induced are then given the test drug, orally, for a few days and the PES study is repeated when steady state conditions are reached. In addition to assessing the inducibility of monomorphic sustained VT, conduction times and refractory periods of the atrium, ventricle and AV node are also determined, to examine the effect of the drug on these cardiac electrophysiological parameters.

Electrophysiological (EP) testing after oral doses is preferable to similar testing after intravenous (i.v.) drug administration, since there may be differences in metabolism and since i.v. dosing may produce blood levels that may not reflect myocardial tissue levels.

In patients with SVT due to AV nodal re-entry or AV re-entry, the anti-arrhythmic effect of the drug, given orally for a few days (until steady state is reached), may be examined by assessing inducibility of SVT both before and following the drug therapy. Single and double extra stimuli at 2–3 pacing cycle lengths are introduced from the right atrium, coronary sinus and RV to induce tachycardia. The tachycardia circuit is defined and the presence of a dual-functional AV nodal pathway or an AV anomalous pathway is confirmed. Programmed electrical stimulation is undertaken at baseline and repeated after oral dosing, and the effect of the drug on conduction times and the refractory periods of the atrium, AV node, ventricle and anomalous AV pathway (antegrade and retrograde) is determined. In patients with Wolff–Parkinson–White Syndrome (WPW), the effect of the drug on ventricular rate during atrial fibrillation (AF) should also be determined. This is particularly important in WPW patients with a short refractory period (antegrade) of the anomalous pathway, since drug therapy may slow ventricular rate to better-tolerated levels, if AF does occur. In patients with paroxysmal AF or atrial flutter, EP testing as a tool for the assessment of antiarrhythmic efficacy is not widely accepted.

Assessment of the Drug's Effect on Cardiac Performance

Systolic Time-intervals

Systolic time-intervals measure phases of LV systole from simultaneous recordings of the electrocardiogram (ECG), the phonocardiogram and the carotid arterial pulse tracing.

A reduction in LV performance is associated with a lengthening of the pre-ejection period and a shortening of the LV ejection time with no alteration of electro-mechanical systole. These changes correlate closely with reduced stroke volume and with reduced LV ejection fraction (LVEF) (Weissler, 1977). Assessment of LV function by measurement of systolic time-intervals has been superseded by other non-invasive techniques such as echocardiography and radionuclide angiography. Nevertheless, this method of assessing LV performance is acceptable for Phase I studies if the facility or expertise for echocardiographic or radionuclide assessment is not available.

Echocardiography

For the assessment of LV performance, M-mode echocardiography is appropriate and reliable in healthy subjects and patients with normal hearts. It is unreliable when there is associated segmental LV wall abnormalities, as is often the case, in patients with coronary artery disease (Fortuin *et al.*, 1971; Pombo *et al.*, 1971; Quinones *et al.*, 1974; Henning *et al.*, 1975). M-mode echocardiography has been largely superseded by two-dimensional (2D) echocardiography.

The development of electronically phased 2D echocardiography with a wide scanning angle and a small transducer allows the capability of obtaining biplane images which are similar to angiographic images obtained following contrast angiography. Studies have shown that there is good correlation between LVEF obtained by the above technique and LVEF obtained by single-plane or biplane contrast LV angiography and/or LVEF obtained by gated cardiac blood-pool imaging (radionuclide ventriculography), despite an underestimation of LV volumes (Schiller *et al.*, 1979; Barrett *et al.*, 1981; Quinones *et al.*, 1981; Starling *et al.*, 1981). One drawback of echocardiography is the inability to obtain high-quality images in 10–20% of subjects (Starling *et al.*, 1981).

Radionuclide Ventriculography

Cardiac performance can be assessed by radionuclide techniques. The two commonly employed techniques are first-pass radionuclide ventriculography, which involves the evaluation of first transit through the circulation, and the gated equilibrium technique, which involves the analysis of the entire blood pool after intravascular labelling. Radiopharmaceuticals labelled with ^{99m}Tc are used for first-pass studies and for blood-pool labelling in equilibrium studies. The first-pass technique, which can measure both LVEF and RVEF, can be performed extremely rapidly. The actual period of data acquisition is less than 30 s. On the other hand, the gated equilibrium study samples and sums up several hundred cardiac cycles. Therefore, cardiac status should be stable during data acquisition. There is excellent correlation between the two methods over a wide range of ejection fractions. The equilibrium study is less prone to error because of transient arrhythmias than is the first-pass technique, where analysis is limited to only a few cardiac cycles. However, if ectopic beats occur more than 20% of the time, the equilibrium study may be of no value unless computational ability exists to screen out data from irregularly occurring cardiac cycles (Zaret and Berger, 1986).

Swan–Ganz Catheterisation

In this invasive method for assessing cardiac performance, a balloon flotation catheter (Swan–Ganz catheter) is inserted percutaneously through a large central venous channel and advanced to the pulmonary artery. Right atrial, RV, pulmonary artery and pulmonary capillary wedge pressure are measured. Cardiac output is determined by the thermodilution technique, and systemic and pulmonary vascular resistances are calculated. This invasive method for assessing cardiac performance carries negligible risks and is used for the assessment of the acute haemodynamic effects of the drug.

Assessment of the Effect of the Drug on Conduction Times and Repolarisation

The effect of the drug on atrioventricular (PR interval), and intraventricular (QRS duration) conduction and ventricular repolarisation (QT interval) can be determined by measuring these surface ECG parameters in investigational drug studies. Class I drugs increase atrioventricular conduction time and intraventricular conduction, with varying effect on ventricular repolarisation times; antiarrhythmic drugs with Class Ia activity increase ventricular repolarisation time; drugs with Class Ib action reduce repolarisation time; and Class Ic drugs do not significantly affect ventricular repolarisation. From the QT and RR interval values, the corrected QT interval, QT_c (corrected for heart rate), is determined. Several formulae are available for this conversion but no formula fits the relationship between QT interval and heart rate as well as Bazett's formula: $QT_c = QT/\sqrt{RR}$ (Ahnve, 1984).

When ECG interval measurements are required, a 12-lead ECG is obtained at 50 mm/s speed. Since QRS begins earliest in leads V_1–V_3 and since these leads also show the highest voltage of T-wave, it has been suggested that one of these leads be used for the measurement of QT interval (Lepeschkin, 1952). However, others have used either the standard lead showing the longest QT interval or any lead showing the longest QT interval (Simonson *et al.*, 1962; Ahnve, 1984). In those instances where several ECG interval measurements are made each day—for example, when the duration of effect on surface ECG parameters is being examined—it may be difficult to obtain 12-lead ECGs several times a day. In such instances printouts from monitoring leads placed in an appropriate (e.g. Lead V_2 or II) position may be used. At least five consecutive sinus cycles should be measured and the figures averaged.

Assessment of the Drug's Effect on Arrhythmia Aggravation

Since most anti-arrhythmic drugs can induce new or aggravate existing arrhythmias, a careful attempt should be made to document the occurrence of arrhythmia aggravation or new arrhythmias (pro-arrhythmic responses). Sinus arrest, second-degree or complete AV block, SVT, atrial flutter or AF and ventricular tachyarrhythmias not seen before may occur during drug therapy. The drug may also increase the frequency of VPCs. Velebit *et al.* (1982) have proposed that the following should constitute a pro-arrhythmic response: (1) a fourfold increase in the frequency of VPCs when compared with control; (2) a tenfold increase in repetitive forms (couplets or runs of VT) when compared with the control values; and (3) the occurrence of recurrent VT that is incessant and difficult to terminate. The proposed criteria for ventricular pro-arrhythmias during EP testing include (a) conversion of non-sustained VT induced during the control test to a sustained VT during drug therapy and (b) induction of sustained VT with a cycle length less than the cycle length of the baseline VT (Poser *et al.*, 1985).

Pro-arrhythmic responses should be categorised uniformly in all studies with the investigational drug. An attempt should be made to determine whether the pro-arrhythmic response is (a) primary, i.e. unrelated to any identifiable arrhythmogenic factor or secondary, i.e. requiring adjunctive factor, or (b) bradyarrhythmic or tachyarrhythmic. The level of certainty that the pro-arrhythmic response is drug-induced and its clinical relevance should also be recorded (Horowitz *et al.*, 1987).

CLINICAL STUDIES

Studies in Volunteers

Clinical studies during early phase (Phase I and Phase II) drug evaluation seek to examine and/or establish (1) the pharmacological effects and anti-arrhythmic efficacy of a range of single and multiple doses; (2) the safety of a range of single and multiple doses; (3) dose–response relationships; (4) appropriate dosing intervals and titration frequency; (5) the cardiac electrophysiology of the drug; (6) suitability for use in different types of cardiac rhythm disorders, e.g. ventricular or supraventricular arrhythmias; (7) the pharmacokinetics of parent drug and metabolites; (8) the drug's capacity for arrhythmia aggravation; and (9) the drug's effect on LV function.

The earliest clinical study designed to examine the safety, pharmacokinetics and pharmacological effects of single doses of a drug is usually undertaken in healthy male volunteers. However, this study may be undertaken in mildly symptomatic patients with frequent VPCs, if the patients studied are otherwise healthy and are not receiving interfering concomitant medication. The lowest dose administered should be a fraction of the dose found effective in animal studies. Subsequent doses may be doubled when the previous dose is low, but at the upper range, smaller increments should be made. Fifteen to twenty subjects should be studied and each subject should receive no more than 3–4 doses.

The drug's effect on cardiovascular and ECG parameters is evaluated by measuring blood pressure, heart rate and surface ECG intervals (PR, QRS, QT). LV function is assessed with the help of 2D echocardiography or by measuring systolic time-intervals. In order to evaluate duration of pharmacological effects (e.g. PR, QRS or QT) measurements are made at several time-points. Venous blood samples are taken at specified times to determine single-dose kinetics. Laboratory tests of haematology and biochemistry parameters are performed before and after dosing. Data from this study will help to determine the safety, pharmacological effects and kinetics of single doses. The plasma drug concentration–effect relationship will also be examined.

Additional single-dose studies in healthy volunteers should be performed. One of these, using both the oral and i.v. formulations, should be undertaken to determine absolute bioavailability, volume of distribution and clearances. A mass balance study to examine the absorption, metabolism and excretion of the parent drug and its metabolites and a study to examine the influence of food on the pharmacokinetics of the drug should also be included.

If polymorphic distribution in the oxidative metabolism of the drug is observed, a kinetic study in extensive and poor metabolisers of debrisoquine, sparteine or dextromethorphan should be undertaken, to demonstrate genetically based polymorphic oxidative metabolism.

The results of the single-dose study will help in choosing suitable doses and dosing interval for a multiple-dose study in healthy volunteers. This study will provide information regarding safety, pharmacological effects and kinetics following multiple dosing. A proportion of subjects in the study should receive matching placebo in a single-blind fashion. Observations/tests similar to those made for the single-dose study should be undertaken. The total number of subjects involved in the Phase I studies will range from 60 to 90, depending on the number of studies to be undertaken, the doses that need to be tested and the degree of intersubject variability.

Studies in Patients

Ascending Single-dose Study in VPC Patients

An ascending single-dose study is undertaken in 15–20 mildly symptomatic patients with high-frequency ventricular ectopy (VPCs ≥30/h based on average of each of two consecutive 24 h Holter tape evaluations). The VPC frequency limits set for entry into the study are high, to reduce day-to-day and hour-to-hour variability to a minimum. Females of childbearing potential, the elderly and children are excluded. To allow an accurate evaluation of safety, pharmacodynamics and pharmacokinetics, concomitant medication allowed is kept to an absolute minimum. A stable baseline for arrhythmia frequency should be established by making observations following the administration of placebo, single-blind, on day 1 of the study. Comparison of anti-arrhythmic and other pharmacological effects of the different doses of the drug used in the study should be made with effects seen following placebo. In addition to measuring blood pressure, heart rate and surface ECG intervals and assessing LV function, the presence and duration of antiarrhythmic effect after each dose should be determined. When a drug does not suppress simple VPCs in a substantial proportion of patients (e.g. Class III drugs), the effect of various doses on surface ECG intervals should be carefully documented in order to allow the selection of suitable doses and dosing interval for subsequent studies.

Multiple-dose Studies in VPC Patients

Data from the ascending single-dose study in patients with frequent VPCs should permit the selection of suitable doses (3–4), appropriate dosing interval and titration frequency for a multiple-dose, dose-range-finding study. This study is also undertaken in patients with frequent VPCs in whom previous anti-arrhythmic medication has been stopped for a period of five drug half-lives or more. The end-points for dose titration are VPC suppression or tolerance, and baseline observations/tests are undertaken on placebo. A sufficient number of patients (40–60) should be studied in order to determine safety, efficacy, pharmacological effects and limited pharmacokinetics. Methodologies used include (1) long-term electrocardiographic monitoring for assessing arrhythmia suppression; (2) exercise tests, to assess the effect of the drug on exercise-induced tachycardia (Class II drugs) and on ventricular arrhythmias; (3) surface ECG interval measurements, to examine the effect on cardiac conduction and on ventricular repolarisation; (4) 2D echocardiography or radionuclide ventriculography, for assessing LV function; and (5) laboratory tests, for evaluating the drug's effect on haematology and biochemistry parameters. Adverse events, symptoms due to ventricular ectopy and pro-arrhythmic responses are recorded.

In patients in whom the investigational drug suppresses ventricular ectopy, a placebo washout phase should be introduced for up to 72 h, with continuous ECG monitoring and regular blood sampling for plasma drug level estimation, in an attempt to determine when arrhythmias return and thereby the minimum therapeutic plasma drug concentration.

The study should be extended to collect long-term efficacy and safety data. At some time during long-term treatment (e.g. 6 months) active medication should be replaced by placebo in a single-blind manner, to examine whether VPCs return to near-baseline levels. This will confirm not only long-term anti-arrhythmic effect, but also the need for continuing drug therapy.

Data from the multiple-dose study will help to determine suitable doses for the study of patients with life-threatening ventricular arrhythmias and will confirm that the titration frequency used was appropriate. It should be emphasised that doses effective in patients with life-threatening ventricular arrhythmias may be lower than the doses effective in suppressing ventricular ectopy.

A double-blind placebo-controlled study of the investigational drug should be undertaken in patients with ventricular ectopy, during Phase II to (1) examine the efficacy and safety of the oral doses used, (2) establish that the drug is significantly better than placebo, and (3) determine the minimally effective and maximally tolerated doses. An open-label long-term follow-up will help to examine the long-term safety of effective doses. The number of patients studied should take into account power for comparing each of the doses against placebo and dropouts from the study. In studies involving three active doses and placebo, 220–240 patients may be required.

In the above study the effect of the drug on the patient's well-being should be assessed, since this information may be required by certain regulatory agencies. Throughout the clinical programme, the effect of the drug on symptoms related to cardiac arrhythmias must be evaluated.

PES Study in Patients with VT/VF

The assessment of the drug's efficacy in patients with VT/VF may be made on the results of invasive (PES) or non-invasive (Holter tape monitoring) testing. Mitchell *et al.* (1987) showed, in a prospective study, that anti-arrhythmic drug therapy selected on the basis of invasive (PES) testing in patients with VT prevented recurrences of VT better than drug treatment selected on the basis of non-invasive testing. The preferred method, therefore, for the preliminary examination of the efficacy of investigational anti-arrhythmic drugs in VT or VF is by PES studies. Forty to sixty patients who have been free of prior anti-arrhythmic medication for at least five drug half-lives should be studied. Where possible, a range of oral doses should be tested, starting with the lowest dose, to provide information on the efficacy and safety of each of the doses. Venous blood samples are collected prior to dosing (trough) and during the EP study, to examine the relationship between plasma drug levels, efficacy, pro-arrhythmias or adverse reactions. The effect of each of the doses on surface ECG interval is also examined, to determine whether some relationship exists between changes in ECG interval and anti-arrhythmic effect. Long-term follow-up of patients in whom the drug suppresses inducibility of VT or slows the VT rate significantly (partial response) is undertaken, with the help of periodical clinic visits. During the long-term follow-up, patients are provided with a suitable device for TTM. Such monitoring will help to identify major rhythm abnormalities, whether due to ineffective therapy or due to aggravation of arrhythmia. During clinic visits, the physician may also wish to monitor the patient's cardiac rhythm with the help of Holter tape recordings. An attempt should also be made to follow non-responders to the drug. Such an attempt is justifiable in patients in whom spontaneous and induced VT are well tolerated and will help to determine whether effective suppression of spontaneous VT can be achieved in patients whose VT is still inducible. The administration of the drug intravenously, during PES testing, is not crucial during the evaluation of the oral formulation. However, an additional aim of an investigational drug programme should be to compare the effects of short-term i.v. and oral treatment on inducibility of VT, in the same patient. If both i.v. and oral regimens suppress inducibility, i.v. administration might be useful in the clinical management of patients during PES.

Studies With the Intravenous Formulation

A number of studies (80–120 patients) should be undertaken, using the i.v. formulation, to examine (1) the pharmacokinetics following i.v. administration; (2) anti-arrhythmic effects and safety of a range of i.v. doses, in patients with frequent VPCs; (3) cardiac EP and haemodynamic effects, in patients with normal LV function undergoing cardiac EP studies; and (4) acute cardiac haemodynamic effects in patients with mild, moderate and severe LV dysfunction.

In the initial study, ascending doses may be administered i.v. as bolus infusions in 10–15 min but for subsequent studies, an initial loading dose infused i.v. should be followed by a maintenance i.v. infusion so that studies undertaken to examine cardiac EP and haemodynamic effects are performed at times when plasma drug levels have plateaued. Observations/tests should include (1) measurement of blood pressure and heart rate; (2) measurement of conduction and ventricular repolarisation times (surface ECG intervals); (3) evaluation of VPC suppression from Holter tape data; and (4) measurement of cardiac EP (intracardiac ECG) and cardiac haemodynamic effects (Swan–Ganz catheterisation).

Studies in Supraventricular Arrhythmias

Although the most important goal of anti-arrhythmic drug development is the registration of the drug for use in life-threatening ventricular arrhythmias, it is usual to initiate studies in supraventricular arrhythmias at the same time. The use of the drug in the following cardiac rhythm disorders should be explored: (1) AV re-entrant tachycardia (WPW and concealed AV anomalous pathway with retrograde conduction); (2) AV nodal re-entrant tachycardia; (3) paroxysmal AF; (4) ectopic atrial tachycardia; and (5) chronic AF and atrial flutter.

Results from cardiac EP studies of the drug will have shown that the drug alters favourably certain cardiac EP parameters and is therefore likely to be effective in supraventricular arrhythmias. For example, the drug may do one or more of the following: increase the AV nodal conduction time; increase the refractory period or delay conduction (antegrade and retrograde) in the anomalous AV pathway; or increase the refractory period of the atrium and/or the AV node. For the two supraventricular re-entrant tachycardia (SVT) indications (AV nodal re-entry and AV re-entry), regulatory agencies may require that two studies be undertaken—one a PES study (during Phase II), involving 40–60 patients, to examine the effect of oral doses of the drug on the inducibility of SVT, followed by long-term follow-up in responders and non-responders; and the other a placebo-controlled study (during Phase III), to compare the effect of the drug on the frequency of spontaneously occurring SVT, with placebo and a marketed compound. Long-term follow-up should cover a period of 1–2 years. For the remaining supraventricular arrhythmia indications, two controlled studies may also be required. Sufficient numbers of patients (up to 200 for each indication) should be studied, to provide experience in a wide patient population. These studies are undertaken during Phase III and active controls are used for comparison.

The design for the PES study in SVT should be similar to the design for the PES study in patients with VT. The effect of the drug on conduction times, refractory period of the atrium, AV node (antegrade and retrograde), AV anomalous pathway (antegrade and retrograde) and the effect on inducibility of SVT is determined. TTM is employed during long-term follow-up, to document recurrence of arrhythmia. In order to show significant drug-induced differences in arrhythmia frequency, patients selected into the study should have experienced at least 3–4 episodes of SVT over a period of 6 months prior to entry into the study. Patients entering long-term follow-up on the investigational drug should include (1) those in whom the drug prevents induction of SVT, (2) those in whom induction is still possible but in whom cardiac EP parameters are favourably altered and tachycardia cycle length is increased by the drug, and (3) those in neither of categories (1) and (2) but in whom spontaneous SVT is well tolerated.

For patients with paroxysmal AF, studies (in up to 200 patients) should be undertaken, to examine the effect of the drug in abolishing and preventing the arrhythmia. The drug should be compared with placebo and active control. TTM should be used during follow-up, in order to assess the drug's effect on arrhythmia frequency.

In patients with chronic persistent AF, controlled studies (in up to 200 patients) should be undertaken, to examine the beneficial effect of drug on ventricular rate. For patients with ectopic atrial tachycardia, a long-term controlled study similar to that for paroxysmal AF should be undertaken, using TTM.

REFERENCES

Ahnve, S. (1984). Correction of the QT interval for heart rate. Review of different formulas and the use of Bazett's formula in myocardial infarction. *Am. Heart J.*, **109**, 568–74

Anderson, J. L., Gilbert, E. M., Albert, B. L., Henthorn, R. W., Waldo, A. L., Bhandari, A. K., Hawkinson, R. W. and Pritchett, E. L. C. (1988). Flecainide for prevention of symptomatic paroxysmal atrial fibrillation. A multicenter double blind, placebo controlled crossover study. [Abst.] *J. Am. Coll. Cardiol.*, **11** (No. 2), 77A

Barrett, M. J., Jacobs, L., Gomberg, J., Horton, L., Wolf, N. M. and Meister, S. G. (1982). Simultaneous contrast imaging of the left ventricle by two-dimensional echocardiography and standard ventriculography. *Clin. Cardiol.*, **5**, 208–13

Brugada, P., Green, M., Abdollah, H. and Wellens, H. J. J. (1983). Significance of ventricular arrhythmias initiated by programmed ventricular stimulation: The importance of the type of ventricular arrhythmia induced and the number of premature stimuli required. *Circulation*, **69**, 87–92

Bucknall, C. A., Brooman, I., Dunckley, G., May, R. and Curry, P. V. L. (1984). Improved cardiac arrhythmia diagnosis by transtelephonic electrocardiography. [Abst.] *Eur. Heart J.*, **5**, Suppl. 1, 1280

Buxton, A. E., Waxman, H. L., Mavchlinski, F. E., Untereker, W. J., Waspe, L. E. and Josephson, M. E. (1984). Role of triple extra stimuli during electrophysiologic study of patients with documented sustained ventricular tachyarrhythmias. *Circulation*, **69**, 532–40

Fortuin, N. J., Hood, W. P., Sherman, M. E. and Craige, E. (1971). Determination of left ventricular volumes by ultrasound. *Circulation*, **44**, 575–84

Henning, H., Schelbert, H., Crawford, M. H., Karliner, J. S., Ashburn, W. and O'Rourke, R. A. (1975). Left ventricular performance assessed by radionuclide angiocardiography and echocardiography in patients with previous myocardial infarction. *Circulation*, **52**, 1069–75

Henthorn, R. W., Waldo, A. L., Anderson, J. L., Gilbert, E. M., Alpert, B. L., Bhandari, A. K., Hawkinson, R. W. and Pritchett, E. L. C. (1988). Flecainide for prevention of paroxysmal supraventricular tachycardia. A multicenter double blind placebo-controlled crossover study. [Abst.] *J. Am. Coll. Cardiol.*, **11** (No. 2), 77A

Horowitz, L. N., Spielman, S. R., Greenspan, A. M. and Josephson, M. E. (1982). Role of programmed stimulation in assessing vulnerability to ventricular arrhythmias. *Am. Heart J.*, **103**, 604–8

Horowitz, L. N., Zipes, D. P., Bigger, J. T., Campbell, R. W. F., Morganroth, J., Podrid, P. J., Rosen, M. R. and Woosley, R. L. (1987). Proarrhythmia, arrhythmogenesis or aggravation of arrhythmia—A status report. *Am. J. Cardiol.*, **59**, 11, 54E–56E

Lepeschkin, E. and Surawicz, B. (1952). The measurement of the QT interval of the electrocardiogram. *Circulation*, **VI**, 378–87

Livelli, F. D. Jr., Bigger, J. T., Reiffel, J. A., Gang, E. S., Patton, J. N., Noethling, P. M., Rolnitzky, L. M. and Giklich, J. I. (1982). Response to programmed ventricular stimulation: sensitivity, specificity and relation to heart disease. *Am. J. Cardiol.*, **50**, 452–8

Mann, D. E., Luck, J. C., Griffin, J. C., Herre, J. M., Limacher, M. C., Magro, S. A., Robertson, N. W. and Wyndham, C. R. C. (1983). Induction of clinical ventricular tachycardia using programmed stimulation: value of third and fourth extra stimuli. *Am. J. Cardiol.*, **52**, 501–6

Michelson, E. L. and Morganroth, J. (1980). Spontaneous variability of complex ventricular arrhythmias detected by long term electrocardiographic recording. *Circulation*, **61**, 690–5

Mitchell, L. B. (1987). A randomized clinical trial of the noninvasive and invasive approaches to drug therapy of ventricular tachycardia. *New Engl. J. Med.*, **317**, 1681–7

Morganroth, J. (1981). In Morganroth, J., Moore, E. N., Dreifus, L. S. and Michelson, E. L. (Eds.), *The Evaluation of New Antiarrhythmic Drugs*. Martinus Nijhoff, The Hague, Boston, London, pp. 103–11

Morganroth, J., Michelson, E. L., Horowitz, L. N., Josephson, M. E., Pearlman, A. S. and Dunkman, W. B. (1978). Limitations of routine long-term monitoring to assess ventricular ectopic frequency. *Circulation*, **58**, 408–14

Podrid, P. J., Graboys, T. B., Lampert, S. and Blatt, C. (1987). Exercise stress testing for exposure of arrhythmias. *Circulation*, **75** (Suppl. III), 60–8

Pombo, J. F., Troy, B. L. and Russel, R. O. Jr. (1971). Left ventricular volumes and ejection fraction by echocardiography. *Circulation*, **43**, 480–90

Poser, R. F., Podrid, P. J., Lombardi, F. and Lown, B. (1985). Aggravation of arrhythmia induced with antiarrhythmic drugs during electrophysiologic testing. *Am. Heart J.*, **110**, 9–16

Pratt, C. M., Francis, M. J. and Slymen, D. J. (1987). Correlation between telephone and ambulatory electrocardiographic recordings. *Cardiol. Bd Rev.*, **4** (7), 78–86

Quinones, M. A., Gaasch, W. H. and Alexander, J. K. (1974). Echocardiographic assessment of left ventricular function with special reference to normalized velocities. *Circulation*, **50**, 42–51

Quinones, M. A., Waggoner, A. D., Reduto, L. A., Nelson, J. G., Young, J. B., Winters, W. L., Ribeiro, L. G. and Miller, R. R. (1981). A new simplified and accurate method for determining ejection fraction with two-dimensional echocardiography. *Circulation*, **64** (4), 744–53

Sami, M., Kraemer, H., Harrison, D. C., Houston, N., Chimasaki, S. and DeBusk, R. F. (1980). A new method for evaluating antiarrhythmic drug efficacy. *Circulation*, **62**, 1172–9

Schiller, N. B., Acquatella, H., Ports, T. A., Drew, D., Goerke, J., Ringertz, H., Silverman, N. H., Brundage, B., Botvinick, E. H., Boswell, R., Carlsson, E. and Parmley, W. W. (1979). Left ventricular volume from paired biplane two-dimensional echocardiography. *Circulation*, **60** (3), 547–55

Schoenfeld, M. H., McGovern, B., Garan, H. and Ruskin, J. N. (1984). Long-term reproducibility of responses to programmed cardiac stimulation in spontaneous ventricular tachycardia. *Am. J. Cardiol.*, **54**, 564–8

Shapiro, W., Canada, W. B., Lee, G., DeMaria, A. N., Low, R. I., Mason, D. T. and Laddu, A. (1982). Comparison of two methods of analyzing frequency of ventricular arrhythmias. *Am. Heart J.*, **104**, 874–5

Simonson, E., Caddy, L. D. and Woodbury, M. (1962). The normal QT interval. *Am Heart J.*, **63** (6), 747–53

Starling, M. R., Crawford, M. H., Sorensen, S. G., Levi, B., Richards, K. L. and O'Rourke, R. A. (1981). Comparative accuracy of apical biplane cross-sectional echocardiography and gated equilibrium radionuclide angiography for estimating left ventricular size and performance. *Circulation*, **63** (5), 1075–84

Vandepol, C. J., Farshidi, A., Spielman, S. R., Greenspan, A. M., Horowitz, L. N. and Josephson, M. E. (1980). Incidence and clinical significance of induced ventricular tachycardia. *Am. J. Cardiol.*, **45**, 725–31

Vaughan Williams, E. M. (1984). A classification of antiarrhythmic actions re-assessed after a decade of new drugs. *J. Clin. Pharm.*, **24**, 129–47

Velebit, V., Podrid, P. J., Lown, B., Cohen, B. H. and Graboys, T. B. (1982).

Aggravation and provocation of ventricular arrhythmias by antiarrhythmic drugs. *Circulation*, **65**, 886–94

Weissler, A. M. (1977). Current concepts in cardiology. Systolic-time intervals. *New Engl. J. Med.*, **296** (6), 321–4

Winkle, R. A. (1978). Antiarrhythmic drug effect mimicked by spontaneous variability of ventricular ectopy. *Circulation*, **57**, 1116–21

Zaret, B. L. and Berger, H. J. (1986). In Hurst, J. W., Logue, R. B., Rackley, C. E., Schlant, R. C., Sonnenblick, E. H., Wallace, A. G. and Wenger, N. K. (Eds.), *The Heart: Arteries and Veins*. McGraw-Hill, New York, pp. 1809–58

24
Phase I Trials on Anti-hypertensive Drugs

John R. Cockcroft* and David J. Webb†

*Dept of Clinical Pharmacology, Royal Postgraduate Medical School, London W12 0NN, UK

†Dept of Pharmacology and Clinical Pharmacology, St George's Hospital Medical School, London SW17 0RE, UK

> *Morals do not forbid making experiments on one's neighbour or on one's self. . . . Among the experiments that may be tried on man, those that can only harm are forbidden, those that are innocent are permissible and those that may do good are obligatory.*
>
> Claude Bernard, 1865

INTRODUCTION

Cardiovascular disease is the major cause of mortality in the western world. Since hypertension has been identified as a potent risk factor for both stroke and myocardial infarction,[1,2] it is not surprising that many drugs which reduce blood pressure are already in widespread clinical use, with more under preclinical investigation, or at the stage of Phase I trials. The results from the major hypertension trials confirm that blood pressure reduction lowers the incidence of stroke, even in mild hypertension, and by the percentage expected for a direct relationship between hypertension and stroke.[3] However, blood pressure reduction has proved singularly disappointing in prevention of myocardial infarction.[4-7]

One of the explanations advanced to explain this failure of anti-hypertensive treatment to prevent myocardial infarction is the additional unwanted effects of such drugs, unrelated to their hypotensive action. For instance, thiazides may indirectly enhance cardiovascular risk by their propensity to cause hypokalaemia,[8] hyperuricaemia,[9] hyperglycaemia[10] and hypercholesterolaemia.[11] More recently, it has been suggested that there may be a common factor responsible for both elevation of blood pressure and the trophic changes associated with vascular damage and atheroma, which are the hallmarks of sustained hypertension.[12] While the hypotensive efficacy and unwanted effects of anti-hypertensive drugs may be identified in Phase I trials, until the factor or factors responsible for vascular hypertrophy and damage are identified, such trials will provide no indication as to whether these drugs are likely to have an impact on vascular mortality.

Anti-hypertensive therapy is currently, therefore, aimed at blood pressure reduction, with the drugs used acting on the major physiological mechanisms and organ systems known to be responsible for maintenance of blood pressure; these include the sympathetic nervous system, the renin angiotensin system, the kidney and vascular smooth muscle. Many early anti-hypertensive drugs were centrally acting and tended to have unacceptable side-effects. Thus the agents currently employed fall into five major categories: diuretics, alpha- and beta-adrenergic receptor blocking drugs, direct acting vasodilators, calcium channel blockers and angiotensin-converting enzyme inhibitors.

A number of novel agents have recently entered Phase I trials. These include: agents which are agonists at presynaptic receptors on adrenergic nerve terminals, stimulation of which reduces noradrenaline release[13]; drugs which open potassium channels in vascular smooth muscle,[14,15] leading to hyperpolarisation and vasodilatation, such as cromakalim; and the renin inhibitors which, apart from their potential as anti-hypertensive agents,[16] offer the possibility of increased insight into the pathogenesis of essential hypertension.[17,18]

OBJECTIVES AND LIMITATIONS OF PHASE I STUDIES

The major objectives in the early evaluation of any anti-hypertensive agent are to obtain pharmacokinetic and pharmacodynamic data, essential for the design of studies in patients. Phase I studies also provide vital information on safety, overall acceptability and tolerability. As hypertensive patients often require more than one drug for adequate control of blood pressure, studies may be designed to obtain information on drug interaction. This may be pharmacokinetic, as in the case of the inhibition of the metabolism of propranolol by cimetidine.[19] Alternatively, this may be pharmacodynamic, as in the case of the profound and occasionally life-threatening first-dose hypotension associated with the use of angiotensin-converting enzyme inhibitors in diuretic-treated patients,[20] or the cardiodepressant effects of the combination of beta-blockers with certain calcium channel blocking drugs, especially those with an effect on the atrioventricular node of the heart.[21]

Potentially serious adverse effects of anti-hypertensive agents may only become apparent when large numbers of individuals are studied, a situation impractical during Phase I trials. Large-scale post-marketing surveillance studies may have a role in this respect. Thiazide diuretics, for example, produce few symptomatic side-effects, but in longer-term clinical evaluation, biochemical disturbances, such as hyperuricaemia, hyperglycaemia, hypercalcaemia, hypercholesterolaemia and hypokalaemia have been identified.[22] Indeed, some adverse effects of these drugs are still emerging, as with impotence, described for the first time during large-scale diuretic treatment during the IPPPSH trial.[23] Such symptomatic side-effects require identification, as treatment with anti-hypertensive agents is often given to individuals who are otherwise healthy, and drugs are given life-long.

PHARMACOKINETICS

Early-phase studies in man can only be undertaken after exhaustive tests in laboratory animals, designed to establish basic pharmacological properties, pharmacokinetics and lethal doses. However, these factors may be subject to considerable interspecies variation, even using primate models, and parameters established using such models may not reliably ... `ict effects in man.[24] To obtain useful pharmacokinetic data, it is necessary ⋃ employ an assay for the drug, and its metabolites, which is both specific and sensitive. Generation of metabolites may depend on the route of administration. Early studies with the beta-blocker propranolol, suggested that the drug was less active when given intravenously. This was subsequently explained by generation of a highly active metabolite 4-OH propranolol in the liver after oral administration. After intravenous dosing, however, 4-OH propranolol was not detectable.[25,26] Many of the ACE inhibitors, with the exception of captopril and lisinopril, are prodrugs, converted to their active form by de-esterification in the liver after oral dosing. Phase I studies with ACE inhibitors may therefore require intravenous administration of prodrug and active metabolite, as well as oral administration of the prodrug formulation.

Despite the ability to measure plasma drug levels, these may not correlate with drug effect. Certainly, early animal experiments with hydralazine showed that its hypotensive effect correlates better with tissue than with plasma drug concentration.[27] This may be particularly relevant in Phase I studies with ACE inhibitors, as here the assessment of pharmacological activity relies heavily on measurement of ACE activity in plasma, and its subsequent reduction following drug administration.[28] Since the majority of circulating angiotensin II is probably produced at a local tissue level in a variety of organs and vascular beds,[29] the effect of an ACE inhibitor on circulating ACE activity may be completely dissociated from its effect on blood pressure. Similarly, if the ACE inhibitor is tightly bound to tissue ACE, then the plasma half-life of the ACE inhibitor may have little relevance to the duration of action of the drug.[30] A better measure of pharmacological activity in these circumstances might be the response to infused angiotensin I.[31]

PHARMACODYNAMICS

As Phase I studies involve healthy normotensive volunteers, the hypotensive effect of a drug will depend on whether it interferes with a physiological mechanism which is important in the maintenance of normal blood pressure. Thus, alpha-receptor blocking drugs, interfering with the sympathetic nervous system, will invariably lower blood pressure in normotensive man. The renin–angiotensin system may be less important in these circumstances, and ACE inhibitors may have little effect on blood pressure despite reduction of circulating ACE activity by greater than 90%. However, the mechanisms maintaining elevated pressures in hypertensive patients may differ from those in normotensive subjects, and thus responses in Phase I trials may not accurately predict the hypotensive effect of a drug in later clinical studies.

When a pharmacological effect is produced by drug administration, it is important to attempt to correlate the plasma concentration with pharmacological response. A strong correlation between concentration and effect implies that the parent compound, rather than a metabolite, is the active agent. This is of particular relevance when subjects develop side-effects or fail to respond to an appropriate dose of the drug. Such information has revealed that certain anti-hypertensive drugs become less effective as their plasma concentration is increased. For example, the alpha-2 receptor agonist clonidine lowers blood pressure by decreasing central sympathetic outflow. However, as its plasma concentration increases, it stimulates alpha-1 receptors peripherally, leading to vasoconstriction which may attenuate its central action.[32]

It is possible that the mechanisms by which drugs lower blood pressure during single dose studies, or short-term administration, differ from those during chronic administration. These differences in response are exemplified by the beta-blocker propranolol which, on acute administration, reduces cardiac output and heart rate, but produces no reduction in blood pressure. However, if treatment is maintained for a longer period, blood pressure gradually falls, while cardiac output and heart rate remain reduced, suggesting a progressive reduction in total peripheral resistance.[25]

Systemic Haemodynamic Studies

Haemodynamic measurements are made after administration of any new drug to man as part of general safety monitoring. However, in the study of an anti-hypertensive drug, such measurements are essential to study efficacy, and may be useful in defining the mode of action of an anti-hypertensive compound. Simple haemodynamic measurements (blood pressure and heart rate) are mandatory, though others, such as cardiac output, pulmonary capillary wedge pressure and total or regional vascular resistance (with forearm blood flow) may be included. Since newer techniques now make non-invasive assessment of a number of these parameters widely available,[33–35] such measurements may in future be used more frequently in Phase I studies.

Drugs which are potent vasodilators are highly effective in reducing blood pressure, but their use may be accompanied by activation of both the sympathetic nervous system and the renin–angiotensin system, leading to tachycardia, and salt and water retention. Minoxidil is a drug which exemplifies these side-effects to the extent that patients nearly always require the counteracting effect of a beta-blocker and diuretic.[36] In systemic studies, the reflex activation of homeostatic physiological mechanisms[37] may even mask the action of potent vasodilator drugs, or may mask the contribution of vasodilatation to a drug's action. Here, studies employing local drug administration may be of particular value (see below).

Local Haemodynamic Studies

Since hypertension is a condition characterised by an increase in peripheral resistance, many anti-hypertensive drugs exert their major effect by relaxation of the resistance arterioles. However, many of these agents may also dilate veins, and this action may contribute to their overall haemodynamic effect.

The direct effect of drugs on the resistance arterioles, without the influence of reflex effects associated with systemic administration, may be investigated by local infusion into individual vascular beds. In this regard, blood flow in the human forearm can be measured simply, reliably and repeatedly, using venous occlusion plethysmography[38] during local infusion of drugs via the brachial artery. Changes in blood flow, at constant perfusion pressure, provide a reliable measure of change in resistance vessel tone. Furthermore, this technique allows the use of drugs at doses producing a local effect within the forearm, but 100-fold lower than those exerting a central or systemic action. Thus forearm perfusion pressure is unaltered, and the non-infused forearm serves as a control for the experiments.[39] Moreover, it is also possible to study the effect of locally infused drugs on the size of dorsal hand veins in man, maintained at a constant congesting pressure by an upper arm cuff. Here, the dose of drug affecting vein size is generally 10-fold lower than in the forearm, and a combination of arterial and local venous techniques allows assessment of whether drugs have a preferential effect on resistance arterioles or veins. Where venodilators are studied, the veins may be preconstricted by local infusion of noradrenaline.[40]

Such techniques have been used to study the capacity of various converting enzyme inhibitors to produce inhibition of local tissue-converting enzyme in the forearm in man[39,41] and, more recently, to study the novel vasodilator cromakalim in man.[42] The effect of this drug in the forearm is shown in Figure 24.1. Cromakalim produces a marked and dose-related increase in blood flow in the infused forearm, with no change in blood flow in the non-infused forearm over the same period. When given into noradrenaline-preconstricted dorsal hand veins in the same subjects, and at equivalent doses, cromakalim has no effect on vein size, showing that its action is arterioselective in man.

SUBJECTS

Age and Sex

Male subjects, exclusively, are used for Phase I testing of anti-hypertensive drugs, usually in the age range 18–50 years. This allows full teratogenicity testing to be delayed until efficacy in Phase I studies has been proven. The exclusion of women,[43] and subjects over 65 years of age, from Phase I studies

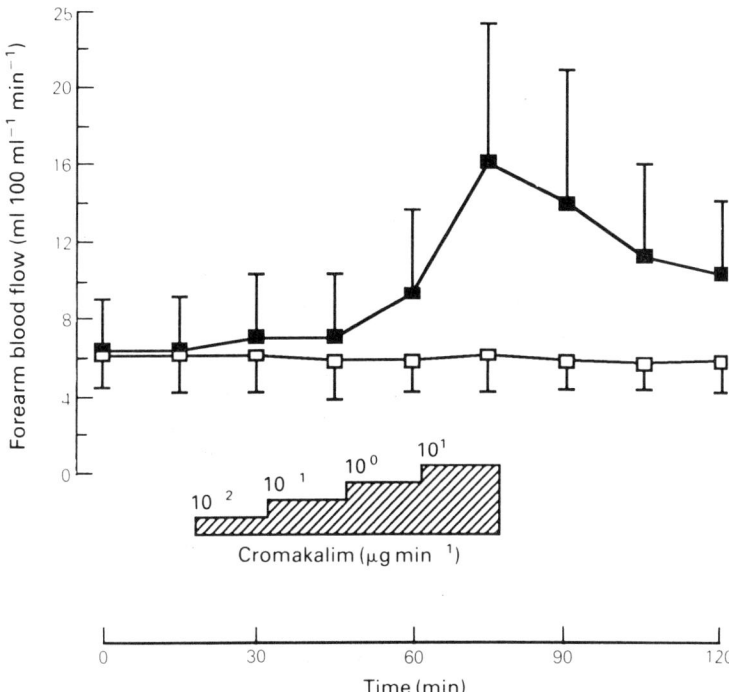

Figure 24.1 Blood flow (ml 100 ml^{-1} min^{-1}) in both the infused (■) and non-infused forearms (□) of eight subjects during intra-brachial artery infusion of incremental doses of cromakalim (0.01–10 μg min^{-1}), preceded, and followed by saline infusion. Values shown are mean ± s.d.

on anti-hypertensive agents is unfortunate, as large numbers of patients who are currently on anti-hypertensive therapy are excluded. It is known that women show significant pharmacokinetic and pharmacodynamic differences from men.[44]

Race

Black subjects often show a different response from caucasians to anti-hypertensive agents. Beta-blockers and ACE inhibitors are often less effective,[45,46] while diuretics are often more effective, in black subjects. Care should be taken when translating the results of early studies to different racial groups.

Smoking

Ideally, non-smokers should be used, as smoking has a pressor effect, by increasing circulating catecholamines[47] acting on both alpha- and beta-adrenergic receptors in the vasculature. In studies with beta-blocking drugs, this might lead to unopposed stimulation of alpha-receptors, and an enhanced pressor effect. The use of selective and non-selective beta-blockers may also produce differing effects on blood pressure in relation to smoking.[48] In addition, smoking may alter the hepatic metabolism of some anti-hypertensive drugs, affecting the results of pharmacokinetic studies.

Alcohol

Excessive alcohol intake has a marked pressor effect in both normotensive and hypertensive subjects.[49-51] Ideally, all alcoholic beverages should be avoided for at least 48 h before and during any study, and as alcohol withdrawal may raise blood pressure,[52] only moderate drinkers should be studied.

Salt Intake

Salt intake may affect blood pressure and the response to drugs. Subjects who are salt depleted develop activation of the renin–angiotensin system, and severe hypotension may follow administration of an ACE inhibitor.[20] Indeed, some studies in normal subjects, employ sodium depletion in order to enhance the effect of such drugs.[53] Subjects on a high salt diet may respond less to ACE inhibitors than to diuretics. In order to assess response in relation to sodium intake, 24 h urinary sodium measurements are often obtained before a study.

Over-the-Counter Preparations

Many over-the-counter proprietary medicines contain potent vasoactive agents. These include non-steroidal anti-inflammatory agents, which are known to cause salt and water retention and may blunt the response to anti-hypertensive agents,[54] and sympathomimetics, which have a pressor effect.[55] For this reason, the investigator should enquire about any use of over-the-counter medicines.

Caffeine

Subjects are usually advised to abstain from caffeine- containing beverages overnight, and on the day of a study. However, in subjects with a usual daily intake of 200 mg caffeine/day (equivalent to 4 cups of 'instant' coffee), withdrawal symptoms may occur between 13 and 23 h after abstinence.[56] Recent studies in patients abstaining from caffeine-containing beverages pre-operatively, have shown a 43% incidence of post-operative headache with caffeine consumption greater than 200 mg/day. The incidence rose to

73% when consumption was greater than 1000 mg/day.[57] Headache, anxiety and irritability, all of which have been associated with caffeine withdrawal, may adversely influence responses in haemodynamic studies. Conversely, however, if unrestricted coffee drinking is permitted, caffeine may produce a pressor effect.[48] The issue of whether caffeine intake should be restricted remains unresolved.

CONCLUSIONS

Phase I studies of anti-hypertensive drugs in healthy subjects are designed to obtain pharmacokinetic and pharmacodynamic data essential to the subsequent design of studies in hypertensive patients. These studies also provide information on safety and tolerability, although serious adverse effects which occur infrequently may not be detected. Effect may not correlate with plasma drug level, and may indicate the need for further investigation of drug action. Short-term effects in Phase I studies may not predict effects in longer-term studies, and responses in normotensive subjects may differ from those in hypertensive patients. In future, the development of non-invasive haemodynamic techniques, and of local drug infusion, may contribute significantly to the understanding of anti-hypertensive drug action.

REFERENCES

1. Framingham Study (1971). Systolic versus diastolic blood pressure and risk of coronary heart disease. *Am. J. Cardiol.*, **27**, 355–3
2. Kannel, W. B. (1975). Role of blood pressure in cardiovascular disease: The Framingham study. *Angiology*, **26**, 1–14
3. Dollery, C. T. (1987). Risk predictor, risk indicator and benefit factors in hypertension. *Am. J. Med.*, **82** (Suppl. 1A), 2–8
4. Australian Therapeutic Trial in Mild Hypertension (1980). Report by the management committee. *Lancet.*, **1**, 1261–7
5. Hpertension Detection and Follow Up Programme Co-operative Group (1979). Five-year findings of the Hypertension Detection and Follow Up Programme I. Reduction in mortality of persons with high blood pressure, including mild hypertension. *J. Am. Med. Assoc.*, **242**, 2562–71
6. Hypertension Detection and Follow Up Programme Co-operative Group (1982). Five-year findings of the Hypertension Detection and Follow Up Programme III. Reduction in stroke incidence among persons with high blood pressure. *J. Am. Med. Assoc.*, **24**, 633–8
7. Medical Research Council Working Party on mild to moderate hypertension (1985). MRC trial of treatment of mild hypertension: principal results. *Br. Med. J.*, **291**, 97–104
8. Hollifield, J. W., Slaton, P. E. and Liddle, G. W. (1975). Some biochemical consequences of diuretic therapy of low renin essential hypertension. Proceedings of the Third Symposium of Hypertension by UCLA at Boca Raton. In Samblin, M. P. (Ed.), *Systemic Effects of Antihypertensive Agents*. Stratton International, New York, pp. 131–52

9. Breckenridge, A. (1966). Hypertension and hyperuricaemia. *Lancet*, **i**, 15–17
10. Murphy, M. B., Lewis, P. J., Kohner, E. M., Schuner, B. and Dollery, C. T. (1982). Glucose intolerance in hypertensive patients treated with diuretic, a fourteen-year follow-up. *Lancet*, **ii**, 1293–8
11. Ames, R. P. (1983). Negative effects of diuretic drugs on metabolic risk factors for coronary heart disease: possible alternative drug therapies. *Am. J. Cardiol.*, **51**, 632–9
12. Lever, A. F. (1986). Slow pressor mechanisms in hypertension: a role for hypertrophy of resistance vessels? *J. Hyperten.*, **4**, 515–24
13. Haeusler, G. (1987). Potential future developments in the field of anti-hypertensive drugs. *Eur. Heart J.*, **8** (Suppl. M), 135–42
14. Buckingham, R. E., Clapham, J. C., Coldwell, M. C., Hamilton, T. C. and Howlett, D. R. (1986). Stereo-specific mechanism of action of the novel anti-hypertensive agent, BRL 34915. *Br. J. Pharmacol.*, **87**, 78p
15. Coldwell, M. C. and Howlett, D. R. (1987). Specificity of action of the novel anti-hypertensive agent, BRL 34915 as a potassium channel activator. Comparison with nicorandil. *Biochem. Pharm.*, **36**, 3663–9
16. Webb, D. J., Manhem, P. J. O., Ball, S. G., Inglis, G., Leckie, B. J., Lever, A. F., Morton, J. J., Robertson, J. I. S., Murray, G. D., Menard, J., Hallett, A., Jones, D. M. and Szelke, M. (1985). A study of the renin inhibitor H142 in man. *J. Hyperten.*, **3**, 653–8
17. Szelke, M., Leckie, B., Hallett, A. *et al.* (1982). Potent new inhibitors of renin. *Nature*, **299**, 555–7
18. Tree, M., Szelke, M., Leckie, B. J. *et al.* (1985). Renin inhibitors: their use in understanding the role of angiotensin II as a pressor hormone. *J. Cardiovasc. Pharmacol.*, **7** (Suppl. 4), S49–S52
19. Haegerty, A. M., Donovan, M. A., Castleden, C. M., Pohl, J. F., Patel, L. and Hedger, A. (1981). Influence of cimetidine on pharmacokinetics of propranolol. *Br. Med. J.*, **282**, 1917–9
20. Hodsman, G. P., Isles, C. G., Murray, G. D., Usherwood, T. P., Webb, D. J. and Robertson, J. I. S. (1983). Factors related to the first dose hypotensive effect of captopril: prediction and treatment. *Br. Med. J.*, **284**, 832–4
21. Packer, M. (1989). Combined beta-adrenergic and calcium-entry blockade in angina pectoris. *New Engl. J Med.*, **320**, 709–18
22. Cockcroft, J. R. and Dollery, C. T. (1989). The diuretic dilemma. In Buhler, F. R. and Laragh, J. H. (Eds.), *The Handbook of Hypertension*, Vol. 13. Elsevier, Amsterdam, in press
23. Stressman, J. and Ben-Ishay, D. (1980). Chlorthalidone-induced impotence. *Br. Med. J.*, **281**, 714
24. Brodie, B. B. and Reid, W. D. (1967). Some pharmacological consequences of species variation in rates of metabolism. *Fed. Proc.*, **26**, 1062–70
25. Paterson, J. W., Connolly, M. E., Dollery, C. T., Hayes, A. and Cooper, R. G. (1970). The pharmacodynamics and metabolism of propranolol in man. *Pharm. Clin.*, **2**, 127–33
26. George, C. F., Fenyvesi, T., Connolly, M. E. and Dollery, C. T. (1972). Pharmacokinetics of dextro, laevo and racemic propranolol in man. *Eur. J. Clin. Pharm.*, **4**, 74–80
27. Keberle, H., Faigle, J. W., Hedwall, P., Riem, W. and Wagner, J. (1973). Plasma concentrations and pharmacological response in animals. In Davies, D. S. and Pritchard, B. N. C. (Eds.), *Biological Effects of Drugs in Relation to Their Plasma Concentrations*. Macmillan, London, 13–24
28. Brunner, H. R., Waeber, B. and Nussberger, J. (1983). Does pharmacological profiling of a new drug in normotensive volunteers provide a useful guideline to

antihypertensive therapy? *Hypertension*, **5** (Suppl. 3), 101–7

29. Campbell, D. J. (1987). Circulating and tissue angiotensin systems. *J. Clin. Invest.*, **79**, 1–6
30. Cohen, L. and Kurz, M. D. (1982). Angiotensin converting enzyme inhibition in tissues from spontaneously hypertensive rats after treatment with captopril or MK421. *J. Pharm. Expl. Ther.*, **220**, 63–9
31. Biollaz, J., Burnier, M., Turini, G. A. *et al.* (1981). Three new long acting angiotensin-converting enzyme inhibitors: relationship between plasma-converting enzyme activity and response to angiotensin I. *Clin. Pharmacol. Ther.*, **29**, 668–70
32. Dollery, C. T., Davies, D. S., Draffan, G. H., Dargie, H. J., Dean, C. R., Reid, J. L., Clare, R. A. and Murray, S. (1976). Clinical pharmacology and pharmaco-kinetics of clonidine. *Clin. Pharmacol. Ther.*, **19**, 11–17
33. Bennett, E. D., Barclay, S. A., Davis, A. L. *et al.* (1984). Ascending aortic blood velocity and acceleration using Doppler ultrasound in the assessment of left ventricular function. *Cardiovas. Res.*, **18**, 632
34. Ihlen, H., Myhre, E., Amlie, J. P. *et al.* (1985). Changes in left ventricular stroke volume measured by Doppler echocardiography. *Br. Heart J.*, **54**, 378
35. Metcalf, M. J. and Rawles, J. M. (1989). Stroke distance in acute myocardial infarction: a simple measurement of left ventricular function. *Lancet*, **i**, 1371–3
36. Dargie, H. J., Dollery, C. T. and Daniel, J. (1977). Minoxidil in resistant hypertension. *Lancet*, **ii**, 515–18
37. Kirchheim, H. R. (1976). Systemic arterial baroreceptor reflexes. *Physiolog. Rev.*, **56**, 100–76
38. Roberts, D. H., Tsao, Y. and Breckenridge, A. M. (1986). The reproducibility of limb flow measurements in human volunteers at rest and after exercise by using mercury in Silastic strain gauge plethysmography under standardised conditions. *Clin. Sci.*, **70**, 635–8
39. Benjamin, N., Cockcroft, J. R., Collier, J. G., Dollery, C. T., Ritter, J. M. and Webb, D. J. (1989). Local inibition of converting enzyme and vascular responses to angiotensin and bradykinin in the human forearm. *J. Physiol.*, **412**, 543–55
40. Robinson, B. F. (1978). Assessment of the effects of drugs on the venous system in man. *Br. J. Clin. Pharm.*, **6**, 381–6
41. Webb, D. J. and Collier, J. G. (1987). Influence of ramipril diacid on the peripheral vascular effects of angiotensin I. *Am. J. Cardiol.*, **59**, 45D–9D
42. Webb, D. J., Benjamin, N. and Vallance, P. (1989). The potassium channel opening drug cromakalim produces arterio-selective vasodilation in the upper limbs of healthy volunteers. *Br. J. Clin. Pharm.*, **27**, 757–61
43. Kinney, E. L., Trautman, J., Gold, J. A., Vessel, E. S. and Zelis, R. (1981). Under-representation of women in new drug trials. *Ann. Int. Med.*, **95**, 495–9
44. Guidicelli, J. F. and Tillement, J. P. (1977). Influence of sex on drug kinetics in man. *Clin. Pharm.*, **2**, 157–66
45. Bühler, F. R., Burkart, F., Lutold, B. E., Kung, M., Marbet, G. and Pfisterer, M. (1975). Antihypertensive beta blocking action as related to renin and age: A pharmacologic tool to identify pathogenic mechanisms in essential hypertension. *Am. J. Cardiol.*, **36**, 653–9
46. Cruickshank, J. K. and Beevers, D. G. (1985). Ethnic and geographical differences in blood pressure. In Bulpitt, C. J. (Ed.), *Epidemiology of Hypertension*. Elsevier, Cambridge, pp. 70–87
47. Cryer, P. E., Hammond, M. W. and Santiago, J. V. (1976). Norepinephrine and epinephrine release and adrenergic mediation of smoking-associated haemodynamic and metabolic events. *New Engl. J. Med.*, **295**, 573–7
48. Freestone, S. and Ramsay, L. E. (1983). Effect of beta-blockade on the pressor

response of coffee plus smoking in patients with mild hypertension. *Drugs*, **25** (Suppl. 2), 141–5

49. Klatsky, A. L., Friedman, T. D., Seiglaub, A. B. and Gerard, M. J. (1977). Alcohol consumption and blood pressure: Kaiser Permanente multiphasic health examination data. *New Engl. J. Med.*, **196**, 1194–200

50. Potter, J. F., Watson, R. D. S., Skan, W. and Beevers, D. G. (1986). The pressor and metabolic effects of alcohol in normotensives. *Hypertension*, **8**, 625–31

51. Potter, J. F., McDonald, I. A. and Beevers, D. G. (1986). Alcohol raises blood pressure in hypertensive patients. *J. Hyperten.*, **4**, 435–41

52. Bannon, L. T., Potter, J. F., Beevers, D. G., Saunders, J. B., Walters, J. R. E. and Ingram, M. C. (1984). Effect of alcohol withdrawal on blood pressure, plasma renin activity, alldosterone, cortisol and dopamine beta-hydroxylase. *Clin. Sci.*, **66**, 659–63

53. Webb, D. J., Cumming, A. M. M., Leckie, B. J. *et al.* (1983). Reduction of blood pressure in man with H142, a potent new renin inhibitor. *Lancet*, **2**, 1486–7

54. Oates, J. A. (1988). Antagonism of antihypertensive drug therapy by nonsteroidal anti-inflammatory drugs. *Hypertension*, **11** (Suppl. 2), 4–6

55. Bravo, E. L. (1988). Phenylpropanolamine and other over-the-counter vasoactive compounds. *Hypertension*, **11** (Suppl. 2), 7–10

56. Griffiths, R. R., Bigelow, G. E. and Liebson, I. A. (1986). Human coffee drinking: reinforcing and physical dependence producing effects of caffeine. *J. Pharmacol. Expl. Ther.*, **239**, 416–25

57. Galletly, D. C., Fennelly, M. and Whitwam, J. G. (1989). Does caffeine withdrawal contribute to postoperative headache? *Lancet*, **i**, 1335

25
Drugs for Heart Failure

Janet E. Rush and Mariell Jessup†*

*Merck Sharp & Dohme Research Laboratories, West Point, PA 19486, USA

†Heart Failure and Transplantation Center, Temple University, 3401 North Broad St, Philadelphia, PA 19140, USA

INTRODUCTION

Assessing a drug for efficacy and safety in heart failure is a challenging task (Guyatt, 1986). For example, six compounds have been considered by the US Food and Drug Administration (FDA) during the 1980s: captopril, enalapril, amrinone, milrinone, lisinopril and isosorbide dinitrate. However, only two (captopril and enalapril) have been approved for oral use in chronic heart failure. The chief difficulties have been: (1) inability to define the optimal dose and dose interval; (2) inability to demonstrate a statistical superiority over placebo or a comparative agent; and (3) assessment of adverse effects and the impact of a drug on the natural course of a fatal disease (Packer and Leier, 1987).

FDA guidelines for heart failure drugs have been drafted, but considerable controversy exists in some areas. The World Health Organization has no published guidelines at present, nor do most other regulatory agencies. Guidelines have been issued for the evaluation of heart failure therapies in Japan. The European Economic Community has published guidelines on cardiac glycosides which may also apply to other inotropic therapies. In the absence of approved published guidelines for the evaluation of drugs for heart failure, it is desirable that any clinical programme for a heart failure claim be discussed with regulatory officials early in the course of the clinical development programme.

The syndrome of congestive heart failure (CHF) is usually seen as a relentlessly progressive, irreversible disease. However, individual patients with CHF may have marked fluctuations in their functional status independent of pharmacotherapy, which may be due to dietary indiscretions, ischaemic episodes or physical conditioning. Depending upon the aetiology of the underlying cardiomyopathy, certain patients (e.g. those with alcoholic cardiomyopathy or viral myocarditis) may improve markedly with the passage of time. These all too frequent observations emphasise the need for placebo-controlled studies, even in Phase II, in order to avoid misinterpretations during early studies which can lead to costly mistakes in the course of clinical development.

Agents used to treat heart failure may be categorised as diuretics, vasodilatory agents or inotropic agents, and often all three classes of drugs are used concomitantly. None of the oral diuretics, widely used in the treatment of CHF, have been approved by the FDA for that purpose. (Diuretics are discussed elsewhere in this volume.) Similarly, oral nitrate therapy, widely used for heart failure has not been sanctioned for such use by the US FDA. Thus, the interesting situation exists that many agents routinely used for the treatment of heart failure have not been approved in the USA for that indication. This, again, attests to the difficulties encountered in developing a drug for patients with CHF.

PATIENT POPULATION

The syndrome of CHF may develop as a consequence of many different insults to the heart, including myocardial infarction, viral myocarditis, long-standing valvular disease or alcoholic cardiomyopathy; in many cases the causative event is unknown and these are designated 'idiopathic'. In general, the same therapeutic approach is used regardless of aetiology; however, it is unknown at the present time whether the aetiology of the patient's CHF affects response to a given therapy. Most therapeutic agents have been evaluated primarily for their effects on left ventricular systolic function. Other aspects of heart failure (diastolic function, right ventricular function) have not been assessed adequately in large-scale trials.

It is important that initial studies in CHF be performed in patients with chronic heart failure (e.g. stable for 3 or more months). Patients with CHF of more recent onset may have an evolution of their clinical syndrome during the study, and it would be impossible to differentiate this from drug effect.

In initial studies in heart failure, the patient population should be as homogeneous as possible. The diagnosis of CHF should be firmly established with the use of an objective parameter such as cardiothoracic ratio by chest X-ray or left ventricular ejection fraction by radionuclide scan, in association with clinical signs and symptoms. In a haemodynamic study, haemodynamic criteria of CHF can be established. Background therapy should be as uniform as possible. If a vasodilatory agent is being evaluated, the patients should be discontinued from any vasodilatory therapy for 1 week or more prior to the study. Concomitant therapies which may affect cardiac output or vascular resistance, such as beta-blockers and certain antiarrhythmic agents, should be discontinued prior to the study period. Patients should be on a controlled sodium intake during the study.

COMPONENTS OF A PHASE I AND PHASE II CLINICAL PROGRAMME

The reader is referred to Chapter 5 for a discussion of techniques which may be used to assess the cardiovascular properties of a new therapy in healthy volunteers. However, it should be emphasised that responses in healthy volunteers may differ significantly from responses of CHF patients (Francis, 1987). After identifying a pharmacological agent (through animal and/or human volunteer studies) with vasodilatory or inotropic properties (or both), and identifying the proper dose and administration schedule to obtain the effect in volunteers, it is wise to plan pharmacokinetic, pharmacodynamic and dose-finding studies in patients with CHF.

Pharmacokinetic Studies

Drug absorption, metabolism and disposition, as well as delivery of the drug to the target tissues, may be altered in CHF patients. The pathophysiological mechanisms for these effects include poor cardiac output with poor tissue perfusion, hepatic congestion with impaired metabolism, decreased renal function, variations in volume of distribution, decreased body fat ('cardiac cachexia'), and oedema of the gastrointestinal tract with impaired absorption (Packer *et al.*, 1980). Recognising the substantial potential for different pharmacokinetic characteristics of a drug in CHF patients compared with healthy volunteers, regulatory agencies may expect to be provided with pharmacokinetic data in CHF patients, including multiple-dose studies. In the absence of multiple-dose pharmacokinetic data, measurement of trough and peak serum levels following chronic therapy may be adequate. Pharmacokinetic and pharmacodynamic interaction studies performed in the target population, especially with widely used agents such as diuretics, digitalis compounds and angiotensin converting enzyme inhibitors, should also be considered.

A focus of the pharmacokinetic studies should be to correlate haemodynamic effects with plasma drug concentrations in both healthy volunteers and CHF patients. This provides useful perspective regarding the degree to which data in healthy subjects can be applied to patients.

The extent to which the heart failure state influences the pharmacokinetic behaviour of a drug will be somewhat dependent on the drug's specific characteristics. For drugs with high membrane permeability, such as lipid-soluble drugs, the rate-limiting step in drug absorption is perfusion of the absorption site. For such compounds, oedema of the gastrointestinal tract and low cardiac output are likely to influence absorption (Barr and Riegelman, 1970).

Another consideration is whether the drug is metabolised by the renal or the hepatic route. In the CHF patient, hepatic blood flow is usually reduced, owing to low cardiac output, and metabolism may be impaired as a result of hepatic congestion. The effects on drug metabolism of changes of liver blood flow depend upon the extraction ratio (Nies *et al.*, 1976). Heart failure patients usually have some decrease in the glomerular filtration rate due to reduced renal perfusion. For drugs that are filtered, the endogenous creatinine clearance is a relatively accurate predictor of drug clearance.

Volume of distribution in the CHF patient will vary, depending upon the severity of the patient's disease and prior therapy. In general, untreated CHF is a state characterised by volume overload and, therefore, with an increased volume of distribution. However, CHF patients who are aggressively diuresed and/or have very low cardiac outputs frequently have such intense peripheral vasoconstriction that the volume of distribution is decreased.

In summary, the pharmacokinetic and pharmacodynamic characteristics of drugs may differ substantially in CHF patients relative to healthy volunteers. Both single- and multiple-dose pharmacokinetic studies should be performed in the target population. In choosing the CHF subjects to be included in pharmacokinet   udies, the severity of CHF should be carefully considered and the specific characteristics of the drug under investigation should be taken into account.

Pharmacodynamic, Dose-finding and Dose–Response Studies

Haemodynamic studies in healthy subjects may be used to define a potential mechanism of action of a drug and to estimate a dose for CHF patients. However, it should be recognised that the altered physiology of CHF may make these patients more sensitive to certain classes of drugs (e.g. vasodilatory agents). In other cases a cardiovascular end-point may not be detected in healthy subjects. Dose-finding studies in CHF patients should thoroughly assess the lower end of the dose range.

The initial studies in CHF patients should be carefully monitored exploratory open-label pharmacodynamic studies. Such studies should be performed in as many patients as necessary to identify two or three safe and effective doses. The number of patients it takes to do this will vary, depending on many factors—e.g. whether an oral or an intravenous formulation is used, the potential toxicities of the drug, and the consistency of response from patient to patient. After these exploratory studies have provided information on two or three safe and effective doses, a formal dose response study should follow (Schmidt, 1988).

A parallel, fixed-dose, double-blind, placebo-controlled design (Figure 25.1) has proved useful in evaluating new drugs and satisfying regulatory agencies. Ideally, this study would assess invasive haemodynamic responses as well as other clinical parameters. It is also important to demonstrate the lack of tolerance with the chosen dose and administration schedule. In general, 2–3 months is an adequate time-frame in which to assess both the development of tolerance and clinical efficacy (Packer *et al.*, 1982). Ideally, invasive haemodynamic measurements should be performed at both the beginning and the end of the study in as many patients as feasible. This makes possible the correlation of haemodynamic measurements, drug levels and the clinical response to chronic therapy. A well-executed study with these three components can be a very convincing argument for the drug's efficacy.

The most reliable dose–response information in CHF is obtained from invasive haemodynamic measurements, since other efficacy parameters such as exercise capacity and physical signs of heart failure are too subjective to be of benefit in assessing dose response. However, patients who are candidates for haemodynamic studies are frequently too ill to exercise on a bicycle or

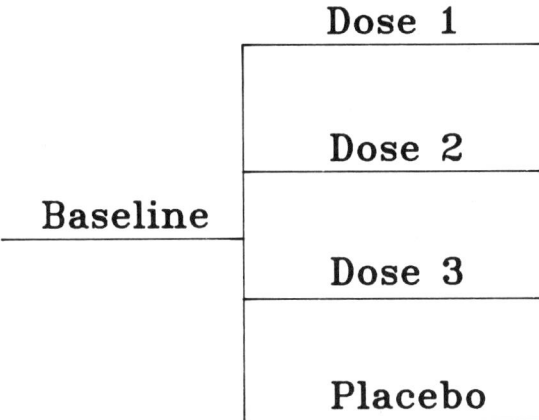

Figure 25.1 Sample design for a dose–response study

treadmill. Nevertheless, regulatory agencies, especially the US FDA, believe that exercise capacity is the efficacy parameter most closely related to clinical benefit, and thus pivotal studies must include an assessment of exercise tolerance. Therefore, it may be difficult for the same study to serve as both a dose–response study and a pivotal efficacy study.

Other Phase II Studies

Three concerns to consider when planning early studies to assess heart failure drugs are:

(1) Studies of cardiovascular effects of a given drug in healthy volunteers may not be predictive of the effect in patients with CHF. For example, an arterial dilatory agent will improve cardiac output only in patients with marked elevations of systemic vascular resistance. In healthy volunteers, compensatory mechanisms limit the degree to which cardiac output can be increased by an arterial dilatory agent. A venodilatory agent may cause reduced cardiac output in a healthy volunteer, yet produce improved exercise tolerance and no change in cardiac output in patients with CHF.

(2) Acute effects in short-term studies of CHF patients may not be predictive of efficacy during long-term administration. This may be due to activation of neurohormonal compensatory mechanisms which will counter-act the acute beneficial effect of the drug (Franciosa *et al.*, 1982; Topic *et al.*, 1982).

(3) Favourable haemodynamic effects may not be translated into clinical benefit (Guyatt, 1985).

Thus, it is recommended that a pilot study be carried out early in the development programme which assesses the drug effect on a critical clinical index of efficacy, e.g. exercise tolerance after chronic (6–12 weeks) therapy, in the target population. Ideally, this study would be double-blind and placebo-controlled, and carried out by an experienced investigator.

Depending upon the characteristics of the drug, it may be wise to obtain additional information in the course of early exploratory studies to evaluate the full range of haemodynamic effects in the CHF patient. For a vasodilatory agent, it may be helpful to know the effect on coronary sinus blood flow. For an inotropic agent, it would be prudent to assess contractility, for example, by using left ventricular end-systolic pressure–volume analysis (Herrmann *et al.*, 1987). Alternatively, contractility can be evaluated by non-invasive techniques (David *et al.*, 1988). In assessing an inotropic drug, it may be useful to determine the effect on myocardial oxygen consumption, since drugs which cause marked increases in myocardial oxygen consumption may be undesirable in certain situations (i.e. acute myocardial infarction). If there is concern about a possible tendency to produce arrhythmias, an electrophysiological study may be considered.

EFFICACY PARAMETERS IN THE CHF PATIENT

Heart failure studies may be lengthy, expensive and difficult to enrol. Thus, it is beneficial to evaluate multiple parameters in each patient rather than incur the inconvenience and expense of additional studies to assess parameters omitted from earlier studies. Many such efficacy parameters are standard procedures and relatively inexpensive to obtain. The parameters listed below should generally be obtained in all studies; the sample size should be based on one or two key parameters. Survival should always be assessed no matter how small or how short the study.

Heart size (measured on chest X-ray)
New York Heart Association class
Physical signs of heart failure
Symptoms of heart failure
Patient's overall assessment of response
Quality of life and ability to perform tasks of daily living
Hospitalisations during therapy
Need for concomitant medications

Examples of other parameters which address both efficacy and mode of action may be measured in selected studies:

Invasive haemodynamic measurements (via pulmonary artery catheter), at rest and during exercise
Exercise duration
Expired gases during exercise (maximal oxygen consumption, anaerobic threshold, oxygen pulse)
Ejection fraction (radionuclide determination preferred), at rest and during exercise

Effect on diastolic function (e.g. using echocardiography plus Doppler flow)
Effect on ventricular arrhythmias (Holter monitor)
Contractility
Coronary sinus blood flow
Myocardial oxygen consumption
Humoral measurements (plasma renin activity, arginine vasopressin, norepinephrine, atrial natriuretic peptide)

These efficacy measurements may not correlate with each other, since each measurement assesses a slightly different aspect of the disease and the patient's response to the therapeutic intervention (Packer, 1987). Some researchers have combined several efficacy parameters into a 'CHF Score' (Lee, 1982). However, there is no composite score which has gained wide acceptance. If a composite score of several parameters is to be used to assess efficacy in a clinical trial, it should be defined prior to the start of the trial and included in the protocol. Regulatory agencies are unlikely to accept composite scores which are developed during the analysis of trial results.

Invasive Haemodynamic Measurements

Haemodynamic measurements should be done by an investigator experienced in evaluating drug effects and knowledgeable regarding the impact of confounding factors such as circadian rhythms, meals (Cornyn *et al.*, 1986), concomitant medications and the effects of study procedures (e.g. insertion of a pulmonary artery catheter). Ideally, haemodynamic studies should be performed under fasting conditions and at the same time of day in all patients. An adequate resting time should be allowed following insertion of any catheters, to ensure a stable baseline. It is frequently useful to evaluate haemodynamic measurements both at rest and during exercise. The haemodynamic effects of a vasodilatory drug depend upon its preferential site of action (Rude *et al.*, 1981).

The usual haemodynamic measurements include pulmonary arterial pressure, pulmonary capillary wedge pressure and cardiac output. Systemic arterial pressure should ideally be measured via an arterial catheter. Measurements can be made more reliably on equipment providing phasic, hard copy printouts. The post-a-wave, end-expiratory wedge pressure may be the most accurate reflection of the pulmonary capillary wedge pressure (Green *et al.*, 1987). The pressure transducer should be located at the level of the right atrium. The measurement with the greatest variability is usually cardiac output determined by thermodilution. This variability can be decreased if all cardiac output determinations are performed by the same individual and if an automatic injection device is used. Cardiac output determinations should be done in triplicate, and a strip chart recorder may be used to evaluate the integrity of the thermal curve.

Haemodynamic measurements should be performed at regular intervals following administration of drug, to assess the peak and the duration of the drug's action. While healthy volunteer studies may be used as a guide, the time-course of action in a CHF patient may differ considerably, owing to impaired absorption and/or metabolism. Low cardiac output may interfere with delivery of the drug to the target tissue, altering the expected pharmacodynamic responses by yet another mechanism.

An invasive haemodynamic study can be quite challenging to perform. In most countries, pulmonary artery catheters are used only in severely ill patients, primarily those who would be classified as New York Heart Association Class IV (dyspnoeic at rest). These patients are frequently unstable, and prone to hypotension and ventricular arrhythmias, and may not be able to tolerate withdrawal of concomitant therapies. Centres selected to perform haemodynamic studies should be experienced in clinical research and committed to strict adherence to the protocol.

Although invasive haemodynamic studies are invaluable for assessing dose response and duration of action, haemodynamic benefits do not necessarily translate into measurable clinical improvements. Drugs which increase cardiac output may fail to improve exercise capacity (Franciosa *et al.*, 1982). Conversely, it is possible to cause improved exercise tolerance without an acute effect on cardiac output (Leier *et al.*, 1983). Changes in pulmonary capillary wedge pressure seem to correlate best with improved exercise tolerance and clinical response (Packer, 1987).

Pilot Exercise Study

The only acceptable aims of successful heart failure therapy are to improve symptoms, increase exercise tolerance and extend survival. Haemodynamic end-points, although they are essential for investigation of the dose response and the drug's duration of action, are actually surrogate end-points. Before launching into a Phase III programme, it is usually desirable to demonstrate efficacy in a small-scale study with improvement of symptoms and exercise tolerance as end-points. This may not be necessary when investigating a drug in a class with known efficacy in CHF, such as an angiotensin converting enzyme inhibitor. In this case it may be desirable to proceed directly to Phase III once the dose and the dose interval have been defined.

There are a number of examples of small-scale successful studies in the literature, using both crossover and parallel designs (Cleland *et al.*, 1985; Franciosa *et al.*, 1985). The advantages and disadvantages of applying the crossover design to CHF patients are discussed by Guyatt (1985). The use of a placebo control may highlight the efficacy of the new compound, although use of an active control will make enrolment proceed more quickly. (The problems with enrolment in a placebo-controlled study may be lessened by unequal randomisation to active drug and placebo.) The study should be double-blind because of the subjective nature of the end-points.

Options to consider in trial design would include the use of a forced-titration scheme which allows patients to start at low doses but prescribes upward titration unless adverse reactions prevent increasing the dose. This approach increases the chances that patients will be receiving therapeutic doses at the end of the trial. A placebo should be used during the baseline period, and a minimum and maximum exercise time should be required for entry into the study (Massie *et al.*, 1985). This will help to exclude patients either too ill to complete a controlled study or too well-compensated to derive benefit from a new therapy. Steps should be taken to ensure the relative uniformity of the patient population with respect to age, degree of systolic dysfunction and exclusion of other diseases which could effect exercise tolerance (pulmonary disease, angina, arrhythmias).

It has been recommended that exercise testing be performed in conjunction with measurement of expired gases (Weber *et al.*, 1982). Effort-dependent variability in exercise capacity is well documented (Lipkin, 1987) and it is especially important to reduce this variability as much as possible in a small pilot study.

An example of the value of measurement of expired gases is provided by a large multicentre placebo-controlled study of enalapril in the treatment of heart failure. After 3 months, the improvement of exercise tolerance in the enalapril group was greater than the improvement in the placebo group, but in the study population as a whole this difference was not statistically significant (Packer, 1988). This result was due to the large improvement noted in the placebo group, which seemed to indicate that the patients were not exercised to their maximum capacity during the baseline period. Three of the investigators measured expired gases, whereas the remaining investigators did not. In the three centres where expired gases were measured, enalapril was statistically superior to placebo (Creager *et al.*, 1985; Franciosa *et al.*, 1985), and there was no appreciable placebo effect. By following the patient's oxygen consumption during the test and evaluating whether the patient passes the anaerobic threshold, it is possible to identify with greater certainty whether the patient has exercised to his maximal capacity (Lipkin, 1987).

If it is impractical to measure expired gases, the Borg scale may be of value to help reduce variability (Borg, 1970). A requirement that all subjects perform three (or, at a minimum, two) exercise tests prior to being randomised to therapy will lessen the chance of an important training effect during the study.

Duration of the study is an important consideration. Successful studies have usually had treatment periods of 2–3 months. Six weeks should be considered the absolute minimum, since considerable improvement can be demonstrated in placebo-treated patients during the first 4 weeks of study therapy (Captopril Multicenter Research Group, 1983). This phenomenon could be due to a training effect as well as other factors such as closer medical supervision, better adherence to dietary restrictions and better compliance with medication.

In summary, for a small pilot exercise study to be successful, it is best performed by an experienced investigator and should measure expired gases as well as exercise duration. The drug-titration schedule should encourage the attainment of therapeutic drug levels in most patients. A double-blind study of 2–3 months' duration is suggested, with an absolute minimum of 6 weeks.

Other Efficacy Measurements

Other more subjective parameters measured during controlled trials may be used to support the efficacy of a given therapy.

New York Heart Association Class

The New York Heart Association (NYHA) criteria, although widely employed, are not very useful in demonstrating efficacy of a study therapy (Guyatt, 1985). Not only are the criteria imprecise and observer dependent (Goldman *et al.*, 1981), but also the categories are so broad that considerable improvement may occur and yet the patient may not change his NYHA class. It is also possible for NYHA class to change if a patient stops performing stressful activities (Goldman *et al.*, 1982). Questionnaires have been developed to more reliably determine NYHA class (Goldman *et al.*, 1981). The quality of the data will be better if collected by the same observer at each visit and if the observer is not responsible for therapeutic decisions (such as drug titration or alteration of concomitant therapy). It is very important to collect information on the patient's NYHA status at baseline, since most agencies regard this as useful information for categorising the patient population studied.

Other Scales of Functional Capacity

No one instrument for assessing the patient's response to therapy has met with uniformly favourable reviews among investigators. Three scales which have been used in CHF patients are the 'Living with Heart Failure' questionnaire (Rector *et al.*, 1987); the 'Yale Scale', also referred to as the Dyspnoea–Fatigue Index (Chalmers *et al.*, 1987); and the Specific Activity Scale (Goldman *et al.*, 1981). 'Living with Heart Failure' is a questionnaire completed by the patient, and the 'Yale Scale' is a rating of the patient's capacity as assessed by health personnel. The Specific Activity Scale is somewhat similar to the New York Heart Association Criteria, except that specific activities are assessed. In using these scales, the following suggestions may improve the quality of the data: (1) Instructions regarding the administration of the instruments should be written and complete. (2) The same observer should administer the scale throughout the study. (3) The observer should not be charged with making therapeutic decisions regarding the patient. (4) The instruments should be administered immediately upon the patient's arrival in the investigator's office. This prevents other factors, such as how well the patient does on the exercise test, from influencing the answers to the questionnaires.

Concomitant Therapy

The management of concomitant therapy is a particularly problematic aspect of heart failure trials (Guyatt, 1985). The problem is most evident with respect to concomitant diuretic therapy. If one group in a randomised trial requires more diuretic during the study, and also shows more improvement in exercise duration than the other group, was the exercise improvement due to the study therapy or due to the change in diuretic dose?

A decision on what concomitant therapy to allow during CHF studies will depend partly upon the labelling desired following approval. Information on concomitant therapy should be collected in detail during the study, since a decrease in the need for concomitant therapy may be an efficacy end-point. It is important to ensure that concomitant therapy is similar in both treatment groups in terms of the nature of the concomitant agents utilised. This is especially important when patients may be taking drugs with vasodilatory or positive or negative inotropic properties.

SUMMARY

Phase I studies for the evaluation of new therapies for heart failure should establish the cardiovascular effects of the new compound in healthy volunteers, and the doses producing those effects. The major goals of Phase II studies in the evaluation of new therapies for heart failure are to identify the appropriate dose and dosing interval in the target population, determine the pharmacokinetic and pharmacodynamic characteristics in CHF, and establish some level of confidence that the new therapy will improve symptoms and exercise capacity during chronic therapy. Invasive haemodynamic studies are useful for the investigation of dose response and duration of action, but favourable haemodynamic changes do not translate uniformly into long-term clinical benefits. Phase II planning should also incorporate a carefully performed pilot exercise study to determine the ability of the new therapy to improve exercise duration during chronic therapy.

REFERENCES

Barr, W. H. and Riegelman, S. (1970). Intestinal drug absorption and metabolism I: Comparison of methods and models to study physiological factors of *in vitro* and *in vivo* intestinal absorption. *J. Pharmacol. Sci.*, **59** (2), 154–63

Borg, G. (1970). Perceived exertion as an indicator of somatic stress. *Scand. J. Rehab. Med.*, **2–3**, 92–8

Captopril Multicenter Research Group (1983). A placebo-controlled trial of captopril in refractory chronic congestive heart failure. *J. Am. Coll. Cardiol.*, **2** (4), 755–63

Chalmers, J. P., West, M. J., Cyran, J., De La Torre, D., Englert, M., Kramar, M., Lewis, G. R. J., Maranhao, M. F. L., Myburgh, D. P., Schuster, P., Sialer, S., Simon, H., Stephens, J. D. and Watson, R. D. S. (1987). Placebo-controlled study of lisinopril in congestive heart failure: a multicentre study. *J. Cardiovasc. Pharmacol.*, **9** (Suppl. 3), S89–S97

Cleland, J. G. F., Dargie, H. J., Ball, S. G., Gillen, G., Hodsman, G. P., Morton, J., East, B. W., Roberton, I., Ford, I. and Robertson, J. I. S. (1985). Effects of enalapril in heart failure: a double blind study of effects on exercise performance, renal function, hormones and metabolic state. *Br. Heart J.*, **54** (3), 305–12

Cornyn, J. W., Massie, B. M., Unverferth, D. V. and Leier, C. V. (1986).

Hemodynamic changes after meals and placebo treatment in chronic congestive heart failure. *Am. J. Cardiol.*, **57**, 238–41

Creager, M. A., Massie, B. M., Faxon, D. P., Friedman, S. D., Kramer, B. L., Weiner, D. A., Ryan, T. J., Topic, N. and Melidossian, C. D. (1985). Acute and long-term effects of enalapril on the cardiovascular response to exercise and exercise tolerance in patients with congestive heart failure. *J. Am. Coll. Cardiol.*, **6** (1), 163–70

David, D., Lang, R. M. and Borow, K. M. (1988). Clinical utility of exercise, pacing, and pharmacologic stress for the noninvasive determination of myocardial contractility and reserve. *Am. Heart J.*, **116** (1, Part 1), 235–47

Franciosa, J. A., Weber, K. T., Levine, T. B., Kinasewitz, G. T., Janicki, J. S., West, J., Henis, M. M. and Cohn, J. N. (1982). Hydralazine in the long term treatment of chronic heart failure: lack of difference from placebo. *Am. Heart J.*, **104** (3), 587–94

Franciosa, J. A., Wilen, M. M. and Jordan, R. A. (1985). Effects of enalapril, a new angiotensin-converting enzyme inhibitor, in a controlled trial in heart failure. *J. Am. Coll. Cardiol.*, **5** (1), 101–7

Francis, G. S. (1987). Hemodynamic and neurohumoral responses to dynamic exercise: normal subjects versus patients with heart disease. *Circulation*, **76** (Suppl. VI), VI-11–VI-17

Goldman, L., Cook, E. F., Mitchell, N., Flatley, M., Sherman, H. and Cohn, P. F. (1982). Pitfalls in the serial assessment of cardiac functional status. How a reduction in 'ordinary' activity may reduce the apparent degree of cardiac compromise and give a misleading impression of improvement. *J. Chron. Dis.*, **35** (10), 763–71

Goldman, L., Hashimoto, B., Cook, E. F. and Loscalzo, A. (1981). Comparative reproducibility and validity of systems for assessing cardiovascular functional class: advantages of a new specific activity scale. *Circulation*, **64** (6), 1227–34

Green, J. A., Nara, A. R. and Gengo, F. M. (1987). Characterization of the dose-concentration-dependent hemodynamic effects of nifedipine in heart failure. *J. Clin. Pharm.*, **27**, 574–81

Guyatt, G. H. (1985). Methodologic problems in clinical trials in heart failure. *J. Chron. Dis.*, **38** (4), 353–63

Guyatt, G. H. (1986). The treatment of heart failure. A methodological review of the literature. *Drugs*, **32**, 538–68

Herrmann, H. C., Ruddy, T. D., Dec, G. W., Strauss, H. W., Boucher, C. A. and Fifer, M. A. (1987). Inotropic effect of enoximone in patients with severe heart failure: demonstration by left ventricular end-systolic pressure-volume analysis. *J. Am. Coll. Cardiol.*, **9** (5), 1117–23

Lee, D. C., Johnson, R. A., Bingham, J. B., Leahy, M., Dinsmore, R. E., Goroll, A. H., Newell, J. B., Strauss, W. and Haber, E. (1982). Heart failure in outpatients. *New Engl. J. Med.*, **306** (12), 699–705

Leier, C. V., Huss, P., Magorien, R. D. and Unverferth, D. V. (1983). Improved exercise capacity and differing arterial and venous tolerance during chronic isosorbide dinitrate therapy for congestive heart failure. *Circulation*, **67** (4), 817–22

Lipkin, D. P. (1987). The role of exercise testing in chronic heart failure. *Br. Heart J.*, **58**, 559–66

Massie, B., Bourassa, M., DiBianco, R., Hess, M., Konstam, M., Likoff, M. and Packer, M. (1985). Long-term oral administration of amrinone for congestive heart failure: lack of efficacy in a multicenter controlled trial. *Circulation*, **71** (5), 963–71

Nies, A. S., Shand, D. G. and Wilkinson, G. R. (1976). Altered hepatic blood flow and drug disposition. *Clin. Pharmacokin.*, **1**, 135–55

Packer, M. (1987). How should we judge the efficacy of drug therapy in patients with chronic congestive heart failure? The insights of six blind men. *J. Am. Coll. Cardiol.*, **9** (2), 433–8

Packer, M. (1988). Clinical trials in congestive heart failure: why do studies report conflicting results? *Ann. Int. Med.*, **109**, 3–5

Packer, M. and Leier, C. V. (1987). Survival in congestive heart failure during treatment with drugs with positive inotropic actions. *Circulation*, **75** (Suppl. IV), IV-55–IV-63

Packer, M., Meller, J., Medina, N., Gorlin, R. and Herman, M. V. (1980). Dose requirements of hydralazine in patients with severe chronic congestive heart failure. *Am. J. Cardiol.*, **45**, 655–60

Packer, M., Meller, J., Medina, N., Yushak, M. and Gorlin, R. (1982). Hemodynamic characterization of tolerance to long-term hydralazine therapy in severe chronic heart failure. *New Engl. J. Med.*, **306** (2), 57–62

Rector, T. S., Kubo, S. H. and Cohn, J. N. (1987). Patients' self-assessment of their congestive heart failure. Part 2: Content, reliability and validity of a new measure, the Minnesota Living with Heart Failure Questionnaire. *Heart Failure*, October/November, 198–209

Rude, R. E., Grossman, W., Colucci, W. S., Benotti, J. R., Carabello, B. A., Wynne, J., Malacoff, R. and Braunwald, E. (1981). Problems in assessment of new pharmacologic agents for the heart failure patient. *Am. Heart J.*, **102** (3, Part 2), 584–90

Schmidt, R. (1988). Dose-finding studies in clinical drug development. *Eur. J. Pharm.*, **34**, 15–19

Topic, N., Kramer, B. and Massie, B. (1982). Acute and long-term effects of captopril on exercise cardiac performance and exercise capacity in congestive heart failure. *Am. Heart J.*, **104** (5, Part 2), 1172–9

Weber, K. T., Kinasewitz, G. T., Janicki, J. S. and Fishman, A. P. (1982). Oxygen utilization and ventilation during exercise in patients with chronic cardiac failure. *Circulation*, **65** (6), 1213–23

26
Antithrombotic and Thrombolytic Drugs

J. Ritter

Dept of Clinical Pharmacology, Guy's Hospital, London Bridge, London SE1, UK

INTRODUCTION

Thrombotic disease (venous thromboembolism, coronary and cerebral arterial thrombosis), collectively accounts for the majority of deaths in developed countries. Several drugs of venerable lineage are used in the prevention of such events, notably heparin and warfarin (and its congeners), which interfere with the coagulation cascade; aspirin, which inhibits platelet aggregation; and streptokinase, which causes fibrinolysis. These drugs were introduced into clinical practice before present regulatory requirements were formulated, but the information that has been gained about their clinical pharmacology forms a basis for evaluating new drugs that act on the coagulation cascade or on platelets.

Some of these new drugs are entirely novel; some are existing enzymes or anticoagulants produced in novel ways such as recombinant DNA technologies in the case of tissue plasminogen activator[1] or the leech polypeptide hirudin (see Reference 2). Recombinant DNA technology offers the prospect of multiple modifications of existing drugs, even when these are extremely complex polypeptides or proteins. Enzyme modification (e.g. acylation) offers further prospects of improving existing drugs,[3] as exemplified by anisoylated plasminogen streptokinase activator complex (APSAC). Many such drugs have been launched recently or are in the process of development. Their introduction into human use follows detailed animal pharmacology and toxicity testing, and extensive *in vitro* experiments on human blood, plasma and platelets. In this chapter, the general objectives of such studies are outlined, and then specifics relating to the kinds of subjects that are most suitable and the tests that may be most useful are considered. The references cited are intended to exemplify the principles involved, and are not exhaustive.

OBJECTIVES OF EARLY PHASE STUDIES

The objects of early phase studies on a new antithrombotic drug are to establish at least the lower part of the dose–response curve, to determine the pharmacokinetics of the drug, and to go some way towards establishing its safety and tolerability. Antithrombotic drugs are often used in combination with each other and with other circulatory drugs. Such drugs frequently have narrow margins of safety and steep dose–response curves. Studies of possible drug interactions are also therefore essential early in the evaluation process.

Pharmacokinetics

Pharmacokinetic studies depend on the availability of a sufficiently sensitive and specific assay for the drug, often by means of high-performance liquid chromatography, and the methodology therefore varies from drug to drug. Initial experimental design will be determined by data from animal studies (particularly primate data, when available). These provide reasonable expectations regarding absorption, bioavailability, routes of elimination and the presence or otherwise of active metabolites. The principles underlying such studies are described in the chapter by S. Toon.

Safety and Efficacy

The most predictable adverse effect of antithrombotic drugs is, of course, haemorrhage. Therefore, a history of bleeding disorder or peptic ulcer disease is sought particularly diligently, and is cause for exclusion of potential volunteers from early phase studies of such drugs. Subjects must be questioned specifically regarding blood loss during repeated-dose studies. Tests of coagulation and haemostasis (see below) assume particular importance among the battery of routine tests performed in assessing the safety of any new drug, and laboratory evidence of occult bleeding (e.g. testing of urine, testing of stool for occult blood) must be sought during repeated-dose studies.

Drugs of which the principal site of action is the coagulation system may also have idiosyncratic effects on platelets. Heparin is an example, since it may cause thrombocytopenia. Conversely, drugs that act mainly on platelets may also affect the coagulation cascade: for instance, aspirin, in addition to its effects on platelets may prolong the prothrombin time when ingested in toxic amounts. Such effects are potentially important, since they presumably increase the risk of haemorrhagic complications. Thus, there is considerable overlap in the tests that are indicated in studying anticoagulant and antiplatelet drugs both to determine their pharmacodynamic profile and in establishing their safety. Fibrinolytic drugs are frequently macromolecules with the potential of causing immune reactions. Therefore, evidence of antibody response is sought by routine immunological methods. This may be particularly important when recombinant DNA technology has been used to produce a modification of a naturally occurring polypeptide to alter its pharmacological properties in some desirable way, since such an alteration may be accompanied by an unexpected change in immunogenicity.

Additionally, there are many more specialised tests that will be indicated in studies of particular drugs on the basis of their known pharmacology. One particularly promising method of studying thrombosis involves platelet labelling and imaging (see, e.g., Reference 4), and this is described in the chapter by H. Sinzinger.

SUBJECTS

For the first use of antiplatelet drugs *in vivo*, subjects should ideally be healthy men taking no other medication and with no history of bleeding tendency or peptic ulcer. It is especially important to proscribe the use of aspirin for at least 10 days before the study. This is because aspirin irreversibly inhibits platelet cyclo-oxygenase, and platelet life span is 7–10 days. Because aspirin is present in so many over-the-counter preparations, independent confirmation of adherence to this requirement is highly desirable. Measurement of thromboxane B_2 (TXB_2) in serum prepared by allowing whole blood to clot in a plain glass tube at 37 °C for 60 min followed by radioimmunoassay of TXB_2 provides a simple check of compliance. Thrombin generated during clotting stimulates platelet thromboxane synthesis, and the usual value of serum TXB_2 prepared in this way and measured by radioimmunoassay is around 300 ng/ml. Aspirin ingestion in usual doses inhibits serum TXB_2 by greater than 99%. Antisera, standards and radioactive ligands are commercially available (e.g. Amersham International, New England Nuclear), and radioimmunoassay of TXB_2 in serum is a simple and appropriate measure of platelet cyclo-oxygenase activity.

Antithrombotic drugs that act on the coagulation cascade, such as heparin or warfarin, may be used for the first time in man in patients experiencing a thrombotic event. However, some recent anticoagulants such as ORG 10172, a low molecular weight heparinoid, have been extensively investigated in healthy human volunteers without untoward morbidity.[5] Drugs that promote dissolution of thrombi (thrombolytic agents) may salvage potentially viable myocardium when administered sufficiently early in the course of myocardial infarction. However, these drugs have been perceived as potentially extremely hazardous. For this reason, very little work on them has been performed in healthy volunteers. Instead, following extensive *in vitro* studies on human plasma and clots, early human studies have been performed on patients with thrombotic diseases, who might therefore be hoped to benefit from their effects. For instance, the first use of tissue-type plasminogen activator in humans was in a woman with extensive ileofemoral and renal vein thrombosis[6] and subsequent early phase evaluation of recombinant tissue type plasminogen activator has been performed in patients experiencing myocardial infarction.[7,8] Similarly, subcutaneous hirudin has been administered to a patient with Kasabach–Merritt syndrome, a disorder characterised by intravascular coagulation, and caused normalisation of platelet count and fibrinogen.[9] An analogous situation exists in early phase evaluation of antimitotic drugs, the inherent toxicity of which precludes their use in healthy volunteers. However, the use of patients does pose special problems. In general, such studies are most usefully performed on extremely well-characterised patients with clear-cut pathology and no coexisting disease, especially disease that predisposes to bleeding such as peptic ulceration and uncontrolled hypertension. In practice, bleeding with thrombolytic drugs is usually related to invasive instrumentation and it may be that, with increasing experience of these agents, their use in healthy volunteers may become ethically justifiable, at least at low doses.

TESTS OF COAGULATION AND COAGULATION FACTOR ACTIVITY

Standard haematological tests provide measures of the effects of anti-thrombotic drugs on the coagulation cascade. Prothrombin time (PT) is prolonged following administration *in vivo* of antagonists of vitamin K, such as warfarin. Partial thromboplastin time (PTT) and whole blood clotting time are prolonged by heparin and other drugs (e.g. low molecular weight heparinoids) that activate antithrombin III or inhibit thrombin directly (e.g. hirudin or argatroban). These tests are performed routinely in most haematology laboratories. Details of the methods are provided by Biggs and MacFarlane.[10] Specific clotting factor activity, such as anti-Xa activity, can be measured by assays based on spectrophotometric determination of the rate of hydrolysis of chromogenic peptide substrates.[11] This has been useful in studies of heparin and heparinoids (see, e.g., Reference 5). As explained above, it is also appropriate to include some of the basic tests (e.g. PT, PTT) in early phase studies of new drugs known to act on platelets (such as prostacyclin analogues (see, e.g., Reference 12) or thromboxane synthase inibitors (see, e.g., Reference 13) to confirm that they are not also affecting the coagulation system directly.

In studies of thrombolytic drugs, laboratory evidence of systemic fibrinolysis is sought. This may include decreases in fibrinogen, plasminogen and clotting factors, and an increase in fibrin degradation products. In the case of thrombolytic drugs such as recombinant tissue plasminogen activator which are relatively thrombospecific, there may be little or no change in these measures. With such drugs, measurements of plasma concentration of the drug which can be related to potency in causing clot dissolution *in vitro* assume considerable importance. Since these drugs are often polypeptides, immunological assays may be appropriate for performing such measurements simply (see, e.g., Reference 14). In contrast to clot-specific agents, drugs such as streptokinase, anisoylated plasminogen streptokinase activator complex (APSAC) or urokinase produce a generalised lytic state, so measurements of coagulation factors and fibrinogen split products provide direct pharmacodynamic evidence of effect. Blood may be collected in tubes containing sodium citrate as anticoagulant (final concentration 10 mM) and aprotinin (final concentration 150 KIU/ml) to counteract proteolysis induced by plasmin *in vitro*. Plasma should be separated promptly (<1 h) and stored at −20 °C. Fibrinogen may be measured by one of several methods, including clotting rate assay[15] or sulphite precipitation.[16] There are also several methods of measuring fibrinolytic products, such as that of Merskey *et al.*[17]

HAEMODYNAMIC MEASUREMENTS

Haemodynamic measurements form an important part in the evaluation of any new drug, because of their implications for safety. Over and above this general concern, there is a particular reason for careful evaluation of such effects in the case of antithrombotic and thrombolytic drugs, because many of these have direct or indirect actions on vascular smooth muscle. Prostacyclin and streptokinase exemplify such vasoactive drugs. Both cause vasodilation— prostacyclin via receptors linked to adenylate cyclase in arteriolar smooth muscle, and streptokinase possibly via kinin generation. Modifications of these drugs which retain their antithrombotic effects, but not their vasodilator action, are being sought. Prostacyclin analogues that are specific for platelets could be therapeutically valuable, but as yet there is no convincing evidence that such specificity is possible. However, APSAC is essentially an inactive prodrug of streptokinase which lacks the acute vasodilator effect of streptokinase itself, enabling it to be given by relatively short intravenous infusion, potentially a considerable advantage (see, e.g., Reference 18).

Haemodynamic measurements of new antithrombotic drugs are therefore of great importance. Simple measurements such as blood pressure and heart rate give essential information. They must be performed carefully under controlled environmental conditions. Automatic devices for recording arterial pressure indirectly, such as the 'Dinamap' (Critikon), are useful in providing an unbiased means of determining blood pressure. Heart rate can be measured accurately from a continuous electrocardiogram. Measurements of blood flow through individual vascular beds may also be valuable in some instances. In particular, measurements in the forearm vascular bed have great potential for use in early phase drug evaluation in man, because minute intra-arterial doses produce effects on local resistance vessels which are reflected in large changes in blood flow, enabling studies to be performed safely with doses well below those needed to produce systemic effects (see, e.g., Reference 19). Drugs are administered through a very-fine-gauge steel cannula, sited in a brachial artery, and blood flow in the forearm is compared with flow through the non-cannulated arm. Flow is measured by use of mercury in silastic strain gauges. Bleeding or haematoma formation is not usually a problem, although experience of administration of antithrombotic drugs by this route is limited.

BLEEDING TIME

Bleeding time is prolonged by drugs that interfere with platelet function (e.g. aspirin) as well as anticoagulants (e.g. heparin and the specific thrombin antagonist, hirudin[20]), and provides a valuable pharmacodynamic measure of drug effect. Bleeding time may also be valuable in identifying potentially useful or hazardous interactions with other cardiovascular drugs. Several methods of performing bleeding time have been described, including ones based on simple disposable devices such as the Simplate II.[21,22] Although conceptually simple, the test must be performed meticulously, and even with the greatest care any individual investigator is likely to encounter substantial variability. For this reason it is essential that such studies be performed blind, preferably on a paired basis with the same investigator throughout. The site of the incision, orientation of the device relative to the forearm and pressure applied to the skin must all be standardised. Subjects should be caffeine-, tobacco- and alcohol-free, and ideally in the post-absorptive state. The environmental temperature must be controlled. Even so, the number of subjects required to demonstrate a doubling of bleeding time may be as many as 20–40.[21–23]

PLATELET COUNT

No clinically useful antithrombotic drugs work by producing thrombocytopenia, but platelet counts are, of course, a routine part of the safety testing profile for any drug undergoing early phase testing. Such counts assume particular importance in recognising potential toxicity of antithrombotic drugs. Conversely, thrombocytopenia is a feature of diffuse intravascular coagulation which may be *corrected* by anticoagulants. Paradoxically, heparin and other anticoagulants such as hirudin[9] may therefore *increase* the platelet count in patients with diffuse intravascular coagulation, providing an indication of the desired effect.

PLATELET ADHESION AND AGGREGATION

There are a variety of methods for studying platelet adhesion (reviewed by Bowie and Owen[24] and Yardumian *et al.*[25]). One method that has been useful in human volunteer studies of heparinoids involves pumping whole blood at a fixed rate through a glass column of microbeads.[26] Currently available antithrombotic drugs do not have marked effects on platelet adhesion to foreign surfaces. Prostacyclin is the most potent endogenous inhibitor of platelet aggregation known,[27] yet it has much less effect on adhesion,[28] possibly accounting for its excellent safety profile in clinical practice.[29] Conversely, diseases in which adhesion is defective, such as von Willebrand's disease and Bernard–Soulier syndrome, are characterised by a severe bleeding diathesis, and it is possible that drugs which interfere with adhesion would prove hazardous. It is noteworthy in this context that nitric oxide, a vasodilator released by endothelial cells (EDRF[30]), which activates guanylate cyclase, inhibits platelet adhesion.[31] Several cardiovascular drugs (including nitroprusside and the organic nitrates) act on guanylate cyclase directly or indirectly, and it is therefore possible that these may potentiate antithrombotic drugs. Such potentially hazardous interactions should be sought in early phase studies.

The effect of drugs on aggregation (i.e. platelet–platelet interaction) may be studied by a variety of methods (see review by Packham *et al.*[32]). One method that has proved useful in human volunteer studies is the turbidometric method described by Born and Cross,[33] or some modification of this, such as the following. Venous blood is drawn gently with an 18-gauge needle to minimise platelet activation during sampling. It is anticoagulated with sodium citrate and subjected to low-speed centrifugation (e.g. 750 *g* for 10 min) at room temperature to produce a turbid suspension of platelets. This is kept at room temperature until a measurement is to be made, when a portion is transferred to a siliconised glass cell containing a Teflon-coated magnetic stirring bar (900 rev/min) and maintained at 37 °C in the light path of an aggregometer (e.g. Payton, Chronolog). Aggregation caused by an agonist is monitored by the change in light transmission detected by a photomultiplier. Changes in light transmission are related to a maximal value which is obtained from platelet-poor plasma prepared from the same blood sample. Alternatively, aggregation can be studied in whole blood by measuring impedance changes[34] or by whole blood platelet counting using an instrument such as the Clay Adams Ultra Flo 100.[35]

Neither method accurately reflects the situation *in vivo*, but either can be valuable in demonstrating that a drug has influenced platelet function. Drugs, such as prostacyclin, that have a short half-life in the circulation may be studied conveniently by whole blood aggregation; alternatively, platelet-rich plasma may be prepared rapidly with an Eppendorf microcentrifuge (see, e.g., Reference 36), enabling evanescent effects to be detected. Useful agonists include adenosine diphosphate (ADP), collagen, thrombin, arachidonic acid, platelet activating factor, or a stable thromboxane mimetic such as U-46619.

The effect of an antiplatelet drug on aggregation caused by these different agonists varies according to its mechanism of action. For instance, thromboxane receptor antagonists selectively inhibit drugs that work by stimulating thromboxane receptors. These include the thromboxane mimetics as well as arachidonic acid, which is converted in the platelets into TXA_2. The secondary, but not the primary, wave of aggregation induced by ADP is partly mediated by TXA_2 and is also inhibited by such drugs. Cyclooxygenase inhibitors or thromboxane synthase inhibitors, by contrast, do not inhibit U-46619-induced aggregation, because they do not block thromboxane receptors, but can inhibit aggregation caused by arachidonic acid, or the second phase of aggregation caused by ADP, which depend on TXA_2 synthesis. In the case of thromboxane synthase inhibitors, however, the effect on arachidonic acid-induced aggregation is variable and unpredictable. This is believed to be because of an accumulation in the cuvette of endoperoxides, such as PGH_2, which may themselves act as agonists on thromboxane receptors and cause aggregation. This can be determined by adding a thromboxane receptor antagonist, such as EPO45[37] to the platelet-rich plasma *in vitro*. Drugs such as prostacyclin increase intracellular cyclic AMP and inhibit aggregation, irrespective of agonist. Clearly, the battery of agonists used in any particular study must be selected according to the known pharmacology of the antithrombotic drug under investigation.

PLATELET SECRETION AND INTRACELLULAR BIOCHEMICAL EVENTS

Platelet secretion is not measured routinely in early phase studies of antithrombotic drugs, although it may be of relevance in particular circumstances. ATP secretion can be measured by means of the lumi-aggregometer.[38] The principle involves detection of light produced when secreted ATP comes into contact with an enzyme system (luciferin–luciferase), which is added to platelet rich plasma in a cuvette. Granule secretion is stimulated by an agonist added to the mixture in the aggregometer. Similarly, biochemical events such as changes in cyclic AMP, cyclic GMP, calcium or inositol lipids are not measured routinely, but may be highly apposite to particular questions posed in relation to individual drugs.

PLATELET ACTIVATION *IN VIVO*

Platelets are very readily activated during blood sampling. Consequently, measurement of platelet-derived products such as TXB_2 in plasma is usually unhelpful in establishing the effect of a drug on platelet activation *in vivo*. One approach that has been used is simultaneous determination by radioimmunoassay of two products, β-thromboglobulin and platelet factor IV (PF IV), which are eliminated from the body at different rates. This may be helpful in situations of very substantial platelet activation, such as extensive deep venous thrombosis or unstable angina pectoris[39] and the approach may be more useful in Phase III studies than in early evaluation of antithrombotic drugs.

A more sensitive indicator for *in vivo* studies in healthy volunteers is provided by the urinary excretion rate of 2,3-dinor TXB_2. This is the major urinary metabolite of TXB_2, and is formed by β-oxidation. Its excretion is increased in disorders associated with platelet activation, including unstable angina, but it is also excreted by healthy subjects in sufficient amounts to permit quantitative studies in volunteers of drugs that inhibit thromboxane production, such as aspirin.[40] The most reliable method for measuring this metabolite is by gas chromatography/mass spectrometry. This method has recently been greatly simplified by the use of immunoaffinity chromatography as a means of extraction and purification of the metabolite from urine.[41,42] Quantification depends on the use of deuterated internal standard, which is added to the urine as soon as the sample is obtained from the subject and which permits losses during storage or extraction to be accounted for accurately. Measurements of other eicosanoid metabolites in urine may be useful with particular drugs. For instance, thromboxane synthase inhibitors increase prostacyclin production in healthy volunteers, and this is reflected in increased urinary excretion of the prostacyclin metabolite 2,3-dinor-6-oxo-$PGF_1\alpha$.[43]

CONCLUSION

Early phase human studies of antiplatelet drugs are best performed in healthy volunteers. Novel anticoagulants have also been evaluated in volunteers as well as patients, whereas thrombolytic drugs have been studied in patients experiencing myocardial infarction or other thrombotic events. Tests of safety and efficacy concentrate on evidence of disordered haemostasis using a combination of *in vivo* and *ex vivo* functional and biochemical techniques.

REFERENCES

1. Pennica, D., Holmes, W. E., Kohr, W. J. *et al.* (1983). Cloning and expression of human tissue-type plasminogen activator cDNA in *E. coli*. *Nature*, **301**, 214–20
2. Wallis, R. B. (1988). Hirudins and the role of thrombin: lessons from leeches. *Trends Pharm. Sci.*, **9**, 425–7
3. Smith, R. A. G., Dupe, R. J., English, P. D. and Green, J. (1981). Fibrinolysis with acyl-enzymes: a new approach to thrombolytic therapy. *Nature*, **290**, 505–8
4. Stuttle, A. W. J., Ritter, J. M., Peters, A. M. and Lavender, J. P. (1988). *In vitro* studies with an antiplatelet monoclonal antibody; P256. *Nucl. Med. Commun.*, **9**, 183–8
5. Bradbrook, I. D., Magnani, H. N., Moelker, H. C. T., Morrison, P. J., Robinson, J., Rogers, H. J., Spector, R. G., van Dinther, T. and Wijnand, H. (1987). ORG 10172: A low molecular weight heparinoid anticoagulant with a long half-life in man. *Br. J. Clin. Pharm.*, **23**, 667–75
6. Weimar, W., Stibbe, J., van Seyen, A. J., Billiau, A., De Somer, P. and Collen, D. (1981). Specific lysis of an iliofemoral thrombus by administration of extrinsic (tissue-type) plasminogen activator. *Lancet*, **ii**, 1018–20
7. Chesebro, J. H., Knatterud, G., Roberts, R. *et al.* (1987). Thrombolysis in myocardial infarction (TIMI) trial, phase I: A comparison between intravenous tissue plasminogen activator and intravenous streptokinase. *Circulation*, **76**, 142–54
8. Sobel, B. E. (1987). Safety and efficacy of tissue-type plasminogen activator produced by recombinant DNA technology. *J. Am. Coll. Cardiol.*, **10**, 40B–44B
9. Markwardt, F. (1988). Seminars in thrombosis and haemostasis (in press)
10. Biggs, R. G., and MacFarlane, R. G. (Eds.) (1966). *Treatment of Haemophilia and Other Coagulation Disorders*. Blackwell Scientific Publications, Oxford
11. Teien, A. N. and Lie, M. (1977). Evaluation of an amidolytic heparin assay method, increased sensitivity by adding purified antithrombin III. *Thrombosis Res.*, **21**, 169–73
12. O'Grady, J. *et al.* (1984). A chemically stable analogue, 9β-methyl carbacyclin, with similar effects to epoprostenol (prostacyclin, PGI_2) in man. *Br. J. Clin. Pharm.*, **18**, 921–33

13. Lewis, P. J. and Tyler, H. M. (Eds.) (1983). Dazoxiben—clinical prospects for a thromboxane synthetase inhibitor. *Br. J. Clin. Pharm.*, **15** (Suppl. 1), 1S–140S
14. Rijken, D. C., Juhan-Vague, I., De Cock, F. and Collen, D. (1983). Measurement of human tissue-type plasminogen activator by a two-site immunoradiometric assay. *J. Lab. Clin. Med.*, **101**, 274–94
15. Vermylen, C., De Vreker, R. A. and Verstraete, M. (1983). A rapid enzymatic method for the assay of fibrinogen: the fibrin polymerization test (FPT). *Clin. Chim. Acta*, **8**, 418–24
16. Rampling, M. W. and Gaffney, P. J. (1976). The sulphite precipitation method for fibrinogen measurement; its use on small samples in the presence of fibrinogen degradation products. *Clin. Chim. Acta*, **67**, 43–52
17. Merskey, C., Lalezari, P. and Johnson, A. J. (1969). A rapid simple sensitive method for measuring fibrinolytic split products in human serum. *Proc. Soc. Exp. Biol. Med.*, **131**, 871–8
18. Ikram, S., Lewis, S., Bucknall, C. *et al.* (1986). Treatment of acute myocardial infarction with anisoylated plasminogen streptokinase activator complex. *Br. Med. J.*, **293**, 768–89
19. Benjamin, N., Cockcroft, J. R., Collier, J. G., Dollery, C. T., Ritter, J. M. and Webb, D. J. (1989). Local inibition of converting enzyme and vascular responses to angiotensin and bradykinin in the human forearm. *J. Physiol.*, **412**, 543–5
20. Kaiser, B. and Markwardt, F. (1986). Antithrombotic and haemorrhagic effects of synthetic and naturally occurring thrombin inhibitors. *Thrombosis Res.*, **43**, 613–20
21. Mielke, C. H., Kaneshiro, M. M., Maher, I. A., Weimar, J. M. and Rapaport, S. I. (1969). The standardized normal Ivy bleeding time and its prolongation by aspirin. *Blood*, **34**, 204–15
22. Babson, S. R. and Babson, A. L. (1978). Development and evaluation of a disposable device for performing simultaneous duplicate bleeding time determinations. *Am. J. Clin. Pathol.*, **70**, 406–8
23. Bick, R. L., Adams, T. and Schmalhorst, W. R. (1976). Bleeding times, platelet adhesion and aspirin. *Am. J. Clin. Pathol.*, **65**, 69–72
24. Bowie, E. J. W. and Owen, C. A. Jr. (1976). Platelet retention and other adhesion-aggregation phenomena. In Day, H. J., Holmsen, H. and Zucker, M. B. (Eds.), *Platelet Function Testing*. Department of Health Education and Welfare, Publication No. (NIH) 78-1087, p. 160
25. Yardumian, D. A., Machie, I. J. and Machin, S. J. (1986). Laboratory investigation of platelet function—a review of methodology. *J. Clin. Pathol.*, **39**, 701–12
26. Hellem, A. J. (1970). Platelet adhesiveness in von Willebrand's disease. A study with a new modification of the glass bead filter method. *Scand. J. Haematol.*, **7**, 374–82
27. Moncada, S., Gryglewski, R., Bunting, S. and Vane, J. R. (1976). An enzyme isolated from arteries transforms prostaglandin endoperoxides to an unstable substance that inhibits platelet aggregation. *Nature*, **263**, 663–5
28. Higgs, E. A., Moncada, S., Vane, J. R., Michael, M. and Tobelem, G. (1978). Effect of prostacyclin (PGI_2) on platelet adhesion to rabbit arterial sub endothelium. *Prostaglandins*, **16** (1), 17–22
29. Pickles, H. and O'Grady, J. (1982). Side effects occurring during administration of epoprostanol (prostacyclin), PGI_2 in man. *Br. J. Clin. Pharm.*, **14**, 177–86
30. Palmer, R. M. J., Ferrige, A. G. and Moncada, S. (1987). Nitric oxide release accounts for the biological activity of endothelium-derived relaxing factor. *Nature*, **327**, 524–6
31. Radomski, M. W., Palmer, R. M. J. and Moncada, S. (1987). Comparative pharmacology of endothelium-derived relaxing factor, nitric oxide and prostacyclin in platelets. *Br. J. Pharm.*, **92**, 181–7

32. Packham, M., Kinlough-Rathbone, R. L. and Mustard, J. F. (1976). Aggregation and agglutination. In Day, H. J., Holmsen, H. and Zucker, M. B. (Eds.), *Platelet Function Testing*, Department of Health Education and Welfare, Publication No. (NIH) 78-187, p. 66

33. Born, G. V. R. and Cross, M. J. (1963). The aggregation of blood platelets. *J. Physiol.*, **168**, 178

34. Cardinal, D. C. and Flower, R. J. (1980). The electronic aggregometer: A novel device for assessing platelet behaviour in blood. *J. Pharm. Meth.*, **3**, 135–58

35. Lumley, P. and Humphrey, P. P. A. (1981). A method for quantitating platelet aggregation and analysing drug-receptor interactions in platelets in whole blood *in vitro*. *J. Pharm. Meth.*, **6**, 153–66

36. Orchard, M. A., Ritter, J. M., Shepherd, G. L. and Lewis, P. J. (1983). Cardiovascular and platelet effects in man of BW245C, a stable mimic of epoprostanol (PGI$_2$). *Br. J. Clin. Pharm.*, **15**, 509–11

37. Jones, R. L., Wilson, N. H., Armstrong, R. A., Peesapaty, V. and Smith, G. M. (1983). Effects of thromboxane antagonists EPO45 on platelet aggregation. In Samuelsson, B., Paoletti, R. and Ramwell, P. W. (Eds.), *Advances in Prostaglandin Thromboxane and Leukotriene Research, Volume II*. Raven Press, New York

38. Ingerman, C. M., Smith, J. B. and Silver, M. J. (1979). *Thrombosis Res.*, **16**, 335–44

39. Sobel, M., Salzman, E. W., Davies, G. C., Handin, R. I., Sweeney, J., Iloetz, R. N. and Kurload, G. (1981). Circulating platelet products in unstable angina pectoris. *Circulation*, **63**, 300

40. FitzGerald, G. A., Oates, J. A., Hawiger, J., Maas, R. L., Roberts, L. J., Lawson, J. A. and Brash, A. R. (1983). Endogenous biosynthesis of prostacyclin and thromboxane and platelet function during chronic administration of aspirin in man. *J. Clin. Invest.*, **71**, 676–88

41. Chiabrando, C., Benigni, A., Piccinelli, A., Carminati, C., Cozzi, E., Remuzzi, R. and Fanelli, R. (1987). Antibody-mediated extraction/negative-ion chemical ionization mass spectrometric measurement of thromboxane B$_2$ and 2,3-Dinor-thromboxane B$_2$ in human and rat urine. *Analyt. Biochem.*, **163**, 255–62

42. Barrow, S. E., Sleightholm, M., Ward, P. and Ritter, J. M. (1989). Cigarette smoking: profiles of thromboxane- and prostacyclin-derived products in human urine. *Biochem. Biophys. Acta*, **993**, 121–7

43. FitzGerald, G. A., Brash, A. R., Oates, J. A. and Pedersen, A. K. (1983). Endogenous prostacyclin biosynthesis and platelet function during selective inhibition of thromboxane synthase in man. *J. Clin. Invest.*, **71**, 1336–43

27
Monitoring of Antithrombotic Activity by Platelet Labelling

H. Sinzinger and P. Fitscha

Atherosclerosis Research Group (ASV) Vienna, Dept of Internal Medicine, Policlinic, Schwarzspanierstr. 17, A-1090 Vienna, Austria

INTRODUCTION

Increased low-density lipoprotein (LDL) influx into the arterial wall, platelet activation and mononuclear cell infiltration are major mechanisms involved in human atherogenesis. Methods for measuring these variables and, hence, the effect of drugs are of importance in the identification of agents which may retard the development of atheroma. In addition, such methods should allow disorders of these mechanisms in the development of atheroma and in associated thromboembolic states to be more clearly understood. Several methods are available for *in vitro* testing of drugs affecting these three mechanisms. However, techniques which permit the monitoring of drug effects *in vivo* and provide *in vivo* information on the interaction of blood components with the vessel wall are rare.

This chapter describes radioisotope techniques which allow *in vivo* monitoring of the above mechanisms which have been implicated in human atherogenesis. Some of these techniques are at an early stage and it has to be remembered that detailed knowledge of their normal physiological ranges may be a necessary prerequisite for identification of drug effects.

Imaging of specific vascular areas using a gamma camera makes it possible to monitor the behaviour of platelets, LDL or monocytes, the last of which can now be labelled without impairing their viability. This also allows pathological conditions to be identified in the vasculature. The insertion of regions of interest (ROI) and measurement of radioactive counts allows quantification and provides information as to the extent of local change.

In order to provide a reference point for measurement in man, it is usual to count radioactivity over any pathological area of interest and also over a control area, after subtraction of background activity. The ratios between the pathological and control areas are termed Platelet Uptake Ratio (PUR) (Sinzinger *et al.*, 1984), Lipid Entry Ratio (LER) (Sinzinger *et al.*, 1989) or Monocyte Entry Ratio (MER).

ROLE OF PLATELETS

By means of platelet labelling it is possible to identify areas of pathologically increased platelet trapping in experimental animals and in man, in addition to measuring platelet kinetics.

Characterisation of Lesions

The presence of active atherosclerotic lesions (Figure 27.1) is characterised by increased platelet trapping, and local uptake may be enhanced by up to 100% compared with unaffected sites in the same patient (Figures 27.2, 27.3). No consistent sex or racial difference in platelet uptake has been reported, although there are differences between various vascular areas and uptake changes with age. The statistical risk factors for atheroma, themselves, have not been shown to affect the rate of vascular platelet uptake.

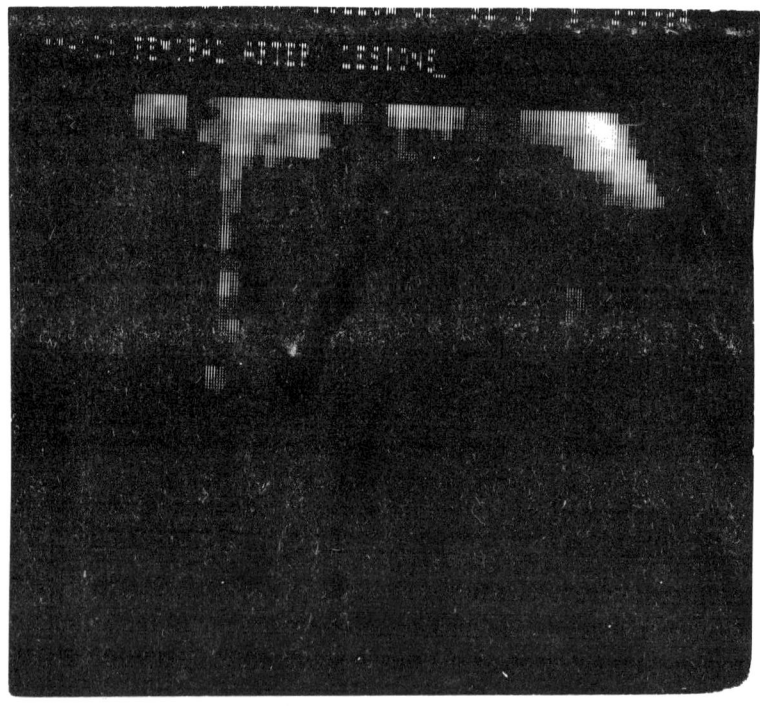

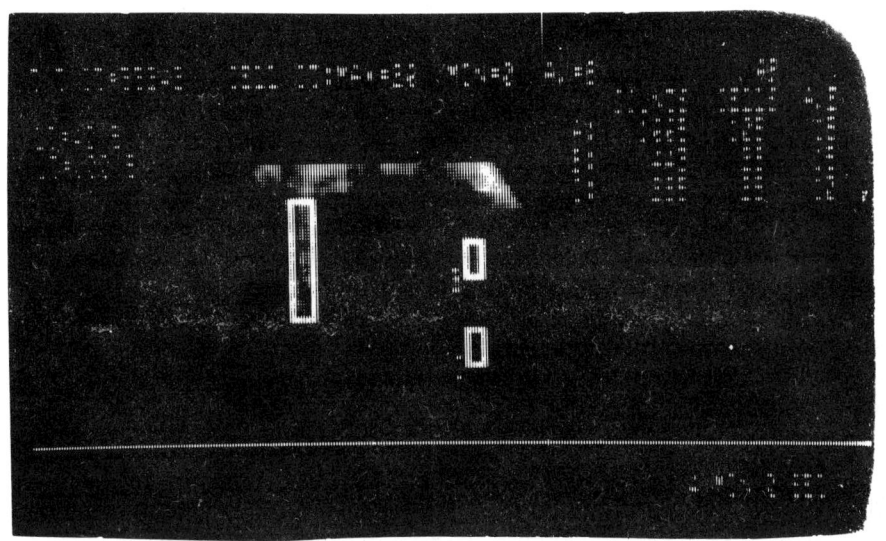

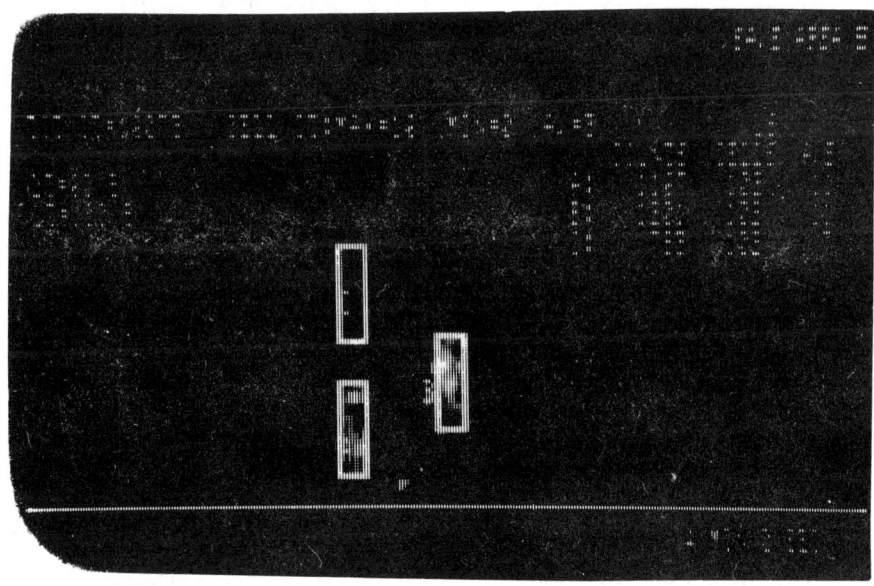

Characterisation of Kinetics

Platelet kinetics are altered in a variety of clinical conditions, whether affecting platelet uptake and destruction or with a primary haematological basis, and imaging together with kinetic data can identify abnormalities as local or systemic. Shortening of platelet survival indicates accelerated consumption. However, the reasons may lie in artefacts during labelling (Heyns *et al.*, 1980), vascular lesions (Heyns *et al.*, 1982) and temporary trapping in the liver, in addition to destruction of the platelets by other mechanisms. Altered platelet membrane composition in hypercholesterolaemia may alter the tracer uptake (Sinzinger *et al.*, 1988a) by the platelets *in vitro* but does not affect the kinetic values obtained. Furthermore, an extremely short platelet survival is often accompanied by a low platelet recovery, which is due to an abnormal platelet population.

Choice of Tracer

^{111}In tracers are preferable to ^{99m}Tc. Indium-labelled tracers have a radioisotope half-life of about 3 days and allow monitoring for up to 7 days after a single labelling procedure. Tracers such as [^{99m}Tc]-oxine ([^{99m}Tc]-*hexa*methyl*propylene*amine*oxime*: [^{99m}Tc]-HMPAO]) are not useful for monitoring of drug effects because of their fast physical decay. However, the data obtained with different complexes such as oxine, oxine-sulphate, mercaptopyridine-*N*-oxide (MPO) and tropolone are similar (Sinzinger *et al.*, 1988a), although only [^{111}In]-oxine is at present available commercially.

Platelet Labelling

The radiolabelling of autologous human platelets (Thakur *et al.*, 1976) may be performed with a kit which has been fully described elsewhere (Sinzinger *et al.*, 1984). Briefly, 16 ml blood is anticoagulated with acid citrate dextrose. After sedimentation and centrifugation, the supernatant platelet-rich plasma is further centrifuged to obtain a platelet pellet. This pellet is resuspended in buffer and incubated with 100 μCi [^{111}In]-oxine-sulphate, tropolone or MPO for 5 min at 37°C (Sinzinger *et al.*, 1981). Finally, the labelled platelets are diluted with autologous platelet-poor plasma and the suspension of radiolabelled platelets is injected intravenously.

Labelling Efficiency and Recovery

Labelling efficiency is an *in vitro* measurement made in an aliquot of blood after labelling, and the value is expressed as a percentage of the total activity which is present in the platelets. About 2 h after reinjection of the labelled platelets, 2 ml blood is drawn for measurement of *in vivo* recovery. The activity is measured in a gamma counter and the activity for the total blood volume is calculated. The relationship of the activity in the labelled platelets to the activity in the blood, expressed as a percentage, is the recovery.

Gamma-camera Imaging

Gamma-camera images are best obtained after 4 min exposure time. Over the site of the lesion being studied, a region of interest is inserted using the computer; after background subtraction the radioactive counts over this ROI are divided by the counts over an identically sized region inserted on the contralateral side and the platelet uptake ratio (PUR) is calculated between the two sites. In addition, spleen–liver imaging and ratio (S/L ratio) measurements are usually made (about 18 h after the reinjection of radiolabelled platelets). The effect of drug on local platelet activity can then be measured daily by imaging before, during and after discontinuing treatment.

Survival Determination

Blood samples are withdrawn two or three times a day for 5 days at least and radioactivity counting allows determination of platelet survival. The disappearance of the radioactivity curve can be further computed according to various models (Fritz *et al.*, 1986). Repeated measures of platelet survival may be performed before, during and after drug intervention (Heyns *et al.*, 1982).

Spontaneous Course

Lesions

Active sites of atheroma with lesions identified by imaging are relatively stable and show minimal changes in activity over periods of at least several weeks unless subject to pharmacological intervention.

Platelet Survival

Abnormal platelet survival values secondary to haematological and immunological disorders may fluctuate, depending on the activity of the underlying disease, whereas abnormalities secondary to atherosclerotic vascular disease are relatively stable.

Influence of Drugs

The influence of drugs on the intensity and persistence of lesions has been described (Sinzinger and Fitscha, 1989). The effects of platelet inhibitory agents, such as aspirin (Kessler *et al.*, 1985), prostaglandins (Sinzinger and Fitscha, 1984) and anticoagulants, have been demonstrated. Effects have not been shown with other compounds (Stratton *et al.*, 1982, 1984), such as sulphinpyrazone and ticlopidine. Similarly, the effects of drugs on platelet survival have been successfully monitored. Prolongation of platelet survival in haematological disorders may also be an indication of beneficial drug effects.

Monitoring for Drug Effects

Monitoring must be carried out over a time-scale appropriate to the expected effects of the drug under investigation. If the aim of the study is to monitor and measure immediate effects, imaging can be performed daily for up to 1 week. Changes within this short period of time can only be expected for intravenous drug application or for anticoagulants. If oral platelet inhibitor drugs or vasoactive substances are to be examined, a measurable effect, if any, may not be apparent until after several weeks of treatment. In these circumstances, a further labelling and monitoring procedure carried out after several weeks of treatment is recommended. For an example of how platelet labelling and imaging have been used in assessing drug effects, see Sinzinger *et al.* (1987).

Mechanisms Monitored

Lesion Imaging

An alteration in the quantity of platelets deposited at the site of a specific lesion or on the surface of implanted grafts (Huang *et al.*, 1981) may be largely due to a change in the thrombogenicity of the vascular surface (Mustard *et al.*, 1984), even in the absence of an endothelial lining, rather than due to changes in platelet function alone.

Platelet Survival

Platelet survival can be influenced by a variety of factors, and a change in platelet survival alone should be interpreted with caution. It is important to exclude other factors which may influence survival measurement, such as platelet damage during labelling and processing, altered consumption in liver and/or spleen, and unrelated clinical events. For example, the presence of a large haematoma may shorten platelet survival time.

Histological Assessment

Histological validation has revealed that normal arteries as well as advanced atherosclerotic lesions show platelet deposition. An increased amount of radioactivity has been demonstrated in areas of parietal microthrombus formation, and radioactive material can be found within arterial wall cells of mononuclear origin, although the platelet itself is no longer present.

Comparison with Other Conventional Techniques

Angiography

Angiography indicates the physical state of the vasculature, where platelet uptake measurements might be expected to reveal more of the dynamics of lesions and of the effects of drug therapy in the short term. However, because these techniques are not measuring the same thing, it is not surprising that in individual patients there has sometimes been a lack of correlation between findings with these two methods.

Magnetic Resonance (MR)

It is expected that, with further development in nuclear magnetic resonance, correlations will be found between the biochemical variables measured in this way and local platelet dynamics. At the present time, however, such information is not available.

Side-effects

Radiolabelling of platelets properly performed is virtually without side-effects. We have experienced no adverse events in the course of more than 5000 human labelling procedures. The radiation dose for one labelling procedure amounts to about 130 mrem, roughly equivalent to the radiation exposure from one chest X-ray.

ROLE OF LDL

Identification of Lesions

Vascular areas with increased LDL entry can be identified by a positive gamma-camera image after LDL radiolabelling (Kaliman *et al.*, 1985; Sinzinger *et al.*, 1986). In normolipaemic subjects the incidence of areas with increased LDL entry is low (<10%); however, the rate increases in patients with severe lesions and multiple risk factors and with age. The number and extent of lesions in patients suffering from hyperlipoproteinaemia is much higher than in normolipaemic patients.

Identification of Kinetics

The systemic kinetics of labelled LDL has not yet been clarified. However, monitoring of kinetics at local vascular sites indicates that this technique provides information as to the integrity of the endothelial lining and the number and activity of foam cells (Sinzinger and Angelberger, 1988).

Choice of Tracer

No tracer combinations are yet commercially available. Iodine-labelled tracers (^{123}I, ^{125}I, ^{131}I) require thyroid gland blockade before and during the procedure; hepatic deiodination (Lee *et al.*, 1983) may also occur. ^{99m}Tc has a very short half-life and is unsuitable for monitoring of systemic kinetics. Other tracers, such as an ^{111}In complex are in an early stage of development.

Low-density Lipoproteins (LDL)

After anticoagulation of 20 ml blood with heparin, autologous LDL (1–3 mg) are separated by means of high-affinity chromatography (Sinzinger *et al.*, 1988b) or ultracentrifugation. Radiolabelling is then carried out using ^{123}I (Sinzinger *et al.*, 1986), ^{125}I (Lees *et al.*, 1983), ^{131}I or ^{99m}Tc (Ginsberg *et al.*, 1985).

Spontaneous Course

Lesions

Lesions visible on imaging are relatively stable over periods of months in the absence of dietary or drug intervention.

Kinetics

Local lesion kinetics allow definition of lesion type in relation to the state of the endothelium and number of foam cells.

Influence of Drugs

Very limited data are available concerning the effects of drugs using radio labelling. Preliminary findings show that diet as well as hypolipidaemic drugs reduces lipid trapping by foam cells, the changes being pronounced enough to be monitored by this technique. This is an area where further development and validation will be important.

Monitoring

Two approaches are available: (1) local measurement of kinetics at vascular sites using gamma-camera imaging; (2) quantitative measurement of hepatic LDL receptors calculated from liver counts.

Mechanisms Monitored

Lesion Imaging

An alteration in lesion intensity corresponds to a decreased or increased entry of LDL into the vessel wall.

Local Kinetics

Changes in local kinetics allow identification of alterations in the surface lining and in the amount of foam cells in the arterial wall. Persistence of LDL in the arterial wall correlates to the content of foam cells, whereas the speed of entry and amount of maximal radioactivity is an indicator of the presence and integrity of the endothelial lining.

Histological Assessment

LDL uptake is only seen in areas rich in foam cells. The entry is higher at the periphery than at the centre of a lesion. Local kinetics have been correlated morphologically with the state of the endothelial lining.

Comparison with Other Conventional Techniques

At the present time no studies have been done to investigate the correlation of results with LDL labelling and conventional techniques of angiography, ultrasound or nuclear magnetic resonance.

Side-effects

The radiation dose from a single labelling is about 100 mrem, equivalent to less than that from one chest X-ray.

ROLE OF MONONUCLEAR ELEMENTS

Preliminary studies demonstrate that human mononuclear cells can be radiolabelled and that their kinetics as well as their entry into the arterial wall can be monitored. A major limitation is their radiosensitivity, which makes it necessary to separate a sufficient number of cells and to titrate radioactivity according to the number of separated cells. In order to achieve a sufficient quantity of cells, concentration and purification steps are essential. Furthermore, special attention has to be paid to the radiosensitivity of the mononuclear elements as well as their functional integrity. These aspects still need further clarification.

ETHICAL CONSIDERATION

There are particular ethical considerations in the use of radiolabelled material in humans for non-diagnostic purposes only. However, the extent of risk in such studies should be seen in perspective: as mentioned earlier, the exposure to radioactivity as a result of a platelet or LDL labelling procedure is less than that from a conventional chest X-ray.

CONCLUSION

The methods for radiolabelling platelets, LDL and monocytes accompanied by gamma-camera imaging should improve our understanding of human atheroma and allow elucidation of the mode of action and prediction of efficacy of atheroma-inhibiting drugs. Drugs intended to inhibit platelet activity should prolong platelet survival and reduce platelet accumulation at local vascular lesions. Drugs affecting lipids should decrease the number and extent of lipid lesions and normalise lipid kinetics at local vascular lesions. It may be that drugs will be identified which affect the behaviour of monocytes and decrease the extent of monocyte invasion of the vessel wall. It is evident that effects on one or other of these mechanisms are not exclusive, and drugs which have beneficial effects in atheroma may well modify several of these measures. Further development and application of these methods should yield important information both as to pathogenesis and also as to the effects of drug intervention.

REFERENCES

Fritz, E., Ludwig, H., Scheithauer, W. and Sinzinger, H. (1986). Shortened platelet half-life in multiple myeloma. *Blood*, **68**, 514–20

Ginsberg, H. V., Vallabhajosula, S., Lee, N. A. and Badimon, J. H. (1985). 99m-Tc-low-density lipoprotein: a new agent for studying lipoprotein metabolism and imaging atherosclerotic lesions *in vivo*. In Nestel, P. J. (Ed.), *7th International Symposium on Atherosclerosis*, Melbourne, A162

Heyns, A. duP., Badenhorst, P. N., Pieters, H., Lotter, M. G., Minnaar, P. C., Duyvene deWit, L. J., Van Reenen, O. R. and Retief, E. P. (1980). Preparation of a viable population of indium-111 labelled human blood platelets. *Thromb. Haemost.*, **42**, 1473

Heyns, A. duP., Lotter, M. G., Badenhorst, P. N., Pieters, H., Nel, C. J. C. and Minnaar, P. (1982). Kinetics and fate of indium-111-labelled platelets in patients with aortic aneurysms. *Arch. Surg.*, **117**, 1170–4

Huang, T. W. and Harker, L. A. (1981). In-111 platelet imaging for detection of platelet deposition in abdominal aneurysms and prosthetic arterial grafts. *Am J. Cardiol.*, **47**, 882–9

Kaliman, J., Sinzinger, H., Bergmann, H. and Kolbe, C. (1985). Value of 123-I-low density lipoproteins (LDL) in the diagnosis of human atherosclerotic lesions. *Circulation*, **72**, 300

Kessler, C., Henningsen, H., Reuther, R., Antalics, I. and Kimmig, B. (1985). Szintigraphie mit 111-In-markierten Thrombozyten: Therapiekontrolle bei Acetyl-salicylsäure (ASS)-behandelten Schlaganfallpatienten. *Nuc. Compact*, **6**, 30–31

Lees, R. S., Lees, A. M. and Strauss, H. W. (1983). External imaging of human atherosclerosis. *J. Nucl. Med.*, **24**, 154–6

Mustard, J. F. (1984). Platelets, endothelium and vessel injury. In *Platelets, Prostaglandin and Cardiovascular Systems*, Abstract Book, Florence, pp. 8–11

Sinzinger, H. and Angelberger, P. (1988). Imaging and kinetics studies with radiolabelled and autologous LDL in human atherosclerosis. *Nucl. Med. Comm.*, **9**, 859–66

Sinzinger, H., Angelberger, P. and Kolbe, H. (1981). Influence of incubation time and temperature on indium-111 oxine uptake by human platelets. *Thromb. Haemost.*, **45**, 295

Sinzinger, H., Angelberger, P., Pesl, H., Flores, J. and Rauscha, F. (1989). Further insights into lipid lesion imaging by means of 123-I-labelled autologous low-density lipoproteins (LDL). *Atherosclosis*, **VIII** (in press)

Sinzinger, H., Bergmann, H., Kaliman, J. and Angelberger, P. (1986). Imaging of human atherosclerotic lesions using 123-I-low-density lipoprotein. *Eur. J. Nucl. Med.*, **12**, 291–2

Sinzinger, H. and Fitscha, P. (1984). Epoprostenol and platelet deposition in atherosclerosis. *Lancet*, **i**, 905–6

Sinzinger, H. and Fitscha, P. (1989). Monitoring of antithrombotic therapy with radiolabelled platelets. *Proc. Book Int. Symp. Radio-lab. Plat.*, Cologne (in press)

Sinzinger, H., Fitscha, P., Kaliman, J., Silberbauer, K. and O'Grady, J. (1987). Development of optimal infusion regimen, for epoprostenol using radiolabelled platelet uptake over atherosclerotic lesions. *Br. J. Clin. Pharm.*, **24**, 607–13

Sinzinger, H., Flores, J., Widhalm, K. and Granegger, S. (1988a). Platelet viability (aggregation, migration, recovery) after radiolabelling of platelets from hypercholesterolemics using various tracers (oxine, oxine-sulphate, tropolone, MPO). *Eur. J. Nucl. Med.*, **14**, 358–61

Sinzinger, H., Kolbe, H. and Strobl-Jäger, E. (1984). A simple and safe technique for sterile autologous platelet labelling using Monovette-vials. *Eur. J. Nucl. Med.*, **9**, 320–2

Sinzinger, H., O'Grady, J. and Fitscha, P. (1988b). Platelet deposition in human atherosclerotic lesions is decreased by low-dose aspirin in combination with dipyridamole. *J. Intern. Med. Res.*, **16**, 39–43

Stratton, J. R. and Ritchie, J. L. (1982). Sulfinpyrazone fails to inhibit platelet deposition on Dacron prosthetic grafts in man. *Circulation*, **66**, 55–61

Stratton, J. R. and Ritchie, J. L. (1984). Failure of ticlopidine to inhibit deposition of 111-indium-labelled platelets on dacron prosthetic surfaces in humans. *Circulation*, **69**, 677–83

Thakur, M. L., Welch, M. J. and Joist, H. (1976). Indium-111 labelled platelets: studies on preparation and evaluation of *in vitro* and *in vivo* functions. *Thromb. Res.*, **9**, 345–57

VI
Assessment of Drug Effects on the Respiratory System

28
Assessment of Respiratory Responses

Timothy W. Evans and Peter J. Barnes

National Heart and Lung Institute, Dovehouse Street, London SW3 6LY, UK

INTRODUCTION

The assessment of responses of the respiratory system to new drugs is dependent upon the particular pathology and condition being treated. The lung can be divided into vascular and parenchymal compartments. Pharmacological manipulation of the pulmonary vasculature is discussed elsewhere. Diseases of the parenchyma involve either the conducting airways, as in asthma or chronic obstructive pulmonary disease (COPD), or the alveoli, interstitium and gas-exchanging membranes, as in pulmonary fibrosis. Drug evaluation in respiratory disease therefore depends upon the assessment of responses to therapies manipulating airflow and airway resistance, lung volumes and gas exchange.

ASTHMA

Physiology

Asthma is a condition characterised by airway hyperresponsiveness to a wide variety of specific and non-specific stimuli, and is defined in physiological terms by variable airway narrowing.[1] Tests of airway function routinely performed are discussed in more detail below, but include spirometry (forced expiratory volume in 1 s, FEV_1; expressed as a percentage of forced vital capacity, FVC) and the maximal expiratory flow–volume curve (MEFV). Peak expiratory flow rate (REFR) is a portable and easy means of assessing airflow, but is influenced particularly by the central airways. More complex tests of airflow limitation include the direct assessment of airflow resistance (specific (airways) conductance, SGAW) by whole body plethysmography. Reductions in all parameters of resistance are observed in acute asthma, but are not diagnostic of the condition in the absence of evidence of reversibility. Consequently, a series of results obtained daily are of value in diagnosis, particularly if they reveal spontaneous changes in airflow limitation or diurnal variation. Widespread airway narrowing and closure also leads to increased lung volumes (total lung capacity, TLC; residual volume, RV; and, therefore, functional residual capacity, FRC). Differences between TLC (measured by plethysmography) and accessible gas volume (measured by helium dilution) indicate gas trapping through mucous plugging of small airways.[2]

In chronic asthma physiological assessment may become more complex, particularly if the diagnosis is not clear. Spirometry or maximum expiratory flow manoeuvres are repeated at intervals sufficient to allow for immediate or delayed responses to the inhaled stimulus and compared with measurements taken during a control period. Assessments of both airway resistance and lung volumes may be repeated before and after bronchodilator therapy, to confirm reversibility. Arbitrarily selected values of 15–20% increases in the selected

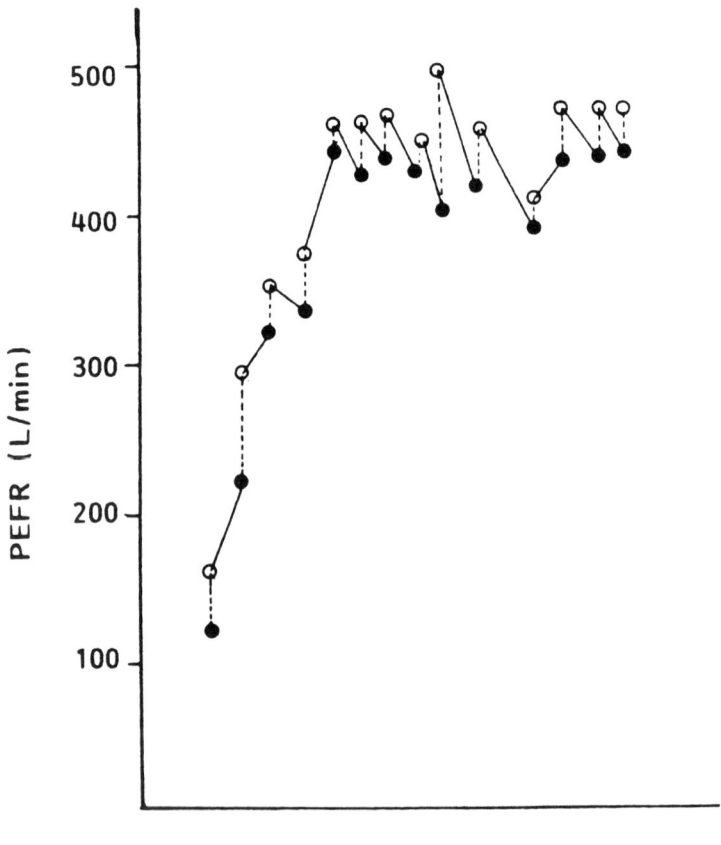

Figure 28.1 Peak expiratory flow rate (PEFR) chart before and after commencement of therapy. Note that initial steep improvement in PEFR is followed by a more gradual response, with obvious variation in bronchoconstriction before (closed circles) and after (open circles) nebulised beta-agonists

index on several occasions may aid diagnosis or the assessment of treatment response, but a sustained improvement over time in PEFR is of greater value[3] (Figure 28.1).

Indices of gas transfer are rarely abnormal in asthma in remission. Carbon monoxide diffusing capacity (DLCO) is mildly reduced, but when corrected for accessible gas volume (KCO), may be increased, suggesting increased distribution of blood flow to ventilated alveoli. Measurements of ventilation/ perfusion matching (V/Q) in mild asthma have suggested two populations of alveoli: those with normal V/Q and those with a grossly reduced V/Q ratio, possibly reflecting alveolar collapse distal to obstructed small bronchi.[4] This may be confirmed by isotope scanning.

More sensitive tests to respiratory physiology such as single-breath tests of the distribution of ventilation, and measurement of closing volume, residual volume and frequency dependence of compliance, are almost always abnormal in asthma and may be reflected in mild hypoxia, but are likely to be of little benefit in the assessment of responses to therapy.

Pathology

In acute asthma reversible airway oedema and mucosal inflammation may be as significant in increasing resistance to airflow as smooth muscle contraction. Studies of the lungs of patients dying in status asthmaticus have revealed intense airway inflammation, with shedding of epithelium and plugging of the bronchi with viscid secretions containing eosinophils and desquamated epithelial cells.[5] Additional changes include thickening of the basement membrane, bronchial smooth muscle hypertrophy and eosinophil accumulation in airway walls and lymph nodes. Studies of bronchial biopsies from volunteers with asthma have shown similar, although less marked, inflammatory changes, suggesting that such changes are present when the condition is relatively mild or in remission.[6] The use of bronchoalveolar lavage in the assessment of asthma has suffered as a result of difficulties in standardisation, but studies suggest that eosinophils are present, often showing signs of degranulation; that an increase in mast cells occurs with increased liability to release histamine; and that the lymphocyte subpopulation may be altered.[7] This latter condition may also be reflected in atopy—the presence of airway and skin hyperresponsiveness to a single or multiple specific allergen(s).

EVALUATION OF DRUG RESPONSES

The assessment of responses to drug therapy depends upon the underlying condition. Changes in parameters of airflow obstruction and lung volumes are commonly used in the measurement of therapeutic responses in asthma. PEFR is particularly useful in the domiciliary setting. Changes in bronchial hyperresponsiveness assessed by challenge testing have been widely used in the evaluation of therapy. In recent years changes in the histological appearances of mucosal biopsies obtained via fibre optic bronchoscopy, and of the cellular composition of bronchoalveolar lavage, have also been used, but at present are research tools.

Lung Volumes and Resistance to Airflow

Spirometry

The ratio between the FEV_1 and the VC or FVC is the simplest and most practical guide to the presence of airflow obstruction. In normal subjects it matters little which of the latter two measurements is used, but in patients with airflow limitation the forced manoeuvre is less than the relaxed measurement, owing to earlier airway closure. However, the first part of the FEV_1 is effort-dependent and the measurement is not particularly sensitive to early changes in small airway function.

Flow–Volume Curves

The measurement of maximum mid-expiratory flow (MMF), also known as the forced expiratory flow between 25% and 75% of FVC (FEF_{25-75}), is a routine measurement in North America, but is less often available in Europe (Figure 28.2). Although MMF offers the theoretical advantage of being less effort-dependent than FEV_1, there is a large variation in values among normal subjects. Nevertheless, the full inspiration needed to produce a complete expiratory flow curve or FVC may in itself affect bronchomotor tone and the use of 'partial' flow–volume curves may be more accurate. Recording airflow at 30% of vital capacity from a forced partial expiratory flow manoeuvre shows good reproducibility under these circumstances and may be used to obtain dose–response curves to bronchodilator or broncho-constrictor substances during drug evaluation[8,9] (Figure 28.3).

Plethysmography

The use of the body plethysmograph to measure resistance to airflow corrected for thoracic gas volume (specific conductance or SGAW) is now widespread. The measurement is made with the subject breathing with gentle efforts at low flow rates. Apart from the difficulties associated with using a body box, results tend to be dominated by changes in large airway calibre. In patients with airways disease SGAW is a reasonable measure of resistance, but in normal subjects it is considerably more sensitive in detecting changes in airway calibre than are forced expiratory manoeuvres.[10]

Bronchial Challenge Testing

Histamine and Methacholine Provocation Testing

Bronchial hyperresponsiveness may reflect airway inflammation, and tests of

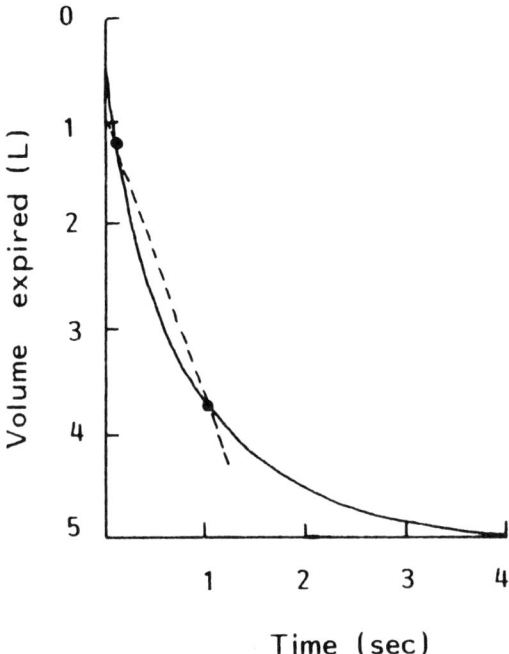

Figure 28.2   Recording on forced expired volume against time, showing the measurement of maximum mid-expiratory flow (MMF), represented by the slope of the dotted line joining points at 25% and 75% of expired vital capacity

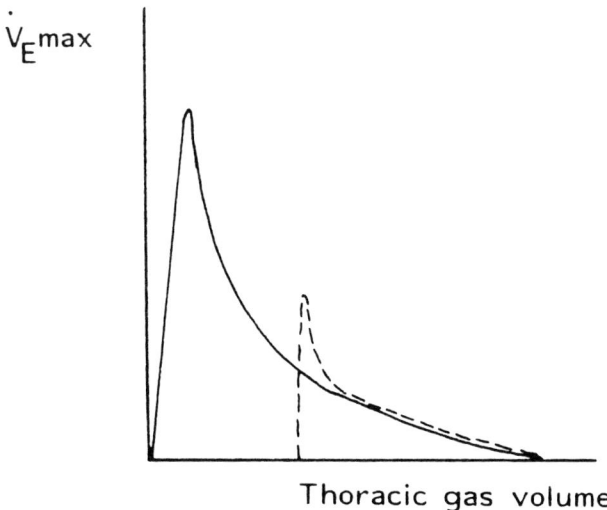

Figure 28.3   Partial flow-volume manoeuvre, showing good reproducibility with expiration from TLC, which may cause reflex bronchodilation (see text)

airway responsiveness may therefore be useful in evaluating the anti-inflammatory actions of drugs, or their protective effects against bronchoconstriction. The bronchial agonist (usually methacholine or histamine) is administered ᴜs an aerosol by inhalation and the bronchoconstrictor response is measured as changes in forced expiratory volumes or flows (maximal or partial) or changes in resistance or specific conductance. Conventionally, increasing doses of the provocative agent are given in a cumulative fashion every 5 min, and responsiveness is defined in terms of the dose required to produce a predetermined degree of bronchoconstriction (PC_{20} or PC_{35}, the provocative concentrations of agonist required to produce a 20% or 35% fall in the measured parameter, usually FEV_1 or specific conductance, respectively).[11] Clearly, the response occurs at a lower provocative concentration in subjects with asthma[12] (Figure 28.4). Good reproducibility of the technique means that comparisons made before and after therapeutic in-

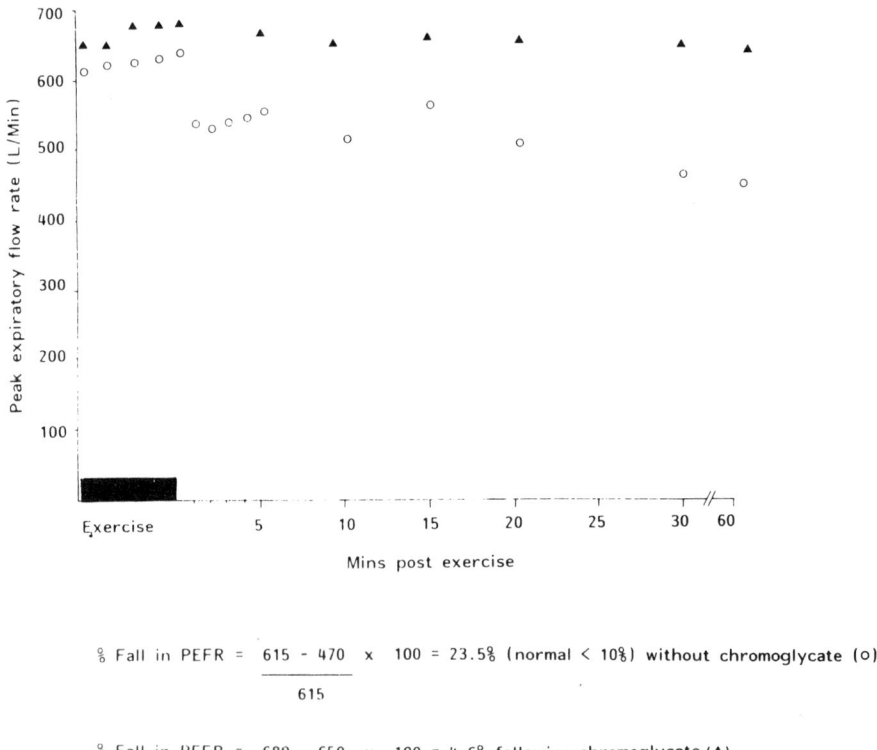

$$\% \text{ Fall in PEFR} = \frac{615 - 470}{615} \times 100 = 23.5\% \text{ (normal} < 10\%) \text{ without chromoglycate (o)}$$

$$\% \text{ Fall in PEFR} = \frac{680 - 650}{650} \times 100 = 4.6\% \text{ following chromoglycate (▲)}$$

Figure 28.4 Exercise-induced asthma test. Note fall in peak expiratory flow rate (PEFR) in asthmatic patient after exercise (open circle). PEFR remains stable in same patient if exercise is preceded by treatment with disodium cromoglycate (closed triangle)

tervention are possible even in normal subjects. However, problems involved in this approach include the comparison of dose–response curves which start from different airway calibres[13] and the uncertainty over the quantity of any inhaled drug reaching the airways. Histamine and methacholine challenges provide similar information although methacholine is generally associated with fewer side-effects, despite being less easy to obtain.

Exercise Challenge

Subjects who present with evidence of airflow limitation after exercise may be defined as having exercise-induced asthma (EIA). The incidence and severity of EIA is influenced considerably by the nature of the provocation test (e.g. running, cycling or swimming) and the conditions under which the exercise is performed, being particularly difficult to standardise in unfit people. This problem has partially been explained by increasing evidence that EIA is influenced by ambient humidity and, to a lesser extent, temperature.[14,15]

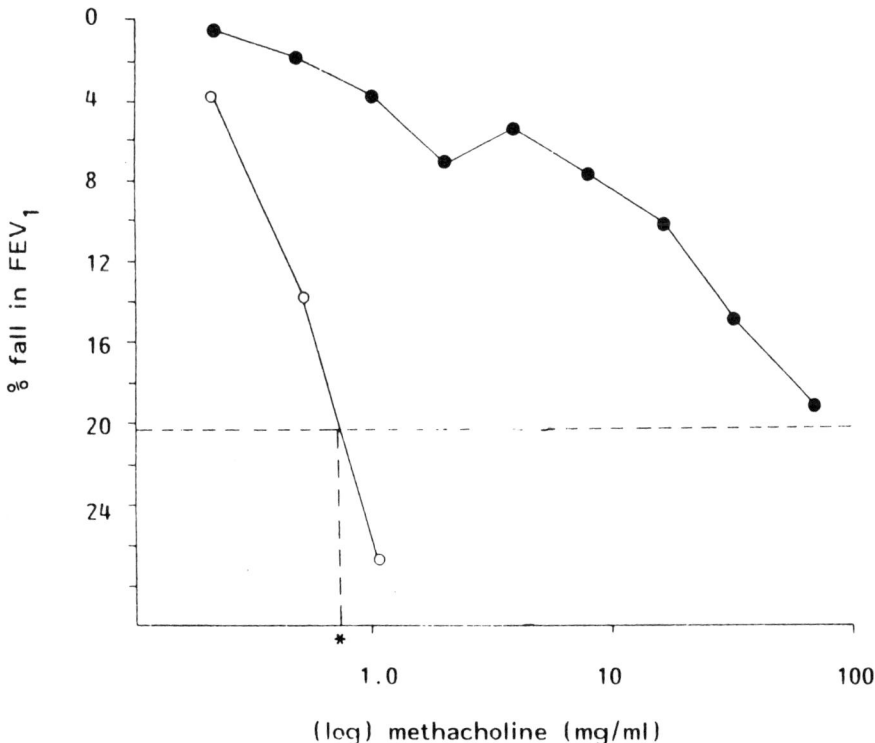

Figure 28.5 Methacholine challenge in normal (closed circles) and asthmatic (open circles) subjects. Note that the provocative concentration of methacholine required to produce a 20% fall in FEV_1 (*) was approximately 0.6 mg/ml in the asthmatic patient, whereas the normal subject did not achieve such a reduction even at the highest dose

Exercise challenge is basically simple to perform, particularly in children, but investigates only a single level of challenge (unlike histamine or methacholine, which measure the precise dose of agonist producing a particular degree of bronchoconstriction) (Figure 28.5).

Cold Air Challenge

In the last few years isocapnic ventilation with cold air, or dry air at room temperature, have been used as bronchial provocation tests in patients with asthma. The factors determining the response to cold air, including CO_2 requirement, tidal volume, respiratory rate, duration of test and inspired air temperature, have recently been standardised, to provide an easily reproducible means of provocation.[16] It is particularly useful in subjects unable to exercise.

Sulphur Dioxide Challenge

In a number of laboratory investigations sulphur dioxide (SO_2) has been shown to induce bronchoconstriction and respiratory symptoms in exercising asthmatics. The range of physiological and clinical responses to inhaled SO_2 has subsequently been assessed, showing a comparative lack of response in normal individuals. Sulphur dioxide inhalation may therefore prove to be useful in assessing the response of asthmatics to various therapies, although it is difficult to set up, owing to difficulties in regulating and measuring inhaled concentrations of SO_2.

Antigen Challenge

In atopic subjects challenge of the skin or airways with allergens to which they are specifically sensitive leads to early and, in a proportion of patients, late 'weal and flare' and bronchoconstrictor responses, respectively. The early reaction is rapid in onset (10–20 min after challenge), resolving over the ensuing 2 h. The late response begins about 6 h after challenge and may last for up to 24 h, during which the airways become non-specifically hyperreactive to stimuli such as histamine and methacholine, which may last up to 2 weeks.[18] Different cellular infiltrations of the airways of experimental models have been observed at the time of maximal early and late responses and are thought to be responsible. Consequently, skin testing and early and late responses may be used as models to assess the efficacy of drugs thought to influence the inflammatory mechanism underlying the allergic response.[19]

Allergen inhalation tests need to be performed under strictly standardised conditions and are not totally without hazard to the patient. The initial dose of allergen administered can be determined from the intensity of a skin-prick reaction. The correlates of responses to antigen inhalation testing have also been established in detail (particularly skin responses and IgE RAST (radioallergosorbent test) levels). Allergen-induced late asthmatic responses are very valuable; the size of the late reaction is indirectly related to the dose of allergen inhaled. Repeated allergen challenge may lead to a chronic increase in bronchial responsiveness and no more than two or three challenges should be performed in any one subject during a drug study.

Bronchoscopy

Information regarding the alveolar cellular and immunological sequelae of antigen challenge can be obtained in asthmatic individuals by introducing a fibre optic bronchoscope into a segmental bronchus and lavaging the lung segment. Analysis of fluid in these circumstances reveals elevated neutrophils, eosinophils and helper T-cells.[20] Presumably, quantification of mediator production would further enhance the useful nature of this approach. Lavage also provides fluid for analysis of cellular content (total cell count, wet eosinophil count, mast cell and macrophage counts) and differential subpopulations (e.g. activated lymphocytes). Bronchial biopsies can be processed and stained for inflammatory cells and immunological markers. However, although these invasive investigations may be a useful means of measuring anti-inflammatory drug effects in the future, they are not performed routinely at present.

Measurements of Microvascular Permeability

Increased microvascular permeability of the bronchial circulation may occur in asthma.[21] Various techniques may be used to detect epithelial and endothelial permeability changes in response to various stimuli. The principle method involves the inhalation of technetium-labelled DTPA and the subsequent measurement of its clearance from the lungs. Quantification of intravenously injected radiolabelled albumin in bronchoalveolar lavage fluid has also been used as an index of endothelial permeability. However, the former investigation is relatively non-specific in cigarette smokers, and the latter may be difficult to interpret in the presence of infection.[22]

CHRONIC OBSTRUCTIVE PULMONARY DISEASE

Assessment of response to drug therapy in COPD overlaps with that of asthma, depending upon the degree of reversibility of airflow obstruction. In these circumstances tests of respiratory function are similar. Assessments of changes in functional residual capacity (FRC) and residual volume (RV) before and after drug therapy may be more helpful in COPD (particularly emphysema) as a reflection of changes in gas trapping. However, the most frequent complaint of patients with COPD is breathlessness, which has until recently been a subjective sensation difficult to measure with any reproducibility. The visual analogue scale of breathlessness upon which patients represent their dyspnoea by marking a 10 cm line representing a scale of 'no breathlessness' to 'extreme breathlessness' has proved remarkably reproducible in these circumstances.[23] The second principle means of assessing progress in therapy for COPD has involved the use of the 12 min walk, in which distance covered, number of stops and breathlessness scale are measured over a 12 min period before and after therapeutic intervention.[24]

INTERSTITIAL LUNG DISEASE

Patients with fibrosing interstitial lung disease have reduced lung volumes and a pronounced impairment of gas transfer. Reduced compliance may lead to changes in closing volume and decreased resistance to airflow.[25] The assessment of changes in the composition of bronchoalveolar lavage and DPTA or gallium isotope scanning as indices of inflammation are as yet incomplete, but may prove to be valuable in the evaluation of the response to therapy.[26]

REFERENCES

1. Boushey, H. A., Holtzman, M. J., Sheller, J. R. and Nadel, J. A. (1980). State of the art: bronchial hyperreactivity. *Am. Rev. Respir. Dis.*, **121**, 389–413
2. Pride, N. B. (1983). Physiology, In Clarke, T. J. H. and Godfrey, S. (Eds.), *Asthma*. Chapman and Hall, London
3. Turner-Warwick, M. (1977). On observing patterns of airflow obstruction. *Br. J. Dis. Chest*, **71**, 73–8
4. Wagner, P. D., Dantzker, D. R., Iacovoni, V. E., Tomlin, W. C. and West, J. B. (1978). Ventilation-perfusion inequality in asymptomatic asthma. *Am. Rev. Respir. Dis.*, **118**, 511–24
5. Dunnill, M. S. (1960). The pathology of asthma with special reference to changes in the bronchial mucosa. *J. Clin. Pathol.*, **13**, 27–33
6. Dunnill, M. S. (1980). *Pulmonary Pathology*. Churchill Livingstone, London, pp. 50–66
7. Gerblich, A. A., Campbell, A. E. and Schuyler, M. R. (1984). Changes in T lymphocyte subpopulations after antigenic bronchial provocation in asthmatics. *New Engl. J. Med.*, **310**, 1349–52
8. Bouhuys, A., Hunt, V. R., Kim, B. M. and Zapletal, A. (1969). Maximum expiratory flow rates in induced bronchoconstriction in man. *J. Clin. Invest.*, **48**, 1159–68
9. Barnes, P. J., Gribben, H. R., Osmanilov, D. and Pride, N. B. (1981). Partial flow–volume curves to measure bronchodilator dose–response curves in normal subjects. *J. Appl. Physiol.*, **50**, 1193–7
10. Gyuatt, A. R. and Alpers, J. H. (1968). Factors affecting airways conductance: a study of 752 working men. *J. Appl. Physiol.*, **48**, 1159–68
11. Snashall, P. D., Gillet, M. K. and Chung, K. F. (1988). Factors contributing to bronchial hyperresponsiveness in asthma. *Clin. Sci.*, **74**, 113–18
12. Woolcock, A. J., Salome, C. M. and Yan, K. (1984). The shape of the dose–response curve to histamine in asthmatic and normal subjects. *Am. Rev. Resp. Dis.*, **130**, 71–5
13. Chung, K. F., Morgan, B. M., Keyes, S. J. and Snashall, P. D. (1982). Histamine dose–response relationships in normal and asthmatic subjects. The importance of

starting airway calibre. *Am Rev. Resp. Dis.*, **126**, 849–54

14. Godfrey, S. (1983). Exercise-induced asthma. In Clark, T. J. H. and Godfrey, S. (Eds.), *Asthma*. Chapman and Hall, London, pp. 57–78

15. Lee, T. H. (1986). Heat loss, osmolarity and the respiratory epithelium. In Kay, A. B. (Ed.), *Asthma: Clinical Pharmacology and Therapeutic Progress*. Blackwell Scientific Publications, Oxford, pp. 393–400

16. Assoufi, B. K., Dally, M. B., Newman-Taylor, A. J. and Denison, D. M. (1986). Cold air test: a simplified standard method for airway reactivity. *Clin. Resp. Physiol.*, **22**, 349–57

17. Linn, William S., Avol, E. L., Peng Ru-chuan, Shamoo, D. A. and Hackney, J. D. (1987). Replicated dose–response study of sulfur dioxide effects in normal, atopic and asthmatic volunteers. *Am. Rev. Resp. Dis.*, **136**, 1127–34

18. Cockcroft, D. W., Ruffin, R. E., Dolovich, J. and Hargreave, F. E. (1977). Allergen-induced increase in non-allergic bronchial reactivity. *Clin. Allerg.*, 7, 503–13

19. Durham, S. R. and Kay, A. B. (1986). Inflammatory cells and mediators in allergen-induced late phase asthmatic reactions. In Kay, A. B. (Ed.), *Asthma: Clinical Pharmacology and Therapeutic Progress*. Blackwell Scientific Publications, Oxford, pp. 33–46

20. de Monchy, J. G. R., Kauffman, H. F., Venge, P., Koeter, G. H., Jansen, H. M., Sluiter, H. J. and de Vries, K. (1985). Bronchoalveolar eosinophilia during allergen-induced late asthmatic reactions. *Am. Rev. Resp. Dis.*, **131**, 373–6

21. Elwood, R. K., Belzberg, A., Hogg, J. C. and Pare, P. D. (1982). Bronchial mucosal permeability in asthma. *Am. Rev. Resp. Dis.*, **125**, 63–7

22. Barrowcliffe, M. P. and Jones, J. G. (1987). Solute permeability of the alveolar capillary barrier. *Thorax*, **42**, 1–10

23. Bond, D. and Lader, M. (1974). The use of analogue scales in rating subjective feelings. *Br. J. Med. Psychol.*, **47**, 211–18

24. McGavin, C. R., Gupya, S. P. and McHardy, G. J. R. (1976). Twelve minute walking test for assessing disability in chronic bronchitis. *Br. Med. J.*, **i**, 822–3

25. Turner-Warwick, M. (1978). *Immunology of the Lung*. Arnold, London

26. Turner-Warwick, M. (1984). Do gallium scans, bronchoalveolar lavage and SACE help monitor activity of chronic sarcoidosis during treatment? In *Proceedings of the 10th International Conference on Sarcoidosis and Other Granulomatous Disorders, Baltimore*

29
Anti-asthmatic Drugs

A. M. Edwards

*Pharmaceutical Division, Fisons Ltd, 12 Derby Road, Loughborough,
Leics LE11 0BB, UK*

DEFINITION OF ASTHMA

Asthma is a chronic disease affecting the bronchial mucosa and bronchial smooth muscle, and characterised by airflow obstruction which varies both with time and as a result of treatment. The obstruction results partly from constriction of the bronchial smooth muscle and partly from swelling of the bronchial mucosa and the presence of bronchial mucus. The swelling of the bronchial musoca is due both to oedema and to cellular infiltration, characteristically with eosinophils but also with polymorphonuclear leucocytes, macrophages and lymphocytes.

Specific trigger factors cause short- and long-term changes in airways calibre. They are airborne and ingested allergens such as house dust, house dust mite, animal danders, pollens, fungal spores and a variety of foodstuffs. Non-specific triggers which cause short-term changes are exercise, cold air and atmospheric pollutants such as car fumes, cigarette smoke and aerosols. Longer-term alterations can be induced by infections both viral and bacterial.

It is not known what the exact relationship is between these trigger factors and the functional alterations of mucosal inflammation and bronchial muscle constriction, but it would seem likely that allergens and infection will produce predominantly inflammation, whereas the non-specific triggers will result in bronchoconstriction. However, as it has been shown that even in mild asthmatic patients requiring little or no treatment a chronic inflammatory state of the bronchial mucosa exists, it is possible that both play a part in most circumstances.

One of the consequences of the inflammatory changes in the bronchial mucosa and characteristic of asthma is that patients show an abnormal bronchoconstrictive response to bronchial challenges with histamine and methacholine. This abnormal response, known as bronchial hyperreactivity or bronchial hyperresponsiveness, is used both to identify potential asthmatic subjects in epidemiological studies and to measure the effects of treatment.

The clinical consequences of these pathological changes and functional disturbances are the characteristic symptoms of asthma—wheeze, shortness of breath, cough, morning tightness—and, in the chronic state, the symptoms limit the ability to carry out normal day-to-day activities and cause disturbances to sleep. These subjective symptoms are associated with measurable changes in airflow, which not only varies seasonally, according to the predominance of allergenic factors, but also shows a characteristic diurnal variation.

MEASUREMENTS OF AIRFLOW LIMITATION

Variable airways obstruction, being a characteristic of asthma, means that measurements of airways function forms an important part of the evaluation of drugs for the treatment of asthma. It is beyond the scope of this chapter to give a detailed evaluation of the various measurements that can be made. In short-term experiments in man, measurements of both large airway function (peak expiratory flow rate, PEFR; forced expiratory volume in 1 s, FEV_1; and forced vital capacity, FVC and also those of small airway function (forced expiratory volume between 25% and 75% of vital capacity, FEF_{25-75}; and partial expiratory flow rate, pEFR) are commonly used, whereas in longer-term experiments, those measurements that can be repeated frequently (PEFR) are most often used.

Measurements of airway function exhibit an exaggerated diurnal variation in asthmatic patients, the amplitude of which varies according to disease severity. In short-term experiments examining possible treatment effects, this factor also has to be taken into account.

The purpose of this introduction is to emphasise three important factors when considering evaluating the effects of anti-asthmatic drugs.

(1) Asthma is a disease of mixed functional pathology in which the key defect—airflow limitation—stems from both inflammatory oedema and muscle bronchoconstriction.

(2) Asthma is a disease in which the pathology, the functional consequences of the pathology and the clinical symptoms are subject to inherent intrapatient and interpatient variability.

(3) All asthmatic patients will be taking some type of medication which will have some effect on the pathology, functional measurements and clinical measurements of their disease. These effects have to be both taken into account and allowed for in any studies.

EVALUATION OF ANTI-ASTHMATIC DRUGS IN MAN

The initial studies of any anti-asthmatic compound in man will be to characterise the absorption, distribution, metabolism and excretion of the compound, and its single-dose and repeated-dose tolerance in healthy volunteers.

The next series of studies will be bronchial challenge studies, which will investigate the ability of the compound to block or attenuate the bronchoconstricting effects of a number of agents, which include inhaled antigen, exercise, sulphur dioxide, sodium metabisulphite, adenosine monophosphate, bradykinin, histamine and methacholine. The relationship between these challenges and asthma is not known, and, as such, they are not predictive of the ability of a drug to be useful in asthma. However, they are useful to explore the pharmacological profile of the compound and to investigate the protective effect of different dose sizes and how long that protective effect lasts.

The definitive studies are short-term (28 days) studies in asthmatic patients. As none of the challenge studies are predictive of clinical efficacy in asthma, these 28 day therapeutic trials are the only useful initial studies. These will be considered in more detail.

Bronchial Challenge Experiments

Full details of the standards to which these studies should be given are provided in more detailed texts (Chai *et al.*, 1975; Eggleston *et al.*, 1979; Cropp *et al.*, 1980; Eiser *et al.*, 1983). The principles that must be followed in any experiment of this type are listed below.

(1) The subjects used in the experiment must be co-operative, be stable, and have given written informed consent to participate in the study.

(2) They should be adult asthmatic patients with baseline pulmonary function as measured by FEV_1 within $\pm20\%$ of their predicted normal.

(3) Their pulmonary function should not fluctuate over the period of the experiment by more than $\pm10\%$. This will exclude patients with severe asthma and those on large doses of medication or medications.

(4) They should not have any other disease and should not have a history (within 6 weeks) of a recent viral or other infection that affects the respiratory tract.

(5) Patients whose asthma is exacerbated by a seasonal allergen (pollens and fungal spores) should not be used in experiments during or near to the time of year when these pollens or fungal spores are prevalent. Similarly, patients allergic to avoidable allergens (cats, dogs, horses) should avoid such contact during the period of the experiment.

(6) Measurements of bronchial hyperreactivity should not vary by more than $\pm10\%$ during the period of the experiment. (Bronchial hyperreactivity is usually determined using bronchial challenges with increasing doses or concentrations of solutions of histamine or methacholine. The level of hyperreactivity is expressed as either the *concentration* of histamine or methacholine, or the *dose* of either substance that on inhalation produces a 20% fall in pulmonary function. These are shown, respectively, as the PC_{20} (histamine:methacholine) or the PD_{20} (histamine:methacholine).)

(7) Where possible, anti-asthmatic treatments that are likely to influence the effects of the challenge should be discontinued before each challenge. Because of the dangers of withdrawing prophylactic treatments such as corticosteroids (oral or inhaled), sodium cromoglycate and sustained-release theophyllines, either patients who are taking these routinely should be

excluded or, if this is not possible, the dose of their treatment and the timing of each dose should be fixed each day and maintained throughout the period of the experiment. (Inhaled beta$_2$-agonists should be discontinued 12 h before each challenge, oral beta$_2$-agonists 24 h before and antihistamines 72 h before.)

(8) Each challenge should be conducted under the same conditions, in the same environment and at the same time each day. The whole experiment, which will usually involve at least four challenges (two controls, active treatment preceding challenge, placebo treatment preceding challenge), should be conducted over as short a time-scale as possible, with at least 3 days but not more than 7 days between each challenge.

(9) The challenges should only be carried out in specialist units or laboratories staffed by personnel who are skilled and experienced in the techniques involved and who are capable of dealing with any medical emergency should it arise. Patients should be kept under observation throughout the period of the experiment and resuscitation equipment should be available to deal with any respiratory or cardiovascular emergency. Patients should not be permitted to leave the laboratory until their pulmonary function has returned to normal predicted values and these values have been sustained for at least 60 minutes. Patients should be sent home with an inhaled bronchodilator with instructions on its use in case an unexpected delayed reaction should occur. Patients should also be issued with a peak flow meter and instructed to take readings regularly (four times daily) throughout the experiment. Any fluctuation from normal would require contact with the doctor conducting the experiment.

(10) The measurements to be used can be any appropriate measurement of pulmonary function that will change as a result of the challenge (FEV_1, PEFR, pEFR, FEF_{25-75}). The severity of the challenge should be chosen that produces a reduction of FEV_1 at its maximum of between 20% and 30%. The two control challenges should be within $\pm5\%$ of each other.

(11) The evaluation of the results will determine the protective effect of the compound as compared with a matching placebo. The treatments should be randomised in a double-blind fashion and given at the same fixed time before the challenge. The protective effect may be expressed as

$$\frac{\text{maximum \% fall in } FEV_{1,\,placebo} - \text{maximum \% fall in } FEV_{1,\,active}}{\text{maximum \% fall in } FEV_{1,\,placebo}} \times 100$$

A drug that provides at least 50% protection in at least 80% of patients is worthy of further trials. For a drug that is going to be administered at 6-hourly intervals, at least 50% protection should still be present at 6 h and for a drug to be administered 12-h, 50% protection should still be present at 12 h.

Conclusion

Bronchial challenge experiments are not predictive of efficacy of a drug in asthma. It is unlikely that the mechanism whereby inhaled antigen induces bronchoconstriction is the same mechanism whereby inhaled sulphur dioxide induces bronchoconstriction. However, such experiments are useful in establishing the pharmacological profile of any compound and also in determining the minimum effective protective dose of a compound and the length of time that protection lasts.

Bronchial challenge experiments are not without their dangers and should only be carried out in specialist units with properly trained staff. Patients should be kept under continual supervision and only allowed home when normal. Patients should be aware of who to contact and how, should any unexpected delayed reaction occur.

SHORT-TERM THERAPEUTIC TRIALS

The short-term therapeutic trial is the definitive experiment that will determine the therapeutic potential of an anti-asthmatic drug. These trials have to be conducted under precisely defined circumstances in carefully selected patients and the remainder of this chapter will define these conditions.

Objectives

The objectives of the study must be clearly stated. In most cases they should be to compare the safety and efficacy of drug X with drug Y in the management of patients with bronchial asthma. Drug X will be the test drug and drug Y will be either a matching placebo or another active treatment.

Trial Design

The trial should be a randomised double-blind parallel group design in which the group treated with the new drug X is compared with the group treated with the control drug Y (placebo or another active treatment).

The test treatment period should be a minimum of 28 days and should be preceded by a baseline period of at least 14 days. During the baseline period, patients will continue to take their existing therapy unchanged.

The test treatment period and the baseline period may be separated by a run-in period of varying length, during which existing therapy may be adjusted.

For these early trials, it is not considered appropriate to use trial designs of the cross-over type, even with a washout period, because of the difficulty in interpreting any changes in a disease with so much inbuilt interpatient and intrapatient variability.

Selection of Patients

The selection of patients for these early trials is of paramount importance. It is likely that in these early studies women of childbearing age will be excluded and the trials will be carried out in men. It is essential that considerable trouble be taken to select patients who are homogeneous with respect to the following variables:

age
type of asthma
  allergic
  non-allergic
length of asthma
  starting in childhood
  starting in adult life
type of treatment currently being taken
  patients on beta$_2$ agonists alone
  patients on theophyllines
  patients on corticosteroids
  patients on sodium cromoglycate
  patients on ketotifen
  patients on nedocromil sodium
severity of asthma as judged by pulmonary function
  performed at the clinic
  performed daily during the baseline period
severity of asthma as judged by symptoms recorded daily by the patient
  asthma at night
  asthma during the day
severity of asthma as judged by bronchial reactivity
reversibility of asthma

Each of these variables will be used in the evaluation of the test treatment and each of them may have some bearing on the response to the test treatment. Unless considerable attention is paid to the selection of patients, ambiguous or equivocal results may be obtained, giving rise to both Type I and Type II errors.

Age

Asthma appears to change with age, with non-allergic mechanisms playing a more important role with increasing age. Asthma which starts in adult life (e.g. over the age of 25 years) may be different from asthma which starts in childhood. Patients should therefore be selected within a fairly narrow age band (not more than 20 years), and for those whose asthma started in childhood, the age range 20–40 years is suitable. If patients with late-onset asthma are selected, the age range 35–55 years is probably more suitable.

Asthma Type

The presence or absence of evidence of an allergic cause is important and it is preferable to select either all allergic patients or all non-allergic patients. The presence of allergy should be confirmed by either skin tests or tests for specific IgE, and there should be historical evidence of the asthma worsening when the patient is exposed to the antigen. Patients with perennial asthma symptoms are preferable to those with seasonal asthma only.

Current Therapy

The treatment a patient is currently receiving will have a major effect on that patient's asthma and their response to any new treatment.

Inhaled beta$_2$-agonists are usually used to treat acute symptoms on an 'as required' basis, and the number of times they have to be used during the day and during the night is an important measure of the severity of their asthma. Some patients use inhaled bronchodilators as their only treatment and may use a regular dose, irrespective of need, with additional doses taken for acute symptoms. The way these various situations are handled is an important part of the design.

The use or not of oral beta$_2$-agonists appears to be of less importance and patients may continue to take them. The daily dose should remain fixed throughout the trial. The same applies to theophylline- or aminophylline-containing tablets in which the dose has not been adjusted to attain certain blood levels.

Patients maintained on *sustained-release theophyllines* with the dose adjusted to achieve certain serum theophylline levels should either be selected on the basis that they all fall into this category or none at all.

Patients using *inhaled corticosteroids* and/or *oral corticosteroids* should be selected because they all take either inhaled or oral, or both, and the dose should have remained constant for the previous 3 months. Patients requiring large doses of oral corticosteroids (greater than 5 mg prednisone or equivalent per day) are best avoided in early trials, as are patients who need repeated courses of oral corticosteroids. Patients taking inhaled corticosteroids should take them within the same dose range. For example, ≤400 μg of beclomethasone dipropionate (BDP) or equivalent per day: 400–800 μg of BDP per day: 800–1200 μg of BDP per day. Patients requiring larger doses than this are best avoided.

With regard to *sodium cromoglycate, ketotifen* and *nedocromil sodium* either all patients may be taking them or none.

All of these treatments may or may not be adjusted as part of the trial design. If they are not to be changed, then the dose and dose frequency must remain fixed throughout the baseline and test treatment periods.

Severity of Asthma

The severity of asthma can be determined by pulmonary function tests, by the judgement of the clinician after questioning the patient or by the patient by recording severity scores.

Full spirometry should be carried out during each clinic visit. During the baseline period, the pulmonary function tests carried out at the clinic should not vary by more than 10% and all patients should be within a 20% band of predicted normal values: i.e. within 80–100% predicted normal or 60–80% predicted normal.

During the baseline period and throughout the trial, patients will be asked to measure and record their peak expiratory flow rate on three occasions each day—immediately after rising in the morning; between 1600 and 1800 hours; and on going to bed. The mean daily peak expiratory flow rate should not vary by more than ±10% during the baseline period and all patients should fall within a 20% band of predicted normal values.

The severity of asthma can be measured by the patient on a daily basis using a simple scale. The following scales have been used extensively in trials and are found to be sensitive and to change with changing severity of the asthma or as a result of treatment.

Daytime asthma

0 No symptoms during day.
1 Occasional wheeze or breathlessness quickly relieved by bronchodilator aerosol.
2 Wheezing or short of breath most of the day but did not interfere with usual activities.
3 Wheezing or short of breath most of the day. Interfered to some extent with usual activities.
4 Asthma very bad. Could not go to work or school or engage in usual activities at all.

Night-time asthma

0 No symptoms.
1 Awoke once in the night because of wheezing or cough. Awake for less than an hour. Did not need to use a bronchodilator aerosol.
2 Awoke once in the night because of wheezing or cough. Awake for less than an hour but needed to use a bronchodilator aerosol to get back to sleep.
3 Awoke once for more than an hour *or* awoke more than once because of wheezing or cough.
4 Awake for most of the night because of wheezing or cough.

Other scales can be found in the literature. Visual analogue scales are not considered to be reliable. Once a scale has been fixed, it should be used in all trials.

Patients may be selected on the basis of mean asthma severity scores during a baseline period. For patients attending hospital clinics, on modern treatment and who are suitable for trials, it is likely that their asthma will be well managed and on these scales mean scores of less than 1 will be recorded. This does not usually give sufficient room for improvement during a short-term trial and the test drug may not show any effect, even if it is an active treatment. This problem will be addressed in the section on the run-in period and the rules for concomitant medication.

Bronchial Reactivity and Reversibility

All asthmatic patients have reactive airways which can be measured by either a histamine or methacholine dose response. This reactivity is also reflected in the response to a single dose of an inhaled bronchodilator. Patients should be within the same broad range of bronchial reactivity and should all have evidence of reversibility to an inhaled bronchodilator $\leq 15\%$.

Methodology

Baseline, Run-in, Concomitant Medication

During the baseline period, patients should be kept on their existing treatment and the necessary daily observations should be made by the patients to ensure that they satisfy the entry criteria. At least two clinic visits should be made for baseline pulmonary function, reversibility and bronchial hyperreactivity readings. In addition, blood and urine samples will be taken for baseline readings.

At the end of the baseline, information will be available to determine whether there is sufficient room for improvement in asthma severity for a new treatment to be shown to be effective. In most hospital clinics this will not be the case and a run-in period will be needed during which a proportion of existing medication will be removed, in order to produce a slight but controlled worsening of asthma symptoms. This is a difficult ethical decision, but provided that stable, co-operative, well-controlled patients who are fully informed and give written consent are included, then the risks are considered to be minimal. Full discussion with a properly constituted ethical committee will be required and adequate arrangements should be made for the patients to be able to contact a medically qualified person at any time of day or night.

The following situations exist:

(1) *Patients on beta$_2$-agonists alone*   Oral beta$_2$-agonists should be stopped at the end of the baseline: inhaled beta$_2$-agonists should be allowed on an 'as needed' basis only and any regular dosing should be stopped for the run-in period.

(2) *Patients on sustained-release theophyllines*   These should be stopped at the end of the baseline period. Patients to be given either immediate-release theophyllines or inhaled beta$_2$-agonists, to be used on an 'as needed' basis.

(3) *Inhaled corticosteroids*   The withdrawal of any corticosteroid treatment has to be undertaken cautiously. Any dose reduction should not be greater than 25% of the starting dose and not more frequently than every 2 weeks. Patients needing daily doses of inhaled corticosteroids in excess of

1200 µg of beclomethasone dipropionate or equivalent should not be included and the suggested dose reduction is as follows:

Starting dose	Reduced dose
1200 µg	1000 µg
1000 µg	800 µg
800 µg	600 µg
600 µg	500 µg
500 µg	400 µg
400 µg	300 µg
300 µg	200 µg
200 µg	150 µg
150 µg	100 µg
100 µg	50 µg
50 µg	0 µg

Patients should be seen weekly during this phase and if there is any evidence of worsening asthma in excess of that required by the protocol, the patient should be withdrawn from the trial and returned to their previous dose of inhaled corticosteroids. All patients to be given inhaled beta$_2$-agonists to be used on an 'as needed' basis.

Criteria for Entry into Test Treatment Period

Criteria need to be defined for when a patient's asthma has sufficiently worsened for entry into the test treatment period. As soon as these criteria have been satisfied, the patient may be entered into the test treatment phase. Likewise, a fixed time should be given for the run-in period (usually 4 weeks) and patients who do not satisfy the criteria by then should be withdrawn from the trial.

Suggested criteria are as follows: a mean daily score for either day or night asthma of 1.5 or greater over 7 days; a mean morning PEFR over 7 days 10–20% lower than that over the last 7 days of the baseline period; a 10–20% increase in the total daily use of inhaled beta$_2$-agonist. These are relatively small changes, but they are quantifiable and are produced as a result of treatment withdrawal and can be reversed within a 28-day period by an effective anti-asthma treatment. Induced changes any greater than these are likely to be associated with unstable asthma, and patients should be withdrawn from the trial.

Measurements of Efficacy

Data will be collected throughout the trial—baseline, run-in, test treatment phases—and will be used to determine whether the test treatment is efficacious.

Primary Variables

Patient's Global Opinion of Efficacy

At the end of the trial, each patient will be asked to score on a 1–5 scale the efficacy of the test treatment they received:

1 Very effective.
2 Moderately effective.
3 Slightly effective.
4 No effect.
5 Made condition worse/withdrawn because of worsening asthma.

Patients' Assessment of Asthma Symptoms

Patients will keep a daily diary card, recording the severity of their symptoms. It is usual to include 4–5 symptoms each on a 0–4 scale.

DAYTIME ASTHMA
0 No symptoms during day.
1 Occasional wheeze or breathlessness quickly relieved by bronchodilator aerosol.
2 Wheezing or short of breath most of the day but did not interfere with usual activities.
3 Wheezing or short of breath most of the day. Interfered to some extent with usual activities.
4 Asthma very bad. Could not go to work or school or engage in usual activities at all.

NIGHT-TIME ASTHMA
0 No symptoms.
1 Awoke once in the night because of wheezing or cough. Awake for less than an hour. Did not need to use a bronchodilator aerosol.
2 Awoke once in the night because of wheezing or cough. Awake for less than an hour but needed to use a bronchodilator aerosol to get back to sleep.
3 Awoke once for more than an hour *or* awoke more than once because of wheezing or cough.
4 Awake for most of the night because of wheezing or cough.

MORNING TIGHTNESS
0 None.
1 Slight. Awoke at usual time. Chest tight but did not need to use bronchodilator aerosol.
2 Awoke at usual time. Chest tight and needed to use bronchodilator aerosol.
3 Awoke earlier than usual because of asthma and needed to use bronchodilator aerosol *once* between waking and measuring morning PEFR. (One dose = two inhalations.)

4 Awoke earlier than usual because of asthma and needed to use broncho-dilator aerosol more than once between waking and measuring morning PEFR.

COUGH (DAY)
0 None.
1 Occasional coughing but not troublesome.
2 Frequent coughing but it did not interfere with usual activities.
3 Frequent coughing, interfering to some extent with usual activities.
4 Distressing cough most of the day.

COUGH (NIGHT)
0 None.
1 Occasional coughing but not troublesome.
2 Frequent coughing but it did not interfere with sleep.
3 Frequent coughing, interfering to some extent with sleep.
4 Distressing cough most of the night.

Daily Peak Flow Readings

Using a suitable portable Peak Expiratory Flow Meter, patients should record their peak expiratory flow rate at least twice and preferably three times a day (on waking; between 1600 and 1800 hours; on retiring to bed). The morning reading should be taken before the first dose of the inhaled bronchodilator of the day.

Daily Use of Inhaled Bronchodilators

The patient should record their use (doses or puffs) of inhaled bronchodilator used each day: the 24 h total and the number of doses used between rising in the morning, retiring at night and during the night.

Secondary Variables

Clinician's Global Opinion of Efficacy

On same scale as patient.

Pulmonary Function Tests

Carried out at each clinic visit: FEV_1; FVC; PEFR.

Clinician's Assessment of Severity of Asthma

At each clinic visit, after examining the patient, examining the diary cards and conducting the pulmonary function tests, the clinician should make an evaluation of the severity of the asthma on that day using the following scale:

1 Very severe.
2 Severe.
3 Moderately severe.
4 Mild.
5 No symptoms.

Number of Patients

The number of patients will need to be fully discussed with the statistician associated with the trial and will depend upon the circumstances. The following considerations are relevant:

In trials which involve the worsening of symptoms during the run-in period, the null hypothesis approach will state that neither treatment will produce an improvement in the asthma. It is unlikely that any improvement that does take place will be to a position better than baseline values. For the variables used, the maximum improvement from run-in is likely to be:

for diary card symptoms	20–30%
for daily PEFR	10–15%
for inhaled bronchodilator use	10–15%
for clinic asthma severity	15–20%
for global efficacy	20% difference

If the comparative treatment is placebo, there will need to be sufficient patients included to detect differences of this magnitude if the active treatment is efficacious. If the comparative treatment is another active treatment, then sufficient patients will be needed to show no difference between the two treatments.

Statistical Methods

The data collected in this type of study consist of daily recordings of symptom severity, PEFR readings, use of inhaled bronchodilators and global opinion of efficacy.

For all diary card data, changes from the last week of baseline or the last week of run-in, as compared with the last 2 weeks of the treatment period, are compared. Two-tailed tests should be used throughout at the 5% level of significance. For full details, readers are referred to a standard reference on statistical evaluation of clinical trials.

Patients who have to be withdrawn from the trial during the test treatment phase owing to worsening of asthma should be included in all analyses, provided that they take at least 7 days of the test treatment. End-point analysis is then undertaken, using the mean of the last 3 days prior to withdrawal.

Setting

These preliminary trials should be conducted in hospital outpatient clinics staffed by clinicians experienced in the management of asthma and with adequate staff to provide 24 h coverage. Special trial clinics should be arranged and there should be close attention to ensuring that all patients know who to contact and how to contact them, should their asthma deteriorate. Arrangements for immediate in-patient care should be available, with the availability of full resuscitation if needed.

CONCLUSION

The early evaluation of anti-asthmatic drugs in man presents a challenge of attention to detail and organisation. The inherent variability of asthma does not lend itself to routine pharmacological examination and the lack of complete understanding as to the mechanisms involved does not allow any short-term or single-dose studies to be predictive. Considerable preclinical knowledge on any new compound has to be obtained to allow up to 4 weeks' administration in man before any assessment of clinical efficacy can be undertaken. The conduct of the first 28 day trials must be meticulous, so that a true assessment can be made before large numbers of patients with what is a potentially dangerous condition are exposed to an untried and unproven treatment.

REFERENCES

Chai, H., Farr, R. S., Froehlich, L. A., Mathison, D. A., McLean, J. A., Rosenthal, R. R., Sheffer, A. L., Spector, S. L. and Townley, R. G. (1975). Standardisation of bronchial inhalation challenge procedures. *J. Allergy Clin. Immunol.*, **56**, 323–7

Cropp, G. J. A., Bernstein, I. L., Bouchsey, H. A., Hyde, R. W., Rosenthal, R. R., Spector, S. L. and Townley, R. G. (1980). Guidelines for bronchial inhalation challenges with pharmacologic and antigenic agents. *ATS News*, Spring, 11–19

Eggleston, P.A., Rosenthal, R. R., Anderson, S. A., Anderton, R., Bierman, C. W., Bleecker, E. R., Chai, H., Cropp, G. J. A., Johnson, J. S., Konig, P., Morse, J., Smith, L. J., Summers, R. J. and Trantlein, J. J. (1979). Guidelines for the methodology of exercise challenge testing of asthmatics. *J. Allergy Clin. Immunol.*, **64**, 642–5

Eiser, N. M., Kerrebijn, K. F. and Quanjer, P. H. (1983). Guidelines for standardisation of bronchial challenges with (non-specific) bronchoconstricting agents. *Bull. Eur. Physiopath. Resp.*, **19**, 495–514

VII
Assessment of Drug Effects on the Central Nervous System

30
Measurement of CNS Effects

B. Musch,* I. Hindmarch† and B. Saletu††

*Clinical Research Dept, Rhône-Poulenc Santé, 20 Ave Raymond Aron, Antony, France 92165

†Human Psychopharmacology Research Unit, Department of Psychology, University of Leeds, Leeds, England

††Section of Pharmacopsychiatry, Department of Psychiatry, University of Vienna, Vienna, Austria

INTRODUCTION

The measurement of CNS effects is particularly relevant for a new drug, not only when this drug is supposed to exert a psychotropic effect, but also for drugs acting on other systems for which possible side-effects or adverse reactions at the level of the CNS need to be investigated and assessed at the earliest stage of development.

Clinical observation and follow-up of subjects administered with a new drug in Phase I and early Phase II will provide very superficial information on the appearance of manifestations such as sedation, drowsiness, sleepiness, excitation, irritability, insomnia, etc. More in-depth assessment of CNS effects demands the use of more structured and objective techniques.

CNS effects can be classified, for practical and descriptive reasons, in terms of effects on behaviour, on vigilance/attention and cognition, on neurophysiological activity of the brain and on neuroendocrinological functions. The measurement of each of these classes of effects involves specific techniques and instruments. We shall review these aspects of measuring CNS effects and separate them into four groups: (1) psychometric testing; (2) neurophysiological and psychophysiological measurements; (3) behavioural assessments; and (4) neuroendocrinological measurements.

It has to be stressed that human psychopharmacology has progressed considerably in the last few decades and has moved from the observation of merely behavioural effects along the axis sedation–excitation to very sophisticated techniques specifically and objectively assessing different CNS functions. The aim of modern human psychopharmacology is twofold: to assess and measure possible CNS toxicity of drugs independently of their therapeutic action, and, in the case of drugs supposed to have a psychotropic effect, to give predictive information on the possible therapeutic effect. It is this latter aim which greatly stimulated research in the field of human psychopharmacology in order to improve the therapeutically predictive value of early administration in humans.

PSYCHOMETRIC TESTING

Pharmacodynamics seeks to establish the relationship between pharmaco-kinetics and behavioural measures. Psychopharmacology has as its basic assumption that the effects of a psychoactive drug will be manifested by the changes produced in overt behaviour. Such changes are regarded as more or less independent of any pharmacokinetic measures and variables.

The major task of psychopharmacologists is to develop sensitive, reliable and valid procedures for assessing drug-induced changes in human behaviour. The development of psychometric systems must be done within an appropri-ate theoretical and methodological framework, and with due regard to the psychophysics of human sensory and response systems. Failure to take adequate account of the theoretical context of a test and failure to consider the psychological aspects and limits of using human subjects invalidate many so-called psychometric 'tests' and do not permit any generalisation of findings and results obtained beyond the close confines of a particular experiment. A review of the psychometric tests available in 1980 (Hindmarch, 1980) showed that many did not consider any basic theoretical or methodological aspects of measurement. Many 'tests' were ingenious and sometimes whimsical, but these were more likely to be unreliable, invalid and insensitive to the effects of psychoactive drugs.

The advent of the microprocessor has caused a burgeoning of computer-based, 'automatic', test systems, the majority of which also fail to consider the essential requirements of validity and reliability. It is not sufficient to create a 'test'.

A psychometric assessment or measure of drug effects in man requires that a test be constructed and developed according to established theoretical, methodological, psychological and pragmatic standards. Tests without a history of reliable usage and without validation against external norms are of no use to those wishing to investigate the psychoactive effects of phar-maceutical agents. On the other hand, there are several psychometric assessments which have been shown to be reliable and valid measures of the CNS activity of a wide range of drugs, including antihistamines, hypnotics, antidepressants, antianxiety agents and nootropics (Hindmarch, 1980, 1981, 1982, 1983, 1984a,b, 1985, 1986). These tests assess many aspects of information processing, sensorimotor co-ordination, short-term or working memory, reaction time, psychomotor functions related to skill behaviours (for example, car driving) and mental arithmetic and logical reasoning. A judicious selection of different tests reflecting different aspects of CNS functions can be made to form a battery of measures which cover the possible range of activities of putative psychotropic agents.

The tests of psychological performance can be presented on micro-processors, as pencil and paper tasks or on specially designed hardware, with or without computer assistance. The results from such assessments can be augmented with scores from subjective rating scales, which, when properly constructed, can give reliable ratings of sedation and/or arousal (Hindmarch *et al.*, 1980; Hindmarch and Gudgeon, 1982; Gudgeon and Hindmarch, 1983; Hindmarch, 1987), mood (Hindmarch, 1979a,b) and sleep (Hindmarch, 1984a, 1975, 1979c, 1984b).

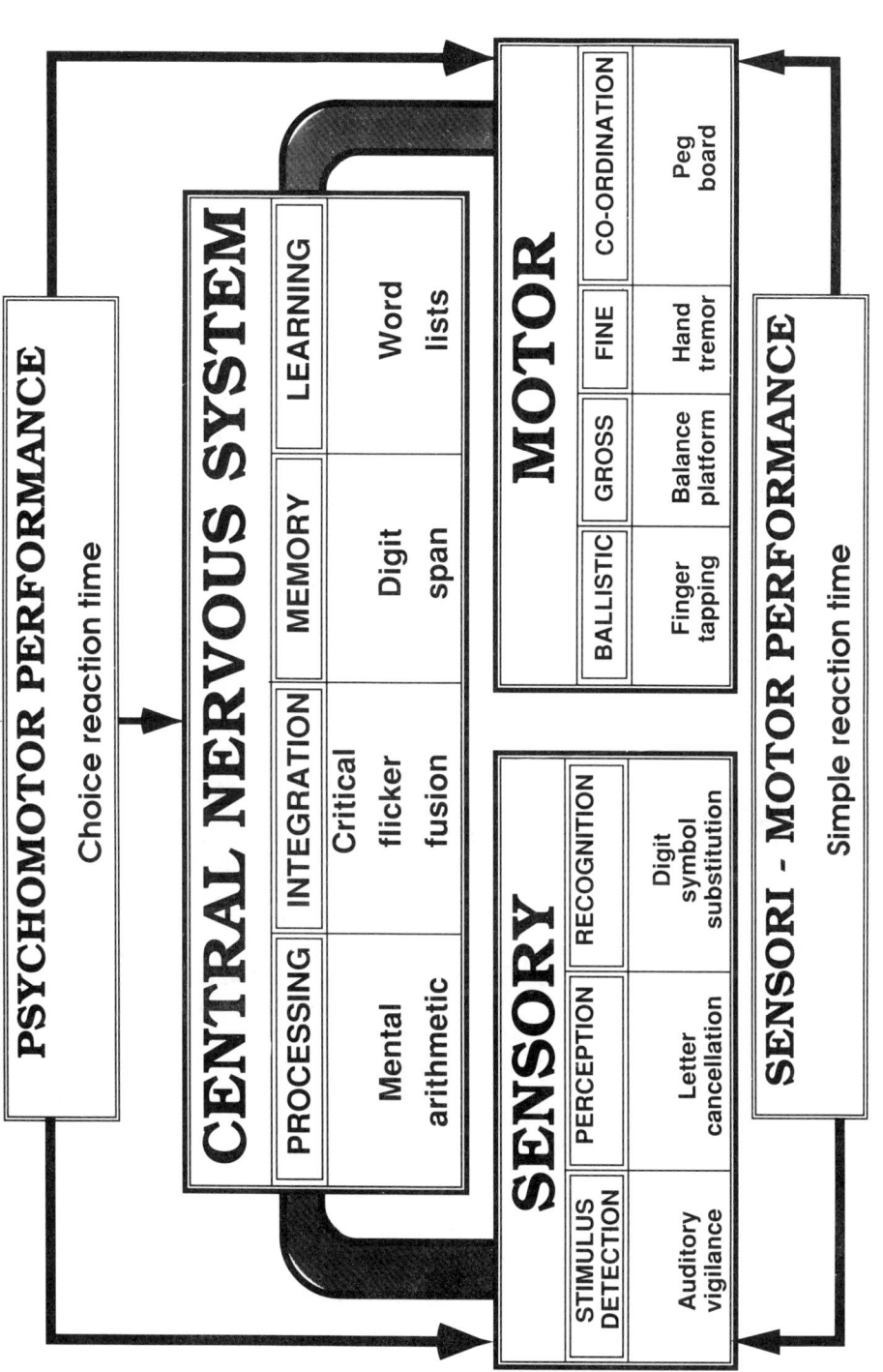

Figure 30.1

A consideration of Figure 30.1 shows that the mode and level of activity of the brain and central nervous system will be dependent upon personality, motivation and memory. It is necessary to examine the extent of the effect of all these factors on the measurement of psychoactive drug-induced changes in behaviour and to see how such influences might be controlled and minimised.

It has been shown (Eysenck, 1963, 1972; Claridge, 1967, 1970) that an inverted-U relationship holds between some personality dimensions, e.g. neuroticism, and performance on sensorimotor tasks such as the pursuit rotor. Interindividual differences in performance, due to personality, are well illustrated in the different psychomotor test scores which have been observed (Malpas *et al.*, 1974; Tansella *et al.*, 1974) in patient and 'normal' volunteer populations. Significant relationships between neuroticism, or anxiety levels, and performance changes with benzodiazepine derivatives have also been reported (Biehl, 1974; Leygonie, 1975) and anxious patients have been shown (Krugman, 1947; Buhler, 1955; Goldstone, 1955; Jones, 1958) to have significantly lower critical flicker fusion thresholds than age-matched 'normals'.

Naturally, the effects of personality on performance become more pronounced at the extremes of affectual dimensions. In studies of the effects of a psychoactive drug in normal volunteers, the interaction of personality and performance can be minimised by screening the subjects through the use of the Middlesex Hospital Questionnaire (Crown and Crisp, 1970), the Eysenck Personality Inventory (Eysenck and Eysenck, 1964) and the Spielberger State–Trait Anxiety Inventory (Spielberger *et al.*, 1968).

Extraneous variables such as the intentions of volunteers, the level of payment, and the expectations of the experimenter and subject can only be controlled by the use of double-blind experimental designs, a careful screening of volunteers, the use of experienced experimenters and a thoroughly reasoned protocol to govern the pragmatics of the test situation.

Drug action on a performance measure can also be affected by the nature of the assessment task. It was impossible to show any decrement of reaction-time performance following temazepam 30 mg or placebo in a car-driving simulator (Fargus and Hindmarch, 1974). However, a significant impairment of reaction time was produced by temazepam 30 mg in contrast to placebo, on a laboratory-based reaction-time task (Hindmarch, 1975). The protocols, dose, regimen and subject populations were similar for both studies, and the contrary results are due to the different test situations. The car-driving simulator presented the task in a high-interest situation: a computer-controlled driving compartment with appropriate noises and movements. On the other hand, the laboratory-based reaction task was a straightforward light and button assembly with little intrinsic interest. The sensitivity of the psychopharmacological measure can be ensured by including a verum, or positive internal control, as well as placebo. For example, amylobarbitone sodium is known to have sedative effects. If such effects are not obvious on an assessment measure following the experimental use of the drug, then it must be assumed that the test is insensitive and no credence can be given to any findings obtained in such an instance.

Tests of psychomotor performance involving the co-ordination of sensory and motor systems, e.g. the pursuit rotor, will be prone to practice and learning effects as, on repeated administration, the subject acquires the skills that facilitate performance. Practice, learning and the effects of memory on performance measures are relatively easy to control. Prior to entry in a study relying on a sensorimotor measure of performance, all subjects must be trained on the task until their 'learning curve' has reached a limiting value and maintained such a value for several trials. When subjects are trained to a criterion, where no further increase in performance can be detected, they can then be admitted to a study. Such pretraining can completely eliminate learning effects, as evidenced in the unchanging placebo responses found in some studies (Taeuber *et al.*, 1979). There would seem to be five aspects of information processing which are worthy of measuring and including in a test battery of psychological function: sensory mechanisms; central integration and processing; motor activity; sensorimotor co-ordination; and mnestic and cognitive functions. The total psychological response to a psychoactive drug is much more complex, involving the interaction of personality, motivational variables, and sociocultural habits and expectations as well as cognitive and psychological aspects of information processing.

An information processing model has been adopted by most researchers as a basis for their particular tests of psychological and cognitive function as represented by measures of attention, memory and information processing. Such representation can be achieved by use of a battery of psychomotor and cognitive tests. While individual researchers might have different approaches, it is evident that most reliable and sensitive tests measure an individual's capacity and/or efficiency to process information. All sensory, motor, intellectual, mnestic and sensorimotor activities involve the cognitive processing of information. Performance indices in each of these domains are governed, in general, by an individual's efficiency in processing information.

As information processing is assigned to a central role in activating affective and behavioural functions (Beck, 1985), it is to be expected that the reduction in the efficiency of information processing should be associated with a lower behavioural responsivity. Differences have been shown (Siegfried *et al.*, 1984) over a wide range of tests of psychomotor ability, cognitive function, memory and crticial flicker fusion threshold between groups of elderly depressed and non-depressed patients. Critical flicker fusion threshold was particularly effective in discriminating between the two patient groups and in reflecting the improvement in global 'cognition and learning' measures following antidepressant therapy in the depressed population. Choice reaction time, paired-associate learning scores and critical flicker fusion threshold measures were found to monitor the cognitive effects of antidepressants in elderly patient populations (Birren *et al.*, 1980; Siegfried, 1987).

It has been demonstrated (Siegfried and O'Connolly, 1986) that psychometric tests are useful in classifying antidepressants, in discriminating between them and in profiling a particular drug's action in the clinical situation.

Psychopharmacological investigations can thus indicate the nature and extent of a drug's psychoactive properties, which in many instances can demonstrate the therapeutic index, the clinical utility and potential and the side-effects of the compound.

NEUROPHYSIOLOGICAL AND PSYCHOPHYSIOLOGICAL MEASUREMENTS

The discovery of more and more sophisticated techniques and instruments to investigate brain activity has allowed the development of objective measurements of CNS effects induced by drugs. In a field where objective techniques are limited, the use of EEG has represented a major achievement in psychopharmacology. Quantitative analysis of the human electroencephalogram in combination with statistical procedures to study drug effects is defined as 'quantitative pharmaco-EEG' (Q-EEG).

As early as the 1930s, EEG changes induced by barbiturates, morphine, cocaine and scopolamine were described. In the mid-1950s systematic EEG studies were applied to the evaluation of drug effects. Modern computer facilities have substantially contributed to the development of modern quantitative pharmaco-EEG.

It soon become clear that every drug with psychotropic properties produces systematic and statistically significant effects on the function of the central nervous system (Fink, 1969; Itil, 1974; Saletu, 1976; Herman, 1982). Furthermore, the discovery that drugs with similar therapeutic effects induced similar CNS changes, resulting in similar Q-EEG profiles, has brought a substantial predictive value to Q-EEG studies.

It has to be added that Q-EEG has many practical advantages: it is easy to apply, painless, and without discomfort for the subjects, and it represents the only non-invasive technique to measure brain functions continuously and repetitively.

With Q-EEG it is possible to classify psychotropic substances and to evaluate objectively their bioavailability at the target organ, the human brain. Specific questions to which Q-EEG can give answers are:

(1) Whether a drug has CNS effect at all as compared with placebo in man.
(2) To which Q-EEG profile category the new drug belongs, by thus predicting to which therapeutic class it may belong.
(3) At which dosage it acts.
(4) At which time it acts.
(5) The equipotent dosages of different galenic formulations.

Methodological Aspects

A typical Q-EEG study will be an acute, double-blind, placebo-controlled trial in healthy normal volunteers, whose number will be determined by the number of doses to be tested (usually three dose levels). A clinically well-known reference drug with similar pharmacokinetic chracteristics will also be used. EEG recordings are usually accomplished by psychometric testing and pharmacokinetic investigations as well as blood pressure and pulse rate evaluation. The classical assessment schedule will be: before drug intake, 1 h, 2 h, 4 h, 6 h and 8 h thereafter. Parenteral administration as well as subacute and chronic administrations will demand different recording periods.

Q-EEG investigations include a 3 min vigilance-controlled EEG (V-EEG), a 4 min resting EEG and a 4 min orienting-response recording.

During the V-EEG recording the technician tries to keep the subject alert; as soon as drowsiness patterns appear at the EEG, the subject is aroused by the technician; during the orienting-response recording the subject has to listen attentively to a meaningless sentence which he is asked to remember at the end of the recordings. At the end of each recording means and sigmas of all EEG variables obtained during V-EEG, resting EEG and EEG reactivity are calculated.

Q-EEG Classification of Psychotropic Drugs

As mentioned above, Q-EEG profiles of psychotropic drugs present similarities and differences which allow classifications of drugs according to their profiles. These similarities parallel similarities in the therapeutic effect of the drugs. At the same time, within each class, differences exist which lead to the identification of subgroups.

Interestingly enough, certain similarities at the Q-EEG analysis exist among different classes which allow speculations about possible overlapping at the clinical level.

The following Q-EEG profiles have been identified.

Neuroleptics

Neuroleptics can be classified as follows:

(1) Sedative, low-potency neuroleptics—chlorpromazine, zotepine, clozapine, dapiprazole.
(2) Non-sedative high-potency neuroleptics—haloperidol.

The first subgroup is characterised by an increase in delta and theta activity, a decrease in alpha activity, and, less frequently, an increase in concomitant fast beta activity; the second subgroup is characterised by a lack of delta augmentation and an increase in alpha and/or alpha-adjacent beta activity.

Another classification was proposed by Itil (1968), who distinguished between neuroleptics of 'major tranquillizer reaction' type and neuroleptics of 'major neuroleptic reaction' type.

A certain overlapping in Q-EEG characteristics exists between neuroleptics and antidepressants, as is the case for clozapine, for which an antidepressant effect has been claimed in patients.

Antidepressants

Antidepressants can be classified as follows:

(1) Thymoleptic profile—imipramine, amitriptyline.
(2) Thymeretic profile—desimipramine.

The first subgroup is characterised by a concomitant increase in slow and fast activities and a decrease in alpha activity; the second, by an increase in alpha activity and an increase in slow and fast activities. The former profile is indicative of sedative properties; the latter, of activating properties. This Q-EEG differentiation agrees well with the existing therapeutic differences of these two types of antidepressants.

Interestingly enough, the desimipramine-type profile is close to that of psychostimulants (Hermann, 1982; Itil, 1982).

Anxiolytics

According to WHO, anxiolytics include tranquillisers and hypnotics and they are represented mainly by the chemical class of benzodiazepines. All benzodiazepines have the same pharmacological properties and they show at Q-EEG analysis a common profile. Nevertheless, differences can be shown at Q-EEG analysis which are in agreement with differences in the clinical activity of these drugs (Poldinger, 1983; Hollister, 1985).

Certain benzodiazepines, such as bromazepam and clobazam, induce in the clinical dosage range no augmentation of slow waves even if administered at high doses (Saletu, 1986). On the other hand, there are benzodiazepines, such as flurazepam, flunitrazepam and triazolam, which produce in the low dose range a 'tranquilliser profile', while in the higher dose range a significant increase in delta activity appears which reflects hypnotic properties (Saletu *et al.*, 1979, 1981, 1985).

Psychostimulants

Psychostimulants such as amphetamine and methamphetamine induce mainly an increase in alpha and alpha-adjacent beta activity together with a trend towards a decrease in slow and fast activities. This profile is interestingly close to that of thymeretic antidepressants and that of nootropics/antihypoxidotics.

Nootropics/Antihypoxidotics

Several molecules belonging to different chemical classes can show a similar clinical activity—namely to improve the noopsychic (intellectual and mnestic functions) and to protect against impairment of 'cerebral biological oxidation' (piracetam, nicergoline, dihydroergotoxine, ifenprodil, vincamine, suloctidil, adrafinil). It is interesting to note that all these drugs generally induce at the Q-EEG analysis a decrease in delta and theta and an increase in alpha and alpha-adjacent beta activity. These changes are indicative of an improvement in vigilance, which is suggested to be the characteristic effect of this group of drugs.

The above-mentioned classification based on Q-EEG profiles gives a global idea of the role of Q-EEG in the early evaluation of psychotropic drugs. It has to be regarded as an empirical classification which does not exclude similarities among profiles of different psychopharmacological classes, and also the fact that Q-EEG characteristics of well-known psychotropic drugs can be shared by non-psychotropic drugs. These considerations explain, on the one hand, the complexity of this methodology, and on the other hand, underline the possible role of Q-EEG in terms of prediction of clinical effects in newly administered drugs, for which in most cases, animal pharmacology is scarcely predictive.

Cerebral Bioavailability and Pharmacokinetics and Pharmacodynamic Relationship

The other roles of Q-EEG concern first of all the possibility of determining objectively and quantitatively the cerebral bioavailability of a psychotropic drug at the level of human brain, and to establish time and dose-efficacy relationships of the drug. Second, because of the fact that plasma pharmacokinetics does not always correspond to 'receptor kinetics' and pharmacodynamic peak effects, Q-EEG can be useful in assessing relationships among these variables.

EEG Imaging of Brain Activity

A further development in the investigation of brain activity is the use of EEG imaging, which allows a topographic representation of EEG brain activity. This new technique is now becoming more and more sophisticated, owing to the fast development of computers and image instruments; its use appears to be a necessary implementation of the classical EEG technique. Some difficulties encountered with the classification of drugs by means of pharmaco-EEG have been thought to be due to the fact that most investigators analysed one or at most only a few leads. Inconsistencies of results suggested the importance of a comprehensive regional topographic approach. In 1951 Walter and Shipton introduced a new toposcopic system.

Further early data on spatiotemporal EEG mapping were published by, among others, Lehmann (1971), Petsche (1973) and Ragot (1978). The first article on the brain electrical activity mapping (BEAM) technique was published by Duffy *et al.* in 1979, followed by Dublinsky and Barlow (1980), Buchsbaum *et al.* (1982) and Etevenon *et al.* (1983). Up to 1983 minicomputers were used; later EEG topograms obtained using microcomputers were described (Sebban *et al.*, 1984).

Topographic pharmaco-EEG images represent a more accurate way of classifying psychotropic drugs in man according to their neurophysiological effects. Furthermore, this new methodology will, it is hoped, increase knowledge about the mode of action of the drugs and the pathophysiology of the brain in psychiatric and neurological disorders.

BEHAVIOURAL ASSESSMENTS

The assessment of behaviour after drug intake is essential, not only in animal pharmacology but especially when a drug is administered to humans. Of course changes in behaviour are only one aspect of the changes that occur in individuals; physiological and biochemical changes usually occur at the same time.

The objective measurement of behaviour, which can be standardised to a certain extent in animals, is difficult in humans. The clinical description of changes in behaviour after drug intake needs to be quantified to allow pooling of data, comparisons and, ultimately, statistical analyses.

In healthy volunteers, the simplest way is to use a comprehensive check list of behavioural and mood effects. Specific and standardised check lists exist such as the one proposed by Nowlis (1965) or by Aitken (1969). Scoring the severity of the effects on a 10 mm line (Visual Analyses Scale) seems to be more sensitive to changes than using fixed-point scales.

The existence of personality inventories such as the Multiphasic Minnesota Personality Inventory (MMPI) has opened the way to further approaches to the evaluation of the interaction: drug—behavioural effects—prediction of therapeutic effects. It is well known that personality can significantly interfere with perception of drug effects in humans. The use of a personality inventory in early studies in healthy volunteers is highly recommended, to allow interpretation and prediction of the drug effects, and to control variables related to the single subject.

The use of personality profiles to predict therapeutic effects has been particularly developed in the field of anxiety and antianxiety drugs; this will be further discussed in the chapter on anxiolytics. The idea behind this approach is to differentiate healthy volunteers on the basis of their personality traits (for instance, 'introvert' against 'extrovert' personalities) and to use their tendency to be more sensitive to the effects of drugs of a particular type (Eynseck, 1957). Barrett and Di Mascio (1966), for instance, by using the Taylor Manifest Anxiety Scale compared the response of 'high anxiety' and 'low anxiety' subjects to three different anxiolytics. Drug response was evident only in 'high anxiety' subjects. Paradoxically, in the same experiment the anxiolytic drugs increased anxiety in the 'low anxiety' subjects. In another study Di Mascio *et al.* (1968) using normal subjects classified as 'high' or 'low' depressed in the MMPI, showed that imipramine exerted a mood-elevating effect only in the 'high depressed' group; an opposite effect was observed in the 'low depressed' group.

In dealing with measurements of behavioural effects after drug intake, it seems worth mentioning the rating scales meant to assess psychopathology. Of course these rating scales are to be used in patients or in any case when a predrug level of psychopathology exists and can be modified by the administration of the drug. Initially, rating scales were constructed as a list of symptoms characterising the clinical picture. The merit of these rating scales lay in helping to standardise the clinical description of the patients and to elaborate structured and semistructured interviews. The discovery of psychotropic drugs gave a major impetus to the development of instruments to measure psychopathology. Specific rating scales for the various psychiatric diseases were developed, to assess changes induced by drugs.

There are many kinds of rating scale and they can be classified in different ways. As mentioned, there are rating scales designed to make diagnoses, such as the St Louis criteria (Feighner *et al.*, 1972). Of course, these rating scales should not be used to measure drug-induced changes.

In terms of their content, scales can be concerned with symptoms, behaviour in the ward, social adjustment, family relationship and functional capacity in occupational environment. The content can also be classified into that which is related to a specific disorder or that which covers all psychiatric syndromes. In the first case it can be mentioned that specific rating scales exist to assess changes in symptoms related to the various psychiatric disorders, especially depression, anxiety and schizophrenia.

Finally, from a very practical point of view, rating scales can be classified according to the users: those scales used by the subject (self-rating) and those requiring an observer who can be skilled (e.g. psychiatrist or psychologist), semi-skilled (e.g. nurse), or unskilled (e.g. patient's relatives). The observer rating scales are now widely used to assess behavioural and psychopathological changes in clinical trials.

As these instruments of measurement are mentioned in the specific chapters concerning the various drugs, we shall consider in this chapter just some methodological principles.

Observer rating scales demand first of all familiarity with and knowledge of the clinical phenomena to recognise mild symptoms, to elicit the information which is needed, to independently score the items and to avoid constant errors such as: reluctance to use the extreme score (i.e. 'severe'); tendency to give a high or low score to one item, and then repeat the same high or low score for the other items; tendency to give high scores at the beginning of a trial and low ones at the end.

Another important bias could be introduced when ratings have to be repeated frequently, because this can induce a tendency to repeat the previous scores, especially towards the end of the trial. If ratings need to be repeated frequently, the self-rating scales or the scales assessing 'state' psychopathology—for instance, the 'state' form of the State–Trait Anxiety Inventory of Spielberger (1978)—are to be preferred.

Self-rating scales offer some practical advantages, such as the fact that they are economical of the time of investigators. Of course, they demand that the patient be capable of completing and understanding the scale. Paykel and Prusoff (1973) observed that older and psychotic patients tended to under-score themselves, whereas younger and neurotic patients overrated.

Another important issue is the correlation between observer rating scales and self-rating scales. Apparently these two types of scales correlate poorly, which seems to indicate that they measure something different.

The above considerations should provide guidance in the choice of the most suitable instruments to assess behavioural changes in volunteers and psycho-pathological changes in patients. There is now an extensive literature on rating scales for assessing psychopathology and it will not be difficult to find an adequate instrument for a specific experimental situation or clinical trial.

NEUROENDOCRINOLOGICAL MEASUREMENTS

The relationship between symptoms referable to the nervous system and endocrine effects has been the object of extensive research for many years. The principle focus of such research has been the anterior pituitary hormone secretion (APHS), as it has been shown that biogenic amines and other neurotransmitters play a fundamental role in the modulation of APHS through an action on the hypothalamic hypophysiotrophic neurons (Fuxe and Hockfelt, 1969). Other investigations have shown that there is a close anatomical relationship between these monoamine systems and the hypothalamic neurons containing releasing factors for APHS (Martin, 1973; McNeil and Sladeck, 1978).

Neurological diseases such as Huntington's chorea and Parkinson's disease, and psychiatric disorders such as schizophrenia and affective illness, are considered to be disorders of neutrotransmission and consequently these disorders might also involve hypothalamic neutrotransmission. Furthermore, if therapeutic actions in these conditions are the result of the drugs' effects on neurotransmitters, it is possible that these effects would be associated with changes in APHS. These changes could be used as an index of the clinical effects or at least of an index of the effects of drugs on neutrotransmission.

It is well known that neuroleptics such as the phenothiazines, butyrophenones, thioxanthenes and benzamide derivatives exert their pharmacological effect by blocking the dopaminergic transmission, at the level of postsynaptic dopamine receptors. This dopamine-blocking ability relates closely to their clinical efficacy in schizophrenic patients (Creese *et al.*, 1976). It is also well known that neuroleptics have effects on the APHS, as shown by the increase in prolactin secretion in animals (de Wied, 1967), in normal subjects (Kleinberg *et al.*, 1971) and in schizophrenic patients (Beaumont *et al.*, 1974). Other pituitary hormones, such as GH, ACTH, LH, FSH and TSH, are affected by neuroleptics (Muller *et al.*, 1977).

Antidepressants cover a wide spectrum of neuropharmacological agents, with different effects on neurotransmission. In general, the administration of antidepressants does not lead to consistent hormonal changes or to endocrinological side-effects.

Benzodiazepine anxiolytics are considered to be free of neuroendocrine effects, although data exist on a possible increasing effect of GH and a decrease in basal and stress ACTH secretion (Syvalhti and Kanto, 1975; Barlow *et al.*, 1979).

It can be concluded that studies on the effects of drugs on APHS represent a useful marker of the effects of drugs on the various neurotransmitters, although certain limitations should be kept in mind:

(1) APHS varies considerably in relation to temporal factors (e.g. menstrual cycle, sleep, etc.).
(2) Feedback exists from target organ hormone secretion.
(3) There is a wide variation in normal levels of these hormones.
(4) Non-specific stimuli may influence APHS at the time of the study (e.g. stress, nutritional state, glucose intake, etc.).

REFERENCES

Aitken, R. C. B. (1969). Measurement of feelings using visual analogue scales. *Proc. Roy. Soc. Med.*, **62**, 989

Barlow, S. M., Knight, A. F. and Sullivan, F. M. (1979). Plasma corticosterone responses to stress following chronic oral administration of diazepam in the rat. *J. Pharm. Pharmacol.*, **31**, 23–6

Barrett, J. E. and Di Mascio, A. (1966). Comparative effects on anxiety of the 'minor tranquilizers' in 'high' and 'low' anxious student volunteers. *Dis. Nerv. Syst.*, **27**, 483–6

Beaumont, P. J. V., Corker, C. S., Friesen, H. G., Gelder, M. G., Harris, G. W., Kolakowska, T. and Mandelbrote, B. M. (1974). The effects of phenothiazines on endocrine function. I. Patients with inappropriate lactation and amenorrhoea. II. Effects in men and post-menopausal women. *Br. J. Psychiat.*, **124**, 413–30

Beck, A. T. (1985). Theoretical perspectives on clinical anxiety. In Turman, A. H. and Maser, J. D. (Eds.), *Anxiety and the Anxiety Disorders*. Erlbaum Associates, London, pp. 183–96

Biehl, B. (1974). The effects of two tranquillizers on driving performance as measured in the normal driving task. *Proceedings 18th Congress of International Association of Applied Psychology*, Montreal

Birren, J. E., Woods, A. M. and Williams, M. V. (1984). Behavioural slowing with age. Causes, organisations and consequences. In Pook, L. W. (Ed.), *Ageing in the 1980s: Psychological Issues*. APA, Washington, D.C.

Buchsbaum, M. S., Rigal, F., Coppola, R., Cappelletti, J., King, C. and Johnson, J. (1982). A new system for gray-level surface distribution maps of electrical activity. *Electroencephalogr. Clin. Neurophysiol.*, **53**, 237–42

Buhler, R. A. (1955). Flicker fusion threshold and anxiety level. *Psychol. Abstr.*, **29**, 701

Claridge, G. S. (1967). *Personality and Arousal*. Pergamon Press, Oxford

Claridge, G. S. (1970). *Drugs and Human Behaviour*. Allen Lane, London

Creese, I., Burt, D. R. and Snyder, S. H. (1976). Dopamine receptor binding predicts clinical and pharmacological potencies of antischizophrenic drugs. *Science, N.Y.*, **192**, 481–3

Crown, S. and Crisp, A. H. (1970). *Manual of the Middlesex Hospital Questionnaire*. Psychological Test Publications, Barnstable

De Wied, C. (1967). Chlorpromazine and endocrine function. *Pharm. Rev.*, **19**, 251–98

Di Mascio, A., Meyer, R. E. and Stifler, L. (1968). Effects of imipramine on individuals varying in level of depression. *Am. J. Psychiat.*, **124**, 55

Dublinsky, J. and Barlow, J. S. (1980). A single dot-density topogram for EEG. *Electroencephalogr. Clin. Neurophysiol.*, **48**, 473–7

Duffy, F. H., Burchfield, J. L. and Lombroso, C. T. (1979). Brain electrical activity mapping (BEAM): a method for extending the clinical utility of EEG and evoked potential data. *Am. Neurol.*, **5**, 309–21

Etevenon, P., Peron-Magnan, P. and Boulenger, J. P. (1986). EEG cartography profile of caffeine in normals. *Clin. Neuropharm.*, **9** (S4), 538–40

Etevenon, P., Peron-Magnan, P., Verdeaux, G., Gaches, J. and Denicker, P. (1983). Electroencephalographie quantitative en neurologie et psychiatrie. Poster 422, 473A. Colloque *Génie Biologique et Médical*, Toulouse, p. 43

Eysenck, H. J. (1957). Drugs and personality. Theory and methodology. *J. Ment. Sci.*, **103**, 119–31

Eysenck, H. J. (1963). *Experiments with Drugs*. Pergamon Press, Oxford

Eysenck, H. J. (1972). *Handbook of Abnormal Psychology*. Pitman Medical, London

Eysenck, H. J. and Eysenck, S. B. G. (1964). *Eysenck Personality Inventory.* University of London Press, London

Fargus, P. C. G. and Hindmarch, I. (1974). A 1,4-benzodiazepine, temazepam: effect on reaction time related to car driving. *IRCS Med. Sci.*, **2**, 1173

Feighner, J. P., Robins, E., Guze, S. B., Woodruff, R. A., Winokur, G. and Munoz, R. (1972). Diagnostic criteria for use in psychiatric research. *Arch. Gen. Psychiatr.*, **29**, 57–67

Fink, M. (1969). *Ann. Rev. Pharmacol.*, **9**, 241

Fuxe, K. and Hokfelt, T. (1969). Catecholamines in the hypothalamus and the pituitary gland. In Ganong, W. F. and Martin, L. (Eds.), *Frontiers in Neuroendocrinology.* Oxford University Press, New York

Goldstone, S. (1955). Critical flicker fusion measurements and anxiety level. *J. Exp. Psychol.*, **49**, 200–2

Gudgeon, A. C. and Hindmarch, I. (1983). Midazolam: Effects on psychomotor performance and subjective aspects of sleep and sedation in normal volunteers. *Br. J. Clin. Pharm.*, **16**, 121S–126S

Herman, W. M. (1982). In Herman, W. M. (Ed.), *Electroencephalography in Drug Research.* Gustav Fischer, Stuttgart, New York, p. 249

Hindmarch, I. (1975). A 1,4-benzodiazepine, temazepam: its effect on psychological aspects of sleep and behaviour. *Arzneimittelforschung*, **25**, 1836–9

Hindmarch, I. (1979a). A preliminary study of the effects of repeated doses of clobazam on aspects of performance, arousal and behaviour in a group of anxiety rated volunteers. *Eur. J. Clin. Pharm.*, **16**, 17–21

Hindmarch, I. (1979b). Some aspects of the effects of clobazam on human performance. *Br. J. Clin. Pharm.*, **7**, 77S–82S

Hindmarch, I. (1979c). Effects of hypnotic and sleep inducing drugs on objective assessments of human psychomotor performance and subjective appraisals of sleep and early morning behaviour. *Br. J. Clin. Pharm.*, **8**, 43S–46S

Hindmarch, I. (1980). Psychomotor function and psychoactive drugs. *Br. J. Clin. Pharm.*, **10**, 1189–209

Hindmarch, I. (1981). Measuring the effects of psychoactive drugs on higher brain function. In Burrows, G. D. and Werry, J. S. (Eds.), *Advances in Human Psychopharmacology II.* JAI Press, pp. 79–106

Hindmarch, I. (1982). Antidepressant drugs and performance. *Bri. J. Clin. Pract.*, **19**, 73–7

Hindmarch, I. (1983). Measuring the side-effects of psychoactive drugs: a pharmacodynamic profile of alprazolam. *Alcohol and Alcoholism*, **18**, 361–7

Hindmarch, I. (1984a). The Leeds Sleep Evaluation Questionnaire (LSEQ) as a measure of the subjective response to nocturnal treatment with benzodiazepines. In Burrows, G. D., Norman, T. R. and Maguire, K. P. (Eds.), *Biological Psychiatry: Recent Studies.* J. Libbey, London, pp. 228–39

Hindmarch, I. (1984b). Psychological performance models as indicators of the effects of hypnotic drugs on sleep. In Hindmarch, I., Ott, H. and Roth, T. (Eds.), *Sleep, Benzodiazepines and Performance.* Springer-Verlag, Heidelberg, pp. 58–69

Hindmarch, I. (1985). Anxiety, performance and anti-anxiety drugs. *Br. J. Clin. Pract.*, **39**, 53–8

Hindmarch, I. (1986). The effects of psychoactive drugs on car handling and related psychomotor ability: a review. In O'Hanlon, J. F. and de Gier, J. F. (Eds.), *Drugs and Driving.* Taylor and Francis, London, pp. 71–82

Hindmarch, I. (1987). Three antidepressants (amitriptyline, dothiepin, fluoxetine), with and without alcohol, compared with placebo on tests of psychomotor ability related to car driving. *Hum. Psychopharm.*, **2**, 177–83

Hindmarch, I. and Gudgeon, A. C. (1982). Loprazolam (HR158) and flurazepam with ethanol compared on tests of psychomotor ability. *Eur. J. Clin. Pharm.*, **23**, 509–12

Hindmarch, I., Parrott, A. C. and Stonier, P. D. (1980). The effects of nomifensine and HOE8476 on car driving and related psychomotor performance. In Stonier, P. D. and Jenner, F. A. (Eds.), *Nomifensine*. Royal Society of Medicine International Congress and Symposium Series No. 25, London, pp. 47–54

Hollister, L. E. (1985). In Smith, D. E. and Wesson, D. R. (Eds.),*The Benzodiazepines, Current Standards for Medical Practice*. MTP Press, Lancaster, p. 87

Itil, T. M. (1974). In Itil, T. M. (Ed.), *Modern Problems of Pharmacopsychiatry*, Vol. 8: *Psychotropic Drugs and Human EEG*, Karger, Basle, p. 43

Itil, T. M. (1982). In Herman, W. M. (Ed.), *EEG in Drug Research*. Gustav Fischer, Stuttgart, New York, p. 131

Jones, O. (1958). Relationship between visual and auditory discrimination and anxiety levels. *J. Gen. Psychol.*, **59**, 111–18

Kleinberg, D. L., Wharton, R. N. and Frantz, A. G. (1971). Rapid release of prolactin in normal adults following chlorpromazine stimulation. *53rd Programme of Endocrine Society Meetings*, San Francisco, p. 126

Krugman, H. (1947). Flicker fusion frequency as a function of anxiety reaction: an exploratory study. *Psychosom. Med.*, **4**, 269–72

Lehmann, D. (1971). Multichannel topography of human alpha EEG fields. *Electroencephalogr. Clin. Neurophysiol.*, **31**, 439–49

Leygonie, F., Rethone, A., Yuleyatak, F. and Yuceyatiak, A. (1975). Anxiolitique nouveau, le clobazam, action sur le sommeil de nuit et le niveau de performance au réveil. *Gaz. Med. France*, **82**, 1303

McNeil, T. H. and Sladek, J. R. (1978). Fluorescence-immunocytochemistry: simultaneous localization of catecholamines and gonadotrophin-releasing hormone. *Science, N.Y.*, **200**, 72–4

Malpas, A., Legg, N. J. and Scott, D. F. (1974). Effects of hypnotics on anxious patients. *Br. J. Clin. Psychiat.*, **124**, 482–4

Martin, J. B. (1973). Neural regulation of growth hormone secretion. *New Engl. J. Med.*, **288**, 1384–93

Muller, E. E., Nistico, G. and Scapagnini, E. (1977). *Neurotransmitters and Anterior Pituitary Function*. Academic Press, New York.

Nowlis, V. (1965). Research with the mood adjective check-list. In Tomkins, S. and Izard, C. (Eds.), *Affect, Cognition and Personality*. Springer-Verlag, New York, p. 352

Paykel, E. S. and Prusoff, B. A. (1973). Response set and observer set in the assessment of depressed patients. *Psychol. Med.*, **3**, 209–16

Petsche, H. (1973). EEG topography. In Remond, A. (Ed.), *Handbook of Electroencephalography and Clinical Neurophysiology*. Elsevier, Amsterdam

Poldinger, W. and Wider, F. (1983). In Langer, G. and Heiman, H. (Eds.), *Psychopharmarka, Grundlagen und Therapie*. Springer-Verlag, Vienna, p. 447

Saletu, B. (1976). *Bibliotheca Psychiatrica*, No. 155. Karger, Basle.

Saletu, B., Grünberger, J., Berner, P. and Koeppen, D. (1985). In Hindmarch, I., Stonier, P. D. and Trimble, M. R. (Eds.), *Clobazam: Human Psychopharmacology and Clinical Applications*, International Congress and Symposium Series, No. 74. Royal Society of Medicine, London, p. 23

Saletu, B., Grünberger, J., Linzmayer, L. and Flener, R. (1981). *Agressologie*, **22**, 5

Saletu, B., Grünberger, J., Volavka, J. and Berner, P. (1979). *Arzneim. Forsch. Drug Res.*, **29**, 700

Saletu, B., Küfferle, B., Grünberger, J. and Anderer, P. (1986). *Pharmacopsychiatrie*, **19**, 36–52

Sebban, C. L., Debouzy, C. L. and Berthaux, P. (1984). EEG quantifié et cartographie numérisée. In Lassen, N. A. and Cahn, J. (Eds.), *Maladies et Médicaments*. Libbey, London, pp. 176–81

Siegfried, K. (1987). Towards a clinical classification of antidepressant profiles. In Hindmarch, I. and Stonier, P. D. (Eds.), *Human Psychopharmacology*, Vol. II. Wiley, Chichester

Siegfried, K. and O'Connolly, M. (1986). Cognitive and psychomotor effects of different antidepressants in the treatment of old age depression. *Int. Clin. Psychopharm.*, **1**, 221–30

Siegfried, K., Jansen, W. and Pahnke, K. (1984). Cognitive dysfunction in depression. *Drug. Dev. Res.*, **4**, 533–53

Spielberger, C. D., Goruch, R. L. and Lushene, R. E. (1968). *Manual for State-Trait Anxiety Inventory*. Florida State University, Tallahassee

Spielberger, C. D., Gorsuch, R. L. and Lushene, R. E. (1970). *Manual for the State-Trait Anxiety Inventory*. Consulting Psychologist Press, Palo Alto

Sylvalahti, E. and Kanto, J. (1975). Serum growth hormone, serum immunoreactive insulin and blood responses to oral and intravenous diazepam in man. *Int. J. Clin. Pharm.*, **12**, 74–82

Taeuber, K., Zapf, R., Rupp, W. and Badian, M. (1979). Pharmacodynamic comparison of the acute effects of nomifensine, amphetamine and placebo in healthy volunteers. *Int. J. Clin. Pharm. Biopharm.*, **17** (1), 32–7

Tansella, M., Zimmermann-Tansella, C. and Lader, M. (1974). The residual effects of N-desmethyldiazepam in patients. *Psychopharmacologica (Berlin)*, **38**, 81–90

Walter, G. and Shipton, H. (1951). A new toposcopic display system. *Electroencephalogr. Clin. Neurophysiol.*, **3**, 281–92

31
Drugs in Epilepsy

J. I. Morrow and A. Richens

Dept of Pharmacology and Therapeutics, University of Wales College of Medicine, Heath Park, Cardiff CF4 4XN, UK

INTRODUCTION

Epilepsy is a chronic condition but one which manifests itself only intermittently. To achieve adequate control of seizures, drugs must be taken continuously and in the long term. Therefore, the development and testing of drugs for epilepsy poses problems peculiar to the condition. It is the purpose of this chapter to anticipate these problems and to discuss potential strategies in early studies on new drugs for epilepsy.

PHASE I STUDIES

Toxicology

Existing antiepileptic drugs (AEDs) are recognised to have effects on the central nervous system (CNS) beyond seizure control. Awareness is growing, in particular, about effects on cognition and behaviour (Schmidt, 1982a; Reynolds, 1983). Although early studies are often not useful in detecting potential adverse effects, because numbers are small and adverse events are usually uncommon, possible CNS effects deserve particular attention in this category of drug, as they are common and often dose-dependent. Therefore, consideration should be given to detailed neurophysiological testing which may accompany early single- and multiple-dose kinetic studies.

Pharmacokinetic Studies

Elimination Half-life

To achieve acceptance as a drug for chronic therapy, it is desirable for a new compound to have a sufficiently long elimination half-life ($t_{\frac{1}{2},el}$) such that once- or twice-daily dosing is all that is required; a half-life in the range of 15–30 h is ideal. In existing therapy sodium valproate has a $t_{\frac{1}{2},el}$ of about 8–15 h and shorter when used concurrently with other AEDs capable of inducing liver enzymes. Yet sodium valproate is in wide usage and is an effective AED even when given less frequently than the $t_{\frac{1}{2},el}$ would suggest is required. This is because the antiepileptic effect of the drug is not a direct reflection of plasma levels: it comes on more slowly and outlasts the presence of the drug. This effect can also be seen with other drugs and may either be due to active metabolites or, in the case of sodium valproate, result because the drug may have a modifying effect on the activity of enzymes responsible for the degradation of inhibition neurotransmitter substances (Sawaya *et al.*, 1975). Therefore, it would be a mistake to reject a new compound simply on the basis of elimination half-life without regard to efficacy.

Hepatic Metabolism

The metabolism of any new compound needs to be strictly defined, with particular regard to hepatic metabolism. Many existing AEDs are recognised to be inducers of hepatic microsomal enzymes and this may have an important bearing on later efficacy studies.

The chronic administration of AEDs capable of inducing liver enzymes may affect the new compound in one of two ways. Drugs with a high first-pass metabolism may have a reduced bioavailability. Felodipine, one of a group of calcium antagonists which have been attracting interest as potential AEDs,

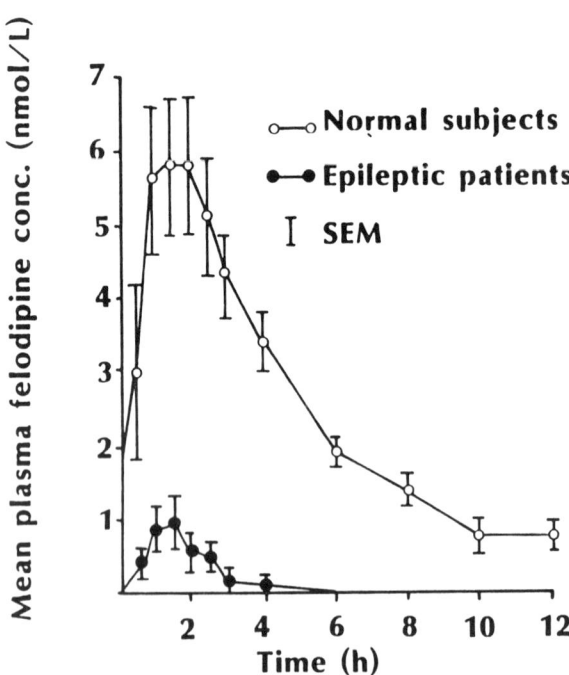

Figure 31.1 Felodipine mean plasma concentrations (from Capewell *et al.*, 1988)

has been demonstrated to have a markedly reduced oral bioavailability as a result of first-pass metabolism when given to patients with microsomal enzyme induction due to chronic AED therapy (Capewell *et al.*, 1988) (Figure 31.1). This suggests that patients on AED therapy may require substantially higher doses of any drug with a high first-pass metabolism in order to achieve plasma levels equivalent to those of non-induced subjects. On the other hand, drugs with restrictive systemic elimination may have a shortened $t_{\frac{1}{2},el}$ in the presence of drugs capable of hepatic induction. Lamotrigine, a novel anticonvulsant, has a mean half-life of 24 h, but in epileptic patients the elimination half-life was reduced to approximately 12 h in those who were taking carbamazepine or phenytoin. If any new compound is subject to hepatic metabolism, then pharmacokinetic studies on volunteers alone may be insufficient to predict the properties of the drug in treated and enzyme-induced epileptic patients. Additional parallel studies on hepatic-induced patients or volunteers may be necessary before proceeding to efficacy studies.

The existing AED phenytoin can be difficult to use, because its metabolism is saturable. To achieve optimum therapy and avoid toxicity requires frequent monitoring and care in dosage adjustment. It would be desirable for any new compound to have simpler and preferably linear kinetics, but in either case the dose–blood concentration relationship should be defined.

Enzyme Induction

Many AEDs are enzyme inducers capable of inducing their own metabolism and the metabolism of other drugs. The $t_{\frac{1}{2},el}$ of carbamazepine in healthy volunteers can be up to 55 h but in chronic dosing 10–20 h is more usual. Similarly, the coadministration of carbamazepine with sodium valproate induces the metabolism of the sodium valproate. It must be determined whether the new compound is capable of inducing its own and/or the metabolism of other drugs. Measurements of antipyrine clearance, plasma glutamyl transpeptidase and urinary 6-hydroxycortisol are standard techniques for assessing this possibility (Park, 1982). If the compound is not an enzyme inducer, it has an advantage over most standard AEDs. If it is, interactions may occur with coadministered AEDs, resulting in reduced amounts of the original drug which may have an important bearing on later efficacy studies.

Enzyme Inhibition

A new compound may be capable of inhibiting the metabolism of other drugs. This may result in a rise in the blood concentrations of coadministered AEDs. In assessing the efficacy of nafimidone, Treiman and Ben-Menachem (1987) noted marked rises in the carbamazepine serum concentration of their patients and similar though less marked rises in the serum concentration of phenytoin (Figure 31.2). A rise in the concentration of the original AED may provide an alternative explanation for a reduction in seizures or result in unacceptable toxicity during the course of later efficacy studies.

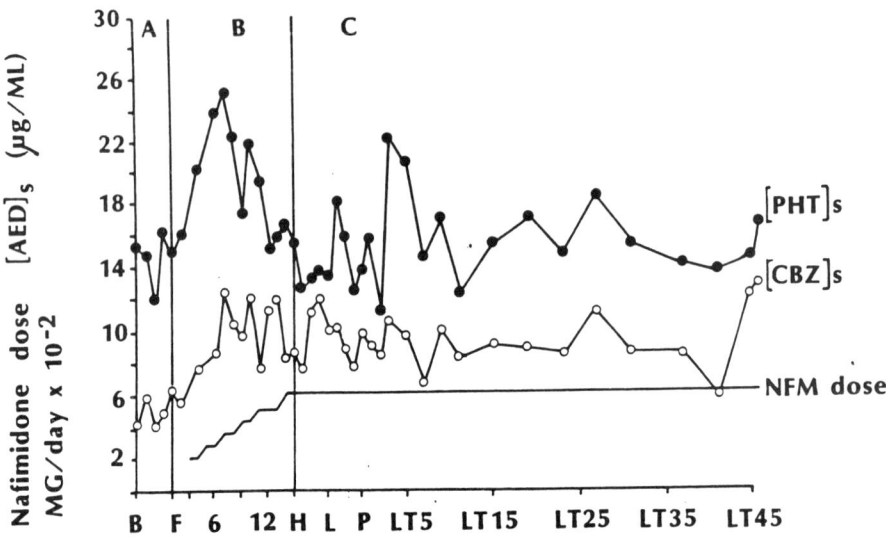

Figure 31.2 Inhibition of carbamazepine (CBZ) and phenytoin (PHT) metabolism by nafimidone. Serum concentration of CBZ and PHT during the course of the study in one patient. Vertical lines divide the data into three segments: baseline (A), where each point represents a weekly visit; hospitalisation (B), where each point represents a hospital day; and outpatient observation (C), where gradations in the axis represent weeks. Nafimidone (NFM) was added during hospitalisation; the dose is indicated by the lines without symbols. CBZ and PHT levels rose rapidly after the addition of NFM, until their doses were lowered to compensate for the inhibition of elimination caused by NFM. CBZ dose was 800 mg/day during A. It was decreased to 300 mg/day during B in response to rising CBZ levels and was then maintained at 300 mg/day throughout C. PHT dose was 400 mg/day during A and was reduced to 200 mg/day during B; 200 mg/day was maintained throughout C. (From Treiman and Ben-Menachen, 1987)

Metabolites

The metabolites of some existing AEDs are known to be active, i.e. have an antiepileptic effect of their own. Primidone is metabolised to phenobarbitone and carbamazepine is metabolised to the active carbamazepine 10,11-epoxide. An active metabolite may alter the antiepileptic profile of the drug, giving rise to an antiepileptic effect which outlasts the presence of the parent drug. The relative concentration of parent drug and metabolites may further vary according to the rate of metabolism. An active metabolite will give rise to difficulties in predicting the efficacy of the drug, particularly in cross-over trials, if blood concentrations of the parent drug alone are monitored.

Protein Binding

The degree of protein binding should be estimated, as this may influence the plasma concentration–effect relationship as well as being a further potential site for drug interaction. If the new compound is bound, *in vitro* binding studies should be performed, as saturable binding may occur and must be defined. Sodium valproate has been demonstrated to displace phenytoin from binding sites (Monks *et al.*, 1978), resulting in a fall in the total plasma concentration but little change in the free concentration (i.e. the efficacy of phenytoin will be unaltered although the plasma concentration has fallen). If a new compound has a similar effect, this may have a bearing on later short-term efficacy and toxicity studies. Consequently, binding interaction studies with phenytoin, sodium valproate, benzodiazepines and other drugs should be performed in any new compound demonstrated to have a significant degree of protein binding.

PHASE II STUDIES

Efficacy studies are not possible in volunteers, as no suitable test has been defined. Therefore, studies of this nature must be carried out on groups of epileptic patients. The stages of development and usage of new AEDs are outlined in Table 31.1.

Table 31.1 Pathway for Phase II evaluation of a new antiepileptic drug

(1) Single-dose efficacy studies
interictal spikes
photosensitivity
spike and wave
cluster seizures
(2) Short pilot efficacy studies
seizure frequency
(3) Double-blind placebo-controlled efficacy studies
cross-over
parallel
(4) Double-blind comparison with reference drug
add-on therapy
(5) Double-blind comparison with reference drug
monotherapy

Single-dose Studies

The intermittent nature of seizures limits the scope of single-dose studies, but several methods of assessing efficacy after a single dose have been devised. These studies have the advantage that they can be carried out at an early stage with minimal toxicological data. However, to show efficacy the new compound must have a quick onset of action, a feature not always necessary in the long-term treatment of epilepsy.

Interictal Spikes

It is recognised that some patients with epilepsy will demonstrate epileptiform spike activity between seizures on an EEG recording. It is possible to quantify these interictal spikes by counting their number over defined periods. It is further recognised that antiepileptic drugs may reduce the number and frequency of these interictal spikes, thus providing a method of evaluation of a new AED at an early stage using a single dose. By comparing spike count at baseline and/or with placebo, a measure of efficacy can be achieved.

Although this method has been used in the early stages of development of new AEDs, its relevance to seizure control may be questioned, because the relationship of interictal spikes to epilepsy remains undefined. It is recognised that interictal spikes may occur in seizure-free patients and patients with active epilepsy may not demonstrate interictal spikes. Therefore, an abolition or reduction in interictal spikes may not necessarily equate with efficacy against seizures. Furthermore, the frequency of interictal spikes may vary widely from patient to patient and in the same patient from minute to minute, resulting in practical problems of assessment.

Photoconvulsive Response

Some patients, particularly those with primary generalised epilepsy, may demonstrate a photoconvulsive response, i.e. photic stimulation may evoke an epileptiform abnormality on an EEG recording. This response can be quantified over the frequency range of photic stimulation which produces it. The efficacy of a new compound can, therefore, be assessed by the abolition of the photoconvulsive response or by a reduction in the frequency range which produces it. However, photosensitive epilepsy is uncommon in adults, and efficacy against a photoconvulsive response does not guarantee efficacy against other forms of epilepsy. Some standard AEDs are highly effective at reducing photosensitivity, e.g. sodium valproate, while other existing effective AEDs are not, e.g. carbamazepine. Therefore, the opposite is also true: failure to abolish a photoconvulsive response does not rule out efficacy against seizures.

Spike and Wave

Children who suffer from absence attacks ('true *petit mal*') may demonstrate paroxysms of spike and wave activity on an EEG recording. The amount of this activity correlates inversely with the degree of seizure control. A reduction in spike and wave paroxysms after a single dose of a new compound may, therefore, be a good indicator for later efficacy studies. However, as for the photoconvulsive response, this form of epilepsy is known to respond to some existing AEDs and not to other AEDs which are effective against commoner types of adult epilepsy. The antiepileptic spectrum of any new drug should, therefore, be previously ascertained from animal studies. The major drawback with this method of assessment is in patient selection. Absence seizures are found almost exclusively in children, and therefore recruitment of sufficient numbers of adult patients will prove difficult. This difficulty is compounded by the fact that this form of epilepsy responds well to conventional AED therapy.

Serial Seizures

To test a single dose of a drug against actual seizures is sometimes possible in patients who are prone to serial or clusters of seizures. In order for a single dose to be effective in this situation, the drug must: (1) have a quick onset of action and (2) be available in a form which can be administered to a patient who may be unable to take oral drugs.

However, the major limiting factor is probably having access to the patient at the time the series of seizures is occurring and before anything else has been administered.

Short Pilot Efficacy Studies (Add-on)

Full animal toxicological data will be required at an early stage, to permit the chronic dosing studies necessary for the full evaluation of any potential AED. However, short-term studies, e.g. of 1 week duration, may be possible with limited toxicological data. These studies will be of 'add-on' type, i.e. the new compound is given in addition to the patient's existing therapy. Seizure type(s) to be studied need to be defined at an early stage and carefully selected.

This type of study may be of either open or placebo-controlled design. The open study is less satisfactory. A placebo response is a recognised phenomenon in epilepsy, as for other conditions. It may occur because patients are recruited because of a high seizure frequency which may only be a temporary phenomenon. In general, an open study will have to be followed by a placebo-controlled study but it may provide a 'feel for the drug' at an early stage. Efficacy can be defined as a reduction in seizures compared with a baseline period.

A placebo-controlled study of short duration may provide evidence of efficacy of a new drug at an early stage. However, to measure a change in seizure frequency over a short period requires subjects to have a high baseline seizure frequency. Patients with frequent seizures suitable for this type of study are often receiving combinations of AEDs and by definition are resistant to them. Therefore, the selection of subjects for this type of study may include a group of patients who will prove resistant to all forms of therapy. Early efficacy studies of this type may be combined with dosing interaction studies and adverse reaction monitoring. Dose regimens may also be tested by expanding the number of study groups so that different dosages may be tested for efficacy and adverse effects. In a recent study (Crawford *et al.*, 1987) patients were randomised to receive 300 mg, 600 mg or 900 mg of gabapentin in addition to their existing therapy. This study demonstrated a dose-dependent effect of the drug compared with baseline levels of seizure frequency. However, the omission of a placebo phase perhaps reduces the power of the study.

Double-blind Placebo-controlled Efficacy Studies

The intermittent nature of seizures means that definitive efficacy studies must be of long duration. Therefore, this type of study will only be permissible after full animal toxicological data have become available.

Early efficacy studies will of necessity be of 'add-on' type, as the use of placebo in patients with active epilepsy could only be justified in the presence of existing AED therapy. Similarly, in order to provide the usual measure of efficacy, i.e. the reduction in number of seizures, only patients with a high seizure frequency are selected for study. The usual seizure frequency used in selecting for this type of study is a frequency of more than four seizures per month. Definition of seizure type is as important. The seizure type(s) selected for study may be chosen with regard to the new compound's potential spectrum of action and also to the practical problem of patient recruitment, i.e. seizure type(s) that may be found sufficiently commonly in the clinic situation. Seizure type must be classified with regard to a recognised seizure classification system, e.g. the International League Against Epilepsy Classification 1981 (Commission on Classification and Terminology of the International League Against Epilepsy, 1981). Whichever classification of seizures is selected, type(s) of seizure must be recorded before and during treatment periods, as a drug may abolish tonic/clonic seizures but other more minor and less functionally disabling seizures may continue. Thus, seizure frequency alone may be little affected, yet the patient has undoubtedly benefited. To take into account the relative functional disability produced by different seizure types, quantitative scales have been devised (Cramer *et al.*, 1983), although they have not been widely used, perhaps because of their cumbersome nature.

The group of patients for study having been selected, how is the drug to be administered? Is there to be a fixed-dose or a variable-dosage regimen? A fixed dose has the advantage of ease of dispensing and shortens the length of the study, but has the disadvantage that in some patients the dose may be too little and in others too great, resulting in toxicity. If a variable-dose regimen is chosen, is the dose to be adjusted according to seizure frequency or to achieve a predetermined blood concentration? In either case, the study will have to be lengthened so that a steady state can be achieved and the study will require the presence of an extra unblinded monitor who can make any necessary dosage adjustments.

The design of double-blind placebo-controlled studies in this category of patient is usually of one of two types—cross-over or a parallel-group design. The former has become the standard method of early assessment of a new AED but objections have recently been raised to this design. A cross-over study has many advantages; a patient group of 20–30 is usually sufficient, as patients act as their own controls. Thus, this type of study can be performed in a single centre. The study consists of an introduction period and two treatment phases separated by a cross-over period. The cross-over period must be of sufficient length to avoid carry-over effects. It is this potential for carry-over effects that is the main drawback to this design. Possible carry-over effects can be tested for by analysis of variance, but if they are shown to have occurred, then the study is invalidated. A parallel-group study has advantages in that it avoids period effects but it must of necessity be a much larger study. Studies of this nature cannot usually be performed in a single centre but must be multicentre, and having a number of different investigators may create its own problems. Both study designs may show an initial reduction in seizures regardless of the treatment, because patients are often chosen when their seizure frequency is particularly high and therefore a reduction is more likely than a worsening of seizure frequency.

Study periods are usually of 2–3 months' duration and efficacy is assessed by reduction in seizure count. Freedom from seizures or a percentage reduction in seizure frequency (e.g. a 50% reduction in seizure frequency) are selected as suitable end-points. Improvement in EEG recordings has also been used to assess efficacy but is unsatisfactory, as interictal EEG changes do not correlate well with seizure control (other than in absence seizures).

The major drawback with these studies is in the selection of patients. Patients with a high seizure frequency resistant to standard AED therapy are of necessity chosen for study. It may be argued that some potential AEDs will be lost because the potential for improvement in these patients is small. In a study of the value of adding a second AED in intractable epilepsy with complex partial seizures (Schmidt, 1982b) it was demonstrated that in only 13% of patients exposed to the second drug did a significant reduction in seizures occur and a similar number of patients actually demonstrated an increase in seizures. However, this finding conflicts with a large number of controlled trials in which a larger reduction in seizure frequency has been demonstrated. Thus, in a group of patients with continuing seizures there may be a proportion who will prove resistant to all forms of therapy, but the size of this proportion remains essentially unknown.

A further refinement to the study design recently used in the study of vigabatrin (Reynolds *et al.*, 1988) may eliminate these multiresistant patients. In this study there was an initial baseline phase followed by an open treatment period on 3 g of vigabatrin. Those patients who did not benefit were then eliminated from the study but those who demonstrated a reduction in seizure frequency were admitted to the double-blind placebo-controlled phase.

Double-blind Comparison with Reference Drug

Efficacy of a new drug can be assessed with reference to a standard AED. Comparison with a reference AED has the advantage over placebo studies in add-on therapy in that those drugs shown to be no more effective than the control group are less likely to be dismissed. Bioequivalence studies of this nature can be of add-on or monotherapy design.

Add-on Therapy

Add-on studies have the advantage that they can usually be performed earlier than monotherapy studies but have the same disadvantages as earlier placebo-controlled add-on studies. They may well be difficult to design, because most patients will have had the reference drug and will have been shown to be poorly responsive to it (which is why they are available for further study). This puts the comparator drug at a disadvantage.

Studies of this nature may be of cross-over or parallel-group design, and the inclusion of a placebo group or phase will increase the power of the study. Indeed, inclusion of a placebo control may be considered essential so that evidence is obtained that both drugs are showing a therapeutic effect. A study which incorporates a placebo phase into a cross-over design so that there are six groups, each of two legs, to encompass all possible combinations of placebo and/or reference AED and/or new AED in two latin squares has many advantages. It can be performed at an early stage and combines both efficacy against placebo with a bioequivalence study as well as allowing for potential carry-over effects.

Monotherapy

Monotherapy studies with a new AED may follow earlier efficacy studies once efficacy of the new drug has been established. Patient selection for this type of study is different from that in earlier studies, in that those suitable are newly diagnosed epileptics and patients previously not receiving AEDs. These trials will usually be of a parallel-group design, patients being randomised to receive either new AED or reference drug. Placebo would usually be considered unethical in this situation. This is certainly the case for tonic/clonic seizures, but for absence, partial seizures of long standing, but previously unrecognised, or even for treatment after a single isolated seizure, there may be a case for comparison with placebo, but this has never been tested.

Monotherapy studies of this nature have a number of notable advantages (for example, less resistant patients and no potential for drug interactions) but these may be balanced by other potential disadvantages. There is a temptation by GPs and others to treat epilepsy once it is suspected, especially in view of the average length of neurology waiting lists! Thus, to attract untreated patients local GPs need to be involved and a 'fast channel' for early referral needs to be established. Many patients treated at an early stage will become seizure-free. It has been estimated that 70–80% of patients treated with modern AED therapy will become seizure-free (Elwes, 1984). The potential to improve on this success rate is, therefore, limited, and to measure small degrees of increased benefit will require large numbers of patients. Even those patients who continue to have seizures may do so at infrequent intervals, so that follow-up will have to be very prolonged.

Toxicological Studies

Throughout all efficacy studies, recording of clinical toxicological data must be thorough. Symptoms and signs should be elicited at regular intervals throughout the study during both placebo and treatment phases. All un-wanted effects should be recorded and an estimate should be made by the physician of their relationship to the drug therapy. Monitoring of electrolyte, blood count, liver function tests, etc., should be standard practice throughout the study period, as should monitoring of the plasma concentrations of coadministered antiepileptic drugs.

More formal studies of drug effects may be carried out simultaneously with efficacy studies, particularly psychometry, mood assessment, cognitive function and psychomotor function. EEG studies may also be performed at intervals.

Those subjects demonstrating benefit from the study drug in an efficacy study may be permitted to continue the drug in the long term. These subjects should continue to be followed so that valuable early data on long-term efficacy and toxicity may be collected.

SUMMARY

Epilepsy is a chronic disease, yet seizures occur only intermittently. Epilepsy is also a heterogeneous disease, in terms of both seizure type and seizure frequency. Therefore, the evaluation of new drugs for epilepsy presents problems peculiar to the condition. Efficacy studies cannot adequately be performed over very short periods and, therefore, full animal toxicological data must be available at an early stage. Similarly, the potential for drug interactions needs to be defined during early studies, as the use of a placebo is usually considered unethical in previously untreated patients and, therefore, early studies, of necessity, are add-on trials in patients who have previously proved poorly responsive to standard AED therapy.

Inevitably, the emergence of new AEDs has been slow. Nevertheless, in recent years there has been a better understanding of the neurophysiological basis of epilepsy and of neurotransmitter substances in particular. This increased knowledge has led to a more logical approach to the development of potential AEDs.

REFERENCES

Capewell, S., Freestone, S., Critchley, J. A. J. H., Pottage, A. and Prescott, L. F. (1988). Reduced felodipine bioavailability in patients taking anticonvulsants. *Lancet*, **2**, 480–2

Commission on Classification and Terminology of the International League Against Epilepsy (1981). Proposal for revised clinical and electroencephalographic classification of epileptic seizures. *Epilepsia*, **22**, 489–501

Cramer, J. A., Smith, D. B., Mattson, R. H., Delgado Escuta, A. V., Collins, J. F. and the VA Epilepsy Co-operative Study Group (1983). A method of quantification for the evaluation of antiepileptic drug therapy. *Neurology (Cleveland)*, **33** (Suppl. 1), 26–37

Crawford, P., Ghadiali, E., Lane, R., Blumhardt, L. and Chadwick, D. (1987).

Gabapentin as an antiepileptic drug in man. *J. Neurol. Neurosurg. Psychiat.* **50** (6), 682–6

Elwes, R. D. C., Johnson, A. L., Shorvon, S. D. and Reynolds, E. H. (1984). The prognosis for seizure control in newly diagnosed epilepsy. *New Engl. J. Med.*, **311** (15), 944–7

Monks, A., Boobis, S., Wadsworth, J. and Richens, A. (1978). Plasma protein binding interaction between phenytoin and valproic acid *in vitro. Br. J. Clin. Pharm.*, **6**, 487–92

Park, B. K. (1982). Assessment of drug metabolism capacity of the liver. *Br. J. Clin. Pharm.*, **14**, 631–51

Reynolds, E. H. (1983). Mental effects of antiepileptic medication—a review. *Epilepsia*, **24** (Suppl. 2), S85–S95

Reynolds, E. H., Ring, H. and Heller, A. (1988). A controlled trial of gamma-vinyl gaba (vigabatrin) in drug resistant epilepsy. *Br. J. Clin. Pract.*, **42** (Suppl. 61), 33

Sawaya, M. L. B., Horton, R. W. and Meldrum, B. S. (1975). Effects of anticonvulsant drugs on cerebral enzymes metabolising GABA. *Epilepsia*, **16**, 649–55

Schmidt, D. (1982a). *Adverse Effects of Antiepileptic Drugs.* Raven Press, pp. 19–24

Schmidt, D. (1982b). Two antiepileptic drugs for intractable epilepsy with complex partial seizures. *J. Neurol. Neurosurg. Psychiat.*, **45**, 1119–24

Treiman, D. M. and Ben-Menachem, E. (1987). Inhibition of carbamazepine and phenytoin metabolism by nafimidone, a new antiepileptic drug. *Epilepsia*, **28**, 699–705

32
Anxiolytics

B. Musch

Dept of CNS Clinical Research, Rhône-Poulenc Santé, 20 Avenue Raymond Aron, 92165 Antony Cedex, France

INTRODUCTION

Establishing the activity of a drug in a clinical condition implies that the disease or the diseases that the drug is supposed to treat are well defined and that a consensus exists on the clinical features that make the condition recognisable as a disease.

Anxiety can be considered a symptom, a syndrome or merely an exacerbation of a normal emotion elicited by danger. The complexity of definition makes the evaluation of potential therapeutic agents against anxiety difficult in man.

Anxiety is an emotion encountered throughout life and its manifestations are inherent to human life; in this respect, 'normal' anxiety represents a warning signal for the mind, as is the case for pain in respect to the body (Villeneuve, 1979). 'Normal' anxiety can help in coping with the environment and lead to better efficiency. When anxiety reaches a degree at which functioning is impaired, it becomes pathological and deserves treatment.

This definition implies that anxiety exists as a continuum from normal to pathological without substantial qualitative distinction. This attitude was reflected in the first edition of the *Diagnostic and Statistical Manual of Mental Disorders (DSM-I)*, which appeared in 1952, where only three anxiety disorder categories were described. Since then research and achievement at both the clinical and pharmacological levels have substantially contributed to a greater specificity and a better clinical definition of anxiety disorders.

In clinical terms a drug can be considered as having anxiolytic properties if it shows efficacy in patients suffering from anxiety as defined by a complex of mental (nervousness, fear, apprehension, tenseness) and physical symptoms (palpitations, sweating, trembling, etc.), which can appear in variable clusters and can constitute different clinical syndromes or disorders.

The development of a new anxiolytic has to take into consideration the general principles applicable to clinical trials of psychotropic drugs as well as specific issues related to anxiety disorders involving definition of selection criteria, assessment of changes, unmet medical need and regulatory requirements.

In defining the clinical development plan for a new anxiolytic, two sets of guidelines have to be taken into account which have been specifically designed for anxiolytic drugs: the FDA *Guidelines for the Clinical Evaluation of Anti-anxiety Drugs* and the WHO (Regional Office for Europe) *Guidelines for the Clinical Investigation of Anxiolytic Drugs*. These documents represent a working reference for clinical researchers and cover the major topics of investigation for new anxiolytics.

PHARMACOLOGICAL TREATMENT OF ANXIETY

Considerations of the clinical development and evaluation of new anxiolytics have to take into account the present status of the pharmacological treatment of anxiety in terms of existing drugs, therapeutic strategies and unmet medical needs. These factors will influence strategies and choices in developing new anxiolytics.

With the introduction of meprobamate in 1955 and the benzodiazepines in the early 1960s, the pharmacotherapy of anxiety entered a new phase and left behind a long period during which the barbiturates and the bromides (together with alcohol and opiates) represented the only pharmacological relief from anxiety. Subsequent progress in pharmacotherapy has considerably modified concepts and ideas concerning diagnosis and pathophysiology of anxiety and other psychiatric disorders. As an example, one can quote the successful use of antidepressants in subtypes of anxiety such as panic disorders which has forced a reconsideration of the nosology of anxiety disorders (Klein, 1981).

Newer anxiolytics have recently been developed: buspirone is the first non-benzodiazepine to reach the market. Existing data suggest lack of dependence potential and of sedation with buspirone; slow onset of action may represent a disadvantage. Alpidem is another non-benzodiazepine anxiolytic recently approved in France; lack of sedation at therapeutic doses together with a rapid onset of action represent its major advantages (Musch *et al.*, 1988).

Antidepressant tricyclics are commonly used in patients with mixed anxiety–depression (Kahn *et al.*, 1986). MAO inhibitors are of some value in treating mixed agoraphobic, phobically anxious and socially phobic patients. Beta-blockers are also used, especially in anxious patients with predominantly somatic complaints (for review see Rickels and Shweizer, 1987).

Benzodiazepines definitely represent the drugs of choice in the pharmacotherapy of anxiety. Although many different benzodiazepines exist for the treatment of anxiety, their differences in terms of efficacy and safety are mainly related to their pharmacokinetic characteristics. Despite their efficacy and established safety, benzodiazepines are not devoid of disadvantages and their use is now under extensive criticism. Benzodiazepines can cause oversedation and impair cognition and memory; their long-term use can induce psychological and physical dependence and patients can experience rebound anxiety and withdrawal symptoms upon discontinuation.

Consequently, two major objectives can be identified for the discovery of new anxiolytic: the possibility of finding (1) pure 'anxiolytic' drugs devoid of 'sedative' effects and (2) anxiolytic drugs which do not induce dependence.

All the existing established anxiolytics possess in animal pharmacology anticonvulsant, muscle-relaxant and hypnosedative properties. In man they are prescribed not only to relieve anxiety, but also, at appropriate dose, as hypnotics, anticonvulsants, myorelaxants or general anaesthetics. This is true for both benzodiazepines and barbiturates. It is commonly believed that with these drugs proper adjustments of doses could induce the desired effect: anxiolytic, sedative or hypnotic. According to the above considerations, the ideal anxiolytic in man (Lehmann, 1969) should have the following characteristics: (1) selective action against anxiety; (2) no action on psychomotor activity or vigilance, or on cognition and memory; (3) no habituation or addiction; (4) lack of toxicity; (5) low dose for an optimum effect. This profile should guide the definition of standard criteria for the evaluation of new anxiolytics.

EARLY TESTING IN HUMANS

The general principles which characterise Phase I studies with potential psychotropics should be followed in the case of a new anxiolytic. These studies will determine human tolerance, pharmacokinetics and metabolism of the new agent.

The safety issue is particularly relevant for anxiolytic drugs, as the risk/benefit ratio has to be particularly favourable in an indication such as anxiety. The assessment of safety for a new drug begins with the first single- and repeated-dose tolerance studies in healthy volunteers. In the case of anxiolytics, as well as with all psychotropics, these early tolerance studies should involve some simple objective tests to measure vigilance and psychomotor coordination. Once the maximum tolerated dose has been established in healthy subjects, more sophisticated clinical pharmacology studies can be performed to assess the possible effects on CNS functions.

As stated above, the possible dissociation between anxiolytic and sedative effect represents a primary objective in the development of new anxiolytics; consequently, it will be necessary to determine carefully to what extent this dissociation can be achieved.

These human pharmacological studies can be classified into three categories: (1) studies assessing psychomotor performances; (2) studies assessing memory; (3) studies assessing CNS effects by means of instrumental neurophysiological techniques (mainly quantitative EEG). Healthy subjects free of anxiety or any other psychiatric conditions are more suitable for these studies than anxious patients.

In any case, it is wise to assess psychomotor performance and memory in patients later in the development of a new anxiolytic, to investigate the impact of the drug on the normal functioning of patients.

Tests in patients should be restricted in number and should be easy to administer. Feasibility is an essential issue in testing CNS effects.

As stated above, these studies are aimed to assess at which doses a new drug can be considered devoid of detrimental effect on psychomotor performance, cognition and memory. Single- and multiple-dose studies, up to a sufficient number of days at which steady state can be obtained, are to be performed using placebo and verum, possibly at doses which can be considered therapeutically active.

Cross-over design rather than parallel groups can better control intrasubject and intersubject variability.

The following tests can be considered particularly useful and are listed according to the function they are supposed to test (Vogel, 1979).

Measures of simple reflexes   finger tapping speed (FTS); simple reaction time (SRT).

Measures of cortical function   critical flicker fusion threshold (CFF). This test appears to be a particularly reliable measure of the changes produced by antianxiety drugs, especially in the sense of a sedative versus stimulant effect (Hindmarch, 1988).

Measures of perceptual motor performance   tracing performance; pursuit meter performance; driving and simulated driving performance; complex performance.

Measures of decision making   sorting performance; choice reaction time.

Tests of concentration   In this group the most commonly used is the Digit Symbol Substitution Test, derived from the Weschler Adult Intelligence Schedule.

Quantitative EEG studies are of some help in establishing sedative effects, time-course of central effects and comparative estimation of EEG profile with existing drugs (Itil, 1979; Saletu, 1987), as are studies employing evoked potentials (Saletu, 1979).

Considering the importance of sleep in daytime well-being, a sleep laboratory study with the new drug in healthy non-insomniac subjects can be of some relevance, especially in terms of comparison with existing anxiolytics which are known to modify sleep patterns.

Phase I studies have to assess pharmacokinetics and metabolism. The ideal anxiolytic should be rapidly absorbed and peak plasma level should be reached soon to ensure a rapid onset of action: anxiety is a clinical condition which needs to be treated rapidly.

Interaction studies represent an important phase in the evaluation of new anxiolytics. Interactions should be studied at both the pharmacokinetic and pharmacodynamic levels. Pharmacodynamic interaction studies are particularly meaningful in the case of psychotropic drugs such as antidepressants and hypnotics, which are frequently associated with anxiolytics. Alcohol interaction studies are mandatory in the case of anxiolytic drugs, because of the widespread alcohol intake among anxious patients.

PREDICTIVE MODELS FOR ANXIOLYTIC ACTIVITY IN HUMANS

Animal models for the screening of drugs are scarcely predictive of the therapeutic effect. Consequently, some research has been devoted to the discovery of techniques in man which, by resembling clinical psychiatric conditions, could represent a predictive model for drug activity in patients. It was at the end of the 1950s and during the 1960s that these techniques were developed, particularly in the field of anxiety by including stress situation or anxious reactions in subjects free of psychiatric diseases. Strategies in developing human models for prediction of antianxiety activity with new drugs have been extensively reviewed by Janke *et al.* (1979).

The first approach was to use 'emotionality', as established by personalities inventories, as a modifier of response to drugs. In this approach subjects for experimental trials were assessed according to their high or low 'neuroticism' level (Barrett and Di Mascio, 1966). Subjects with a high level of 'neuroticism' were more sensitive to antianxiety drugs. Similar to the approach of 'neuroticism–emotionality' as modifier of drug response is the theory elaborated by Eysenck (1963) on the role of extraversion–intraversion in predicting individual drug-response differences.

A second strategy consisted of inducing with different stimuli or 'stressers' a situation of 'stress' in which subjects show a high level of 'emotionality' or 'anxiety' which can be sensitive to the effects of drugs. Several stressers were used: noise; ride on a ferris wheel (Laties, 1959); film stressers (Pillard and Fisher, 1967), such as autopsy film; anticipation of painful events (Uhr and Miller, 1959). Findings from this type of study are not really supportive of the predictive value of these stress-induced anxiety models—in fact, several studies did not show significant changes under stress conditions and the drug effect was not specific for anxiolytic drugs but was common to several sedative drugs.

More recently in the development of the new anxiolytic alpidem, life-stress-induced anxiety was used as a condition in which to test the effect of single doses of the drug. Stress situations were represented by cardiac catheterisation, minor surgical operation and gastroscopy. Patients were free of anxiety disorders and were assessed prior to and 2 h after drug intake. The level of anxiety was assessed by the patient and by the investigator on a series of visual analogue scales. Drug–placebo differences were observed on the scales measuring anxiety and tension but not on those measuring drowsiness and sedation (Musch *et al.*, 1988). These studies can be useful to predict activity and therapeutic dose range, and in any case represent real situations of drug prescription.

STUDIES IN ANXIOUS PATIENTS

Clinical studies in anxious patients are performed in Phase II and Phase III of the clinical development plan. Pilot open studies (early Phase II) are not mandatory in the case of anxiolytic drugs, as anxiety is often self-limiting and sensitive to 'placebo effect'. Nevertheless, open pilot studies, if attentively performed, can be of some utility, especially in terms of early identification of possible side-effects.

The factors that are to be taken into account for Phase II studies can be classified: diagnosis; design; duration of treatment; assessment.

Diagnosis

According to WHO guidelines, the diagnostic criteria to be followed in selecting the patients are quite general: 'patients selected should be suffering from anxiety syndrome of sufficient severity to warrant treatment'.

In the FDA guidelines, considering that anxiety has many different meanings, more specific descriptive diagnostic criteria are suggested: 'anxiety refers to states of manifest anxiety; these states are characterised by the following:

Subjective experiences:

1. Feeling nervous, jittery, jumpy.
2. Feeling fearful, apprehensive, anxious, panicky.
3. Fears of fainting, screaming, losing control, crowds, places, disaster, death.
4. Avoiding certain places, things, or activities because of fear.
5. Feeling tense or keyed up.

Muscular or motor phenomena:

6. Tense, aching muscles.
7. Trembling, shaking.
8. Restlessness, fidgeting.

Autonomic phenomena:

9. Heart beating fast or pounding; chest pain.
10. Trouble catching breath, air hunger, smothering, lump in throat, choking.
11. Sweating, especially armpits, palms, soles of feet.
12. Cold, clammy hands.
13. Dry mouth.
14. Dizziness, faintness, lightheadedness, weakness.
15. Tingling feelings in hands or feet.
16. Stomach "gas", nausea, upset stomach.
17. Frequency or urgency of bladder or bowels.'

Patients selected for trials should show the first two manifestations plus at least three others in the list above. The FDA recommends that quantitatively defined criteria should accompany the qualitative criteria, in the sense that initial scores which exceed certain levels (for instance, in a rating scale) should be stated among the inclusion criteria to document the severity of the illness.

An important diagnostic problem mentioned by the FDA guidelines is the mixture of anxiety and depression. Diagnostic criteria exist to classify patients as primarily anxious or primarily depressed.

FDA diagnostic criteria are an attempt to give a practical and operational approach to the problem of diagnosis and patient selection to researchers dealing with clinical trials in anxiety. They represent a more practical approach than the *DSM-III-R*. Nevertheless, the *DSM-III-R* deserves some comment for its importance in the evolution of the clinical concept of anxiety.

Fyer *et al.* (1987) have extensively reviewed the issue of differential diagnosis and assessment of anxiety. The authors underline how 'the conceptual direction of anxiety research over the past 30 years has been toward ever increasing specificity', as can be observed by looking into the conceptual evolution of anxiety in the *DSM*. In the first version of the *DSM* (*DSM-I*, 1952) only three anxiety disorder categories were identified. In the 1960s research in the field of phobia and panic attacks allowed a more specific differentiation between generalised anxiety and other anxiety disorders (Klein, 1981).

As a consequence of this research activity, the Feighner diagnostic criteria published in 1972 (Feighner *et al.*, 1972) produced operational definitions of anxiety neuroses, phobic and obsessive compulsive disorders.

In 1978 Spitzer *et al.* in their Research Dignostic Criteria split anxiety neuroses into panic and generalised anxiety disorders and included four subtypes of phobic disorder (agoraphobia, simple, social, mixed). The third edition of the *DSM*, in 1980, adopted the principles of this nosology, with three further conceptual specifications concerning agoraphobia as a separate disorder, simple and social phobia as two separate disorders and post-traumatic stress disorder as a new entity.

The recent *DSM-III-R* identifies the following anxiety disorders:

Panic disorder with agoraphobia   300.21
Panic disorder without agoraphobia   300.01
Agoraphobia without history of panic disorder   300.22
Social phobia   300.23
Simple phobia   300.29
Obsessive Compulsive Disorder (or Obsessive Compulsive
   Neurosis)   300.30
Post-traumatic Stress Disorder   309.89
Generalised Anxiety Disorder   300.02
Anxiety Disorder not otherwise Specified   300.00

It is of particular relevance for conducting clinical trials in anxiety that in the *DSM-III-R* Generalised Anxiety Disorder (GAD) is no longer considered to be in the anxiety residual category. The *DSM-III-R* requires excessive or unrealistic worry about two or more life circumstances, 6 associated anxiety symptoms out of 18, and a duration of at least 6 months. The issue of 6 month duration is a critical one in term of patient selection for clinical trials. If it is true that the original GAD 4 week duration criterion overlapped with the diagnosis of adjustment reaction, 6 months' duration is a very restrictive criterion which reduces the number of anxious patients who can be recruited if the *DSM-III-R* criteria for GAD are chosen in the protocol: it is difficult to find patients with 6 month duration of their anxiety symptoms who are still suitable for a drug trial. Consequently, it is now considered acceptable to reduce the duration of the disorder to 1 month while using the *DSM-III-R* diagnostic criteria for GAD.

The development of structured interview schedules has contributed to the improvement of reliability of anxiety disorder diagnosis. These interview schedules are of great importance but their use in the practical conditions of a clinical trial in anxiety is not evident.

In conclusion, diagnostic criteria for anxious patients exist and they should be clearly stated in the protocol, to allow conclusions and results interpretations on drug response in different subgroups.

Design

As mentioned above, uncontrolled pilot studies of small sample size can be of some importance in exploring dose activity and side-effects. Subsequently, results from pilot studies will be confirmed or refuted only by controlled double-blind studies. Placebo control is mandatory in the initial double-blind studies, especially in the dose-finding ones. Later in the development active control with or without placebo control will also be used.

Anxiety is a clinical condition particularly sensitive to the 'placebo response' phenomenon, which can affect 60–70% of responders in the placebo-treated group. In this situation the chance of showing a statistically significant difference in the drug effect between placebo and the experimental drug is only theoretical.

In general, because of the fluctuating nature of anxiety, parallel-group design is preferable to cross-over design, although it will imply the use of greater sample size. In dose-finding studies a fixed-dose parallel-group design is preferable to flexible-dose design, to facilitate statistical analysis and interpretation of results.

Sample size should involve 30–50 patients per medication group, according to the FDA guidelines. It is our personal experience that because of the high placebo response effect, especially in studies involving general practitioners and using parallel groups, groups of less than 50 patients will be unlikely to show drug–placebo differences.

In comparative studies involving active control, even greater sample size will be necessary to show differences. The FDA guidelines are strict in stating the number of controlled studies required: five studies with at least 30–50 patients per medication group, given a probability of the drug–placebo response of at least 5%.

Duration of Treatment

The duration of drug administration adequate to show an anxiolytic effect may vary from days to weeks. Basically, a study period of 2–4 weeks should be adequate, although it is recommended that one of the first Phase II studies involve 6 weeks of drug administration.

A drug-free period prior to the study medication is recommended, to exclude pharmacological interactions, and it should take into account the pharmacokinetic characteristics of the previous medication.

Assessments

Several instruments exist nowadays to assess drug-induced changes in anxious patients. It will be difficult to be comprehensive in quoting them.

It is important to remember that some general principles should always be kept in mind when selecting specific measures: feasibility, inter-rater reliability, validity, comprehensiveness of content and sensitivity to changes. Validity should refer also to translations of rating scales into languages different from the original one, considering that trials in anxiety are frequently conducted on a multicentre, multinational basis, to allow recruitment of adequate sample size.

We consider that assessment of efficacy in anxious patients, as is the case in clinical trials with other psychotropic drugs, should involve one global judgement rating in which the overall clinical change of the patient is assessed. For this purpose the Clinical Global Impression (CGI) appears to be particularly useful, easy to use, and sufficiently standardised to be used in several trials to allow 'meta-analysis' of global efficacy based on data collected in different studies. This instrument involves two items scored on a 7 point scale: severity of illness and global improvement. A third item, called 'therapeutic index', is a two-dimensional scale assessing side-effects and therapeutic effect at the same time (ECDEU, 1976).

If is common to see in many protocols that global assessments such as the CGI are used at each visit during a study. We personally think that these global assessments should be used only at the end of the study, in order to give an overall evaluation of the changes in the clinical status of the patients; otherwise the risk exists of referring the changes only to the previous visit and to give a relative judgement and not a judgement referred to the prestudy situation.

Specific instruments for measuring anxiety and drug-induced changes in anxious symptoms exists.

Initially, the measurement of anxiety was based on the Minnesota Multiphasic Personality Inventory (MMPI) (Hathaway and McKinley, 1942). In order to obtain more specific measures of anxiety, several scales were derived from MMPI to deal specifically with anxiety, such as the Taylor Scale of Manifest Anxiety (Taylor, 1951), consisting of 50 MMPI items, the Welsh Anxiety Scale (Welsh, 1956) and the Finney Anxiety Scale (Finney, 1965).

Of a certain historical and methodological importance was the introduction in 1970 of the State–Trait Anxiety Inventory by Spielberger *et al.* (1970). In this scale two separate measures were given for 'state-anxiety' and 'trait-anxiety' according to the theory of Cattel and Scheier (1960). This self-rating scale is particularly adequate in the case of 'symptomatic' volunteers or in 'situational anxiety'.

The above-mentioned scales reflect the 'unidimensional' view of anxiety in which anxiety is seen as a continuum from normal to pathological anxiety. They do not seem particularly sensitive to drug-induced changes.

Parallel to the evolution of the concept of a discontinuity between normal and pathological anxiety, new assessment instruments were developed to quantify levels of pathology in patients with different anxiety disorders. These instruments can be divided into two categories: observer's rating scales and patient's self-reporting scales.

In the first category the most frequently used rating scales are: Hamilton Anxiety Scale (Hamilton, 1959); Brief Outpatient Psychopathology (Free and Guthrie, 1969); Physicians' Questionnaire (Rickels and Howard, 1970); Covi Anxiety Scale (Lipman, 1982); Symptom Rating Test (Kellner and Sheffield, 1973).

Of these, the most widely employed scale is the Hamilton scale. This was one of the first scales to be designed to assess severity of illness in a specific diagnostic group; it contains 13 items which can be grouped for factor-analysis in somatic and psychic factors. It is considered to be the most sensitive to the effects of treatment. Assessment of symptoms covers the clinical state for the last week and therefore should not be performed too frequently. Furthermore, although one item is related to phobias, additional instruments should be used to specifically investigate phobias and panic attacks, if needed.

The second category is represented by patients' self-rating scales, which seem to be particularly adequate for trials in anxiety where patients are usually co-operative and able to self-administer these scales, and where it is important to use scales which are economical of the time of investigators. The trials are usually conducted in outpatients and by general practitioners.

Whether or not these instruments correlate adequately with observer-rated instruments is a matter for discussion (Arfwidsson *et al.*, 1974): Hamilton (1987) underlined that these scales are poorly correlated with observers' scales, because they tend to measure something different, and that they should be regarded as complementary rather than as substrates for observers' scales.

The most commonly employed patients' rating scales are: Profile of Mood States (McNair *et al.*, 1971); General Health Questionnaire (Goldberg and Hillier, 1979); Hopkins Symptom Checklist—HSCL-90 (Derogatis *et al.*, 1974). Of these HSCL-90 is the most used. This self-rating scale covers a wide range of symptoms from which nine subscales (including obsessive–compulsive, depression and anxiety) have been obtained. Apparently the sensitivity resides chiefly in the anxiety and somatisation clusters (Lipman *et al.*, 1969).

Another method of assessment of some interest is the use of target symptom ratings. These ratings provide a 'tailormade' instrument for the individual patient: the prominent symptoms presented by the patients are rated for their intensity before and through the course of treatment. The key symptoms can be selected by the patient or the investigator and assessed by the corresponding observer. Problems of analysis are encountered with this method, especially due to the difficulty in mixing different symptoms.

It has to be mentioned that specific rating scales exist for the different anxiety disorders such as the Panic and Anxiety Attack Scale and the Marks–Sheerhan Phobia Scale (Sheerhan, 1982).

Patient assessment should also take into consideration measures of social adjustment by patient follow-up after re-entry into the community, with emphasis on assessment of prophylactic and maintenance effects of long-term drug treatment.

This survey of assessment methodology in anxiety trials is necessarily incomplete, but gives an idea of the complexity of the assessment of drug-induced changes in anxious patients.

DEPENDENCE AND ABUSE POTENTIAL

The assessment of the dependence and abuse potential of a new drug is a major challenge, especially in the field of anxiolytic drugs. It is well established that barbiturates can induce physical and psychological dependence. Recently this phenomenon has been recognised also for high doses of benzodiazepines given for a prolonged period of time. It has recently been observed that even low therapeutic doses for prolonged periods of time or even for only 4–6 weeks (Fontaine *et al.*, 1984) may produce physical dependence, as is shown by the appearance of withdrawal symptoms (Peturs-son *et al.*, 1981; Tyrer *et al.*, 1983).

Earlier and more marked withdrawal seems to be observed with benzo-diazepines of short half-life (Rickels *et al.*, 1974) although the incidence of patients experiencing withdrawals is similar after benzodiazepines of short and long half-life. Gradual discontinuation seems to reduce the incidence and severity of withdrawal symptoms.

In man the dependence potential is difficult to assess. Nevertheless, some advice can be given on development of a strategy to predict dependence potential with a new drug for anxiety.

The following factors should be taken into account.

Tolerance The development of tolerance to the pharmacological effect over time is one of the causal factors in the drug-dependence phenomenon. Changes in doses over time in studies where a flexible dosage is employed should be accurately recorded, to assess tolerance, especially in long-term trials.

Predictive human models Drug addicts and alcoholics can be used to assess whether the new drug is 'liked' by these subjects and used as a substitute for their usual 'drug'. Cole *et al.* (1982), using users of recreational sedatives, showed that buspirone had a negative abuse potential with respect to metaqualone and diazepam. Griffith *et al.* (1986) found similar results in alcohol-dependent patients, using three different doses of buspirone, 10 mg, 20 mg and 40 mg, and diazepam at 10 mg and 20 mg.

Withdrawal and rebound phenomena The appearance of withdrawal and rebound phenomena should be accurately investigated in clinical trials with anxiolytics, especially in long-term studies. A post-drug assessment period of up to 2–4 weeks should be included in the protocol and should involve:

record of newly observed signs and symptoms;
record of medical actions (for instance, need to restore anxiolytic treatment);
efficacy assessment as during experimental treatment;
use of withdrawal rating scale such as Ashton scale (Ashton *et al.*, 1984); Tyrer Withdrawal Scale (Tyrer *et al.*, 1981); Lader Tranquilliser Withdrawal Scale (Lader *et al.*, 1987).

Considering that the need for a gradual withdrawal to avoid withdrawal symptoms is typical of drugs such as benzodiazepines, studies are suggested in which gradual withdrawal is compared with abrupt withdrawal. The absence of withdrawal or rebound phenomena after both gradual and abrupt withdrawal supports the suggestion of low dependence potential (Lader and Frcka, 1987).

All these approaches can be of some help in predicting the dependence potential and abuse liability of a drug, although only long-term clinical use can give a precise answer.

A new drug which could show anxiolytic properties without oversedation and minimal or no potential for dependence and abuse will definitely represent a breakthrough in the pharmacotherapy of anxiety.

REFERENCES

Arfwidsson, L., D'Ella, G. and Laurell, B. (1974). Can self-rating replace doctors' rating in evaluating anti-depressive treatment? *Acta Psychiat. Scand.*, **50**, 16–22

Ashton, C. M. (1984). Benzodiazepine withdrawal an unfinished story. *Br. Med. J.*, **288**, 1135–40

Barrett, J. E. and Di Mascio, A. (1966). Comparative effects on anxiety of the 'minor tranquilizers' in 'high' and 'low' anxious student volunteers. *Dis. Nerv. Syst.*, **27**, 483–6

Cattell, R. B. and Scheier, J. H. (1960). *The Meaning and Measurement of Neuroticism and Anxiety*. Ronald Press, New York

Cole, J. O., Hecht Orzack, M., Beake, B., Bird, M. and Bartal, Y. (1982). Assessment of the abuse liability of buspirone in recreational sedative users. *J. Clin. Psychiatry*, **43**, 69–74

Derogatis, L. R., Ronald, S., Rickels, K., Uhlenhuth, E. H. and Covi, L. (1974). In Pichot, P. and Olivier-Martin, R. *Psychological Measurements in Psychopharmacology*. Karger, London

ECDEU Assessment Manual DHEW Publication No. (ADM), 1976

Eysenck, H. J. (1963). In Eysenck, H. J. (Ed.), *Experiments with Drugs*. Pergamon Press, Oxford, pp. 1–24

Feighner, J. P., Robins, E., Guze, S. B., Woodruff, R. A., Winokuz, G. and Munoz, R. (1972). Diagnostic criteria for use in psychiatric research. *Arch. Gen. Psychiat.*, **26**, 57–67

Finney, J. C. C. (1965). *Psychol. Rep.*, **17**, 707–13

Fontaine, R., Chouinard, G. and Annable, L. (1984). *Am. J. Psychiat.*, **141**, 848–52

Free, S. M. and Guthrie, M. B. (1969). *J. Clin. Pharm.*, **9**, 187–94

Fyer, A. J., Mannuzza, S. and Endicott, J. (1987). In Meltzer, H. Y. (Ed.), *Psychopharmacology: The Third Generation of Progress*. Raven Press, New York, pp. 1177–91

Goldberg, D. P. and Hillier, V. F. (1979). A scaled version of the General Health Questionnaire. *Psychol. Med.*, **9**, 139–45

Griffith, J. D., Jasinski, D. R., Casten, G. P. and McKinley, G. R. (1986). Investigation of the abuse liability of buspirone in alcohol dependent patients. *Am J. Med.*, **80** (Suppl. 3B), 30–5

Hamilton, M. (1959). The assessment of anxiety states by rating. *Br. J. Med. Psychol.*, **32**, 50–5

Hamilton, M. (1987). In Hindmarch, I. and Stonier, P. D. (Eds.), *Human Psychopharmacology, Measures and Methods*, Vol. 1. John Wiley, Chichester, pp. 1–17

Hathaway, S. R. and McKinley, J. C. (1942). *The Minnesota Multiphasic Personality Inventory*. University of Minnesota Press, Minneapolis

Hindmarch, I. (1988). Critical Flicker Fusion Frequency (CFF): the effects of psychotropic compounds. *Pharmacopsychiatria*, **15**, 44–8

Itil, T. M. and Huque, M. (1979). In Fielding, S. and Lal, H. (Eds.), *Anxiolytics*. Futura, New York, pp. 281–315

Janke, W., Debus, G. and Longo, N. (1979). In Boisser, J. R. (Ed.), *Differential Psychopharmacology of Anxiolytics and Sedatives* (Modern Problems of pharmacopsychiatry). Karger, Basle, pp. 13–98

Kahn, R. J., McNair, D. M., Lipman, R. S., Covi, L., Rickels, K., Downing, R., Fisher, S. and Frankenthaler, L. M. (1986). *Arch. Gen. Psychiat.*, **43**, 79–85

Kellner, R. and Sheffield, B. F. (1973). A self-rating scale of distress. *Psychol. Med.*, **3**, 88–100

Klein, D. F. (1981). In Klein, D. F. and Rabkin, J. G. (Eds.), *Anxiety: New Research and Changing Concepts*. Raven Press, New York, pp. 235–263

Lader, M. and Frcka, G. (1987). Subjective effects during administration and on discontinuation of zopiclone and tumazepam in normal subjects. *Pharmacopsychiatria*, **20**, 67–71

Lader, M. and Olajide, D. (1987). A comparison of buspirone and placebo in relieving benzodiazepine withdrawal symptoms. *J. Clin. Psychopharm.*, **7**, 11–15

Laties, V. G. (1959). Effects of meprobamate on fear and palmar sweating. *J. Abnorm. Soc. Psychol.*, **59**, 155–61

Lehman, H. E. (1969. In Cerletti and Bove (Eds.), *The Present Status of Psychotropic Drugs*. Excerpta Medica, Amsterdam, pp. 168–75

Lipman, R. S. (1982). *Psychopharm. Bull.*, **18**, 69–77

Lipman, R. S., Rickels, K., Covi, L., Derogatis, L. R. and Uhlenhuth, E. H. (1969). Factors of symptom distress. Doctor ratings of anxious neurotic outpatients. *Arch. Gen. Psychiat.*, **21**, 328–38

McNair, D. M., Lorr, M. and Droppleman, L. F. (1971). *Manual: Profile of Mood States*. Educational and Industrial Testing Services, San Diego

Musch, B., Morselli, P. L. and Priore, P. (1988). Clinical studies with the new anxiolytic alpidem in anxious patients: an overview of the European experiences. *Pharm. Biochem. Behav.*, **29**, 803–6

Petursson, H. and Lader, M. H. (1981). Benzodiazepine dependence. *Br. J. Addict.*, **76**, 133–45

Pillard, R. C. and Fisher, S. (1967). Effects of chlordiazepoxide and secobarbital on film induced anxiety. *Psychopharmacologia*, **12**, 18–23

Rickels, K., Csanalosi, I., Chung, H., Case, W. G., Pereira-Ogan, J. A. and Downing, R. W. (1974). *Am. J. Psychiat.*, **131**, 25–30

Rickels, K. and Howard, K. (1970). *Psychopharmacologia.*, **17**, 338–44

Rickels, K. and Schweizer, E. E. (1987). In Meltzer, Y. (Ed.), *Psychopharmacology: The Third Generation of Progress*. Raven Press, New York, pp. 1193–203

Saletu, B. (1979). In Fielding, S. and Lal, H. (Eds.), *Anxiolytics*. Futura, New York, pp. 317–41

Saletu, B. (1987). In Hindmarch, I. and Stonier, P. D. (Eds.), *Human Psychopharmacology, Measures and Methods*, Vol. 1. John Wiley, Chichester, pp. 173–200

Sheerhan, D. V. (1982). *New Engl. J. Med.*, **307**, 156–8

Spielberger, C. D., Gorsuch, R. L. and Lushene, R. E. (1970). *Manual for the State-Trait Anxiety Inventory*. Consulting Psychologist Press, Palo Alto

Spitzer, R. L., Endicott, J. and Robins, E. (1978). *Arch. Gen. Psychiat.*, **35**, 773–82

Taylor, J. A. (1951). *J. Exp. Psychol.*, **42**, 183–8

Tyrer, P., Rutherford, D. and Huggett, T. (1981). Benzodiazepine withdrawal symptoms and propanolol. *Lancet*, **1**, 520–2

Uhr, L. and Miller, J. G. (1959). Experimentally determined effects of envylcamate on performance, autonomic response, and subjective reactions under stress. *Ann. J. Med. Sci.*, **240**, 204–11

Villeneuve, A. (1979). In Boisser, J. R. (Ed.), *Differential Psychopharmacology of Anxiolytics and Sedative* (Modern Problems of Pharmacopsychiatry). Karger, Basle, pp. 1–12

Vogel, J. R. (1979). In Fielding, S. and Lal, H. (Eds.), *Anxiolytics*. Futura, New York, pp. 343–73

Welsh, G. S. (1956). In Welsh, G. S. and Dahlstrom, W. G. (Eds.), *Basic Readings on the MMPI in Psychology and Medicine*. University of Minnesota Press, Minneapolis, pp. 264–81

33
Hypnotics

G. R. McClelland and P. J. Summerfield

Medical Affairs Dept, Roche Products Ltd, PO Box 8, Welwyn Garden City,
Herts AL7 3AY, UK

INTRODUCTION

The term 'hypnotic' is derived from the Greek *hypnos*, meaning 'sleep'. A
hypnotic drug produces drowsiness and promotes the onset and maintenance
of sleep. The sleep induced by hypnotic drugs does not resemble the artificial
state of suggestibility known as hypnosis. Sedation, sleep and general
anaesthesia are generally regarded as being part of the same continuum of
central nervous system depression. Thus, high doses of most hypnotic drugs
can induce general anaesthesia.

As hypnotics are capable of producing a general central nervous system
depression, they are often indicated for the treatment of anxiety, epilepsy and
disorders of increased muscle tone, and to produce amnesia and general
anaesthesia. However, this chapter will concentrate on the use of hypnotics in
the treatment of sleep disorders.

There are many ways in which sleep disorders (dysomnias) have been
classified. The four general headings used by the *Diagnostic and Statistical
Manual* (*DSM-III-R*) produced by the American Psychiatric Association, and
by the World Health Organization in the *International Classification of
Diseases* (*ICD-9CM*) and 'Guidelines for the clinical investigation of psychotropic drugs' (1986), are as follows: (1) disorders of initiation of and
maintaining sleep (insomnia); (2) disorders of excessive somnolence (hyper-
somnia); (3) disorders of the sleep–wake cycle; (4) dysfunctions associated
with sleep, sleep stages or partial arousals (parasomnia). Hypnotics are
suitable for study in the treatment of insomnia only.

The pharmacological treatment of insomnia, and the social abuse of such
compounds, dates back many centuries, and initially included opiates and
alcohol. Towards the end of the nineteenth century more specific compounds,
such as bromide, chloral hydrate, paraldehyde and urethane, were introduced. At the beginning of the twentieth century the barbiturates were
discovered, and formed the main treatment of insomnia for the next 60 years.

In the early 1960s chlordiazepoxide was introduced, rapidly followed by a
large number of other benzodiazepines. Their acute efficacy and safety meant
that the benzodiazepines quickly displaced the barbiturates as the treatment
of choice for insomnia. However, the existing hypnotics do produce a
pharmacological tolerance (i.e. a progressive reduction in efficacy with

duration of dosing), which limits their continued use in the treatment of insomnia for prolonged periods (Kales *et al.*, 1977). Existing benzodiazepines have also been reported widely to produce a rebound insomnia and other physiological and psychological disturbances (Kales *et al.*, 1983; Lader and Lawson, 1987), upon withdrawal.

Several new hypnotics are currently in the late stages of clinical development, and include compounds which are structurally unrelated to benzodiazepines or barbiturates, but are agonists at the benzodiazepine receptor complex, such as zolpidem and zopiclone. Further benzodiazepines, such as midazolam and quazepam, are also being developed as hypnotics.

This chapter will describe the particular investigations that need to be performed in the early clinical evaluation of new hypnotics, both in healthy, non-patient volunteers and in patients.

PHARMACOKINETIC ASSESSMENT

The ideal hypnotic for the treatment of most insomnias would be a drug which produces a rapid onset of sleep, promotes the maintenance of sleep for a short period and then allows an immediate return to normal wake activity. At present no such compound is available. Some insomnias, such as insomnia related to psychiatric disorders, may require a different pharmacodynamic profile, involving a prolonged anxiolytic action but with minimal daytime sedation.

Pharmacokinetic data are therefore particularly valuable in the early clinical evaluation of hypnotics. A new hypnotic for potential use in the treatment of situational or transient insomnia must have a reasonable oral bioavailability, with a rapid rate of absorption. Measurement of plasma concentration will reveal distribution to the highly vascular tissues. The brain is a highly vascular organ and hypnotics should be able to cross the blood–brain barrier with ease. Thus, plasma concentration should parallel brain concentration.

After absorption the drug is distributed to the poorly vascularised tissues, such as voluntary muscle, and then eliminated by metabolism and excretion. The duration of pharmacodynamic activity is generally determined by the drug concentration in the brain, with the therapeutic effect ceasing when the concentration falls below a threshold. If this threshold is passed during the distribution phase, then the pharmacodynamic effect of a single dose will be short. If the threshold is passed during the elimination phase, then the pharmacodynamic effect should parallel the elimination half-life.

Another pharmacokinetic variable, important in the early volunteer studies, is the possibility of accumulation. Hypnotics are often taken for periods of days, if not weeks, and therefore drugs with a long elimination half-life will accumulate.

The formation of active metabolites may be particularly important to both the duration of drug effect and the possibility of accumulation. Flurazepam, for instance, has a plasma half-life of 2–3 h; however, its active metabolite

N-desalkyl flurazepam has a half-life of approximately 100 h (Jochemsen *et al.*, 1983). It may therefore be useful to measure plasma concentrations of active metabolites early in a hypnotic's clinical development.

Such pharmacokinetic data are not always predictive of the incidence or severity of residual daytime impairment (Harvey, 1985). For instance, temazepam has an elimination half-life of approximately 10 h, yet a 20 mg oral dose has been reported to cause no residual sequelae after overnight ingestion (Nicholson, 1986). Thus, pharmacokinetic data on the parent compound can provide valuable supporting information in early volunteer studies. However, they cannot replace the use of sensitive, objective, pharmacodynamic assessments.

PHARMACODYNAMIC ASSESSMENT—HEALTHY VOLUNTEERS

It is difficult to extrapolate from healthy volunteers to patients with most psychotropic drugs, as the intended therapeutic effect is difficult to identify by an action in an unimpaired subject. Hypnotics are probably the easiest of psychotropic drugs to study in normal subjects, as the intended therapeutic action (sedation) can be observed and quantified. Assessment of central nervous system function is therefore worth while at an early stage in clinical development.

Psychomotor Function

It is important that the objective and subjective measurements of central nervous system function be sensitive and reproducible. There are many tests that have been used to assess sedation in man. Hindmarch (1980), in a relatively limited review, lists over 50 such tests. It is inappropriate to use only one or two tests which measure a restricted range of central nervous system functions. A full battery of tests should be employed to cover the range of functions, and ought to include assessment of alertness, cognitive function, reaction times and memory (WHO, 1986).

Different tasks are more sensitive than others to different psychotropic drugs. McClelland and Jackson (1987) studied a range of psychotropic drugs on a broad battery of tests, and found that the two drugs studied with hypnotic properties, amylobarbitone and oxazepam, could be differentiated clearly from other classes of psychotropics. The objective tests most sensitive to these hypnotics were choice reaction time, a rapid information processing task and a manipulative motor task: least sensitive were digit span and elapsing time estimation.

The effect of amylobarbitone on a rapid information processing task, which involved the identification of concurrent pairs of letters of the alphabet which were being visually presented singly at the rate of one per second, is shown in Figure 33.1. Both motor (as shown by the response time) and cognitive (as

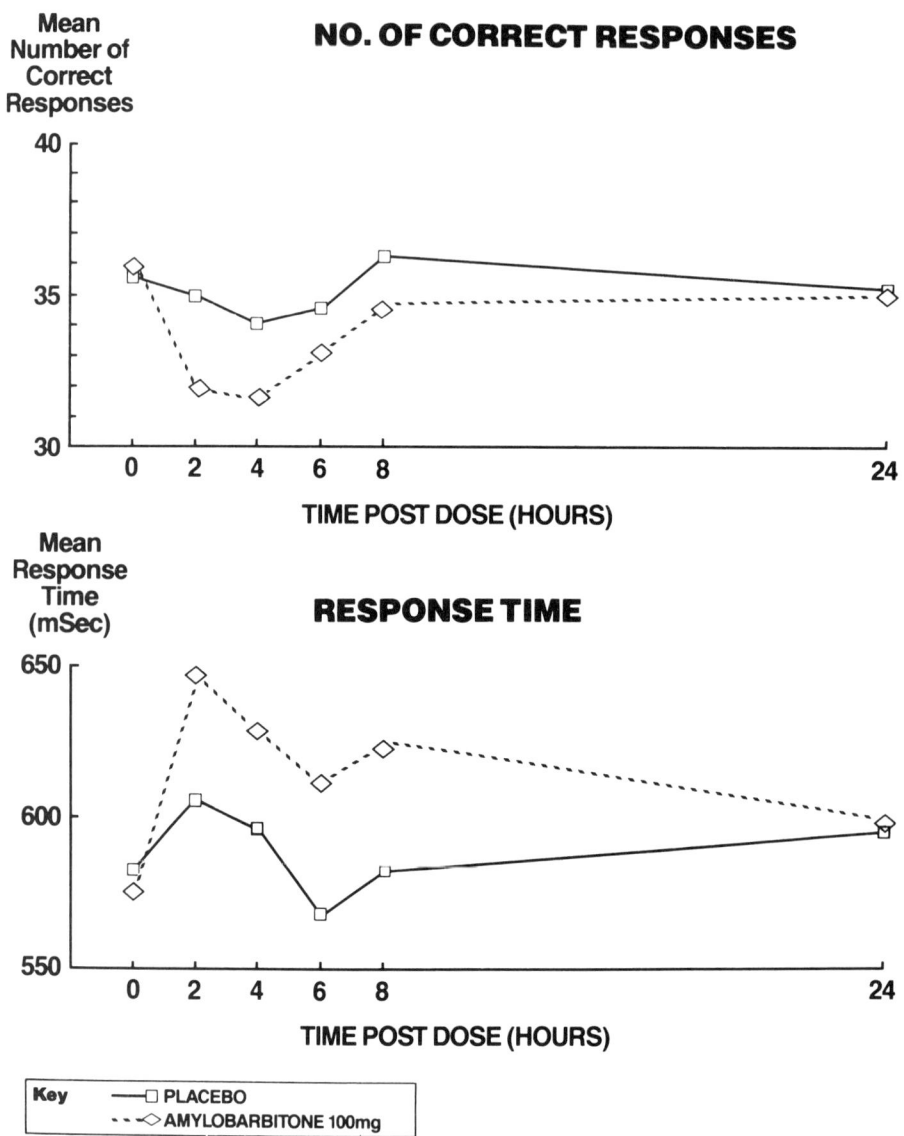

Figure 33.1 The effect of amylobarbitone on a rapid information processing task, after oral administration to 12 normal volunteers (from McClelland and Raptopoulos, 1986)

shown by the number of correct responses) function were clearly impaired in a time-dependent fashion.

Subjective assessments, particularly visual analogue scales (i.e. a 10 cm horizontal line with opposite adjectives at either end, and the subject having

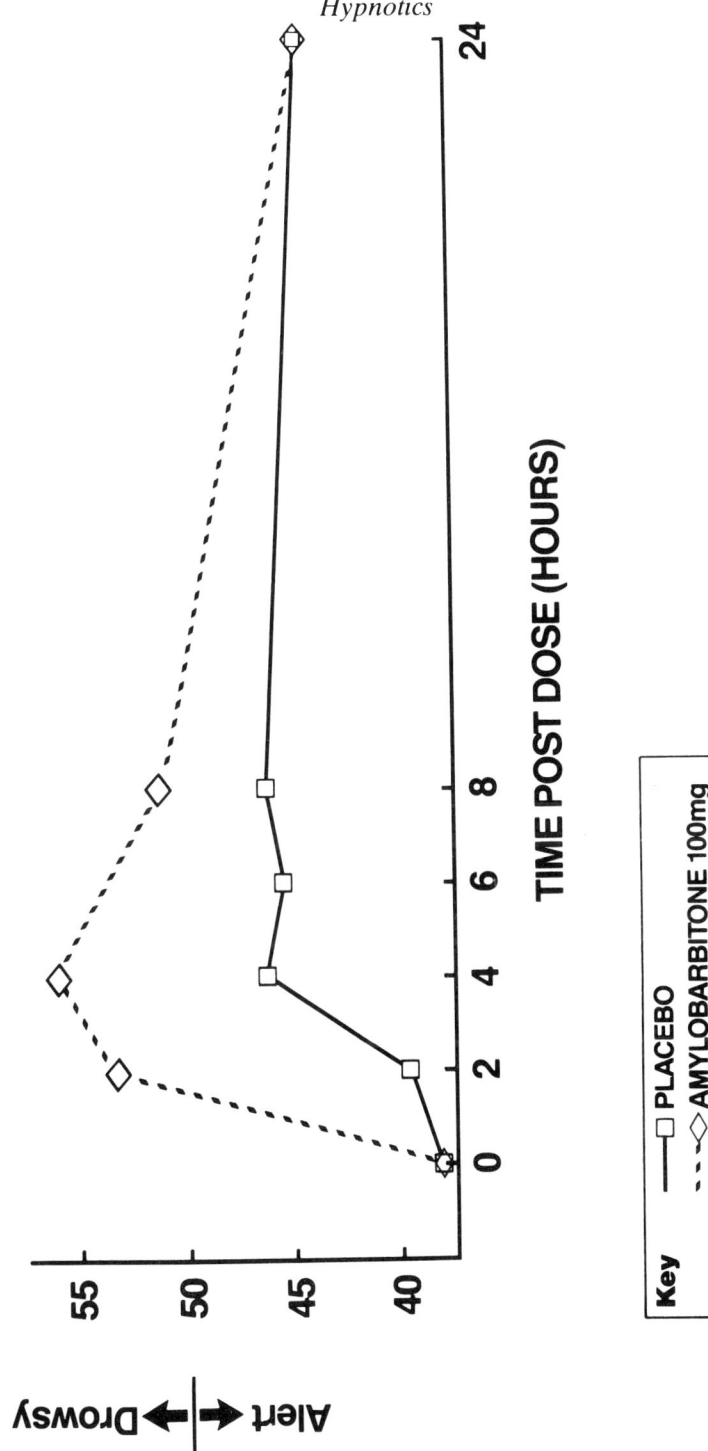

Figure 33.2 The effect of amylobarbitone on a bipolar visual analogue scale for alert/drowsy after oral administration to 12 normal volunteers (from McClelland and Raptopoulos, 1986)

to mark the line at a point which represents their current feeling), are often more sensitive to sedative drug effects than objective measures (Bond and Lader, 1973). It is, therefore, important that subjective measures be included in any test battery (Hindmarch, 1980). Figure 33.2 shows the effect of amylobarbitone on a bipolar visual analogue scale for alert/drowsy. The time-course of this subjective effect parallels the objective effects shown in Figure 33.1.

These objective and subjective measures of central nervous system function are clearly useful in providing information on the onset and duration of sedative effect. They can also be used to produce dose–response curves such that the minimum effective dose is established. Another advantage with the use of a test battery is that any new potential psychotropic drug can be compared with standard drugs previously studied. Thus, further support to preclinical data suggesting potential therapeutic utility in the treatment of insomnia can be provided.

Mode of Action

Information on the possible mode of action of new hypnotics can be gained during these early clinical studies, by using specific pharmacological tools. Flumazenil is a specific benzodiazepine receptor antagonist, with little, if any, intrinsic activity in normal subjects (Brogden and Goa, 1988). Flumazenil can be used to prevent or reverse the effects of a new hypnotic, and thus reveal any central benzodiazepine receptor agonistic activity.

Electroencephalography

The computer-analysed (or quantitative) electroencephalogram (EEG) has been used to study psychotropic drugs following the pioneering work of Fink (1969) and Itil (1974) during the 1960s. Several workers have now confirmed that the EEG can be used to classify psychoactive drugs (Herrmann, 1982) by their action on the different EEG frequencies, and study the time-course of central nervous system effect (Fink, 1982). There are examples, such as nomifensine, where the EEG changes do not correlate with pharmacokinetics (Saletu *et al.*, 1982). However, this work by Saletu and co-workers on nomifensine and benzodiazepines showed that psychometric measures correlated with the EEG rather than the pharmacokinetics, thus emphasising the relative importance of pharmacodynamic assessment of psychotropic drugs.

Sleep Studies

Sleep studies in healthy volunteers can provide useful data, prior to patient studies. The relative homogeneity of the normal volunteer population, and possible reduced study anxiety levels, does mean that studies of hypnotics on sleep can be performed with fewer subjects than in an insomniac patient population. Such studies should include basic measures such as onset of sleep, speed of awakening, number of night-time awakenings and volunteers' subjective assessment of sleep quality. Subjective measures particularly useful are visual analogue scales, as in the Leeds Sleep Evaluation Questionnaire (Parrott and Hindmarch, 1978). EEG recordings can provide objective measures of the onset and offset of sleep, time spent in each of the four sleep stages and amount of REM sleep.

Normal Elderly

Insomnia is more commonly reported in the elderly than the young (Bixler *et al.*, 1979) and they are twice as likely to be receiving a hypnotic (Lader, 1986). In addition, ageing is associated with an increased sensitivity to, and prolongation of activity of, most psychotropic drugs (Lader, 1986). It is, therefore, important to compare the pharmacokinetics and pharmacodynamics of new hypnotics in normal elderly subjects with those in young subjects.

Studies of a possible induction of hepatic drug-metabolising enzymes and of plasma protein binding may be necessary where there are chemical, pharmacological or clinical reasons for believing that an interaction could occur.

Safety

Included in all studies with new hypnotics should be routine physical and cardiovascular assessments, meticulous recording of adverse events and standard laboratory analyses of blood and urine.

Other areas that require specific investigation for new hypnotics include the existence of any 'hangover' effect (i.e. impaired performance the morning after night-time administration). Such studies should employ a battery of tests of performance similar to those used in the acute measurement of volunteers.

Ataxia is a common side-effect of many hypnotics and may be related to an increase in potentially hazardous falls, particularly in the elderly (Swift, 1984; Ray *et al.*, 1987). Body sway can be objectively measured by various methods including a balance platform, and is sensitive to the effects of alcohol and benzodiazepines (McClelland, 1989). The inclusion of an objective measurement of body sway in early volunteer studies may, therefore, determine the extent of this undesirable side-effect.

Tolerance, Rebound and Withdrawal

Hypnotics can produce pharmacological tolerance with repeated administration and rebound actions upon withdrawal. Studies to investigate such potential problems can be performed in normal subjects. However, even the desired therapeutic effects of hypnotics are not always clearly shown in normal subjects (Stanley *et al.*, 1987), let alone any possible tolerance or rebound (Lee and Lader, 1988). An explanation provided by Lee and Lader for their inability to demonstrate rebound with the benzodiazepines quazepam and triazolam was that such effects are difficult to demonstrate in normal subjects, in contrast to insomniacs. The use of standardised, validated, sensitive rating scales, such as that developed by Merz and Ballmer (1983), might provide valuable information on withdrawal potential in volunteers.

Interaction Studies

Hypnotics are commonly taken with other drugs, particularly in the elderly. It is likely that hypnotics will have an additive effect with other drugs having a sedative action, and with alcohol. However, interactions between hypnotics and drugs other than alcohol and psychotropics are uncommon, and of little clinical significance (Lader, 1986).

The main interaction study that must be performed is with alcohol, so that the extent of interaction can be determined.

PHARMACODYNAMIC ASSESSMENT—PATIENTS

Study Design

The initial studies in patients will be performed in young insomniacs who are in all other respects healthy. Such studies start with the intensive monitoring of the effects of single doses before progressing to repeated administration. The main purpose of these initial studies is to define the therapeutic range for investigation in later Phase II and Phase III studies.

The inclusion of healthy elderly subjects in early studies will enable the elderly to be included in late Phase II studies. As the elderly often receive several other medications, it is also important to assess any possible drug interactions before commencing large multicentre trials. While most interaction studies can be performed in animals and any potential interaction can be assessed in normal subjects, some interaction studies have to be performed in patients (e.g. interaction with digoxin).

As with most psychiatric conditions, there is a significant placebo response in the treatment of insomnia (Spinweber and Johnson, 1982). It is, therefore, vital that a matched placebo be included in most, if not all, patient studies. A positive control in the form of an established hypnotic will assist in the evaluation of relative efficacy and safety.

The two main designs used in clinical trials are parallel and cross-over. Each has advantages and disadvantages. In the treatment of insomnia there is often a significant carry-over effect between the two arms of cross-over studies, and this results in the efficacy data from the second period being excluded from statistical analysis, thus effectively reducing the study to a parallel design. It is, therefore, proposed that the optimal general trial design of hypnotics is a parallel study of two (or more) doses of the hypnotic, against placebo and a standard.

Studies performed in sleep laboratories are often restricted to short duration of dosing; however, in clinical practice hypnotics are often pre-scribed for up to 1 month and some patients do receive long-term treatment for many months or years. The main clinical trials should be performed with treatment periods of up to 4 weeks. However, it has been recommended that studies of prolonged treatment, for up to a year, be performed (WHO, 1986).

Tolerance

During periods of prolonged treatment, tolerance to the efficacy of a hypnotic can develop. The reduction in efficacy can appear after just 2 weeks' treatment (Kales *et al.*, 1977). Therefore, careful monitoring of efficacy during repeat-dose studies is important.

Withdrawal Reactions and Rebound Insomnia

Upon cessation of any drug treatment, rebound effects are not uncommon. This is also true of hypnotics, and it has been suggested by Lader and Lawson (1987) that for benzodiazepines rebound insomnia is related to rebound anxiety and withdrawal syndromes. Others (e.g. Feely and Haigh, 1988) have suggested that tolerance and dependency result from the same adaptive mechanisms. However, Reynolds *et al.* (1988) have shown that administration of the benzodiazepine clobazam can result in a tolerance to its anticonvulsant property but not produce dependence (i.e. withdrawal reactions). Thus, tolerance is independent of dependence.

It is, therefore, important that studies with new hypnotics assess both tolerance and dependence. The most frequently reported effects of existing hypnotics upon withdrawal, apart from rebound insomnia, include: anxiety, depression, somatic symptoms such as muscle trembling and muscle pain, malaise, weight loss, sweating, perceptual disturbance, sensory intolerance, hallucinations, psychosis and seizures (Schmauss *et al.*, 1987; Duncan, 1988).

The occurrence of any of these withdrawal reactions must be carefully monitored for any new hypnotic. The Food and Drugs Administration in the USA recommends 3 nights' monitoring after cessation of treatment, to assess any rebound insomnia (FDA, 1977). However, longer periods (at least 2 weeks) of monitoring are required, to study all aspects of potential withdraw-al problems.

Spontaneous reporting of withdrawal symptoms may lead to great differ-ences between investigators in frequency of occurrence. Therefore, a standar-dised method of assessment is advisable, such as the Withdrawal Symptom Scale which has been developed by Merz and Ballmer (1983) and used both in a normal population and, together with the Withdrawal Symptom Question-naire (developed by Dr Peter Tyrer), in benzodiazepine-treated patients (Schmauss *et al.*, 1987).

Pharmacokinetic and Pharmacodynamic Assessments

Since hypnotics are widely used in the elderly, many patients will be suffering from some degree of impairment of renal and/or hepatic function. As a minimum, it is necessary to study the pharmacokinetics of any hypnotic in groups of patients with well-characterised hepatic and renal impairment. The pharmacodynamic measures used in patient studies, both objective and subjective, are essentially those discussed earlier for non-patient volunteers.

Sleep studies in the laboratory are clearly an important part of the early patient studies; however, for longer-term studies it is impractical to keep patients in a laboratory, and it may be necessary to have a longer baseline period for patients than with volunteers. It will also be necessary to characterise the type and extent of insomnia each patient suffers from. It can be argued that laboratory studies do provide an artificial environment, and although studies with the patient at home must rely on subjective assessments, this is the clinical situation. One way in which this difficulty in obtaining objective sleep measures in clinical trials can be solved is to use ambulatory EEG recorders either with standard visual inspection or with automated analysers.

REFERENCES

Bixler, E. O., Kales, A., Soldatos, C. R., Kales, J. D. and Healey, S. (1979). Prevalence of sleep disorders in the Los Angeles metropolitan area. *Am. J. Psychiat.*, **136**, 1257–62

Bond, A. J. and Lader, M. H. (1973). The residual effects of flurazepam. *Psychopharmacology*, **32**, 223–35

Brogden, R. N. and Goa, K. L. (1988). Flumazenil. A preliminary review of its benzodiazepine antagonist properties, intrinsic activity and therapeutic use. *Drugs*, **35**, 448–67

Duncan, J. (1988). Neuropsychiatric aspects of sedative drug withdrawal. *Hum. Psychopharm.*, **3**, 171–80

FDA (1977). *Guidelines for the Clinical Evaluation of Hypnotic Drugs*. US Government Printing Office, Washington D.C.

Feely, M. P. and Haigh, J. R. M. (1988). Differences between benzodiazepines. *Lancet*, **i**, 1460

Fink, M. (1969). EEG and human psychopharmacology. *Ann. Rev. Pharmac.*, **9**, 241–58

Fink, M. (1982). Quantitative pharmaco-EEG to establish dose–time relations in clinical pharmacology. In Herrmann, W. M. (Ed.), *Electroencephalography in Drug Research*. Gustav Fischer, Stuttgart

Harvey, S. C. (1985). Hypnotics and sedatives. In Goodman Gilman, A., Goodman, L. S., Rall, W. and Murad, F. (Eds.), *The Pharmacological Basis of Therapeutics*, 7th edn. Macmillan, New York

Herrmann, W. M. (1982). Development and critical evaluation of an objective procedure for the electroencephalographic classification of psychotropic drugs. In Herrmann, W. M. (Ed.), *Electroencephalography in Drug Research*. Gustav Fischer, Stuttgart

Hindmarch, I. (1980). Psychomotor function and psychoactive drugs. *Br. J. Clin. Pharm.*, **10**, 189–209

Itil, T. M. (1974). Quantitative pharmacoelectroencephalography. Use of computerised cerebral biopotentials in psychotropic drug research. In Itil, T. M. (Ed.), *Modern Problems of Pharmacopsychiatry*. Vol. 8: *Psychotropic Drugs and the Human EEG*. Karger, Basle

Jochemsen, R., van Boxtel, C. J., Hermans, J. and Breimer, D. D. (1983). Pharmacokinetics of 5-benzodiazepine hypnotics in the same panel of healthy subjects. In *Clinical Pharmacokinetics of 5-Benzodiazepine Hypnotics*. R. Jochemsen Doc.Disc. J. H. Pasmans, The Hague

Kales, A., Bixler, E. O., Kales, J. D. and Scharf, M. B. (1977). Comparative effectiveness of nine hypnotic drugs: sleep laboratory studies. *J. Clin. Pharm.*, **17**, 207–13

Kales, A., Soldatos, C. R., Bixler, E. O. and Kales, J. D. (1983). Rebound insomnia and rebound anxiety: A review. *Pharmacol.*, **26**, 121–37

Lader, M. H. (1986). The use of hypnotics and anxiolytics in the elderly. *Int. Clin. Psychopharm.*, **1**, 273–83

Lader, M. H. and Lawson, C. (1987). Sleep studies and rebound insomnia: methodological problems, laboratory findings and clinical implications. *Clin. Neuropharm.*, **10**, 291–312

Lee, A. and Lader, M. (1988). Tolerance and rebound during and after short-term administration of quazepam, triazolam and placebo to healthy human volunteers. *Int. Clin. Psychopharm.*, **3**, 31–47

McClelland, G. R. (1989). Body sway and psychoactive drugs: a review. *Hum. Psychopharm*, **4**, 3–15

McClelland, G. R. and Jackson, D. (1987). Automated testing of the effects of drugs on cognitive function. Presented at *XIth International Meeting of Pharmaceutical Physicians, Brighton*

McClelland, G. R. and Raptopoulos, P. (1986). Paroxetine and amylobarbitone, effects on psychomotor performance. *Br. J. Clin. Pharm.*, **22**, 227P–228P

Merz, W. A. and Ballmer, W. (1983). Symptoms of barbiturate/benzodiazepine withdrawal syndrome in healthy volunteers: standardised assessment by a newly developed self-rating scale. *J. Psychoactive Drugs*, **15**, 71–84

Nicholson, A. N. (1986). Hypnotics and transient insomnia. In O'Hanlon, J. F. and de Gier, J. J. (Eds.), *Drugs and Driving*. Taylor and Francis, London

Parrott, A. C. and Hindmarch, I. (1978). Factor analysis of a sleep evaluation questionnaire. *Psychiat. Med.*, **8**, 325–9

Ray, W. A., Griffin, M. R., Schaffner, W., Baugh, D. K. and Melton, L. J. (1987). Psychotropic drug use and the risk of hip fracture. *New Engl. J. Med.*, **316**, 363–9

Reynolds, E. H., Heller, A. J. and Ring, H. A. (1988). Clobazam for epilepsy. *Lancet*, **ii**, 565

Saletu, B., Grünberger, J., Taeuber, K. and Nitsche, V. (1982). Relation between pharmacodynamics and -kinetics: EEG and psychometric studies with cinolazepam and nomifensine. In Herrmann, W. M. (Ed.), *Electroencephalography in Drug Research*. Gustav Fischer, Stuttgart

Schmauss, C., Apelt, S. and Emrich, H. M. (1987). Characterization of benzodiazepine withdrawal in high and low dose dependent psychiatric in-patients. *Brain Res. Bull.*, **19**, 393–400

Spinweber, C. L. and Johnson, L. C. (1982). Effects of triazolam (0.5 mg) on sleep, performance, memory and arousal threshold. *Psychopharmacology*, **76**, 5–12

Stanley, R. O., Tiller, J. W. G. and Adrian, J. (1987). The psychomotor effects of single and repeated doses of hypnotic benzodiazepines. *Int. Clin. Psychopharm.*, **2**, 317–23

Swift, C. G. (1984). Postural instability as a measure of sedative drug response. *Br. J. Clin. Pharm.*, **18**, 875–905

WHO (1986). Guidelines for the clinical investigation of psychotropic drugs (WHO). *Pharmacopsychiatria*, **19**, 395–9

34
Antidepressants

Judith L. Siegel,* Zofia E. Dziewanowska† and Harriet Laine*

*Clinical Investigation/Neuropsychiatry, †Clinical Research and Development, Hoffmann-LaRoche Inc., Nutley, NJ 07110-1199, USA

INTRODUCTION

As detailed in the *Diagnostic and Statistical Manual of Mental Disorders III-R* (*DSM-III-R*), major depressive illness, a syndrome of unknown pathophysiology, includes both psychological and physiological characteristics.[1] It has been estimated that 5–6% or roughly 10 million Americans suffer from depression each year.[2] The standard pharmacological treatment of depression, either tricyclic antidepressants (TCAs) or monoamine oxidase inhibitors (MAOIs), fails completely in 30–40% of patients and does not fully control the symptoms in others.[3,4] The more recently developed heterocyclic drugs show no greater efficacy.[4] Additionally, all current therapies are associated with variable side-effects that either limit the tolerated dose within an individual (e.g. anticholinergic effects, sedation) or prevent their use in an entire group of individuals (e.g. cardiotoxicity).[5] A strong need remains for the development of antidepressant drugs that have greater overall efficacy associated with a more broadly acceptable side-effect profile.

At the time a potential antidepressant compound is selected for human testing, certain basic information should be available, including: (1) good characterisation of the potential mechanism of action based on effects on brain neurotransmitters *in vitro* and *in vivo*, (2) promising results in animal screens with proven predictability of antidepressant activity in humans, and (3) animal toxicology to support the basic safety of the new compound. This chapter will describe those early steps that can be taken during clinical testing to determine whether the antidepressant candidate will actually become a viable drug. We have chosen to focus on those issues we believe to be most critical in the decision-making process.

Clinical testing of an antidepressant, like testing of any drug candidate, is conducted in three phases, each designed to answer certain questions and build up confidence in both the safety and the efficacy of the new drug. Phase I testing is designed to establish the safety and tolerability of the new drug, usually in healthy volunteers. Phase II testing is designed to establish the efficacy of the drug in the intended patient population and Phase III testing is designed to extend the demonstration of both safety and efficacy in large populations.

PHASE I TESTING

Historically, Phase I testing in healthy volunteers has been limited to defining safety and tolerability after both single and multiple doses of the test drug. However, this strategy is inefficient in its use of these subjects in defining the potential efficacy, pharmacodynamics and pharmacokinetics of the drug. The potential efficacy and pharmacodynamic effect of a new diuretic, for instance, can be easily assessed by measuring urine output after various doses. The issue is not so clear with psychotropic drugs, where efficacy can really be assessed only in the depressed patient population. However, careful testing in healthy volunteers during Phase I can be useful in beginning to define those other properties of the new drug (both positive and negative) that can help in the decision about whether it will be a viable candidate for development. The overall concepts to be described below, while not unique to the study of antidepressant drugs, have been tailored here to determine those factors that are of critical importance.

A caveat to the above is that the tolerability of psychotropic drugs can differ between healthy volunteers and the intended patient population. It is not uncommon for patients to tolerate significantly higher doses than healthy subjects. Therefore, care should be taken when generalising effects, such as sedation and motor impairment, are obtained at certain doses. However, certain other safety aspects such as cardiotoxicity can be easily generalised.

What types of studies can be done during the Phase I testing of a new antidepressant to provide as much information as possible from single- and multiple-dose studies in healthy volunteers? Summarised below are various types of assessments, some of which can be incorporated into the standard single- and multiple-dose tolerance studies and some of which require separate study. While the information provided by all these assessments can be useful in describing the new antidepressant's profile, all need not necessarily be completed before a decision about whether or not to proceed to Phase II. In any complete Phase I programme, data obtained from the first studies of single doses should be used when designing the later multiple-dose studies.

Safety

Since one of the primary goals in the selection of a new antidepressant drug is to create a better safety profile than exists for current therapies, the definition of the side-effects of the test drug is crucial. For instance, major use-limiting side-effects such as cardiotoxicity of a new tricyclic or heterocyclic, or tyramine potentiation of a MAOI, should be determined. A standard 12-lead electrocardiogram can be used to assess potential cardiotoxicity, such as conduction defects (evidenced as QRS widening). Additionally, other potentially bothersome side-effects such as anticholinergic effects (e.g. dry mouth, blurred vision, constipation), sedation and motor impairment, or hypotensive effects, should be defined. These effects should be studied over the entire range of tolerated doses; special note should be taken of the onset and duration of the symptoms. The side-effect profile obtained after single doses should then be compared with that obtained when the same doses are given multiple times. Do the effects become less intense or wane altogether? Does the onset or duration of the effect change? A decision can then be made as to whether the profile that is obtained is acceptable and offers any benefit over existing therapies. Additionally, information should be obtained on the effect of the new drug on various laboratory parameters. A standard panel is adequate at this point in testing.

Information gained about the side-effect profile of the drug during Phase I can also be used to further optimise the dosing regimen for the Phase II studies. For example, if the new antidepressant produces sedation, one strategy could be to give the largest daily dose at night or to give the only dose at night. If side-effects wane with repeated dosing, a dose titration schedule to achieve optimal dose levels can be developed.

Sometimes, standard drugs of a similar therapeutic class (e.g. imipramine, phenelzine) are tested at one or two therapeutic doses, in parallel groups of subjects during the Phase I studies, in order to obtain a direct comparison of side-effects. This comparison may allow another type of early assessment of whether the new antidepressant meets the desired tolerance profile. More often, however, the new drug is tested on its own, to develop its profile before comparing it with other drugs.

Pharmacokinetics

As with any drug, a preliminary evaluation of the pharmacokinetic parameters should be done during Phase I to start to understand the fate of the drug in the body. Information on the time to achieve peak plasma levels and their magnitude after each dose may provide some insight into the onset and intensity of side-effects. Preliminary definition of such parameters as biological half-life $(t_{\frac{1}{2}})$ after both single and multiple doses can aid in the rational development of future dose regimens.

The major effect compartment for antidepressants is in the brain, not plasma, from which samples for pharmacokinetic determinations are taken. Therefore, care should be taken not to infer duration of antidepressant activity from plasma half-life. The two may not be correlated. Further, while information on drug plasma levels attained after given doses is important, strong correlations between plasma level and antidepressant activity have not been demonstrated. This, again, probably reflects the disparity between brain and plasma activity of antidepressant drugs.

Pharmacodynamics

The Phase I studies in healthy volunteers can also be used (1) to attempt to reproduce the biochemical effects of the new antidepressant that were determined in animals and (2) to describe its effect profile on a variety of dimensions that reflect extensions of its pharmacological activity. Although the methodologies currently available are not without flaws, their combined results can contribute in a significant way to the overall understanding of the drug's effects.

The preclinical biochemical assessment of antidepressant drugs usually focuses on the evaluation of interactions with various biogenic amines. Most antidepressants function to increase the central availability of these amines by either decreasing their rate of metabolism (MAOIs) or inhibiting their rate of reuptake into presynaptic nerve terminals (TCAs or serotonin reuptake inhibitors).

Similar biochemical assessments can be done in healthy volunteers, to attempt to confirm this mechanism of action. However, there are no direct methods available for study of brain levels of the biogenic amines in humans. Those indirect methods that are available (e.g. measurement of cerebrospinal fluid levels of amines and metabolites, measurement of urinary excretion of metabolites) are not sensitive. Results from the assessment of the peripheral effects of antidepressants (e.g. pressor responses to peripherally administered tyramine, norepinephrine or phenylephrine during antidepressant therapy; uptake of monoamines or serotonin into platelets) are also variable. And, unfortunately, none of the above demonstrations of similar biochemical functions has proved predictive of strong antidepressant efficacy in humans. These studies are probably more useful when done together with a clinical trial in an appropriate patient population when changes in levels of amines and metabolites can be correlated with change in severity of depression.

Certain neuroendocrine abnormalities have been associated with depression (e.g. hypersecretion of cortisol and growth hormone, disturbance in the rhythm of ACTH secretion). Levels of these hormones return to normal upon remission of disease. The effects of new antidepressant drugs on the neuroendocrine system can be evaluated in both single- and multiple-dose studies in healthy volunteers. Plasma concentrations of hormones such as prolactin, growth hormone or cortisol can be measured and the results can be compared with a known drug from the same class. Again, the results may be interesting, but have not proved predictive of antidepressant activity. These types of studies, too, are better reserved for later trials in patient populations where changes in neuroendocrine function can be correlated with change in severity of depression.

Electroencephalographic and brain imaging (e.g. PET) studies have been used in healthy volunteers to help characterise the pattern of brain activity and localise the area of distribution in brain, respectively. These results are then compared with results from a known drug, to predict similarity of activity. The methodologies available are still being perfected and as yet have limited predictive capacity.

There are many other dimensions of the pharmacological effects of antidepressant drugs that are potentially important in determining a new drug's viability. Many sensitive tests have been developed to assess the more subtle psychomotor (DSST, Reaction Time, Vigilance, Tracking), cognitive (Serial Subtraction, Reading) and memory (Picture Card Recall, Recall of Word Lists, Digit Span) effects produced by psychoactive drugs. Phase I is an ideal time to gather information on a drug's overall activity based on batteries of these tests: studies in patient populations can be too complicated and time-consuming. The initial choice of which tests to be used in the single-dose study should be based on the preclinical profile of the antidepressant. Results of the single-dose study can then be used to select areas with a need for further testing (e.g. memory impairment, sedation, motor incoordination). Results of these tests can give valuable clues as to potential problem areas, such as an inability to concentrate after a given dose, impairment of co-ordination that could negatively affect either the safety of the patient or patient acceptability. They can also give clues as to potential positive attributes, such as enhancement of memory or vigilance.

Taken together, the results of Phase I studies should provide sufficient information to allow for a clear decision as to whether to continue development of the drug. A decision to discontinue can be made because of gross safety or tolerability problems or more subtle problems such as an unacceptable (although not unsafe) side-effect/pharmacodynamic effect profile. Decisions to continue should be supplemented by preliminary information on pharmacokinetics and pharmacodynamic effects that can be used to help to design the next phase of studies.

PHASE II TESTING

Once the decision has been made to continue development, the drug is tested in the intended population, to determine its efficacy and to start to define the effective dose range. Will the compound be safe and tolerated in the targeted population? Will it be more efficacious than placebo at tolerable doses? Will it be as good as a comparative drug with either increased efficacy or a better side-effect profile? These are the broad questions to be answered during this phase of investigation. Several more specific questions must also be asked. Who is the study population to be treated? How can efficacy be measured? How long should treatment last? How should doses be determined? What study design should be used? Studies should be designed that will result in answers to these questions.

WHO IS THE POPULATION?

Depression is not a single disease but, rather, a varied group of symptoms that manifest themselves differently in different people. An antidepressant has not yet been developed that can effectively treat all forms of this illness. It is crucial that decisions be made regarding what subset(s) of the population belonging to the large category of depression would be likely to benefit from treatment with the new drug before starting clinical testing. Before entry into a study, it is essential to develop as accurate a diagnostic picture as possible of every patient chosen for treatment. The diagnostic tool used, whether or not it is one of the standards (e.g. *DSM-III-R*, *International Classification of*

Diseases — 9[1,6]), should be able to identify as closely as possible those patients belonging to that population that has been selected as potentially benefiting from the drug. Anything less than an accurate diagnosis of each patient in the study population may create a heterogeneous group in which efficacy may be impossible to demonstrate, leading to incorrect interpretation of study results.[7]

For instance, if the drug to be tested is targeted to treat patients with a major depressive episode, each patient should clearly meet the diagnostic criteria set out in *DSM-III-R*. Other types of patient inclusion and exclusion criteria that could affect response to a drug, such as use of concomitant medications or presence of concurrent diseases, should also be delineated.

In an attempt to confirm clinical diagnosis, some researchers have used biological markers. Three have met with the most success: failure of cortisol secretion to be suppressed by dexamethasone, blunted response of thyrotropin to thyrotropin releasing hormone, and a reduced latency for first period of rapid eye-movement sleep. Although the specificity and sensitivity of all have been questioned, biological markers can increase the level of confidence in a compound by supporting results found in clinical studies.[8,9]

Since the main goal of Phase II is to determine whether the new antidepressant is efficacious (that is, provide a decrease in the severity of depression), the patient population selected must be chosen so that amelioration of disease is not only possible, but also demonstrable. In patients with extremely mild depressions amelioration is probable, but difficult to demonstrate because of low severity at the start of treatment. Moreover, efficacy in this population will not give convincing evidence of the utility of the drug in the broader group of depressed patients. The demonstration of efficacy in extremely severe or therapy-resistant depressions, while easy to demonstrate because of high initial severity scores, is unlikely. Failure of the drug to demonstrate efficacy in this group of patients does not preclude its utility in the broader group of depressed patients. It is, therefore, generally useful to choose patients who are at least moderately depressed for the initial studies of new antidepressants.

An important consideration is whether the initial population chosen for study should consist of inpatients or outpatients. Inpatients tend to have more, and more fully expressed, symptoms; a research study can be more easily controlled in a hospital setting. For practical reasons, however, it might be best to enrol outpatients with full awareness of the potential problems, such as non-compliance, use of concomitant medications or the fact that the drug may not be efficacious in patients with more severe disease. In either case, the knowledge of the drug at this point should be used to choose the appropriate target population. In most cases, initial Phase II trials are begun with outpatients. Inpatient trials start later, after some initial demonstration of efficacy.

WHAT CAN BE MEASURED?

Once the appropriate study population has been chosen, the tools to measure the clinical end-points, e.g. severity of illness and its change during treatment, must be chosen. The severity of depression cannot be measured directly, as can, for example, the severity of hypertension. Subjective assessment and behavioural rating scales have become the traditional tools used to assess the severity of depression. Although the specifics may differ, the goal of these scales is to provide for an initial assessment of the severity of the illness and a means to define change.

The choice of assessments to be used in a study depends, in large part, on what types of information are desired or required. Using different types of scales, such as an interview-based scale (e.g. Hamilton Rating Scale for Depression, Ham-D[10]), a multi-item self-rated scale (e.g. Hopkins Symptom Checklist[11]) and a physician- or patient-rated global scale (e.g. Clinical or Patient Global Impression Scale[11]) will allow simultaneous assessment from several perspectives. Early in development, when the nature of response in the patient population is unknown, the use of a variety of scales will help to delineate the overall profile of response. Regardless of which scales are used, however, to ensure confidence in the results, they should have established reliability and validity.

In addition to providing information on the overall severity of depression, through a breakdown of individual items most rating scales can also provide more specific clues concerning the major components of the depression. Changes in major symptoms, affective or behavioural components, can also be determined. Rating scales might allow further definition of a drug's more specific effects and determination of the most appropriate patient population for treatment, whether these be patients who are mainly agitated or patients who are mainly withdrawn.

The criteria upon which to base the assessment of efficacy must be delineated before starting a Phase II study. What changes in the severity of depression, as assessed by which tool, will be the minimum acceptable to demonstrate efficacy and provide convincing evidence that development of the drug should continue? When designing a trial, criteria should be set not only for the minimum total score necessary for entry at baseline, but also for the minimum amount of decrease coupled with a maximum total score at the end of treatment acceptable to demonstrate efficacy. The HAM-D has become one of the most widely accepted methods of assessing the efficacy of new antidepressants. Usually, a minimum baseline score of 20 on the 21-item version of the HAM-D is required for entry. In this rating scale a minimum decrease of 50% or greater should usually be set, to define efficacy. In early trials decreases in the HAM-D and any other rating tools should be carefully reviewed, to determine whether a consistent overall picture of amelioration of depression emerges.

Because amelioration of depression is sensitive to placebo effects, a placebo washout period of 1–2 weeks should precede the baseline assessment, to exclude placebo responders and help ensure that changes during treatment reflect a drug effect.

HOW LONG TO TREAT?

There has been some question as to the appropriate length of treatment necessary to demonstrate a convincing antidepressant effect. It has been argued that a clinical study should include 4–6 weeks of active drug administration (preceded by a 2 week placebo washout period), since it might take more than 4 weeks for all benefits to occur.[12] In earlier Phase II studies, where the immediate questions of efficacy and dose and dose range are more relevant, a 4 week trial might be sufficient.[13] However, since one of the goals of Phase II studies is to test a compound most rigorously for efficacy, trials of 6 weeks' duration have become more common. The first 2 weeks are usually used to escalate the dose to therapeutic levels; the remaining 4 weeks allow therapy at this maximal dose.

THE QUESTION OF DOSE AND DOSE REGIMEN

There are two issues related to the question of dose: how to define an effective dose and how to define a functional dose range. Results of animal toxicology and Phase I studies will define dose limits that should be safe. However, Phase I studies are done in healthy volunteers; most likely, patients will tolerate higher doses. To maximise the probability of finding efficacy, doses should be increased to the maximum of the tolerated dose range. The efficacious dose range will, it is hoped, lie somewhere within the limits of the tolerated range.

One strategy for attaining this goal is to use a fixed/flexible dose escalation study design. All patients are started at the same low dose level (one that has minimal or no side-effects and may not be efficacious), which is then increased by a fixed amount at specified times during the next 2 weeks. A patient may stop the dose escalation before the maximum dose is reached if side-effects occur (in which case the dose may be decreased to a tolerated level), or if the physician determines that a given dose level is providing adequate efficacy in that patient. The final dose is maintained for the next 4 weeks of treatment unless the occurrence of side-effects requires further dose decreases. In this manner patients are individually escalated to the upper end of the dose range, which is presumably more efficacious. Those patients who cannot tolerate higher doses, or in whom lower doses proved helpful, can be used to explore the mid-range of doses.

The analysis of the study can then define those doses that were efficacious. In this manner a functional dose range can begin to be determined. Future studies can use the dose range defined in this study, or can utilise fixed-dose groups based on this range. It is prudent, before starting Phase III, to conduct a dose–response study utilising fixed-dose groups and a placebo control, to start to define no-effect, minimum-effect and plateau-effect doses.

As stated earlier, the dosing regimen should be based on the pharmacokinetic parameters determined during Phase I as well as any pertinent pharmacodynamic information.

THE QUESTION OF STUDY DESIGN

Care must be taken to design studies that will provide information sufficient to allow decisions on the future development or discontinuation of the potential antidepressant. Decisions must be made as to whether small, open-label pilot studies, conducted by carefully selected psychiatrists, or large, well-controlled double-blind studies, are most appropriate. The results of small pilot studies may begin to give a feeling for the drug effects, but cannot be relied upon to demonstrate definitive efficacy. Large studies, although requiring considerable time and resources, provide stronger demonstrations of efficacy or lack thereof.

If larger double-blind studies are chosen, decisions must also be made as to the type of control methods employed. Placebo-controlled trials will give information concerning efficacy of the new antidepressant. Positive-control trials (that use a widely accepted antidepressant such as imipramine) will give information about the comparability of the drugs. The most powerful study design is one in which both a placebo (to show efficacy) and a positive control (to show comparability) are employed. Of course, a positive-controlled trial should not be attempted until a fairly good idea of the effective dose range of the new drug is available, so that appropriate doses of each can be chosen.

By the end of Phase II, strong evidence should be available to allow an accurate decision regarding how to proceed into Phase III. Answers to the questions initially posed relative to safety and efficacy in the target population, safety and efficacy relative to a standard drug, and definition of an effective dose range will provide the building blocks for a strong Phase III programme.

REFERENCES

1. American Psychiatric Association (1987). *Diagnostic and Statistical Manual of Mental Disorders*, 3rd edn, revised (*DSM-III-R*). Washington, D.C.
2. Regier, D. A., Myers, J. K., Kramer, M. *et al.* (1984). The NIMH epidemiologic catchment area program. *Arch. Gen. Psychiat.*, **41**, 934–41
3. Thompson, T. L. II and Thomas, M. R. (1986). Depression: medical interface with psychiatry and treatment advances. *J. Clin. Psychiat.*, **47**, 10 (Suppl.), 31–6
4. Hollister, L. E. (1987). Strategies for research in clinical psychopharmacology. In Meltzer, H. Y. (Ed.), *Psychopharmacology: The Third Generation of Progress*. Raven Press, New York, pp. 31–8
5. Cole, J. O. (1988). The drug treatment of anxiety and depression. *Med. Clin. N. Am.*, **72**, 815–30
6. US Department of Health Human Services (1980). *International Classification of Diseases*, 9th revision. DHHS Publication No. (PHS) 80-1260
7. Montgomery, S. A. (1981). Measurement of serum drug levels in the assessment of antidepressants. In Lader, M. H. and Richens, A. (Eds.), *Central Nervous System*. Macmillan, London
8. Linkowski, P., Mendlewicz, J., Kerkhofs, M. *et al.* (1987). 24-Hour profiles of adrenocorticotropin, cortisol, and growth hormone in major depressive illness: effect of antidepressant treatment. *J. Clin. Endocrinol. Metab.*, **65**, 141–52

9. Schatzberg, A. F., Rothschild, A. J., Gerson, B. *et al.* (1985). Towards a biochemical classification of depressive disorders. IX. DST results and platelet MAO activity. *Br. J. Psychiat.*, **146**, 633–7
10. Hamilton, M. (1960). A rating scale for depressions. *J. Neurol. Neurosurg. Psychiat.*, **23**, 56–62
11. NIMH (1976). *ECDEU Assessment Manual for Psychopharmacology*, revised edn. Publication No. (ADM) 76-338. Rockville, Maryland
12. Quitkin, F. M., Rabkin, J. G., Ross, D. *et al.* (1984). Duration of antidepressant drug treatment. *Arch. Gen. Psychiat.*, **41**, 238–45
13. Prien, R. F. and Levine, J. (1984). Research and methodological issues for evaluating the therapeutic effectiveness of antidepressant drugs. *Psychopharm. Bull.*, **20**, 250–7

35
Antipsychotic Agents

T. H. Corn and J. R. M. Haigh

Neuroscience Research Centre, Merck Sharp & Dohme Research Laboratories, Terlings Park, Harlow, Essex CM20 2QR, UK

INTRODUCTION

Since the introduction of chlorpromazine and haloperidol more than 30 years ago, a great many agents have been used for the treatment of psychotic illness. These agents all seem to share the property of antagonist activity at dopamine receptors; indeed, many will have been selected for development either because they bind to dopamine receptors or because they are active in a dopamine-specific behavioural assay. The result is an array of drugs with very similar properties: efficacy against acute psychotic illness combined with the neuroleptic effects of short-term extrapyramidal movement disorders and long-term, disabling, essentially untreatable tardive dyskinesia. The use of the term 'antipsychotic', rather than 'neuroleptic', to describe these drugs is in many ways a reflection of the hope that new agents may be developed in which the apparently inevitable link between antipsychotic and neuroleptic activity will be broken.

STUDIES IN HEALTHY VOLUNTEERS

Healthy volunteers are assumed to have normal physiological and mental status, and are thus a suitable population in which to establish the pharmacokinetic and pharmacodynamic properties of novel compounds. However, without better models it is difficult to predict antischizophrenic activity from studies in these subjects (Hollister, 1972). In this respect, volunteer studies are relatively less useful in the development of psychoactive drugs than in many other therapeutic areas, merely serving to establish the safety and tolerability of candidate compounds. This is increasingly true of the newer antipsychotics, when even the assessment of activity in terms of dopamine receptor blockade may no longer be appropriate.

Objectives of Phase I Studies

The objectives of Phase I studies are as follows:

(1) To determine the safety and tolerability of the candidate compound when given in single and limited multiple doses.
(2) To define the pharmacokinetic characteristics of the compound.
(3) To establish suitable dose regimens for use in early therapeutic studies.
(4) To establish the mechanism of action of the compound in man from evidence of dose-related pharmacological/adverse effects.

Assessment of Safety and Tolerability

Establishing human safety and tolerability for a novel compound often begins with a placebo-controlled, single-rising-dose study and the consequent determination of a maximally tolerated dose. Preclinical behavioural data provide the basis for choosing an appropriate dose range. The precise assessment of adverse events will depend upon the hypothesised mechanism of action (a matter requiring comprehensive preclinical information), but, in addition to standard safety measures, other factors more directly associated with typical antipsychotic drugs should be carefully monitored. Sedation, akathisia (Braude *et al.*, 1983), acute dystonic reactions (about which the volunteer should be warned) and effects on cognition can all be rated by subjective and objective means. The extent to which some of these symptoms are mediated via dopamine receptor antagonism is unknown, but obviously their absence would represent an advantage compared with most current antipsychotic therapies.

Preliminary assay of plasma drug (and, if necessary, metabolite) levels in a single-dose study dictates the regimen used for initial multiple-dose safety studies. The emphasis is again on monitoring adverse experience, but this time at steady state drug concentration. Evidence of untoward symptoms, depending upon their severity, would argue against the continued development of the compound, or at least necessitate evidence of superior efficacy in the later stages of development.

An additional study, which is occasionally advocated, employs a single-dose cross-over design with another psychotropic drug to enable a direct comparison of tolerability in a battery of psychometric tests. However, the choice of relevant doses can be confounding and restrict any valid interpretation.

Pharmacokinetic Characteristics

The principles and techniques of pharmacokinetic analysis, in both single and multiple doses, are the same for antipsychotic as for any other drugs and are described elsewhere in this volume. Standard pharmacokinetic assessment is often undertaken as part of the safety studies, whereas more specialised methods employing radiolabelled drug or an intravenous preparation can be performed at a later stage.

Biological Activity

The problem of assessing potential antipsychotic activity in normal volunteers is recurrent. When drug development for psychotic illness was restricted to dopamine receptor antagonists, the measurement of dose-related changes in plasma prolactin level was standard in Phase I studies. Such an approach is naturally less useful now that different receptor mechanisms are being sought, even though these systems often affect dopaminergic behaviours. However, measures such as an effect on prolactin secretion do not guarantee anti-psychotic potential (Mielke *et al.*, 1977); they merely confirm a pharmacological characteristic in man which is thought to be important in the aetiology or alleviation of schizophrenia.

Despite these problems, normal volunteers are used increasingly as research subjects, owing to the relative scarcity of large numbers of suitable psychotic patients and the difficulty of justifying placebo, or withholding established treatment, in trials where the efficacy of the candidate has not been proved. Consequently, methods of utilising volunteers to permit inferences about drug effects in patients have been described (Pillard and Fisher, 1978). One approach is to select volunteers with traits which approximate to patient symptoms, such as Type A or Type B personalities (Heninger *et al.*, 1965). Another is to use volunteers in whom an altered mental state has been induced by stress, drugs or environmental conditions. Ethical considerations become pertinent here, and as yet none of these techniques has been satisfactorily validated.

Neurophysiological Effects

While there is little chance of identifying true antipsychotic activity in normal volunteers, it is possible to investigate the neurophysiological effects of candidate drugs, most importantly on the electroencephalogram (EEG) (Roubicek, 1980). The waking EEG can be directly affected by chemical alterations in the brain; even the subtle changes characteristic of psychoactive compounds can be measured by digitalised computer analysis. Often the type and degree of short-term EEG changes seen in volunteers are predictive of the long-term clinical effects of a compound. The association between EEG and behaviour has led to the development of 'quantitative pharmaco-EEG', a technique for predicting the clinical profile of a drug from experimental trials in normal volunteers (Itil, 1974). This is only possible because reports indicate that changes in EEG induced by psychoactive drugs do not depend upon a defined pathology. This also provides a method for measuring the time-course of drug effect. Evoked potentials (EP) probably offer a more sensitive method of measuring antipsychotic effect (Shargass and Straumanis, 1978). Changes in EP induced by single doses of psychotropic drugs in volunteers may enable prediction of the clinical effects of unknown agents, although some evidence would advocate caution in this respect (see Saletu *et al.*, 1973).

STUDIES IN SCHIZOPHRENIC PATIENTS

Objectives of Phase II Studies

The objectives of Phase II studies are as follows:

(1) To establish that the postulated mechanism for the candidate compound results in clinical efficacy, with acceptable safety, in the treatment of acute schizophrenia.

(2) To determine the optimal dose regimen in the treatment of acute schizophrenia.

(3) To study the activity of the compound in chronic schizophrenia with a view to establishing prevention of relapse; efficacy against negative symptoms; and absence of long-term adverse reactions (particularly tardive dyskinesia).

Ethical Considerations

It is increasingly necessary to provide an ethical justification for the use of novel agents (with unknown and unpredictable efficacy) and placebo in patients suffering from acute schizophrenia, when conventional drugs are known to be reasonably efficacious and safe in the short-term control of symptoms. The use of novel agents can be justified by the limitations of conventional therapy, the unknown risks of the novel agent being offset by the possibility of unique efficacy against the underlying pathology of schizophrenia. The variability of schizophrenia and the relatively poor sensitivity of rating scales, further compromised by observer bias, provide the scientific and ethical imperative for the conduct of controlled clinical trials. The inclusion of a placebo-treated group in such trials ensures that the minimum number of patients are exposed to the novel drug before a definitive statement about the drug's efficacy is made. If, in addition, adequate safeguards for the individual patient are provided, such as informed consent, rescue medication and ability to withdraw from the trial, the use of novel agents and placebo in schizophrenia can be justified to the satisfaction of most authorities. This issue is dealt with in detail by Spilker (1987).

Open-label Studies

The principal reasons for performing open-label studies are to assess in schizophrenic patients the safety and tolerability of doses previously defined as safe and tolerable in normal subjects, and to indicate dose regimens suitable for initiating later Phase II studies. Such open studies are not appropriate for the measurement of antipsychotic efficacy, although, unfortunately, they are often used for this purpose. The lack of 'blindness' makes it virtually impossible to overcome observer bias. In addition, design is often weakened by the limited use of rating scales, usually the Brief Psychiatric Rating Scale (BPRS; see below), which, when used alone, is not sufficiently rigorous (Boza and Retondo, 1985). The inappropriate extrapolation and interpretation of efficacy data from open-label studies may even be destructive if premature conclusions cannot be substantiated in later placebo-controlled trials. A good example of this is provided by the purported antischizophrenic activity of cholecystokinin (see Montgomery and Green, 1988).

Ethically, however, limited open-label studies are necessary before large-scale, definitive efficacy trials are initiated in schizophrenic patients. Design is variable, but numbers need not be large and duration should be of at least 4 weeks.

Safety assessment should be performed in a manner comparable with the volunteer studies, and, indeed, many of the same problems exist—for example, what parameter to titrate against in a dose-ranging study. Other issues which are common to both open-label and placebo-controlled studies, such as entry criteria, will be discussed below.

Placebo-controlled Studies in Acute Schizophrenia

The importance of performing adequately controlled studies cannot be overemphasised. Proof that a novel treatment has efficacy at least equivalent to that of a standard antipsychotic drug requires a large number of patients. However well constructed, placebo-controlled trials of suitable duration will provide answers from smaller numbers and should be performed at the earliest possible stage of development so that the fewest patients are exposed to a potentially ineffective treatment. In certain cases, the hesitancy to do this coupled with poor study design has resulted in many patients needlessly receiving unproved drugs (see Montgomery and Green, 1988). A variety of issues concerning the design of such studies are worthy of further consideration (see also Spilker, 1987).

Entry Criteria

In order to recruit a homogeneous, but not atypical, population of patients with acute schizophrenia, it is important to have well-defined entry criteria. Many different kinds of instrument are available for assessing schizophrenic patients, including standardised diagnostic criteria, structured interviews and rating scales (Tables 35.1–35.3). Investigators may select assessment procedures depending upon their goals, but most commonly assessment now involves the use of *DSM-III-R* (Table 35.1). However, 'chart diagnosis' is rarely sufficient for research purposes, and patients should also be evaluated by some form of structured clinical interview (Table 35.2), so that information can be obtained in a uniform manner. It is also appropriate to ensure that patients reach a minimum level of severity of illness (for example, BPRS of greater than 45 with a score of at least 4 on two of the following BPRS items: conceptual disorganisation, suspiciousness, hallucinatory behaviour and unusual thought content). Moreover, with a complex illness such as schizophrenia, evaluations should be made by trained individuals with experience of assessing the presence and severity of symptoms. In this way the chances of recruiting stable patients with negative symptoms, non-responders or patients with relatively little measurable acute schizophrenia are minimised.

Study Design

Ideally studies should be of double-blind, parallel-group design, employing at least four groups, so that non-overlapping dose regimens of the drug can be compared with placebo and with a standard drug (e.g. haloperidol) in the same trial. Thus, evidence of efficacy and dose response can be provided by a single study. A cross-over design is inappropriate, owing to the episodic nature of the disease and the possibility of sequence effects whereby a patient's psychotic state may be appreciably affected by the response to the initial treatment. Patients should be hospitalised and given a drug-free washout period (single-blind with placebo) before treatment, to enable the assessment of baseline parameters and illness severity (Mielke *et al.*, 1977). This period, of at least 1 week, can be extended if extrapyramidal symptoms persist, or else patients can be excluded.

Duration

Placebo-controlled studies in acute schizophrenia should last a minimum of

Table 35.1 Diagnostic criteria for assessing schizophrenia

Criteria	Reference
Washington University Criteria	Feighner *et al.* (1972)
Research Diagnostic Criteria (RDC)	Spitzer *et al.* (1978)
Diagnostic and Statistical Manual of Mental Disorders (DSM-III-R)	Diagnostic Committee, American Psychiatric Association (1987)

Table 35.2 Structured interviews for assessing schizophrenia (see Andreasen, 1987)

Present State Examination (PSE)/CATEGO
Schedule for Affective Disorders and Schizophrenia (SADS)[a]
Diagnostic Interview Schedule (DIS)[b]
Structured Clinical Review for DSM-III (SCID)[b]
Comprehensive Assessment of Symptoms and History (CASH)

[a] For use in conjunction with RDC.
[b] For use in conjunction with *DSM-III-R*.

Table 35.3 Rating scales for schizophrenia

Scale	Reference[a]
Brief Psychiatric Rating Scale (BPRS)	Overall and Gorham (1962)
Nurses' Observation Scale for Inpatient Evaluation (NOSIE)	Honigfeld and Klett, (1965)
Clinical Global Impression Scale (CGI)	
Nurses' Global Impression Scale (NGI)	
Scale for the Assessment of Thought, Language and Communication	
Affect Rating Scale	
Scale for Emotional Blunting (SEB)	Abrams and Taylor (1976)
Scale for Assessment of Negative Symptoms (SANS)	
Scale for Assessment of Positive Symptoms (SAPS)	
Schizophrenia Subscale of the PSE (SS-PSE)	
Subscale of the Comprehensive Psychopathological Rating Scale	Montgomery *et al.* (1978)

[a] See Andreasen (1987) unless otherwise cited.

4–6 weeks for adequate assessment of antipsychotic efficacy; studies of less than 1 week, and in some cases only one dose (Tamminga *et al.*, 1986), are unrealistic.

Concomitant Treatment

The evaluation of novel antipsychotic drugs is often compromised by the concomitant use of other neuroleptics which are known to be effective. This represents a serious methodological flaw, as it greatly reduces the capacity of a study to demonstrate efficacy. However, in a placebo-controlled trial there is an ethical requirement for a 'rescue' treatment in the event that a patient becomes extremely distressed. This dilemma is best resolved by allowing the use of a defined 'rescue' medication (often a neuroleptic of short half-life, e.g. droperidol) and employing the amount of usage of this medication as an outcome measure.

Sample Size

To draw valid conclusions, it is essential to recruit adequate numbers of patients to give the study statistical power. The presence of a placebo group does not necessarily overcome the problem of very small numbers, so that either the treatment effect has to be quite marked, to demonstrate a significant difference between groups, or else the measures of change in illness severity have to be extremely sensitive. Negative results from small studies are of little value when the trial is unlikely to detect a real difference (Type II error). The problem of sample size is compounded if the intention is to stratify the treatment groups. Stratification might reasonably be based upon factors such as age, sex, previous neuroleptic treatment and the actual diagnosis of schizophrenia (e.g. acute versus acute exacerbation of chronic); however, such issues are often not addressed until later stages of development.

Efficacy Measures

Although structured interviews and diagnostic criteria are used to make diagnoses and identify symptoms in patients, rating scales are used to measure the change in clinical status with time. Numerous scales are available for research in schizophrenia (Table 35.3). The use of scales which are known to be relatively insensitive has limited the ability of investigators to detect potentially important treatment differences. The BPRS is the most frequently used (usually in conjunction with a global rating scale) but was not designed specifically to measure the severity of schizophrenia and can fail to detect differences highlighted by other scales (Pugh *et al.*, 1983). This has led both to the development of alternative scales, such as the subscale of the Comprehensive Psychopathological Rating Scale, which was devised specifically to be more sensitive to treatment-induced change (Montgomery *et al.*, 1978), and to improvements to the BPRS itself (Bech *et al.*, 1986). Consistency between investigators in the use of these scales is also extremely important, particularly in a multicentre trial, and investigator training sessions and 'quality control' procedures are appropriate in this context. Although the repeated use of such rating scales is necessary throughout studies of this type, they do not represent the only available outcome measures. For instance, the need for additional sedatives might vary between groups, as might the number of patients who drop out. For this latter reason it is often appropriate to perform these studies on an 'intention to treat' basis.

Assessment of Adverse Reactions

The object of controlled studies is to define an optimal dose regimen, characterised by antipsychotic efficacy greater than placebo and at least comparable with a standard. However, it must be remembered that a safety profile superior to that of the standard is also a desirable goal, particularly for drugs with novel mechanisms. For this reason, much store is set by the assessment of adverse events. Besides routine measurement of standard safety parameters, for which rating scales are occasionally reported (Levine and Schooler, 1986), emphasis is placed on evidence of extrapyramidal symptoms and, in particular, tardive dyskinesia (events which may unblind the study). The aim of all novel antipsychotic drugs is to minimise these adverse effects. Rating scales for the assessment of extrapyramidal disorders (Simpson and Angus, 1970; Mindham, 1976) are often different from those used conventionally in conjunction with idiopathic Parkinson's disease. In addition, specific scales for tardive dyskinesia can be employed (Schooler and Kane, 1982) but are only appropriate for prolonged trials.

Controlled Studies in Chronic Schizophrenia

Conventional antipsychotic drugs are effective in acute schizophrenia, and are capable to some extent of preventing the recurrence of acute schizophrenia in chronically ill patients (Crow, 1986). Their weakness in clinical practice is their lack of activity against negative or residual symptoms of schizophrenia and their ability to produce disabling movement disorders: parkinsonism, akathisia and tardive dyskinesia. In addition, their capacity to impair cognitive function is a significant problem for most, if not all, patients. It is in the treatment of chronic schizophrenia that therapeutic opportunities are to be found. Most novel treatments are submitted for regulatory approval with evidence of efficacy only in acute schizophrenia. Increasingly, it will become important to provide evidence of unique efficacy in the early stages of antipsychotic drug development.

Prevention of Relapse

Early evidence of novel clinical activity in this indication could be gained in a parallel-design clinical study in which patients with chronic schizophrenia, maintained on neuroleptic treatment but suffering from early tardive dyskinesia, are randomised to treatment with the novel agent, with a standard neuroleptic agent or with a placebo. The outcome variables which should be studied are simply the recurrence of acute symptoms and the presence of movement disorders measured as described above. Trial duration would need to be of the order of 6 months.

Treatment of Negative or Residual Schizophrenia

There is at present no effective pharmacological therapy for the negative symptoms of schizophrenia (chronic worsening emotional blunting, social withdrawal, eccentric behaviour, illogical thinking and loosening of associations). Conventional neuroleptic agents have only marginal efficacy, and any novel agent with significant efficacy will revolutionise the treatment of this illness. It is, therefore, appropriate to undertake preliminary clinical work in this indication as soon as possible in the development of a novel compound; moreover, it should be stated clearly that there is currently no *a priori* reason to conclude that failure to show efficacy in acute schizophrenia predicts lack of efficacy in residual schizophrenia.

DSM-III-R provides a set of diagnostic criteria for Schizophrenic Disorder Residual Type which would allow recruitment of a suitable patient population. These individuals are likely to be receiving chronic neuroleptic treatment, but, assuming the absence of significant drug interactions, a novel agent without effect on dopamine receptors could be added to existing therapy in a study in which patients are randomised to novel antipsychotic or placebo. Negative symptoms could be monitored by use of an appropriate rating scale such as the Scale for Assessment of Negative Symptoms (Table 35.3). Treatment would need to be continued for at least 3 months because of the normally fluctuating nature of negative symptoms. Evidence of efficacy in an 'add-on' study of this type, together with evidence of efficacy in the prevention of relapse, would suggest a novel and clinically important efficacy profile. It would also justify larger studies in which patients newly recovered from an episode of acute schizophrenia could be randomised to maintenance treatment with the novel agent or conventional neuroleptic and studied over an extended time period for relapse, for development of negative symptoms and for development of tardive dyskinesia.

CONCLUSION

The development of a new dopamine receptor antagonist for the treatment of acute schizophrenia poses no great challenge to clinical research. This particular road is well trodden, with more than 15 such drugs currently on the market in the UK. The challenge for the clinical psychopharmacologist lies in the development of the drugs now emerging for which no pharmacological precedent exists—for example, drugs with effects on serotonin- and cholecystokinin-mediated systems. These drugs, whose efficacy in acute schizophrenia is less easy to predict, will need to be subjected to extensive well-controlled Phase II investigation in acute schizophrenia justified ethically by the promise of superior efficacy and safety in the long term. This is an extremely challenging task, which must begin as early as possible in the development of a novel antipsychotic drug if unique antischizophrenic properties are to be identified which will signal a new era in the treatment of this disabling disorder.

REFERENCES

Abrams, R. and Taylor, M. A. (1976). A rating scale for emotional blunting. *Am. J. Psychiat.*, **135**, 226–9

Andreasen, N. C. (1987). In Meltzer, H. Y. (Ed.), *Psychopharmacology: The Third Generation of Progress*. Raven Press, New York, pp. 1087–94

Bech, P., Kastrup, M. and Rafaelsen, O. J. (1986). Minicompendium of rating scales for states of anxiety, depression, mania, schizophrenia with corresponding DSM III syndromes. *Acta Psychiat. Scand.*, **326**, 32–7

Boza, R. A. and Retondo, D. J. (1985). Is cholecystokinin therapeutic in clinical schizophrenia. *J. Clin. Psychiat.*, **46**, 485–6

Braude, W. M., Barnes, T. R. and Gore, S. M. (1983). Clinical characteristics of akathisia. A systematic investigation of acute psychiatric in-patient admissions. *Br. J. Psychiat.*, **143**, 139–50

Crow, T. J., MacMillan, J. F., Johnson, A. L. and Johnstone, E. C. (1986). The Northwick Park study of first episodes of schizophrenia. II. A randomised controlled trial of prophylactic neuroleptic treatment. *Br. J. Psychiat.*, **148**, 120–7

Diagnostic Committee, American Psychiatric Association (1987). *Diagnostic and Statistical Manual of Mental Disorders (DSM-III-R)*. American Psychiatric Association, Washington D.C.

Feighner, J. P., Robins, E. and Guze, S. B. (1972). Diagnostic criteria for use in psychiatric research. *Arch. Gen. Psychiat.*, **26**, 57–63

Heninger, G., Di Mascio, A. and Klerman, G. L. (1965). Personality factors in variability of response to phenothiazines. *Am. J. Psychiat.*, **121**, 1091–4

Hollister, L. E. (1972). Prediction of therapeutic uses of psychotherapeutic drugs from experiences with normal volunteers. *Clin. Pharm. Ther.*, **13**, 803–8

Honigfeld, G. and Klett, J. C. (1965). The Nurses' Observation Scale for inpatient evaluation. A new scale for measuring improvement in chronic schizophrenia. *J. Clin. Psychol.*, **21**, 65–71

Itil, T. M. (1974). *Psychotropic Drugs and the Human EEG*. Karger, Berlin

Levine, J. and Schooler, N. R. (1986). SAFTEE: A technique for the systematic assessment of side effects in clinical trials. *Psychopharm. Bull.*, **22**, 343–81

Mielke, D. H., Gallant, D. M. and Kessler, C. (1977). An evaluation of a new antipsychotic agent, sulpiride: effects on serum prolactin and growth hormone levels. *Am. J. Psychiat.*, **134**, 1371–5

Mindham, R. H. S. (1976). Assessment of drug induced extrapyramidal reactions and of drugs given for their control. *Br. J. Clin. Pharm.*, **3**, 395–400

Montgomery, S. A. and Green, M. C. D. (1988). The use of cholecystokinin in schizophrenia: a review. *Psychol. Med.*, **18**, 593–603

Montgomery, S. A., Taylor, P. and Montgomery, D. (1978). Development of a schizophrenia scale sensitive to change. *Neuropharmacology*, **17**, 1061–2

Overall, J. E. and Gorham, D. R. (1962). The brief psychiatric rating scale. *Psychol. Rep.*, **10**, 799–812

Pillard, R. C. and Fisher, S. (1978). In Lipton, M. A., Di Mascio, A. and Killam, K. F. (Eds.), *Psychopharmacology: A Generation of Progress*. Raven Press, New York, pp. 783–90

Pugh, C. R., Steinert, J. and Priest, R. G. (1983). Propranolol in schizophrenia: a double blind, placebo controlled trial of propranolol as an adjunct to neuroleptic medication. *Br. J. Psychiat.*, **143**, 151–5

Roubicek, J. (1980). In Hoffmeister, F. and Stille, G. (Eds.), *Psychotropic Agents*, Part 1. Springer-Verlag, Berlin, pp. 177–223

Saletu, B., Saletu, M. and Itil, T. (1973). Effect of tricyclic antidepressants on somatosensory evoked potential in man. *Psychopharmacology*, **29**, 1–12

Schooler, N. R. and Kane, J. M. (1982). Research diagnosis for tardive dyskinesia (RD-TD). *Arch. Gen. Psychiat.*, **39**, 486–7

Shargass, C. and Straumanis, J. J. (1978). In Lipton, M. A., Di Mascio, A. and Killam, K. F. (Eds.), *Psychopharmacology: A Generation of Progress*. Raven Press, New York, pp. 699–710

Simpson, G. M. and Angus, J. W. S. (1970). Drug induced extrapyramidal disorders. *Acta Psychiat. Scand.*, **45**, 11–19

Spilker, B. (1987). In Meltzer, H. Y. (Ed.), *Psychopharmacology: The Third Generation of Progress*. Raven Press, New York, pp. 1659–66

Spitzer, R. L., Endicott, J. and Robins, E. (1978). Research Diagnostic Criteria. *Arch. Gen. Psychiat.*, **35**, 773–82

Tamminga, C. A., Littman, R. L., Alphs, L. D., Chase, T. N., Tuaker, G. K. and Wagman, A. M. (1986). Neuronal cholecystokinin and schizophrenia: pathogenic and therapeutic studies. *Psychopharmacology*, **88**, 387–91

VIII
Assessment of Drug Effects on the Gastrointestinal System

36
Measurement of Gastrointestinal Effects

K. H. Antonin and P. R. Bieck

*Humanpharmakologisches Institut, Ciba-Geigy GmbH, Waldhörnlestr.,
7400 Tübingen 1, West Germany*

INTRODUCTION

Most drugs are administered orally, and the gastrointestinal tract is frequently exposed to high concentrations of substances given with the aim of acting at low concentrations elsewhere in the body. It is known that a number of drugs influence physiological and morphological patterns, and may lead to clinically important problems. Drugs alter gastrointestinal motility and secretion, and cause mucosal lesions throughout the alimentary tract. Absorption of drugs is a complex process influenced by the type of formulation, by the origin and surface of gastrointestinal mucosal membranes and by physicochemical properties of the luminal contents. For the measurement of drug effects on the gastrointestinal tract, a wide variety of methods is used which originate from different specialities, such as anatomy, physiology, chemistry, biochemistry, clinical medicine and radiology. These methods are summarised in this chapter with regard to the measurement of motility, secretion, drug absorption, drug safety and assessment of drug efficacy in diseases. In pharmacological studies in humans, consideration should first be given to the magnitude of the expected effect. On this basis a rational choice of methods can be made. However, it should be recognised that often the most sensitive and accurate measurements are also difficult to perform.

MOTILITY

Highly sensitive and well-standardised techniques are available for the recording and quantification of motility and for the measurement of passage of liquid and solid substances through the gastrointestinal tract.

Oesophagus

Fluoroscopy

The effect of size and shape of tablets or capsules on oesophageal transit time can be measured with barium sulphate-containing formulations visualised by fluoroscopy. The time needed for the formulations to reach the stomach is measured with a stop-watch (Channer and Virjee, 1986).

Scintigraphy

The transit of swallowed materials through the oesophagus can also be quantified with radionuclides. The subject is positioned under a gamma scintillation camera coupled to a computer system. Fluid mixed with [^{99m}Tc]-sulphur colloid as radioactive marker or drug formulations impregnated with the same marker are swallowed. From time–activity curves, the transit time through the oesophagus is calculated. These methods provide an objective parameter for the evaluation of treatment effects (Stacher, 1985; Horowitz *et al.*, 1987).

Manometry

Effects of drugs on oesophageal motility are assessed by manometry. Multilumen catheter systems are used with side holes continuously perfused and filled with water. The manometric catheter is attached to an external transducer, an infusion pump, a preamplifier/amplifier and, finally, a polygraph recorder (Soffer *et al.*, 1988). The system is introduced into the stomach and then slowly withdrawn until pressure of the lower oesophageal sphincter can be recorded.

Direct pressure measurements are also done by strain gauge probes connected directly to the preamplifier.

Long-term pH Monitoring

Documentation of gastro-oesophageal reflux with long-term pH monitoring has been shown to be of considerable value, not only in diagnosis and management of this disease, but also for evaluation of drug effects. Several types of pH-sensitive electrodes, such as glass, antimony, plastic and iridium or tethered radiotelemetric pills, are available. Computerised replay units with visual display and printout facilities are used for recording and calculation of the number of reflux episodes and cumulative duration of high acidity (Branicki *et al.*, 1982; Atkinson, 1987; Emde *et al.*, 1987).

Stomach

Fluoroscopy

The use of liquid barium sulphate or other radio-opaque markers gives only qualitative estimates of the time needed for nearly complete emptying of liquids and subjective impressions on contractility. Barium meals are emptied similarly to liquids with an emptying half-time of 15–20 min. The generally accepted 6 h limit of normal emptying from the stomach gives only an approximate estimation of motility (Smith and Feldman, 1986).

Scintigraphy

Radionuclear methods are very useful to assess gastrointestinal motility. ^{99m}Tc is the most commonly used isotope. Technetium meals consist of chicken liver, egg preparations and cereals. Indigestible solids have been studied with ^{131}I bound to cellulose. The ^{111}In and ^{113}In isotopes, bound to diethylenetriaminepentaacetic acid (DPTA), can be used as liquid markers in dual liquid and/or solid gastric emptying measurements. The gastric emptying of liquids or solids is expressed as fraction of radioactivity remaining in the stomach plotted against time. Half-time $(t_\frac{1}{2})$ of emptying is calculated from such emptying curves (Trotman and Misiewicz, 1982; Malagelada *et al.*, 1984; Minami and McCallum, 1984; Santander *et al.*, 1988). Indium and technetium are not well absorbed by the gastric mucosa. They emit gamma rays at different frequencies. The use of a gamma camera and a computer enables simultaneous analysis and monitoring of liquid and solid phase emptying (Collins *et al.*, 1983; Horowitz *et al.*, 1987). This method does not take into account gastric secretion or duodenogastric reflux. Therefore, residual stomach volumes or the quantity emptied from the stomach cannot be assessed.

Abdominal Ultrasound

Gastric emptying can be measured accurately with ultrasound techniques. However, measurement is technically difficult and time-consuming and cannot be used in obese subjects or in the presence of excessive air in the stomach. These limitations and the fact that ultrasound techniques are only suitable for measurement of liquid emptying, have prevented widespread acceptance (Bateman and Whittingham, 1982; Holt *et al.*, 1986).

Impedance Techniques

The measurement of changes of electrical impedance in the epigastric region after ingestion of liquids of low conductivity allows an accurate determination of liquid emptying. Four electrodes are used, two on the anterior and two on the posterior trunk. One pair of electrodes measures current flow and the second pair is used for recording. The subjects lie flat on their backs and a liquid of low electrical conductivity (orange-flavoured Quosh) is administered. As gastric emptying proceeds, transabdominal impedance alters. The changes are plotted, and give an index of emptying rate. Comparison with scintigraphy demonstrated a close correlation, indicating that the method is a valid measurement of gastric emptying. The impedance techniques are inexpensive and well reproducible, and might gain wider acceptance as experience increases (McClelland and Sutton, 1985).

Electrogastrography

With the electrogastrogram, abnormalities of gastric electrical rhythm can be monitored. Silver–silver chloride electrodes are placed on the skin of the epigastrium and on a limb as reference lead (Stern *et al.*, 1987). An excellent correlation with surgically placed electrodes has been shown (Hamilton *et al.*, 1986).

Manometry

Intraluminal pressure changes in the stomach are measured either with perfused catheters or with probes containing transducers. Each method has advantages and disadvantages. Perfusion catheters are cheaper, but thicker and less well tolerated. The constant infusion of fluid into the lumen may affect motility. Transducers are more expensive, but thinner and better-tolerated. They also cause fewer perturbations of the luminal environment. Pressure wave activity is quantified by a motility index based on amplitude and frequency of the phasic pressure waves (Trotman and Misiewicz, 1982; Santander *et al.*, 1988). During fasting, the different phases of the migrating motor complex are recorded. Phase I is characterised by the absence of any spike activity, Phase II by a period of irregular contractile activity followed by a characteristic propagated burst of contractions (Phase III).

To ensure registration of an adequate number of migrating motor complexes, as well as postprandial activity, the monitoring time should be at least 6 h or longer.

Biliary Tract

Fluoroscopy

Fluoroscopy is a standard method of visualising the gall bladder and biliary duct after oral or intravenous administration of a contrast medium. The contrast medium is concentrated in the gall bladder and produces an image that can be quantified as an accurate estimation of gall bladder volume.

The kinetics of bile duct flow can be studied with cholangiography. Motility of the bile duct and of the sphincter of Oddi can be visualised by cineradiography. However, fluoroscopy in healthy subjects is rarely used, because of considerable radiation exposure.

Scintigraphy

Gall bladder emptying in response to cholagogic stimuli is measured in volunteers and patients with scintigraphy. ^{99m}Tc-labelled diethyl phenylcarbamomethyl iminodiacetate ([^{99m}Tc]-HIDA) is injected intravenously. The gall bladder area is identified and mapped on control scans. Gall bladder activity in subsequent views is expressed as a percentage of the initial values. Activity is plotted against time to obtain a gall bladder emptying curve (Lanzini *et al.*, 1987; Mackie *et al.*, 1987).

Ultrasonography

Ultrasonography is commonly used to study effects of drugs or hormones on gall bladder or bile duct function. Gall bladder volume is determined from a series of cross-sectional images. Volume is calculated as sum of a series of cylinders (Marzio *et al.*, 1987). Volume can also be derived from measurements of gall bladder length and diameter (Hansen and Felgenträger, 1987).

Manometry

The effects of drugs or hormones on intraluminal pressure changes or motor activity of the bile duct are assessed in patients with T-tube drains (McFarland *et al.*, 1984). In healthy subjects a duodenoscope with side view is used. During endoscopy a manometric catheter or a strain gauge probe is passed through the biopsy channel of the endoscope and inserted into the bile duct. Manometric examinations are done before and after administration of the test drug or hormones (Funch-Jensen *et al.*, 1987).

Small Intestine, Large Bowel, Rectum

Manometry

The technique of pressure measurement in the small intestine with perfused tubes is essentially that of oesophageal or stomach manometry (Santander *et al.*, 1988). To measure motor activity of the colon, a manometric catheter is introduced by advancing it together with a colonoscope (Narducci *et al.*, 1987). Prolonged manometric studies of small and large bowel motility are an important tool in the investigation of drug effects in intestinal motility disorders (Camilleri *et al.*, 1986).

Telemetry

Bowel motility can be assessed by ingestible radiotelemetric pills for long periods of time. Pressure changes can be measured with a pressure-sensitive radiotelemetric pill. It consists of a capsule with pressor sensor, a miniature battery and a transmitting coil. The signals are transmitted as pulses at very low power, and are detected by aerials placed on the body surface of the subject. The radiotelemetric pill is tethered with a fine thread and attached to the mouth. It can be located in any area and stationed at a fixed location in the gastrointestinal tract. It has been shown that radiotelemetric pills give information comparable with that provided by intubation systems (Thompson *et al.*, 1980; Trotman and Misiewicz, 1982).

Transit Time in the Upper Intestinal Tract

Fluoroscopy

The transit of non-disintegrating solid dosage forms containing a radio-opaque compound, such as barium sulphate or small steel balls, can be followed by X-ray examinations. However, the necessity of simultaneous administration of barium sulphate suspension, in order to visualise the intestinal tract, may cause difficulties in locating radio-opaque bodies against the background.

Scintigraphy

Detailed information about transit through stomach and small intestine is provided by labelling a meal or solid dosage forms with a gamma-emitting isotope (Davis *et al.*, 1984; Malagelada *et al.*, 1984; Camilleri *et al.*, 1986). The passage through the gastrointestinal tract is monitored with a gamma camera linked to a computer. ^{99m}Tc is the most commonly used isotope. If, in addition, another isotope such as ^{111}In is used, the passage of solids and liquids, or of two drug formulations, can be measured simultaneously. Images of the distribution of radioactivity in the abdominal regions are collected over time and stored in the computer. The stomach is identified first and the colon last. Radioactive counts outside of stomach and colon are assumed to be in the small intestine.

The proportion of total radioactivity present in the stomach, small intestine and colon is determined at any given time during the study. Profiles of gastric emptying, colonic filling and small bowel residence are constructed from the data (Davis *et al.*, 1986; Read *et al.*, 1986).

Salicylazosulphapyridine

Mouth-to-caecum transit time can be measured by the use of salicylazosul-phapyridine. This drug practically is not absorbed in the upper part of the gastrointestinal tract. It is metabolised by the microbial flora in the large bowel to sulphapyridine, which is rapidly absorbed. The time lag until detection of sulphapyridine in plasma or saliva gives an estimate of the transit time from mouth to caecum. In normal fasting subjects this is around 3.5–5 h (Kellow *et al.*, 1986; Antonin *et al.*, 1988).

Hydrogen Breath Test

The appearance of hydrogen in expired air after ingestion of a non-absorbable carbohydrate is the basis for measurement of small bowel transit time. In humans H_2 is produced by bacterial fermentation of carbohydrates in the gastrointestinal tract. In healthy subjects this occurs only in the colon (Bond and Levitt, 1975). H_2 diffuses from bowel to blood at a constant rate and is eliminated from the body by exhalation. A standard dose (10–20 g in 100 ml water) of a non-absorbable carbohydrate, usually lactulose, is given orally. Lactulose is a disaccharide consisting of fructose and galactose, which is not split by brush border disaccharidases. H_2 production occurs almost entirely in the colon by fermentation by colonic bacterial flora. End-expiratory samples of air are collected at 10 min intervals and hydrogen concentrations are determined by gas chromatography or selective and sensitive electrochemical cells. Transit time is defined as time from ingestion of lactulose to a rise in breath H_2 concentration of at least 20 p.p.m. (Trotman and Misiewicz, 1982; van Wyk *et al.*, 1985). Lactulose is an osmotic purgative and will interfere with intestinal motility. It cannot be regarded as a physiological marker of transit. Therefore, test meals rich in carbohydrates are provided as alternatives (Read *et al.*, 1985).

Colonic Transit Time

Colonic motility and transit time are measured by scintigraphic methods. Through a thin tube, positioned in the caecum, a nonabsorbable radionuclide ($[^{111}In]$-DTPA) is instilled. Passage through the colon is monitored by a gamma camera (Krevsky *et al.*, 1986).

Total Transit Time

Fluoroscopy

In this test 20 radio-opaque ring-shaped markers are ingested on day 1, 20 rod-shaped pellets on day 2 and 20 plastics rods containing metal balls on day 3. On day 4 the abdomen is X-rayed and the markers that are retained in the gastrointestinal tract are counted. The number is plotted against the time elapsed from ingestion to visualisation. The intersection with the time axis is defined as gastrointestinal transit time (Jaup *et al.*, 1985; Hallerbäck *et al.*, 1988).

Transit time through the gut can also be measured by collecting and analysing one stool specimen. Twenty radio-opaque markers are given with breakfast to a subject on three consecutive days. Different, but comparable, markers are used each day. The first stool specimen on day 4 is collected and the markers are counted fluoroscopically. The average transit time can be calculated from the number of each type of marker found and the time of ingestion to defecation (Cummings and Wiggins, 1976).

Scintigraphy

Scintigraphic methods, as described above, are used to measure total gastrointestinal transit time of meals or controlled-release dosage forms (Davis *et al.*, 1984, 1986; Malagelada *et al.*, 1984).

Conclusion

Carefully designed scintigraphic studies are the most accurate and sophisticated methods to measure transit through the gastrointestinal tract. The SASP test and radio-opaque marker studies are simple and inexpensive methods. Scinitigraphic techniques allow accurate measurements of the gastrointestinal transit, dispersion and dissolution of orally given new drug formulations (Spiller, 1986). The currently available instrumentation for gastrointestinal manometry provides effective means for the clinical investigation of motor functions in health and disease and for the measurement of drug effects. Radiotelemetric probes allow a greater degree of mobility and comfort for the subjects studied. Long-term pH recording of oesophagus or stomach increased knowledge of the pathology of gastro-oesophageal reflux and gastroduodenal ulcer disease and is useful in the evaluation of new treatments for these disorders.

SECRETION

In addition to the transport of materials through the gastrointestinal tract, water and electrolyte fluxes due to secretion and/or reabsorption in the different regions may be significantly influenced by drugs. On the other hand, water flux may also facilitate dissolution and absorption of drugs.

Small Intestine

Intubation techniques are used to investigate the effects of drugs on water and electrolyte transport in the human small intestine. Double-lumen or multilumen perfusion tubes with occluding balloons and infusion and collection holes are swallowed and positioned fluoroscopically. A glucose electrolyte solution is infused with a peristaltic pump through the infusion hole and aspirated through the collection hole (Moriarty *et al.*, 1986).

Bile

Quantification of biliary excretion and enterohepatic circulation of drugs and their metabolites in man is difficult, as the biliary tract is not readily accessible.

T-tube Drainage or Nasobiliary Tubes in Patients

Most biliary excretion studies have been performed in patients with T-tube drainage following cholecystectomy or other biliary tract surgery (Rollins and Klaassen, 1979; Terhaag and Hermann, 1986). They can also be performed in patients with nasobiliary tubes. However, patients are not ideal for such studies. They usually have hepatobiliary disease, with or without extrahepatic cholestasis. Bile flow and bile salt output are diminished for 2–4 weeks after surgery. Most biliary drainage tubes are not designed to totally divert bile flow. Therefore, it is not known whether bile collection is complete or not. Interruption of normal enterohepatic circulation of bile and bile constituents markedly alters bile output and composition (Rollins and Klaassen, 1979).

Intubation Techniques in Healthy Subjects

In order to overcome the difficulties encountered in patients, healthy human volunteers are studied by use of gastrointestinal tubes. Single- or double-lumen nasoduodenal tubes are positioned with the aspiration site just distal to the ampulla of Vater. Bile samples are obtained by continuous or intermittent aspiration of duodenal fluid, which is rich in bile (Lind *et al.*, 1987).

Multiluminal tubes are positioned in the duodenum and perfused with a liquid lipid diet in order to keep the gall bladder contracted and a non-absorbable marker to quantify bile collection. This procedure appears to be more reliable for quantification than the T-tube drainage technique. However, enterohepatic circulation cannot be interrupted completely, when needed, and bile collection is difficult if the drug being studied is administered orally (Dujovne *et al.*, 1982).

A balloon-occludable multiluminal duodenal tube has been used successfully for studying biliary excretion of drugs. The tube is passed into the duodenum and a balloon is inflated distal to the ampulla of Vater. It allows proximal aspiration and distal reinfusion of bile. With this method enterohepatic circulation can be maintained at the desired level, as the amount of aspirated bile can be reinfused into the intestine (Askin *et al.*, 1978).

Conclusion

Intubation techniques for the study of drug effects on fluid or electrolyte secretion in the intestine or on bile flow are not widely used. They are complicated, costly and time-consuming. Investigations in patients with T-tubes can give qualitative indications of biliary drug excretion.

DRUG ABSORPTION

Most orally administered drugs are designed to be absorbed from the upper gastrointestinal tract. However, absorption of drugs is a complex process. There are several physiological and pathological factors affecting absorption, such as motility, gastrointestinal diseases, certain foods or the formulation of a drug. On the other hand, development of new dosage formulations that release drug slowly through the entire length of the gastrointestinal tract requires systematic studies of the absorptive capacity of all parts of the gastrointestinal tract.

Intubation Techniques

Drug absorption in man can be investigated by intubation techniques. Absorption rates are estimated from the rate of disappearance of drug from the gut lumen. Non-absorbable markers such as polyethylene glycol (PEG) are used to enable corrections for changing volumes due to fluid fluxes. Thin flexible tubes are swallowed by the subjects and placed in different levels of the gastrointestinal tract. After administration of the test drug and the markers, gastric and intestinal contents are collected at frequent intervals (Hirtz, 1987).

Gastric absorption of drugs is studied after occlusion of the pylorus with two balloons. Absorption from the ileum is examined with multiluminal tubes and with an occlusive balloon. The balloon is inflated after intubation, to isolate the intestinal segment to be studied. Secretions from the proximal intestine are aspirated continuously by a tube above the balloon. The drug is infused together with the marker just below the balloon and luminal fluid is aspirated 30 cm distal from this side (Hirtz, 1987).

To study drug absorption in the colon, a tube is swallowed and its distal end is positioned into the caecum under radiological control. Drug is administered through the tube, and the rate of absorption is calculated from plasma concentration profiles (Hirtz, 1987). With intubation techniques it is possible to characterise the absorption of drugs in all segments of the gastrointestinal tract. However, it is complicated, costly and time-consuming, and, therefore, cannot be used extensively.

HF Capsule

A high-frequency capsule (HF capsule) has been developed to study absorption characteristics in man. With the HF capsule extent and rate of drug absorption from all sites of the gastrointestinal tract can be investigated. A smooth plastic capsule (12×8 mm) contains a small latex balloon (1 ml) filled with drug and the release mechanism. The capsule is taken together with a small oral dose of contrast medium, to enable the radiological localisation in the intestines. The release mechanism is triggered with a short impulse from a high-frequency generator, to release the drug in a defined segment of the gastrointestinal tract. From plasma concentration profiles, the rate of absorption can be calculated (Staib *et al.*, 1986; Schuster and Hugemann, 1987).

Application of Drugs into the Large Bowel During Colonoscopy

Colonoscopy has become a routine procedure in diagnosis and treatment of colonic diseases. Development of instruments that are easier to handle made the procedure shorter and more acceptable. Dissolved drug can be placed into distinct areas under visual and fluoroscopic control through instrumental channels in the colonoscope, within 5–20 min (Antonin and Bieck, 1987).

The large intestine must be very well cleaned prior to endoscopy. This led to criticism of the assessment of absorption capacity of the large bowel under 'non-physiological' conditions. However, colonoscopy proved to be a simple, well-tolerated and suitable method for Phase I studies with new compounds or drug formulations. Colonoscopy allows quantification of relative colonic bioavailability of a drug. Disadvantages are discomfort to the volunteers, the necessity of a clean colon and exposure to X-rays. Colonoscopy should only be performed by skilled endoscopists.

Patients with Artificial Stoma

Drug absorption by the colonic mucosa can be investigated in patients with intestinal stoma, if no stenosis is present. Stomas can be used in two ways to study drug absorption. First, intestinal contents of the upper parts of the gastrointestinal tract can be collected from end stomas. After oral drug intake, the portion of the dose not absorbed can be recovered. This gives an indication of the extent of absorption occurring between mouth and stoma. Studying patients with end stomas at different levels of the gastrointestinal tract may give hints towards location and extent of absorption. With this method it is possible to obtain information on effective bactericidal intracolonic concentrations after oral antimicrobial drug application (Antonin and Bieck, 1987) or on therapeutic intracolonic drug concentrations with new oral formulations of 5-amino salicylic acid (Riley *et al.*, 1988). Second, drugs can be introduced into the distal gastrointestinal tract in patients with a loop stoma. The absorptive capacity between stoma and anus can be assessed by measurements of drug concentrations in body fluids (Antonin and Bieck, 1987). Investigations with artificial stomas must be performed in hospitalised patients. They are not inconvenient to the patients. However, the absorptive capacity of only one part of the gastrointestinal tract can be assessed.

Buccal Absorption

To quantify buccal absorption of drugs, an external closed-perfusion cell design can be used (Barsuhn *et al.*, 1988). The flow cell, which allows perfusion of a 1.8 cm^2 area, is placed against the buccal mucosa and fixed with an extended clamp. Drug solutions are recirculated through the perfusion apparatus by use of a reciprocating pump.

Conclusion

The development of a dosage formulation with extended drug release requires basic knowledge of the absorption of compounds throughout the entire gastrointestinal tract. Intubation techniques are highly sophisticated and permit exact characterisation of the absorption processes in all segments of the gastrointestinal tract. However, intubation techniques are complicated, costly, time-consuming and a burden for the study subject. Therefore, they cannot be used routinely. HF capsules may become the most useful method for the investigation of rate and extent of drug absorption from all regions of the gastrointestinal tract. However, at present this technique is not generally available. Limits of this method lie in repeated X-ray controls, the sometimes difficult placement of a drug into the capsule and the fact that the capsule can be used only one time. Colonoscopic application of drugs in healthy volunteers seems to be a simple, well-tolerated and suitable method for studying drug absorption from the colon. Investigation of drug absorption in patients with artificial stomas can give a qualitative impression of the absorptive capacity of the part of the gastrointestinal tract investigated.

DRUG SAFETY

Many drugs can induce gastrointestinal lesions. These may be related to the pharmacological mechanism of action or to direct toxicity due to high local drug concentrations. More than 20 drugs or classes of drugs associated with gastrointestinal toxicity are known (Dukes, 1987). The need to understand the problems and to estimate the risks of drug treatment stimulated development of human models of gastric mucosal injury (Hawkey *et al.*, 1987).

Gastric Electrical Transmural Potential Difference

The concept of a gastric mucosal barrier emerged from animal studies showing that the mucosa is relatively impermeable to back-diffusion of hydrogen ions, and that permeability increases after response to aspirin and other nonsteroidal antiphlogistic drugs (NSAIDs), ethanol or bile salts. This is followed by a fall in potential difference across the mucosa.

Gastric potential difference is measured most frequently by the method of Andersson and Grossman (1965). The potentials are measured from electrolyte bridges (1.5% agar; 3 mol/l KCl) between gastric mucosa—luminal or gastric electrode—peripheral vein—reference electrode. The luminal electrode is a double-luminal gastric tube, the reference electrode an infusion tube with a butterfly needle placed into a forearm vein. Both tubes are filled with KCl-agar. The luminal and the reference electrodes are attached to separate Erlenmeyer flasks, containing 3 mol/l KCl solution and two calibrated calomel electrodes. The potential differences are monitored continuously with an analogue recorder until a stable baseline potential has been established. After the test substances are instilled, measurements are made until potentials return to baseline. During examination, the volunteers lie in a stable left lateral position. The tip of the luminal tube should be positioned in gastric juice (Laule *et al.*, 1982; Fimmel *et al.*, 1984; Hogan, 1988).

Measurement During Gastroscopy

The electrical potential difference can be measured under visual guidance between a stomach microelectrode and an intravenous reference electrode connected to a millivoltmeter during gastroscopic examinations. pH is measured by an intragastric microelectrode and the junction potential is calculated by the Henderson–Hasselbach equation, taking into account the measured pH. This junction potential is subtracted from the potential difference. The corrected potential difference values can be used to evaluate drug effects in different parts of the stomach (Højgaard *et al.*, 1987).

DNA Content of Cellular Exfoliation

Injuries causing loss of epithelial cells can be quantified by measuring cellular exfoliation in gastric washings. Cells differ in their lysing properties and cannot be reliably quantified by counting alone. Therefore, the DNA content in gastric washings has been used as an index of cellular exfoliation. DNA can be quantified by a modification of the diphenylamine method, which is not affected by the presence of sialic acid (Ruppin *et al.*, 1981; Fimmel *et al.*, 1984). The method is relatively time-consuming and insensitive. Prolonged periods of storage at low temperatures are necessary for the precipitation of DNA.

An alternative approach is a radioimmunoassay that is sensitive and quickly done. Serum from patients with systemic lupus erythematosus is used as the source for anti-DNA antibodies (Hurst *et al.*, 1984).

With such techniques, signs of increased cellular exfoliation can be found in patients with atrophic gastritis or gastric ulcerations and in volunteers challenged with ethanol, bile or aspirin. Cellular exfoliation is reduced after treatment with carbenoxolone and prostaglandin E.

This technique does not distinguish between increased loss and increased production of epithelial cells. It seems likely that the higher DNA content of gastric washings observed after single acute challenges with aspirin or taurocholate is due to enhanced loss of epithelial cells, but the higher DNA content of washings after chronic dosing may reflect also increased production of DNA.

Secretion of Bicarbonate

Human gastric and/or duodenal bicarbonate secretion is an important protective factor, preventing gastroduodenal damage. Therefore, bicarbonate is measured to determine the influence of drugs on its secretion (Feldman *et al.*, 1984; Isenberg *et al.*, 1986; Selling *et al.*, 1987). A double-luminal gastro-duodenal tube is positioned under fluoroscopic control, and the pylorus is occluded with two balloons. This prevents any escape of gastric juices into the duodenum and reflux of duodenal contents into the stomach. The duodenum is occluded by a distal balloon creating an isolated duodenal segment. Duodenal secretions are aspirated and bicarbonate secretion is measured by a back-titration method (Isenberg *et al.*, 1986)

Mucosal Blood Flow—Laser Doppler Flowmetry

Endoscopic laser Doppler flowmetry is used to evaluate the effects of drugs or hormones on gastric blood circulation in man. During gastroscopy, a fibre-optic probe is introduced through the biopsy channel of the instrument. The probe contains optic fibres for transmission of laser light to the gastric wall and fibres for collecting the reflected light. Recordings are made from specifically defined areas of the stomach and plotted with a linear recorder. Laser Doppler flowmetry measures relative flow, and the flow values are expressed in units of relative flux (Kvernebo *et al.*, 1986; Lunde *et al.*, 1988).

Gastroscopy

Gastroscopic studies are performed in healthy subjects (Lanza, 1984; Hogan, 1988) or in patients who are treated with drugs that damage the mucosa (Caruso and Bianchi Porro, 1980; Larkai *et al.*, 1987). Before start of the trial, a baseline examination is performed. An absolute exclusion criterion is the presence of any oesophageal, gastric, or duodenal lesions. Endoscopic examinations are performed at the end of each treatment period (no later than 24 h after the last drug administration). They are repeated when severe gastrointestinal symptoms or severe lesions occur. The procedure for this is standardised. After fasting for 10–12 hours, the volunteers receive local anaesthesia of the faucet and posterior pharyngeal wall with xylocaine spray. Gastroscopy is done with the volunteer lying in the left lateral position.

All lesions are described at each stage of the examination and are documented by photography or film or using a video-camera. Television, together with tape recording, permits not only documentation, but also instant analysis. Lesions are graded according to scales (Lanza, 1984). Artefacts caused by the endoscope are not recorded. It is advantageous if the same investigator performs all endoscopic examinations in a study.

Advantages of endoscopy are the directness of visualisation and the possibility of obtaining biopsies.

Some open questions about the use of gastroscopy are:

(1) In about 15–30% of healthy, asymptomatic volunteers gastric lesions are observed during the initial examination (Akdamar *et al.*, 1986). However, in the literature pretreatment data are often not given. Placebo-treated subjects have low gastric injury scores in these studies. It is suggested, therefore, that all volunteers are endoscopically examined before inclusion into such a study. The design should be cross-over and placebo-controlled. This would lead to the necessary sound database of results from healthy asymptomatic volunteers.

(2) The treatment period is frequently too short to reveal changes that might appear with chronic administration.

(3) There is no universally accepted scale for quantification of mucosal damage. Therefore, studies cannot be easily compared. Most often used are estimates of macroscopic changes. Most rating scales attempt to assess the size of the lesions. However, how many small lesions are equivalent to a large one? Or how should petechiae scored?

(4) Endoscopic studies are usually performed in young and healthy sub-

jects. This population is different from that in which peptic ulcers and complications caused by NSAIDs occur.

Colonoscopy

Colonoscopy, probably because of discomfort, is not widely used for the evaluation of possible harmful effects of drugs on the large bowel. In the past, relatively little attention has been given to the question of side-effects of drugs in this segment of human gut (Somerville and Hawkey, 1986; Rampton, 1987). The reason is that most drugs are completely absorbed in the upper intestinal tract after oral administration. They will not reach the large bowel. However, the development of dosage forms that release drug over extended periods of time raises the question as to whether, and to what extent, the mucosa of the large bowel can be damaged.

Faecal Blood Loss

Red blood cells are tagged with radiolabelled sodium chromate ($Na[^{51}Cr]O_4$) and the blood is injected back to the same subject. Gastrointestinal micro-bleeding (ml/day) is determined by the amount of radioactive chromium in three successive 24 h stool specimens collected thereafter (Lussier *et al.*, 1983).

[^{51}Cr]-EDTA Excretion in Urine

Changes in intestinal permeability caused by diseases or NSAIDs in healthy subjects and patients is assessed by measuring the radioactivity in 24 h urines after oral administration of [^{51}Cr]-EDTA. After an overnight fast, the test solution of [^{51}Cr]-EDTA is administered. Urine is collected for 24 h after ingestion and aliquots are assayed in a scintillation counter (Bjarnason *et al.*, 1983, 1986).

Pepsinogen in Blood

Changes in gastric permeability caused by diseases or drugs can be assessed by measuring concentrations of pepsinogen I and pepsinogen II in serum of healthy subjects and patients (Chuong *et al.*, 1986; Hengels, 1987). Serum pepsinogen concentrations are measured by use of radioimmunoassays. A positive correlation between the increase of pepsinogen concentrations and incidence and severity of gastric lesions has been reported (Hengels, 1987). The author concludes that serum pepsinogen determination may be a useful non-invasive technique for early detection of drug-induced gastric side-effects.

Buccal Assay

A new method for studying the potential of drugs to irritate the gastrointestinal tract has recently been reported. Drugs in aqueous gels are applied to the buccal mucosa in small disposable cups. The open face of the cup is in contact with the buccal mucosa of the lip for 1 h. At defined intervals during and after application, subjective sensations and changes in the mucosal surface are recorded. Scales are used for scoring and an irritation index is calculated (Place *et al.*, 1988). The buccal assay is useful only in examining the contact irritation potential of drugs and formulations under most unfavourable conditions, as in cases of adherence of drugs to the oesophageal mucosa.

Conclusion

The gastrointestinal tract is most prone to serious side-effects of drugs. Therefore, human models of gastrointestinal injury are needed in early phases of drug development. For basic research on mucosal damage, measurements of mucosal blood flow or bicarbonate secretion are useful. First data on the development of clinically significant signs of toxicity are obtained by endoscopy. Macroscopic lesions can be detected and may be used as predictors for the risk of major adverse effects during long-term treatment in patients. Measurement of mucosal potential difference is an indirect method and seems useful in the assessment of acute injury. However, after multiple dosage there is no correlation between changes of potential difference and gastroscopic findings (Antonin *et al.*, 1985). Cellular desquamation as measured by DNA content in gastric washings, faecal blood loss as measured by ^{51}Cr labelling, changes of intestinal permeability as measured by urinary excretion of [^{51}Cr]-EDTA or analysis of pepsinogen in serum are not widely used.

OTHER METHODS

Collection of Saliva

To determine anticholinergic effects of drugs, salivary secretion rate can be measured. Basal and stimulated saliva can be collected with cups occluding the orifices of distinct salivary ducts (von Knorring and Mörnstad, 1986). The secretion rate is expressed in ml/min. Mixed salivary secretion from all glands can be quantified with rolls of cotton wool between lips and gingiva and under the tongue. The rolls are weighed before and one or two minutes after application. Salivation can be stimulated by having the subjects chew on a small ball of Parafilm. Drug concentrations in saliva are often proportional to concentrations in plasma. This led to the use of saliva for therapeutic drug monitoring or pharmacokinetic studies (Graham, 1982). Measuring saliva concentrations of drugs can prevent unnecessary blood loss, especially during pharmacokinetic studies in patients. A prerequisite for the use of saliva is a constant range of concentrations between saliva and plasma.

Induced Diarrhoea

For the evaluation of antidiarrhoeal drugs in healthy volunteers, diarrhoea can be induced by castor oil (LaCorte *et al.*, 1982), by synthetic prostaglandin analogues such as misoprostol, or by prolonged infusion of vasoactive intestinal polypeptide (Kane *et al.*, 1983). The number and character (formed, soft or watery) of bowel movements are noted. The stool is weighed and analysed for sodium, potassium, chloride, bicarbonate and osmolality. Subjective side-effects such as flatulence or abdominal cramps are rated for severity (mild, moderate or severe).

Prostaglandins in Biopsies

NSAIDs inhibit cyclo-oxygenase activity. Suppression of endogenous pros-taglandin synthesis in gastric mucosa has been implicated as a possible mechanism of NSAID-induced gastric lesions. Therefore, the effect of NSAIDs on gastric mucosal prostaglandin synthesis was measured and a correlation with effects on the mucosa was sought. During gastroscopy, biopsies were obtained and prostaglandin concentrations of the mucosal biopsy specimens were measured by radioimmunoassay (Goldin *et al.*, 1988; Levine *et al.*, 1988). NSAIDs reduce gastric prostaglandin synthesis without regard to presence or absence of mucosal damage. There was no correlation between degree of suppression of prostaglandin concentrations and endoscopic evidence of mucosal damage.

Gastrointestinal Hormones

Gastrointestinal functions are modulated by complex hormonal and neural interrelationships. The gastrointestinal hormones are a family of polypeptides produced by endocrine cells in the gastrointestinal tract. These hormones regulate specific biological functions of stomach, small and large intestine, endocrine and exocrine pancreas, liver and biliary system, in order to optimise physiological conditions for digestion, absorption and motility (Norman and Litwack, 1987). Measurement of hormones, such as gastrin or pancreatic polypeptide, is used to assess the effects of nutrients or drugs. As radioimmunoassays for most gastrointestinal hormones are not yet generally available, such measurements are mostly used for diagnostic purposes in specialised centres.

INFLAMMATORY BOWEL DISEASES

The aetiology of ulcerative colitis and Crohn's disease remains unknown, and no specific therapy exists. Palliative therapy with several non-specific agents has evolved. However, advances in drug therapy should be evaluated critically (Korelitz, 1980; Riis, 1980). Clear criteria for diagnosis and judgement of therapeutic efficacy are needed(Hodgson, 1982).

Clinical Assessment

The diagnosis of inflammatory bowel disease is usually made on the basis of clinical symptoms. In order to assess clinical actitivity, indices were developed (Hodgson, 1982). Recently, a new index including morphological alterations has been reported (Maier *et al.*, 1988).

Laboratory Parameters

Laboratory findings are very helpful in diagnosis and control of treatment. Acute-phase proteins or orosomucoid concentrations correlate well with disease activity. Hypoproteinaemia and hypalbuminaemia are often present, resulting from excessive enteric protein loss. [^{51}Cr]-EDTA excretion in urine, as described above (Bjarnason *et al.*, 1986) and ^{111}In autologous leucocyte scanning in faeces (Saverymuttu *et al.*, 1983b) have been used to assess disease activity. Identification and quantification of leukotrienes and prostaglandins in tissue, faeces and urine have also been used (Rampton and Hawkey, 1984; Lauritsen *et al.*, 1988).

Endoscopic Assessment

Endoscopy is the most accurately diagnostic tool in inflammatory bowel disease. Inspection of the altered mucosa allows a direct judgement about severity and extent of the inflammatory processes.

Histological Assessment

Biopsies during endoscopy can offer an objective assessment of the severity of the inflammatory process and will confirm the diagnosis.

Radiography

Radiographic examinations may be useful in confirming diagnosis, extent of disease and complications such as strictures or fistulas. However, there is a poor correlation between clinical indices and radiographic images.

Scintigraphy

^{111}In autologous leucocyte scanning is used for the assessment of extent of the disease as well as therapeutic efficacy. White blood cells are separated from venous blood and incubated with ^{111}In. The labelled cells are reinjected intravenously. Radioactivity over the abdomen is scanned with a gamma camera (Saverymuttu *et al.*, 1983a). However, there is poor correlation between scan scores and other indices of disease activity (Park *et al.*, 1988).

Conclusion

For therapeutic trials in inflammatory bowel diseases, the quality of test methods is of crucial importance. Clinically specific symptoms should be assessed and graded by use of standardised indices together with laboratory parameters. Endoscopic and histological findings are useful for the demonstration of an effective treatment regimen.

REFERENCES

Akdamar, K., Ertan, A., Agrawal, N., McMahon, F. G. and Ryan, J. (1986). Upper gastrointestinal endoscopy in normal asymptomatic volunteers. *Gastrointest. Endosc.*, **32**, 78–80

Andersson, S. and Grossman, M. J. (1965). Profile of pH, pressure and potential difference at gastroduodenal junction in man. *Gastroenterology*, **49**, 364–71

Antonin, K. H. and Bieck, P. (1987). Evaluation of the colonic drug absorption in patients with an artificial intestinal stoma and by colonoscopy in normal volunteers. In Rietbrock, N., Woodcock, B. G., Staib, A. H. and Loew, D. (Eds.), *Methods in Clinical Pharmacology* No. 7. Vieweg-Verlag, Braunschweig, pp. 39–51

Antonin, K. H., Britzelmeier, C. and Kohlstetter, K. (1985). Gastric potential difference: A method to establish gastric mucosal integrity in man after longterm treatment with gastric irritants. *Naunyn-Schmiedeberg's Arch. Pharm.*, **329** (Suppl.), R100

Antonin, K. H., Jedrychowski, M. and Bieck, P. R. (1988). Effects of codeine phosphate on gastric motility and mouth-to-cecum transit-time in humans measured by sulfapyridine appearance in saliva after oral salicylazosulfapyridine. *Hepatogastroenterology*, **35**, 186

Askin, J. R., Lyon, D. I., Shull, S. D., Wagner, C. I. and Soloway, R. D. (1978). Factors affecting delivery of bile to the duodenum in man. *Gastroenterology*, **74**, 560–5

Atkinson, M. (1987). Monitoring oesophageal pH. *Gut*, **28**, 509–14

Barsuhn, C. L., Olanoff, L. S., Gleason, D. D., Adkins, E. L. and Ho, N. F. H. (1988). Human buccal absorption of flurbiprofen. *Clin. Pharm. Ther.*, **44**, 225–31

Bateman, D. N. and Whittingham, T. A. (1982). Measurement of gastric emptying by real-time ultrasound. *Gut*, **23**, 524–7

Bjarnason, I., O'Morain, C., Levi, A. J. and Peters, T. J. (1983). Absorption of ^{51}chromium-labeled ethylenediaminetetraacetate in inflammatory bowel disease. *Gastroenterology*, **85**, 318–22

Bjarnason, J., Williams, P., Smethurst, P., Peters, T. J. and Levi, A. J. (1986). Effect of non-steroidal anti-inflammatory drugs and prostaglandins on the permeability of the human small intestine. *Gut*, **27**, 1292–7

Bond, J. H. and Levitt, M. D. (1975). Investigation of small bowel transit time in man utilizing pulmonary hydrogen (H_2) measurements. *J. Lab. Clin. Med.*, **85**, 546–55

Branicki, F. J., Evans, D. F., Ogilvie, A. L., Atkinson, M. and Hardcastle, J. D. (1982). Ambulatory monitoring of oesophageal pH in reflux oesophagitis using a portable radiotelemetry system. *Gut*, **23**, 992–8

Camilleri, M., Brown, M. L. and Malagelada, J. R. (1986). Impaired transit of chyme in chronic intestinal pseudoobstruction. Correction by cisapride. *Gastroenterology*, **91**, 619–26

Caruso, I. and Bianchi Porro, G. (1980). Gastroscopic evaluation of anti-inflammatory agents. *Br. Med. J.*, **280**, 75–8

Channer, K. S. and Virjee, J. P. (1986). The effect of size and shape of tablets on their esophageal transit. *J. Clin. Pharm.*, **26**, 141–6

Chuong, J. J. H., Fisher, R. L., Chuong, R. L. B. and Spiro, H. M. (1986). Duodenal ulcer—incidence, risk factors, and predictive value of plasma pepsinogen. *Dig. Dis. Sci.*, **31**, 1178–84

Collins, P. J., Horowitz, M., Cook, D. J., Harding, P. E. and Shearman, D. J. C. (1983). Gastric emptying in normal subjects—a reproducible technique using a single scintillation camera and computer system. *Gut*, **24**, 1117–25

Cummings, J. H. and Wiggins, H. S. (1976). Transit through the gut measured by analysis of a single stool. *Gut*, **17**, 219–23

Davis, S. S., Hardy, J. G. and Fara, J. W. (1986). Transit of pharmaceutical dosage forms through the small intestine. *Gut*, **27**, 886–92

Davis, S. S., Hardy, J. G., Taylor, M. J., Whalley, D. R. and Wilson, C. G. (1984). A comparative study of the gastrointestinal transit of a pellet and tablet formulation. *Int. J. Pharm.*, **21**, 167–77

Dujovne, C. A., Gustafson, J. H. and Dickey, R. A. (1982). Quantitation of biliary excretion of drugs in man. *Clin. Pharm. Ther.*, **31**, 187–94

Dukes, M. N. G. (Ed.) (1987). *Side Effects of Drugs, Annual 11*. Elsevier, Amsterdam, New York, Oxford

Emde, C., Garner, A. and Blum, A. L. (1987). Technical aspects of intraluminal pH-metry in man: current status and recommendations. *Gut*, **28**, 1177–88

Feldman, M. and Colturi, T. J. (1984). Effect of indomethacin on gastric acid and bicarbonate secretion in humans. *Gastroenterology*, **87**, 1339–43

Fimmel, C. J., Müller-Lissner, S. A. and Blum, A. L. (1984). Bile salt induced, acute gastric mucosal damage in man: Time course and effect of misoprostol, a PGE analogue. *Scand. J. Gastroenterol.*, **19** (Suppl. 92), 184–8

Funch-Jensen, P., Kruse, A. and Ravnsbaek, J. (1987). Endoscopic sphincter of Oddi manometry in healthy volunteers. *Scand. J. Gastroenterol.*, **22**, 243–9

Goldin, E., Stalnikowicz, R., Wengrower, D., Eliakim, R., Fich, A., Ligumsky, M., Karmeli, F. and Rachmilewitz, D. (1988). No correlation between indomethacin-induced gastroduodenal damage and inhibition of gastric prostanoid synthesis. *Aliment. Pharm. Ther.*, **2**, 369–75

Graham, G. G. (1982). Noninvasive chemical methods of estimating pharmacokinetic parameters. *Pharm. Ther.*, **18**, 333–49

Hallerbäck, B., Glise, H., Karlsson, F. and Tegnebjer, M. (1988). Beta-adrenoceptor blockade does not modify gastrointestinal transit time in healthy volunteers. *Scand. J. Gastroenterol.*, **23**, 817–20

Hamilton, J. W., Bellahsene, B. E., Reichelderfer, M., Webster, J. G. and Bass, P. (1986). Human electrogastrograms. Comparison of surface and mucosal recordings. *Dig. Dis. Sci.*, **31**, 33–9

Hansen, W. E. and Felgenträger, B. (1987). Bestimmung der Gallenblasengrösse mit

Ultraschall—Methoden und Ergebnisse. *Leber, Magen, Darm*, 166–72

Hawkey, C. J. (1987). Review: acute human models of gastric mucosal injury. *Aliment. Pharm. Ther.*, **1**, 593–606

Hengels, K. J. (1987). Eignet sich die Serum-Pepsinogen-Bestimmung zur Früherkennung gastraler Nebenwirkungen nichtsteroidalder Antirheumatika? In Simon, B. (Ed.), *Nichtsteroidale Antirheumatika und Gastrointestinaltrakt*. Schattauer Verlag, Stuttgart, New York, pp. 35–40

Hirtz, J. (1987). Intubation techniques for the study of the absorption of drugs in man. In Rietbrock, N., Woodcock, B. G., Staib, A. H. and Loew, D. (Eds.), *Methods in Clinical Pharmacology*, No. 7. Vieweg-Verlag, Braunschweig, pp. 3–11

Hodgson, H. J. F. (1982). Assessment of drug therapy in inflammatory bowel disease. *Br. J. Clin. Pharm.*, **14**, 159–70

Hogan, D. L. (1988). Damage and protection of the gastric mucosa. A multiparameter assessment. *Am. J. Med.*, **84** (Suppl. 2A), 35–40

Højgaard, L., Andersen, J. R. and Krag, E. (1987). A new method for measurement of electrical potential difference across the stomach wall. Clinical evaluation of the gastric mucosal integrity. *Scand. J. Gastroenterol.*, **22**, 847–58

Holt, S., Cervantes, J., Wilkinson, A. A. and Wallace, K. J. H. (1986). Measurement of gastric emptying rate in humans by real-time ultrasound. *Gastroenterology*, **90**, 918–23

Horowitz, M., Maddox, A., Harding, P. E., Maddern, G. J., Chatterton, B. E., Wishart, J. and Shearman, D. (1987). Effect of cisapride on gastric and esophageal emptying in insulin-dependent diabetes mellitus. *Gastroenterology*, **92**, 1899–907

Hurst, B. C., Rees, W. D. W. and Garner, A. (1984). Cell loss from human, canine, and guinea pig gastric mucosa measured by DNA radioimmunoassay. *Clin. Sci.*, **66**, 701–8

Isenberg, J. I., Hogan, D. L., Koss, M. A. and Selling, J. A. (1986). Human duodenal mucosal bicarbonate secretion. Evidence for basal secretion and stimulation by hydrochloric acid and a synthetic prostaglandin E_1 analogue. *Gastroenterology*, **91**, 370–8

Jaup, B. H., Abrahamsson, H., Stockbruegger, R. W., Rosengren, K. and Dotevall, G. (1985). Effect of selective and non-selective antimuscarinics on rectosigmoid motility and gastrointestinal transit. *Scand. J. Gastroenterol.*, **20**, 1101–9

Kane, M. G., O'Dorisio, T. M. and Krejs, G. J. (1983). Production of secretory diarrhea by intravenous infusion of vasoactive intestinal polypeptide. *New Engl. J. Med.*, **309**, 1482–5

Kellow, J. E., Borody, T. J., Phillips, S. F., Haddad, A. C. and Brown, M. L. (1986). Sulfapyridine appearance in plasma after salicylazosulfapyridine. Another simple measure of intestinal transit. *Gastroenterology*, **91**, 396–400

Korelitz, B. I. (1980). Therapy of inflammatory bowel disease including use of immunosuppressive agents. *Clin. Gastroenterol.*, **9** (2), 331–49

Krevsky, B., Malmud, L. S., D'Ercole, F., Maurer, A. H. and Fisher, R. S. (1986). Colonic transit scintigraphy. A physiologic approach to the quantitative measurement of colonic transit in humans. *Gastroenterology*, **91**, 1102–12

Kvernebo, K., Lunde, O. C., Stranden, E. and Larsen, S. (1986). Human gastric blood circulation evaluated by endoscopic laser Doppler flowmetry. *Scand. J. Gastroenterol.*, **21**, 685–92

LaCorte, W. S. J., McMurtrey, J. J., Chapman, J., Gotzkowsky, S., Chang-Chien, S., Ryan, J. R. and McMahon, F. G. (1982). A simple controlled method for the clinical evaluation of antidiarrheal drugs. *Clin. Pharm. Ther.*, **31**, 766–9

Lanza, F. L. (1984). Endoscopic studies of gastric and duodenal injury after the use of ibuprofen, aspirin and other nonsteroidal anti-inflammatory agents. *Am. J. Med.*, **77** (Suppl. 1A), 19–24

Lanzini, A., Jazrawi, R. P. and Northfield, T. C. (1987). Simultaneous quantitative measurements of absolute gallbladder storage and emptying during fasting and eating in humans. *Gastroenterology*, **92**, 852–61

Larkai, E. N., Smith, J. L., Lidsky, M. D. and Graham, D. Y. (1987). Gastroduodenal mucosa and dyspeptic symptoms in arthritic patients during chronic nonsteroidal anti-inflammatory drug use. *Am. J. Gastroenterol.*, **82**, 1153–8

Laule, H., Lücker, P. W., Altmayer, P. and Eldon, M. A. (1982). Gastric potential difference as a model in clinical pharmacology: assessment of gastric mucosal response to aspirin. *Eur. J. Clin. Pharm.*, **22**, 147–51

Lauritsen, K., Laursen, L. S., Bukhave, K. and Rask-Madsen, J. (1988). *In vivo* profiles of eicosanoids in ulcerative colitis, Crohn's colitis, and *Clostridium difficile* colitis. *Gastroenterology*, **95**, 11–17

Levine, R. A., Petokas, S., Nandi, J. and Enthoven, D. (1988). Effects of nonsteroidal, antiinflammatory drugs on gastrointestinal injury and prostanoid generation in healthy volunteers. *Dig. Dis. Sci.*, **33**, 660–6

Lind, T., Andersson, T., Skanberg, I. and Olbe, L. (1987). Biliary excretion of intravenous [^{14}C]omeprazole in humans. *Clin. Pharm. Ther.*, **42**, 504–8

Lunde, O. C., Kvernebo, K. and Larsen, S. (1988). Evaluation of endoscopic laser Doppler flowmetry for measurement of human gastric blood flow. Methodologic aspects. *Scand. J. Gastroenterol.*, **23**, 1072–8

Lussier, A., Tétreault, L. and Lebel, E. (1983). Comparative study of gastrointestinal microbleeding caused by aspirin, fenbufen, and placebo. *Am. J. Med.*, **75**, 80–3

McClelland, G. R. and Sutton, J. A. (1985). Epigastric impedance: a non-invasive method for the assessment of gastric emptying and motility. *Gut*, **26**, 607–14

McFarland, R. J., Corbett, C. R. R., Taylor, P. and Nash, A. G. (1984). The relaxant action of hymecromone and lignocaine on induced spasm of the bile duct sphincter. *Br. J. Clin. Pharm.*, **17**, 766–8

Mackie, C. R., Baxter, J. N., Grime, J. S., Hulks, G. and Cuschieri, A. (1987). Gall bladder emptying in normal subjects—a data base for clinical cholescintigraphy. *Gut*, **28**, 137–41

Maier, K., von Gaisberg, U. and Kraus, B. (1988). Colitis ulcerosa—Aktivitätsindex zur klinischen und histologischen Klassifikation der Entzündungsaktivität. *Schweiz. med. Wschr.*, **118**, 763–6

Malagelada, J. R., Robertson, J. S., Brown, M. L., Remington, M., Duenes, J. A., Thomforde, G. M. and Carryer, P. W. (1984). Intestinal transit of solid and liquid components of a meal in health. *Gastroenterology*, **87**, 1255–63

Marzio, L., Capone, F., Neri, M., di Felice, F., Celiberti, V., Mezzetti, A., Giorgi, D. and Cuccurullo, F. (1987). Effect of cholinergic agonists and antagonists on gallbladder volume in fasting man. *Eur. J. Clin. Pharm.*, **33**, 151–3

Minami, H. and McCallum, R. W. (1984). The physiology and pathophysiology of gastric emptying in humans. *Gastroenterology*, **86**, 1592–610

Moriarty, K. J., O'Grady, J., Rolston, D. D. K., Kelly, M. J. and Clark, M. L. (1986). Effect of prostacyclin (PGI$_2$) on water and solute transport in the human jejunum. *Gut*, **27**, 158–63

Narducci, F., Bassotti, G., Gaburri, M. and Morelli, A. (1987). Twenty-four hour manometric recording of colonic motor activity in healthy man. *Gut*, **28**, 17–26

Norman, A. W. and Litwack, G. (1987). *Hormones*. Academic Press, Orlando, pp. 322–54

Park, R. H. R., McKillop, J. H., Duncan, A., MacKenzie, J. F. and Russell, R. I. (1988). Can ^{111}indium autologous mixed leucocyte scanning accurately assess disease extent and activity in Crohn's disease? *Gut*, **29**, 821–5

Place, V., Darley, P., Baricevic, K., Ramans, A., Pruitt, B. and Guittard, G. (1988). Human buccal assay for evaluation of the mucosal irritation potential of drugs. *Clin. Pharm. Ther.*, **43**, 233–41

Rampton, D. S. (1987). Non-steroidal anti-inflammatory drugs and the lower gastrointestinal tract. *Scand. J. Gastroenterol.*, **22**, 1–4

Rampton, D. S. and Hawkey, S. J. (1984). Prostaglandins and ulcerative colitis. *Gut*, **25**, 1399–413

Read, N. W., Al-Janabi, M. N., Bates, T. E., Holgate, A. M., Cann, P. A., Kinsman, R. I., McFarlane, A. and Brown, C. (1985). Interpretation of the breath hydrogen profile obtained after ingesting a solid meal containing unabsorbable carbohydrate. *Gut*, **26**, 834–42

Read, N. W., Al-Janabi, M. N., Holgate, A. M., Barber, D. C. and Edwards, C. A. (1986). Simultaneous measurement of gastric emptying, small bowel residence and colonic filling of a solid meal by the use of the gamma camera. *Gut*, **27**, 300–8

Redfern, J. S., Lee, E. and Feldman, M. (1987). Effect of indomethacin on gastric mucosal prostaglandins in humans. Correlation with mucosal damage. *Gastroenterology*, **92**, 969–77

Riis, P. (1980). A critical survey of controlled studies in the treatment of ulcerative colitis and Crohn's disease. *Clin. Gastroenterol.*, **9** (2), 351–69

Riley, S. A., Tavares, I. A., Bennett, A. and Mani, V. (1988). Delayed-release mesalazine (5-aminosalicylic acid): coat dissolution and excretion in ileostomy subjects. *Br. J. Clin. Pharm.*, **26**, 173–7

Rollins, D. E. and Klaassen, C. D. (1979). Biliary excretion of drugs in man. *Clin. Pharmacokin.*, **4**, 368–79

Ruppin, H., Person, B., Robert, A. and Domschke, W. (1981). Gastric cytoprotection in man by prostaglandin E_2. *Scand. J. Gastroenterol.*, **16**, 647–52

Santander, R., Mena, I., Gramisu, M. and Valenzuela, J. E. (1988). Effect of nifedipine on gastric emptying and gastrointestinal motility in man. *Dig. Dis. Sci.*, **33**, 535–9

Saverymuttu, S. H., Lavender, J. P., Hodgson, H. J. F. and Chadwick, V. S. (1983a). Assessment of disease activity in inflammatory bowel disease: a new approach using ^{111}In granulocyte scanning. *Br. Med. J.*, **287**, 1751–3

Saverymuttu, S. H., Peters, A. M., Lavender, J. P., Pepys, M. B., Hodgson, H. J. F. and Chadwick, V. S. (1983b). Quantitative fecal indium 111-labeled leukocyte excretion in the assessment of disease in Crohn's disease. *Gastroenterology*, **85**, 1333–9

Schuster, O. and Hugemann, B. (1987). Course of development of the HF-capsule— variations and method-related typical findings. In Rietbrock, N., Woodcock, B. G., Staib, A. H. and Loew, D. (Eds.), *Methods in Clinical Pharmacology*, No. 7. Vieweg-Verlag, Braunschweig, pp. 28–37

Selling, J. A., Hogan, D. L., Aly, A., Koss, M. A. and Isenberg, J. I. (1987). Indomethacin inhibits duodenal mucosal bicarbonate secretion and endogenous prostaglandin E_2 output in human subjects. *Ann. Int. Med.*, **106**, 368–71

Smith, H. J. and Feldman, M. (1986). Influence of food and marker length on gastric emptying of indigestible radiopaque markers in healthy humans. *Gastroenterology*, **91**, 1452–5

Soffer, E. E., Kumar, D., Mridha, K., Das-Gupta, A., Britto, J. and Wingate, D. L. (1988). Effect of pirenzepine on oesophageal, gastric, and enteric motor function in man. *Scand. J. Gastroenterol.*, **23**, 146–50

Somerville, K. W. and Hawkey, C. J. (1986). Non-steroidal anti-inflammatory agents and the gastrointestinal tract. *Postgrad. Med. J.*, **62**, 23–8

Spiller, R. C. (1986). Where do all the tablets go in 1986? *Gut*, **27**, 879–85

Stacher, G. (1985). Oesophageal motility, oesophageal transit, and gastro-oesophageal reflux—a methodological overview. *Hepato-gastroenterology*, **32**, 299–304

Staib, A. H., Loew, D., Harder, S., Graul, E. H. and Pfab, R. (1986). Measurement of theophylline absorption from different regions of the gastro-intestinal tract using a remote controlled drug delivery device. *Eur. J. Clin. Pharm.*, **30**, 691–7

Stern, R. M., Koch, K. L., Stewart, W. R. and Vasey, M. W. (1987). Electrogastrography: current issues in validation and methodology. *Psychophysiology*, **24**, 55–64

Terhaag, B. and Hermann, U. (1986). Biliary elimination of indomethacin in man. *Eur. J. Clin. Pharm.*, **29**, 691–5

Thompson, D. G., Wingate, D. L., Archer, L., Benson, M. J., Green, W. J. and Hardy, R. J. (1980). Normal patterns of human upper small bowel motor activity recorded by prolonged radiotelemetry. *Gut*, **21**, 500–6

Trotman, I. and Misiewicz, G. (1982). Methods in human alimentary motility. *Br. J. Clin. Pharm.*, **14**, 757–63

Van Wyk, M., De Sommers, K. and Steyn, A. G. W. (1985). Evaluation of gastrointestinal motility using the hydrogen breath test. *Br. J. Clin. Pharm.*, **20**, 479–81

Von Knorring, L. and Mörnstad, H. (1986). Saliva secretion rate and saliva composition as a model to determine the effect of antidepressant drugs on cholinergic and noradrenergic transmission. *Neuropsychobiology*, **15**, 146–54

37
Anti-ulcer Drugs

Colin Broom

SKF Research Ltd, The Frythe, Welwyn, Herts AL6 9AR, UK

INTRODUCTION

The development of potent antisecretory drugs, namely the H_2 receptor antagonists, has undoubtedly been the greatest therapeutic advance of the last 15 years. Further development of antisecretory drugs with differing profiles, including H^+/K^+ ATPase inhibitors, is likely to continue, and therefore this chapter focuses primarily on such drugs. Anti-ulcer drugs with different mechanisms of action are likely to be developed, although the methodology of their evaluation is less clear.

ANTISECRETORY AGENTS

The antisecretory effect of drugs can be assessed by use of different methodologies. Several non-invasive tests have been described, although none have been widely accepted. Methods involving the passage of a nasogastric tube or electrode are those of choice.

The study population for the initial evaluation of antisecretory effect are usually healthy volunteers. Subsequently, studies are performed in duodenal ulcer patients in remission, and the data generated are commonly applied to patients with active duodenal ulceration, as well as to patients with reflux oesophagitis and gastric ulceration.

General experience has shown that the findings in young healthy volunteers, who often have quite high acid outputs, usually hold true for the patient population, although ulcer patients, on average, secrete more acid than do a control population (Merki *et al.*, 1988a).

It must be remembered that the antisecretory data derived from the different methodologies are not directly comparable and it is important that there be clarity over the presentation and subsequent interpretation of the data.

Methodological Aspects

The two major methods of determining antisecretory effect are by the aspiration of gastric contents and by monitoring gastric pH via an intragastric electrode.

Aspiration of Gastric Secretion

The technique of aspiration of gastric secretion remains the 'gold standard' for the assessment of antisecretory effect of drugs. This technique has long been established in clinical use (Baron, 1978). It is important that a nasogastric tube be well positioned in the antrum of the stomach, either under fluoroscopic control or using the water recovery test (Hassan and Hobsley, 1970; Findlay *et al.*, 1972). Aspiration may be performed manually with a syringe or, alternatively, using continuous or intermittent aspiration with a suction pump. Regular attention is required to ensure that the nasogastric tube does not become obstructed and does not damage the gastric mucosa.

Basal gastric acid secretory rate is variable (Faber and Hobsley, 1977) and has a circadian rhythm in both healthy subjects and patients (Moore and Englert, 1970; Moore and Halberg, 1986). Aspiration is often technically difficult because of the relatively small volumes secreted, especially when antisecretory drugs are being evaluated. The variability in secretory rate can be overcome to a significant extent by using a stimulant of gastric acid secretion. A number of agents have been used over the years, including histamine, histamine analogues and the H_2 receptor agonist impromidine; however, these have significant disadvantages in terms of tolerability. Penta-gastrin (Peptavlon, ICI), which is a synthetic peptide incorporating the active C-terminal tetrapeptide sequence of gastrin, is now the most widely used and acceptable stimulant, especially when used in low dose by continuous intravenous infusion. An infusion rate of $0.6 \ \mu g \ kg^{-1} \ h^{-1}$ is a near-maximal stimulatory dose for the majority of healthy subjects, although a higher dose level may be required in ulcer patients (Wormsley, 1972; Petersen and Myren, 1975). Steady state stimulation of secretion normally takes 30 min to attain. Early experience with pentagastrin, predominantly at higher dose levels, indicated fading of secretory response with time; however, in the majority of subjects fading is unlikely, perhaps over periods as long as 7 h with currently used dose levels (Petersen *et al.*, 1984; Chin *et al.*, 1986). Maintaining the hydration of subjects with intravenous fluids during extended aspiration is important, to replace the fluid lost from the stomach.

Aspirated secretion is normally collected into 15 min collection periods and the total volume is noted before an aliquot is titrated to pH 7 with 0.1 M sodium hydroxide to determine hydrogen ion concentration. The total acid output during each period can then be calculated.

Other technical aspects associated with aspiration methods include whether to correct for contamination of gastric secretion by saliva or duodenal fluids, and whether to allow for loss of secretion through the pylorus. Although methods of correction are available (Whitfield and Hobsley, 1979), they are, in general, not used.

The onset and peak effect of intravenously administered drugs on steady state pentagastrin-stimulated acid output can be clearly seen and followed for a period of a few hours (Figure 37.1). When drug is given orally, time must be

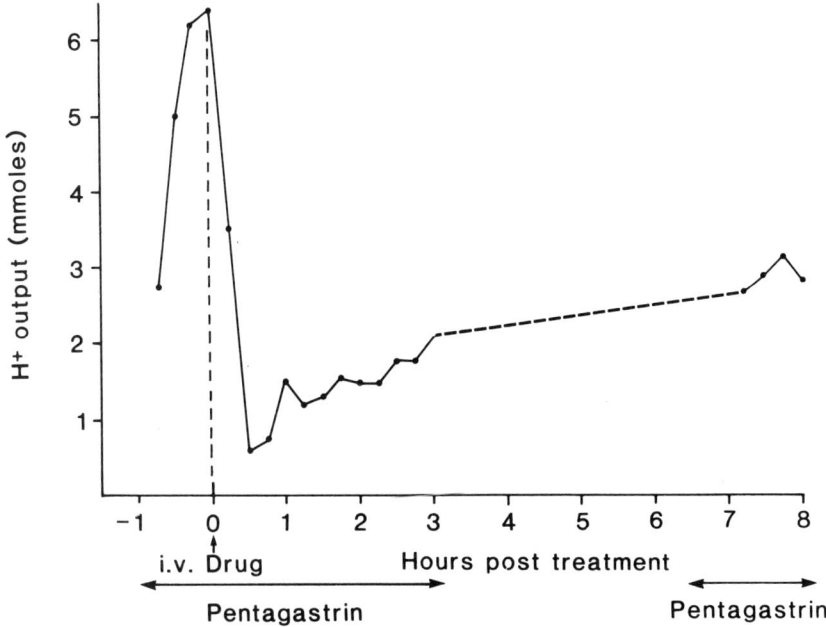

Figure 37.1 Inhibition of pentagastrin-stimulated acid output following an intravenous antisecretory agent

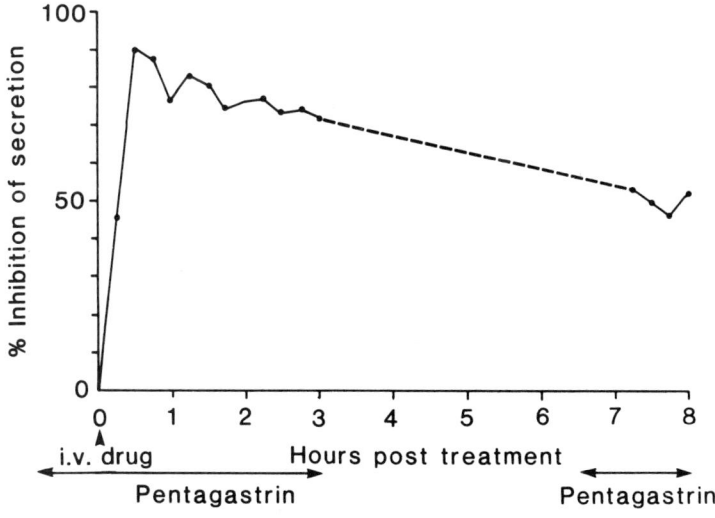

Figure 37.2 Percentage inhibition of pentagastrin-stimulated acid output following an intravenous antisecretory agent

allowed for it to leave the stomach before stimulation and aspiration can begin. The effect of drug is usually compared with a placebo study day and the percentage inhibition of acid secretion is presented. Alternatively, the pretreatment peak level of stimulated secretion can be used as the baseline (Figure 37.2), although this is less satisfactory than using a placebo study day.

There are more physiological stimulants of gastric secretion, including the 'spit and chew' technique, which measures cephalic, vagally mediated stimulation of gastric secretion caused by chewing and tasting food. Ingested food, usually as a standardised homogenised meal, or peptone meal, can also be used. These stimuli are more difficult to standardise, and with the aspiration method blocking of the tube with food particles can occur. Thus, measurement of the total volume of secretion is often not feasible, and therefore determination can be of pH only and not total acid output. The aspirate can be returned to the stomach, but this practice often makes subjects feel nauseated.

Total acid output may be calculated following food stimulation if an intragastric titration technique is used (Fordtran and Walsh, 1973). In this method and subsequent variants, intragastric pH is maintained at an arbitrary pH of around 5 units by the instillation of 0.1 M sodium hydroxide down a nasogastric tube. The acid output of the stomach can be calculated from the amount of sodium hydroxide required over specified periods.

Aspiration techniques also allow the measurement of other constituents of gastric secretion, such as pepsin and intrinsic factor.

Continuous Intragastric pH Monitoring

Although measurement of pH can be made on aspirated samples of gastric secretion, pH may be more conveniently monitored by means of a nasogastric pH electrode. Gastric pH data obtained by this technique may be considered to be closer to physiological reality, since the intragastric contents are not interfered with by aspiration or by instillation of alkali. Additionally, food and drink may be taken and volunteers or patients can be ambulatory. There is now considerable experience with this methodology (Bumm and Blum, 1987). It has been compared with established methods (Fimmel *et al.*, 1985) and appears to have good sensitivity and reproducibility when prolonged pH monitoring is required (Merki *et al.*, 1988b).

A small glass electrode is usually used, although other types, such as an antimony electrode, have been tried. It is connected to a recording device by means of an insulated and protected wire. Radiotelemetry has also been used to relay the signals from the electrode to a recording device. The electrode tip is usually positioned in the body of the stomach under fluoroscopic control or positioned by advancing the pH electrode by 8 cm or so from the point at which an acid pH was first registered (the region of the gastro-oesophageal sphincter). The length that the electrode is inserted is noted and used on future study days.

The pH data measured by the intragastric electrode can be collected either onto magnetic tape or into a solid state recording system. The advantage of the latter system is that the electronically stored data can be transferred more rapidly to a computer, but the disadvantage is that data are more easily lost than with a tape-based system.

There are now a number of commercially available systems for continuous pH monitoring, and although originally intended for clinical use in the diagnosis of gastro-oesophageal reflux, most are applicable, although not necessarily ideal, for the continuous monitoring of intragastric pH. Important aspects to be considered are the reliability of the electrodes and recording devices and, in the case of solid state memory systems, whether data can be inadvertently lost because of technical problems such as battery failure and poor connections. Computer software is now becoming available to allow the collected data to be presented and analysed.

Clearly, the major disadvantage of continuous pH recording is the inability to measure changes in volume of secretion. Also, there is marked intersubject and intrasubject variability in pH measurements, and relatively larger numbers of subjects, i.e. greater than 12, are often required to determine a slight effect on pH. With this number of subjects the technique may be sensitive enough to detect consistent changes in pH of greater than 0.1 pH units over a 24 h period, although the sensitivity may be considerably less over shorter periods of time (Merki *et al.*, 1988b). In general, this technique is more suited to differentiating between different drugs or doses of drugs that exert a marked antisecretory effect; the reasons for this are explained in the next section.

Presentation and Interpretation of Antisecretory Data

The data from the above methodologies can be presented in a number of ways. However, first it is important to understand the meaning of the following parameters of gastric acid secretion.

Gastric Acid Output

The total acid output measured over a given time, which is the *volume* of secretion $\times$ H^+ ion concentration.

pH or H^+ Ion Activity

In biological fluids the pH is negatively related to the log of the H^+ ion activity (effective concentration of H^+ ions at the surface of the measuring electrode).

$$pH = -\log(H^+ \text{ activity})$$

H^+ Concentration

Usually determined by titration to pH 7 with alkali. This is usually greater than the H^+ activity in gastric secretion, owing to the buffering of some H^+ ions by intragastric contents.

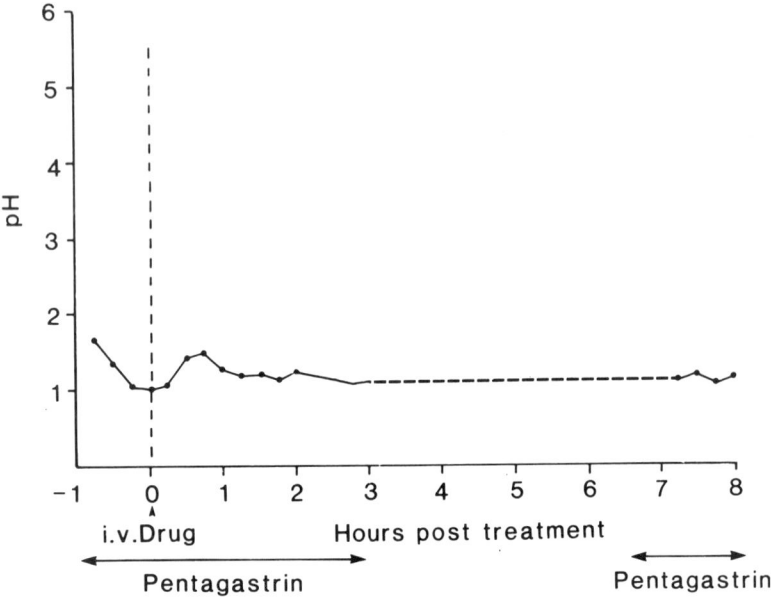

Figure 37.3   Inhibition of pentagastrin-stimulated secretion as measured by pH, following an intravenous antisecretory agent

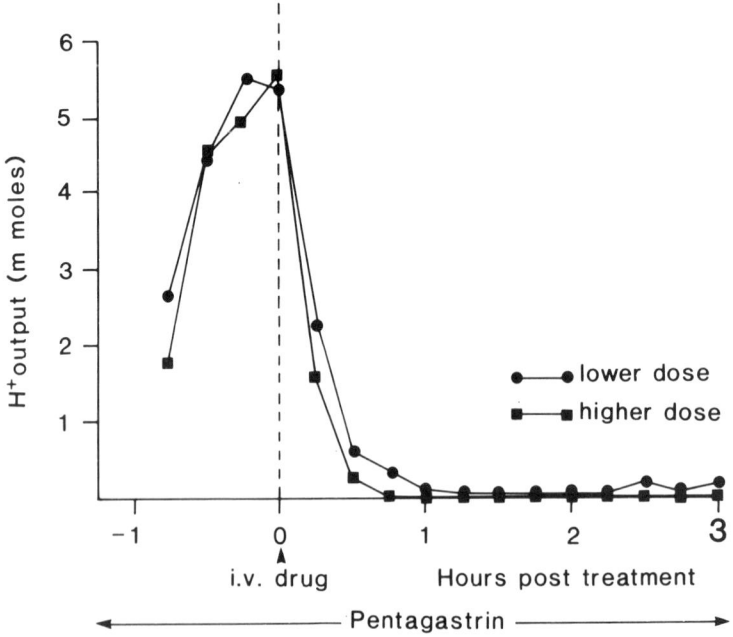

Figure 37.4   Inhibition of pentagastrin-stimulated acid output following an intravenous antisecretory agent

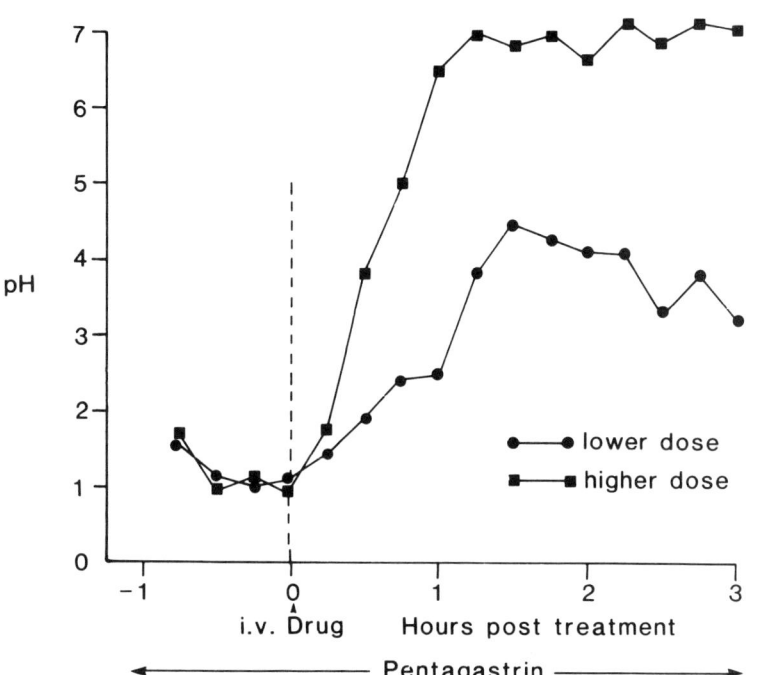

Figure 37.5 Inhibition of pentagastrin-stimulated secretion, as measured by pH following an intravenous antisecretory agent

The figures illustrate the potential misinterpretation of presented data. In the example illustrated in Figures 37.1 and 37.2, pentagastrin-stimulated acid secretion has been inhibited by the intravenous infusion of an antisecretory agent which has produced an early peak inhibition of nearly 90%. If the pH data are presented (Figure 37.3), this dramatic early effect on acid output is less obvious. Approximately 50% inhibition of output is still present between 7 and 8 h but is undetectable by pH measurement. Converting the pH to H^+ activity would suggest a more pronounced peak antisecretory effect than that seen with pH, but the degree of background noise associated with *in situ* pH measurement would still make the inhibition between 7 and 8 h undetectable.

On the other hand, when inhibition of acid output is increased to greater than 95%, as shown in Figure 37.4, it becomes more difficult to differentiate between doses by measurement of acid output. Figure 37.5 illustrates the same data measured by pH, where a very clear demarcation between the two doses can be seen.

Aspiration or pH Monitoring

Low levels of antisecretory effect, particularly if mediated predominantly through changes in volume of secretion, can be more easily detected from methodologies using aspiration to determine acid output. At higher doses of drug, where near-abolition of gastric secretion occurs, pH monitoring has many advantages. The implication of this for drug development is that it is often easier to initially evaluate an antisecretory agent by measuring stimulated acid output, before choosing a relevant, and relatively high, antisecretory dose to evaluate further, using pH monitoring.

Evaluation of the Adverse Biological Effects of Antisecretory Agents

The adverse-event profile associated with most antisecretory agents is excellent. However, potential longer-term effects are related to anacidity in the stomach. This includes overgrowth of bacteria within the anacidic stomach and also the stimulation of gastrin release. It has been debated whether both these factors could, in the longer term, lead to the development of tumours in man, particularly enterochromaffin-like cell hyperplasia and gastric carcinoids. Such tumours are rarely seen in patients suffering from pernicious anaemia, which is associated with anacidity, increased bacterial growth within the stomach and high plasma gastrin levels (far higher than have been seen with treatment using antisecretory agents). The clinical use of more potent and longer-acting antisecretory agents such as ATPase inhibitors or insurmountable H_2 receptor antagonists will lead to higher gastrin levels than those seen with currently available H_2 receptor antagonists. This aspect of their action needs to be evaluated, although, following short-term treatment with the ATPase inhibitor omeprazole, the elevation of gastrin is modest in comparison with those in pernicious anaemia (Lanzon-Miller *et al.*, 1987).

Pharmacological Aspects of Different Antisecretory Drugs

Most experience has been with the reversible H_2 receptor antagonists cimetidine and ranitidine. Other reversible H_2 receptor antagonists are being developed, some with shorter duration of action, such as nizatidine, and some longer-acting drugs, such as sufotidine. Irreversible, insurmountable H_2 receptor antagonists may come back into development, having previously been rejected because of gastric tumours in animals, which are now thought to be probably related to lifelong gastric anacidity.

Irreversible ATPase inhibitors, such as omeprazole, have a different mechanism of action from that of H_2 receptor antagonists. They bind irreversibly to actively secreting H^+/K^+ ATPase enzymes. Since not all these enzymes are active at any one time, repeat dosing with this rapidly eliminated drug is required before a pharmacodynamic steady state is attained (Howden *et al.*, 1984). The potential additive effect of repeat dosing should always be borne in mind not only with irreversible ATPase inhibitors, but also with other antisecretory drugs with longer elimination half-lives where accummulation with increased plasma levels is likely.

CYTOPROTECTIVE AGENTS

Some controversy surrounds the use of the term 'cytoprotection'. However, it is clear, particularly in animal studies, that some drugs such as prostaglandin analogues protect the gastric mucosa from the injury inflicted by noxious stimuli, and this protective effect is independent of any inhibition of acid secretion. In man the results of therapeutic studies conducted with prostaglandin analogues are generally disappointing because the ulcer healing rate in most studies appears to be consistent with the antisecretory effects of these drugs, with no clear evidence of an additive effect due to a cytoprotective mechanism.

The mechanism of the 'cytoprotective' effect is unclear; however, there are probably a number of factors that contribute to the resistance of the mucosa to noxious agents. These include the properties of the mucous layer, the alkaline non-acid secretion of the mucosa and rapid regeneration of mucosa. There is considerable interest in this type of drug, particularly for the prevention of non-steroidal anti-inflammatory induced ulceration.

Demonstration of a protective effect of drugs on the gastric mucosa has been attempted in man by a number of techniques. These include the inhibition of aspirin-induced gastric bleeding, the assessment of the endoscopic appearance of the mucosa and inhibition of changes in mucosal potential difference (Hogan *et al.*, 1987).

The mechanism of 'cytoprotection' has also been studied, and a number of techniques have been described whereby the production of alkaline secretion in the stomach or duodenum has been quantified (Rees *et al.*, 1982) and defective secretion of bicarbonate in the duodenum of ulcer patients suggested (Isenberg *et al.*, 1987). All these methodologies could, theoretically, be adapted to test the effect of drugs. Indeed, one drug, misoprostol, has been shown to stimulate mucus secretion in man (Wilson *et al.*, 1986), and also duodenal bicarbonate secretion in man (Isenberg *et al.*, 1986).

If antisecretory activity of a 'cytoprotective' drug can be identified, those dose levels producing minimal or slight acid inhibition may be taken forward for clinical evaluation in patients. Drugs with no antisecretory effect are clearly more difficult to evaluate in early studies, which will primarily need to establish tolerability before therapeutic studies in patients.

ANTIMICROBIAL AGENTS

Campylobacter pylori is a Gram-negative bacillus which may be found beneath the mucous layer of the human stomach. Although similar organisms have been previously described, and mostly ignored, recent interest has been stimulated by the demonstration of an association with gastritis and ulceration.

Drugs that have been available for a number of years, with known anti-ulcer effect, e.g. colloidal bismuth subcitrate, have quite recently received a resurgence of interest with the finding that they eradicate, at least temporarily, *Campylobacter pyloridis* from the gastric mucosa of ulcer patients. The role of *Campylobacter* in contributing to peptic ulcer disease is currently unclear; however, it is likely that further drugs will be developed with antibacterial properties in the hope that they will be effective in healing ulcers and will reduce the relapse rate that occurs following the cessation of treatment with antisecretory agents. The method by which such drugs will be studied is likely to include *in vitro* techniques to assess the effect against *Campylobacter pyloridis*, although this does not seem to correlate well with *in vivo* activity. It may then be possible to progress to study either the effect of drug on carrier rates in selected volunteers or the patient population, using endoscopic biopsy techniques (Marshall *et al.*, 1987), or using non-invasive methods (Bell *et al.*, 1987) to detect the urea splitting properties of the bacteria.

CONCLUSIONS

There is considerable uncertainty over the correct methodologies to adopt in the early evaluation of anti-ulcer drugs with cytoprotective or antibacterial activity. The evaluation of various methodologies will continue in the hope that future experience will lead to a feasible pathway for early, efficient evaluation. The early evaluation of antisecretory drugs is somewhat clearer, although different drug categories require variations from what has become a relatively well-trodden path for competitive H_2 receptor antagonists. The initial evaluation of antisecretory activity is highly predictive of the therapeutic activity in later studies (Jones *et al.*, 1987), and, therefore, the accurate early phase evaluation of drug effect is of utmost importance.

REFERENCES

Baron, J. H. (1978). *Clinical Tests of Gastric Secretion*. Macmillan, London

Bell, G. D., Weil, J., Harrison, G. *et al.* (1987). ^{14}C-urea breath analysis, a non-invasive test for *Campylobacter pylori* in the stomach. *Lancet*, i, 1367–8

Bumm, R. and Blum, A. L. (1987). Lessons from prolonged gastric pH monitoring. *Aliment. Pharm. Ther.*, 1, 518S–526S

Chin, T. W. F., MacLeod, S. M. and Mahon, W. A. (1986). Absence of tachyphylaxis in gastric acid secretion during pentagastrin infusion. *J. Clin. Pharm.*, 26, 281–5

Faber, R. G. and Hobsley, M. (1977). Basal gastric secretion, reproducibility and relationship with duodenal ulceration. *Gut*, 18, 57–63

Fimmel, C. J., Etienne, A., Cilluffo, T. *et al.* (1985). Long term ambulatory gastric pH monitoring; validation of a new method and effect of H_2-antagonists. *Gastroenterology*, 88, 1842–51

Findlay, J. M., Prescott, R. J. and Sircus, W. (1972). Comparative evaluation of water recovery test and fluoroscopic screening in positioning a nasogastric tube during gastric secretory studies. *Br. Med. J.*, IV, 458–61

Fordtran, J. S. and Walsh, J. H. (1973). Gastric acid secretion rate and buffer content of the stomach after eating. *J. Clin. Invest.*, **52**, 645–57

Hassan, M. A. and Hobsley, M. (1970). Positioning of subject and nasogastric tube during a gastric secretion study. *Br. Med. J.*, **1**, 458–60

Hogan, D. L., Thomas, F. J. and Isenberg, J. I. (1987). Cimetidine decreases aspirin-induced gastric mucosal damage in humans. *Aliment. Pharm. Ther.*, **1** (5), 383–90

Howden, C. W., Forrest, J. A. and Reid, J. L. (1984). Effect of single and repeated doses of omeprazole on gastric acid and pepsin secretion in man. *Gut*, **25**, 707–10

Isenberg, J. I., Hogan, D. L., Koss, A. K. and Selling, J. A. (1986). Human duodenal mucosal bicarbonate secretion. *Gastroenterology*, **91**, 370–8

Isenberg, J. I., Selling, J. A., Hogan, D. L. and Koss, M. A. (1987). Impaired proximal duodenal bicarbonate secretion in patients with duodenal ulcer. *New Engl. J. Med.*, **316** (7), 374–9

Jones, D. B., Howden, C. W., Burget, D. W. *et al.* (1987). Acid suppression in duodenal ulcer; a meta analysis to define optimal dosing with antisecretory drugs. *Gut*, **28**, 1120–7

Lanzon-Miller, S., Pounder, R. E., Hamilton, M. R. *et al.* (1987). Twenty-four hour intragastric acidity and plasma gastrin concentrations before and during treatment with either ranitidine or omeprazole. *Aliment. Pharm. Ther.*, **1**, 239–51

Marshall, B. J., Warren, R., Francis, G. *et al.* (1987). Rapid urease test in the management of *Campylobacter pyloridis*-associated gastritis. *Am. J. Gastroenterol.*, **82**, 200–10

Merki, H. S., Fimmel, C. J., Walt, R. P. *et al.* (1988a). Pattern of 24 hour intragastric acidity in active duodenal ulcer disease and in healthy controls. *Gut*, **29**, 1583–7

Merki, H. S., Witzel, L., Walt, R. P. *et al.* (1988b). Day to day variation of 24 hour intragastric acidity. *Gastroenterology*, **94**, 887–91

Moore, J. G. and Englert, E. (1970). Circadian rhythm of gastric acid secretion in man. *Nature*, **226**, 1261–2

Moore, J. G. and Halberg, F. (1986). Circadian rhythm of gastric acid secretion in man with active duodenal ulcer. *Dig. Dis. Sci.*, **31**, 22–9

Petersen, B., Christiansen, J., Kirkegaard, P. and Skov Olsen, P. (1984). The stability of gastric acid secretion during prolonged pentagastrin stimulation in man. *Clin. Sci.*, **66**, 99–101

Petersen, H. and Myren, J. (1975). Pentagastrin dose-response in peptic ulcer disease. *Scand. J. Gastroenterol.*, **10**, 705–14

Rees, W. D. W., Botham, D. and Turnberg, L. A. (1982). A demonstration of bicarbonate production by the normal human stomach *in vivo*. *Dig. Dis. Sci.*, **27**, 961–6

Whitefield, P. F. and Hobsley, M. (1979). A standardised technique for the performance of accurate gastric secretion studies. *Agents and Actions*, Vol. 9/4. Birkhauser Verlag, Basle, pp. 327–32

Wilson, P. E., Quadros, E., Rajapaksa, T. *et al.* (1986). Effects of misoprostol on gastric acid and mucus secretion in man. Dig. Dis. Sci., **31** (2), 1265–95

Wormsley, K. G. (1972). Responses to pentagastrin in man. *Acta Hepato-Gastroenterol.*, **19**, 120–4

IX
Assessment of Drug Effects on the Kidney

38
Diuretics

J. McMurray* and J. McEwen†*

*Dept of Clinical Pharmacology, † Drug Development (Scotland) Ltd, Ninewells
Hospital and Medical School, Dundee DD1 9SY, UK

INTRODUCTION

Diuretics act on the kidney to increase urine output and electrolyte excretion.
Particularly since the introduction of chlorothiazide (Novello and Sprague,
1957) and frusemide (Kleinfelder, 1963), they have become very widely used.
Many millions of prescriptions are written each year and it is estimated that
diuretics are prescribed for one in four medical patients (Roberts and
Daneshmend, 1981; Whelton and Watson, 1986). Nevertheless, currently
available drugs are often far from ideal, and new products are continually
under development (Hutcheon and Martinez, 1986).

CLEARANCE

Clearance is a concept crucial to the evaluation of diuretics (Levinsky and
Levy, 1973): it is defined as the volume of plasma completely cleared of a
given substance in unit time (Smith, 1956). Renal clearance is derived by
dividing total urinary excretion by the plasma concentration during the
collection interval: it expresses the input–output relationship for any endogenous or exogenous substance and measures renal excretory function (Maack,
1986). Clearance techniques are used to determine glomerular filtration rate
(GFR), renal plasma flow (RPF) and renal tubular function. Many assumptions have to be made, however, in calculating clearance, and precautions
should be taken to ensure validity (Levinsky and Levy, 1973; Seldin and
Rector, 1973; Schuster and Seldin, 1985; Maack, 1986).

NORMAL RENAL WATER AND ELECTROLYTE HANDLING

Proper characterisation of a diuretic also requires an understanding of basic
renal physiology (Seldin and Giebisch, 1985). Approximately 180 l of filtrate
per day are produced by the kidney, of which 99% is reabsorbed by the renal
tubules. Figure 38.1 shows the contribution of the postglomerular nephron to
the reabsorption of sodium (Jacobson, 1981). Different tubular segments

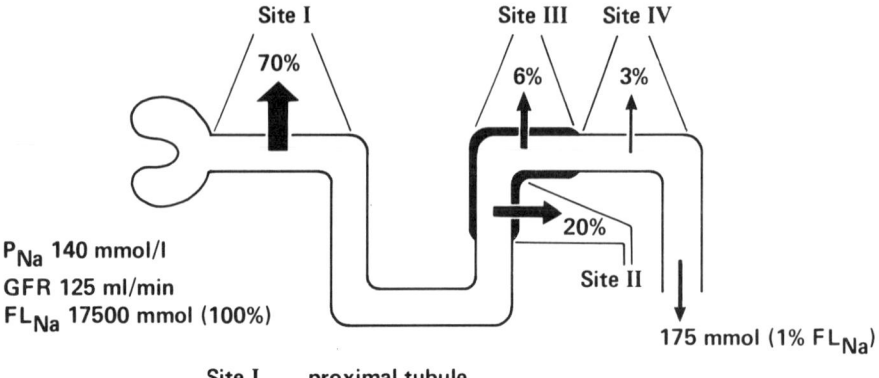

Site I   proximal tubule
Site II   ascending limb of the loop of Henle
Site III   cortical diluting segment
Site IV   distal tubule

Figure 38.1 Principal sites of sodium reabsorption and of diuretic action in the nephron

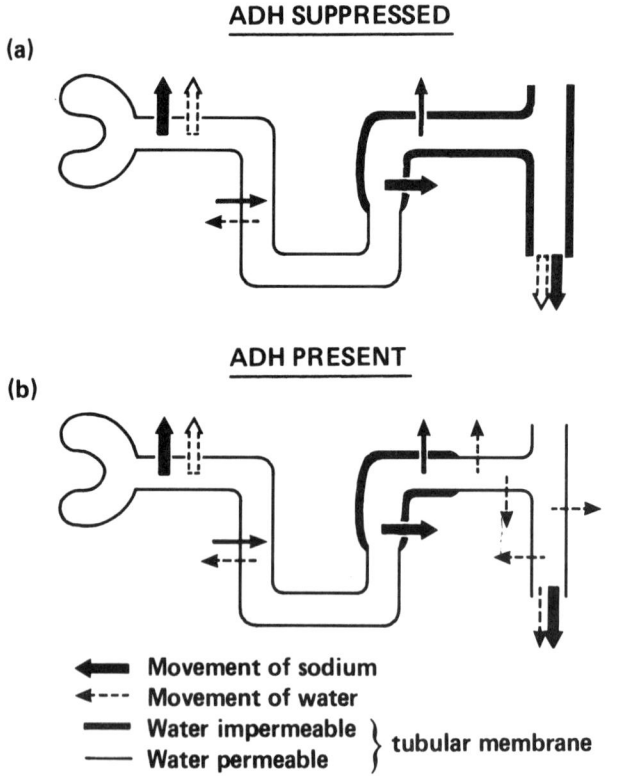

Figure 38.2 Water and sodium transport in the nephron in the presence (b) and absence (a) of ADH

have quantitatively different importance, which becomes relevant when predicting the potential magnitude of effect of a given diuretic. Figure 38.2 illustrates the factors influencing water reabsorption and excretion by the kidney (Puschett, 1981; Roy and Jamison, 1985). Any given solute or osmolar load requires an obligatory water loss. Further water loss ('free water') is determined by the presence or absence of antidiuretic hormone (ADH), also referred to as arginine vasopressin (AVP). Fluid leaving the proximal tubule is isotonic with plasma; it enters the descending limb of the loop of Henle, where solute is added and an insignificant amount of water is extracted. The ascending limb of the loop of Henle (ALH) is impermeable to water, but solute is reabsorbed in this segment, causing a relative dilution of the tubular fluid and generation of 'solute-free water', measured as free water clearance C_{H_2O}. A quantitatively much less important cortical diluting segment also operates in the early distal tubule. After this point, in the absence of ADH (Figure 38.2a), tubular fluid will be excreted without further reabsorption of water as dilute urine. However, when ADH is present (Figure 38.2b), the nephron distal to the ALH becomes highly permeable to water, which then passes from the tubular lumen into the hyperosmolar medullary interstitium. This hypertonicity is largely due to the transport of solute out of the loop of Henle: transport of solute from the cortical diluting segment does not contribute to hyperosmolality. Extraction of water from the lumen of the distal nephron in the presence of ADH results in 'free water reabsorption' (denoted as $T^c_{H_2O}$) and the production of concentrated urine.

MODE OF ACTION OF DIURETICS

Diuretics in current use can be broadly classified into four groups (Hendry and Ellory, 1988). *Loop diuretics* such as frusemide act on the thick ascending limb of the loop of Henle, inhibiting a $Na^+/K^+/Cl^-$ cotransporter in the luminal membrane. *Thiazides* largely act on the early portion of the distal tubule, inhibiting a Na^+/Cl^- cotransporter. *Potassium-sparing diuretics* act on the later portion of the distal tubule, as aldosterone antagonists (e.g. spironolactone) or, with agents such as amiloride, inhibiting transepithelial sodium uptake: consequent hyperpolarisation of apical cell membranes reduces the driving force for K^+ exit into the lumen. *Osmotic diuretics* increase the osmolality of tubular fluid, inducing additional obligatory water loss.

EXTRARENAL ACTIVITY

Some of the beneficial effects of diuretics in heart failure and hypertension seem to be the result of direct vasodilator activity. After frusemide treatment in acute pulmonary oedema, the left atrial pressure falls before the onset of diuresis (Dikshit *et al.*, 1973); frusemide has also been shown to increase vascular capacitance in the human forearm (Biamino *et al.*, 1975). Evidence for a prostaglandin-induced effect of frusemide on vasculature which itself depends upon functioning kidneys has been presented by Johnson *et al.* (1983). In the case of thiazides, following an initial shrinkage in plasma volume, responding hypertensive patients show a fall in peripheral resistance after several weeks of treatment (van Brummelen *et al.*, 1980).

PHARMACOKINETICS

Although measurement of circulating plasma concentrations of diuretics can sometimes be necessary (for example, assessment of absorption and bioavailability), urinary drug levels are of greater pharmacodynamic significance, since most diuretics influence electrolyte transport from within the lumen of the renal tubule (Homeida *et al.*, 1983). However, Brater (1983) has pointed out that the time-course of drug delivery to the active site is itself also a determinant of response—thus, oral doses, maintaining concentrations in urine at the low end of the dose–response curve for a longer period, can produce a greater sodium excretion rate than intravenous doses which give higher urinary levels for a shorter time. Pharmacokinetic factors can also account in part for diuretic resistance: for example, in patients with severe renal insufficiency the accumulation of endogenous organic acids can block secretion of loop diuretics into the tubular lumen (Rose *et al.*, 1977); in severe nephrotic syndrome, substantial amounts of frusemide can be bound to the excess urinary protein appearing in this disorder, preventing drug access to the tubular epithelium (Smith *et al.*, 1985).

Extensive 'depot' binding of chlorthalidone to erythrocyte carbonic anhydrasc (Fleuren *et al.*, 1977) may contribute to its long duration of action.

PHARMACODYNAMIC ASSESSMENT

In order to characterise a new diuretic, it is necessary to determine its site of action in the nephron and to assess its relative potency and efficacy (Goldberg, 1973; Roberts and Daneshmend, 1981; Puschett, 1986). Effects on GFR and RPF should also be measured.

Nephron Sites of Action

Glomerular Filtration Rate

The extent of tubular reabsorption of sodium alters in response to changes in tubular delivery of sodium ('glomerulo-tubular balance'). Before ascribing any increase in urinary sodium excretion to blockade of tubular reabsorption, it is necessary to allow for any increase in the filtered load (FL) of sodium:

this requires awareness of changes in GFR. Many conditions in which diuretics are indicated are themselves characterised by reduced GFR— another reason to identify drug-induced changes in GFR (McMurray and Struthers, 1987).

Although it is not ideal, only inulin (or the related substance polyfructosan) is really suitable for repeated measurements of GFR in man. This requires an intravenous infusion, stable plasma levels and, assuming no urinary catheterisation, accurate bladder emptying. A protocol for inulin administration in normal subjects is shown in Table 38.1 (Liedtke and Duarte, 1980; Kampmann and Molholm Hansen, 1981).

Table 38.1 Estimation of inulin clearance

Loading dose:	50 mg/kg in 100 ml of 0.9% saline over 10 min
Maintenance infusion rate:	30 mg/kg in 0.9% saline at 0.5–2 ml/min
Optimum serum concentration:	200–250 mg/l
Normal range:	male 127–130 ml min^{-1} $(1.73\,m^2)^{-1}$ female 118–120 ml min^{-1} $(1.73\,m^2)^{-1}$

Renal plasma flow and renal blood flow (RBF) should also be measured— first, because knowledge of RPF helps interpretation of changes in glomerular and tubular function; and second, because an increase in RBF is a desirable therapeutic objective in many illnesses treated by diuretics (McMurray and Struthers, 1987).

Para-aminohippurate (PAH) clearance is frequently used to measure RPF and RBF in man, although this again has some limitations (Schuster and Seldin, 1985; Maack, 1986). PAH clearance varies with its plasma concentration, so a constant plasma level is imperative. A protocol for PAH clearance is given in Table 38.2 (Liedtke and Duarte, 1980).

Table 38.2 Estimation of PAH clearance

Loading dose:	8 mg/kg of stock solution (20% PAH) over 1–2 min
Maintenance infusion rate:	15 mg/kg in 0.9% saline at 0.5–2 ml/min
Optimum serum concentration:	20–25 mg/l
Normal range:	male 650–660 ml min^{-1} $(1.73\,m^2)^{-1}$ female 585–595 ml min^{-1} $(1.73\,m^2)^{-1}$

Segmental Tubular Function

Site I

The proximal tubule accounts for the major part (70%) of sodium reabsorption. However, it is not easy to document inhibition of sodium reabsorption in this segment, because enhanced reabsorption in more distal segments compensates for increased sodium delivery. Two main approaches have been used to overcome this problem.

First, sodium entering the ALH in the absence of ADH is absorbed there, so increased free water clearance should be detected. If the fractional excretion of sodium in the urine (C_{Na}/GFR) is added to fractional free water clearance (C_{H_2O}/GFR), a rough index of fractional proximal tubular outflow is obtained. This calculation can be further refined—first, by allowing for the exchange of potassium with sodium in the more distal nephron (Seldin and Rector, 1973); and second, by substituting chloride for sodium in the original calculation. Sodium bicarbonate represents a non-reabsorbable load to the ALH; thus, after a drug such as acetazolamide (Danovitch and Bricker, 1976),

$$\frac{C_{Cl} + C_{H_2O}}{GFR}$$

is a truer representation of distal delivery than

$$\frac{C_{Na} + C_{H_2O}}{GFR}$$

In the presence of ADH, increased sodium delivery to the ALH should result in increased free water reabsorption.

The second approach is to measure the excretion rate of ions cotransported with sodium in the proximal tubule (Seldin and Rector, 1973; Schuster and Seldin, 1985). Phosphate is mainly reabsorbed in the proximal tubule and is frequently used as a marker for proximal tubular sodium reabsorption (Goldberg, 1973; Roberts and Daneshmend, 1981; Puschett, 1986). More recently lithium has been proposed as a proximal marker (Thomsen, 1984), although this has not gained widespread acceptance (Navar and Schafer, 1987): lithium may itself alter proximal tubular function.

Measures of a proximal effect of a diuretic are summarised in Table 38.3.

Table 38.3 Indices of increased proximal tubular outflow

(1)	$\uparrow \dfrac{C_{Na} + C_{H_2O}}{GFR}$
(2)	$\uparrow \dfrac{U_{(Na+K)}V}{P_{Na} \cdot GFR} \times 100 + \dfrac{C_{H_2O}}{GFR} \times 100$
(3)	$\uparrow \dfrac{C_{Cl} + C_{H_2O}}{GFR}$
(4)	$\uparrow \dfrac{C_{PO_4}}{GFR}$
(5)	$\uparrow \dfrac{C_{Li}}{GFR}$

U = urinary concentration, P = plasma concentration, V = urine volume

Site II

The ALH reabsorbs about 20% of FL_{Na} (Kokko, 1984; Odlind, 1984), and complete inhibition of electrolyte transport in this segment can cause a large diuresis and natriuresis, since distal compensatory reabsorption is more limited (Anderton and Kincaid-Smith, 1971). Because of the importance of the ALH in urinary concentration and dilution, blockade of this site will cause a large reduction in free water reabsorption and usually a decrease in free water clearance; the fall in the latter may be small if the cortical diluting segment continues to function (Davies and Wilson, 1975; Lant, 1981). Since the loop of Henle also reabsorbs a significant fraction of the filtered load of magnesium and calcium, loop diuretics also increase urinary calcium and magnesium excretion.

Site III

Approximately 6% of filtered sodium is reabsorbed in the cortical diluting segment. Blockade of sodium transport in this site can, therefore, only cause a moderate saliuresis. Free water clearance is decreased but free water reabsorption does not change, as solute transport in this segment does not contribute to medullary hypertonicity (Table 38.4).

Table 38.4 Localisation of diuretic action by effect on solute-free water clearance and reabsorption

Site of action	$T^c_{H_2O}$		C_{H_2O}	
I	↑	↑	↑	↑
II	↓	↓	—	↓
III	—		↓	
IV	—		—	

Site IV

As only 3% of sodium reabsorption occurs in the distal tubule and collecting duct, inhibition at this site can only cause a small diuresis and natriuresis. A proportion of sodium is reabsorbed here in exchange for potassium (under the regulation of aldosterone) and hydrogen ions (Shackleton *et al.*, 1986). A diuretic acting proximal to this segment will increase sodium exchange with potassium and hydrogen; such diuretics cause a kaliuresis and metabolic alkalosis (Puschett, 1985). In contrast, diuretics blocking sodium transport in this segment cause hyperkalaemia and metabolic acidosis (Shackleton *et al.*, 1986).

Potency

Differences in diuretic response on a molar basis can strictly only be interpreted as differences in potency and efficacy if drugs have the same site of action. For example, an efficacy of 1.0 at site III will still produce less natriuresis than an efficacy of 0.5 at site II (Weiner, 1986).

A second important factor when assessing potency is the time-course of diuretic action. Loop diuretics induce a large and rapid saliuresis and diuresis within 3 h, followed by rebound sodium retention from 12 to 24 h—the so-called 'undershoot' (Hamdy *et al.*, 1984; Reyes and Leary, 1987; McMurray and Struthers, 1988). This is not a feature of thiazide diuretics. Consequently, a single 24 h urine collection underestimates the peak natriuretic effect of loop diuretics, so the net 24 h response may be less than thiazide diuresis. This underlines the importance of the time factor and re-emphasises the difficulties of interclass comparisons. Frequent urine collection is necessary for comprehensive profiling of a diuretic agent.

A further important factor is the physiological state of the subjects studied (Roberts and Daneshmend, 1981; Wilcox, 1987). First, their pre-existing sodium and volume status will influence the magnitude of the response; second, natriuretic and diuretic effects of treatment will activate compensatory homeostatic mechanisms (McMurray and Struthers, 1988). Consequently, sodium and water should be replaced during the study to reveal the true pharmacological effect of the drug (Burke *et al.*, 1972), particularly if repeated drug administration is planned.

PROTOCOLS FOR DIURETIC EVALUATION

In order to select appropriate and safe doses for efficacy studies, some form of ascending-dose design is required when first doses are given to man (McEwen, 1989), to ensure acceptable tolerability and to determine whether the pharmacokinetic profile is similar to that in laboratory animals used in pharmacology and toxicology (McEwen, 1988).

Once a dosage of a new diuretic has been selected for full evaluation, two types of protocol are needed: first, assessment of effects on segmental nephron function; second, evaluation of potency (Puschett, 1981; Roberts and Daneshmend, 1981). Opportunity should also be taken to characterise pharmacokinetics during these experiments, in order to define concentration–response relationships. Healthy and relatively young male volunteers are usually studied first.

Segmental Nephron Function Protocol

This protocol localises the site of action following acute single doses, and has two limbs: maximal hydration and dehydration. A minimum of four sessions are needed, preferably at weekly intervals—a water-loaded balanced cross-over of placebo and active drug, and a similar dehydration cross-over. Responses versus placebo are better than comparisons with predrug baseline, which is rarely a true steady state.

Subjects should receive a standardised diet for 72 h before each treatment (for example, 140 mmol sodium, 80 mmol potassium, 20 mmol calcium and 10 mmol magnesium per day). Compliance and balance should be documented with daily 24 h urine collection. No alcohol or xanthine drinks are permitted in the 36 h preceding the study: normal exercise and sleep patterns should be followed. Subjects should be fasted from midnight prior to the study morning. The study should take place in a temperature-controlled room (24 °C), avoiding stressful noises, interruptions or conversations. Subjects should remain seated or supine during the study, standing only to void urine. A standardised light lunch and evening meal should be given: smoking is forbidden.

In the maximal hydration protocol, comfortable infusion lines for inulin/ PAH and saline are placed, together with a venous sampling cannula, at the beginning of each treatment morning. A 20 ml/kg oral water load is then given over 20 min, followed by voiding at 20 min intervals. Each volume of urine is measured (with an aliquot saved) and an equal volume of water, plus 1 ml/min for insensible loss, is then given orally. Alternatively, urinary sodium and water loss can be replaced intravenously. After 90 min a relatively high urine flow, around 10–12 ml/min, should be obtained. At this point urine osmolality should be checked to ensure that it is below 80 mosm/kg, to check that ADH is suppressed. Venous blood should be sampled at the mid-point of each collection period for clearance calculations. The experimental drug may then be administered, with continued urine and blood collections as before. Urine collections for activity need only be continued until the peak diuretic effect has passed, although later collections may help to characterise the duration of activity and the pharmacokinetic profile of parent compound and metabolites.

The dehydration protocol is technically more difficult. Instead of water loading at the start of the study, an infusion of AVP 0.5 mU kg^{-1} min^{-1} is given, plus 3% sodium chloride solution (not mannitol) at a rate which gives a urine output of at least 4 ml/min. The experimental procedure is otherwise the same as the hydration protocol, although 30 min clearance periods (or longer) may allow more complete and accurate bladder emptying.

In both protocols, urine and blood are collected for determination of the clearance of inulin, PAH, sodium, potassium, calcium, magnesium, phosphate, urate, chloride and osmoles. Recent examples of such protocols are given by Steinmuller and Puschett (1972); Teredesai and Puschett (1979); Brooks *et al.* (1984); McNabb *et al.*, (1984); Cuvelier *et al.* (1986); McMurray and Struthers (1988); McMurray *et al.* (1989).

Protocol for Dose-ranging and Potency

For this protocol the same selection of subjects, prestudy precautions and environment should be adopted. In a balanced cross-over design, a placebo day and enough active days to construct a dose–response curve should be performed, together with one or more doses of a diuretic from the same class, ideally with 7 days between study days. Restoration of pretreatment sodium balance should be ensured by 3 days of standardised diet and confirmed by measurement of body weight and 24 h sodium excretion. Inulin and PAH clearance should be measured, at least for the first 6–8 h of each session. Following drug administration, urine should be collected: suggestions for a loop diuretic are half-hourly to 2 h, hourly to 6 h, two-hourly to 12 h, then 12–24 h; for a thiazide diuretic, 0–3, 3–6, 6–9, 9–12 and 12–24 h collections are suggested. Blood should be taken at the mid-point of each collection period as before.

Sodium and water replacement for urinary losses is important: this can be gauged either from pilot studies or by measurement of the sodium content of each urinary sample. Hourly rates of solute excretion should be tabulated, comparing placebo with each active day. Response may also be presented as percentage of filtered load excreted. Examples of studies of this type are given by Hamdy *et al.* (1984), Reyes and Leary (1987) and Brater *et al.* (1987).

INVESTIGATION OF POSSIBLE ADVERSE EFFECTS

Many potential adverse effects are unlikely to be detected in single-dose studies, so chronic dosing will also be necessary once an appropriate active dose has been selected. The major predictable adverse effects of non-potassium-sparing diuretics are listed in Table 38.5. These are due both to the direct action of the diuretic agent (e.g. hyponatraemia) and the compensatory homeostatic responses invoked by these drugs (e.g. hyperuricaemia).

Table 38.5 Predictable adverse effects of non potassium-sparing diuretics

Hyponatraemia	Glucose intolerance
Hypokalaemia	Metabolic alkalosis[a]
Hypomagnaesaemia	Allergic reactions[b]
Hyperuricaemia	Ototoxicity
Hyperlipidaemia	

[a] Metabolic acidosis with carbonic anhydrase inhibitors.
[b] Including skin rashes, haematological abnormalities and interstitial nephritis.

Hypokalaemic potential may be predicted from the potency measurements outlined above. A plot of natriuretic effect versus kaliuretic effect for the test drug under investigation and one or more established diuretics from the same class gives some estimation of the hypokalaemic potency of the new agent (Puschett and Rastegar, 1974).

In addition to routine measurement of blood glucose, an oral glucose tolerance test should be performed before and after chronic dosing to fully assess the effect of any new diuretic on carbohydrate handling.

Measurement of urate and its handling by the body is complicated: it is discussed in detail by Roberts and Daneshmend (1981) and Mejia and Steele (1986). For example, diuretics may augment urate excretion acutely, but with chronic dosing most decrease urate clearance. A strict standardised diet is essential for any assessment of urate handling.

Ototoxicity is a rare complication of loop diuretics; high-tone audiometry should be considered in the evaluation of such agents.

To exclude direct nephrotoxic effects, screening for microalbuminuria should be performed to exclude glomerular damage; beta-microglobulin or NAG may similarly indicate tubular damage.

Since many adverse effects may occur over months or even years, careful evaluation during treatment of patients will also be a prerequisite in the safety profiling of any new agent (Roberts and Daneshmend, 1981).

REFERENCES

Anderton, J. L. and Kincaid-Smith, P. (1971). Diuretics I: Physiological and pharmacological considerations. *Drugs*, **1**, 54–81

Biamino, G., Wessel, H. J., Noring, J. and Schroder, R. (1975). Plethysmographische und *in-vitro* Untersuchungen uber die vasodilatorische Wirkung von Furosemid (Lasix). *Int. J. Clin. Pharm. Biopharm.*, **12**, 356–68

Brater, D. C. (1983). Determinants of the overall response to furosemide: pharmacokinetics and pharmacodynamics. *Fed. Proc.*, **42**, 1711–13

Brater, D. C., Leinfelder, J. and Anderson, S. A. (1987). Clinical pharmacology of torasemide, a new loop diuretic. *Clin. Pharm. Ther.*, **42**, 187–92

Brooks, B. A., Lant, A. F., McNabb, W. R. and Noormohamed, F. H. (1984). Renal actions of a uricosuric diuretic, racemic indacrinone, in man: comparison with ethacrynic acid and hydrochlorothiazide. *Br. J. Clin. Pharm.*, **17**, 497–512

Burke, T. J., Robinson, R. R. and Clap, J. R. (1972). Determinants of the effect of furosemide on the proximal tubule. *Kid. Int.*, **1**, 12–18

Cuvelier, R., Pellergrin, P., Lesne, M. and Van Ypersele de Strihou, Ch. (1986). Site of action of torasemide in man. *Eur. J. Clin. Pharm.*, **31** (Suppl.), 15–19

Danovitch, G. M. and Bricker, N. S. (1976). Influence of volume expansion on NaCl reabsorption in the diluting segments of the nephron: a study using clearance methods. *Kid. Int.*, **10**, 229–38

Davies, D. L. and Wilson, G. M. (1975). Diuretics: mechanisms of action and clinical application. *Drugs*, **9**, 178–226

Dikshit, K., Vyden, J. B., Forrester, J. S., Chatterjee, K., Prakesh, R. and Swan, H. J. C. (1973). Renal and extrarenal hemodynamic effects of furosemide in congestive cardiac failure after acute myocardial infarction. *New Engl. J. Med.*, **288**, 1087–90

Fleuren, H. L. J. and van Rossum, J. M. (1977). Nonlinear relationship between plasma and red blood cell pharmacokinetics of chlorthalidone in man. *J. Pharmacokinet. Biopharm.*, **5**, 359–75

Goldberg, M. (1973). The renal physiology of diuretics. In Orloff, J., Berliner, R. W. and Geiger, S. R. (Eds.), *Handbook of Physiology: Renal Physiology*. American Physiologic Society, Washington D.C., pp. 1003–31

Hamdy, R. C., Vinson, M., Robbins, A. D., Struthers, L. P. L., Chapman, S. F., Norris, R. J. and Shaw, H. L. (1984). Diuretic potency of loop, thiozide and potassium-sparing agents: a reappraisal of relative activity. In Puschett, J. B. and Greenberg, A. (Eds.), *Diuretics: Chemistry, Pharmacology and Clinical Applications*. Elsevier, Amsterdam, pp. 403–6

Hendry, B. M. and Ellory, J. C. (1988). Molecular sites for diuretic action. *T.I.P.S.*, **9**, 416–21

Homeida, M., Roberts, C. and Branch, R. A. (1977). Influence of probenecid and spironolactone on furosemide kinetics and dynamics in man. *Clin. Pharm. Ther.*, **22**, 402–8

Hutcheon, D. E. and Martinez, J. C. (1986). A decade of developments in diuretic drug therapy. *J. Clin. Pharm.*, **26**, 567–79

Jacobson, H. R. (1981). Functional segmentation of the mammalian nephron. *Am. J. Physiol.*, **241**, F203–F218

Johnston, G. D., Hiatt, W. R., Nies, A. S., Payne, N. A., Murphy, R. C. and Gerber, J. G. (1983). Factors influencing the early nondiuretic vascular effects of furosemide in man. *Circ. Res.*, **53**, 630–5

Kampmann, J. P. and Molholm Hansen, J. (1981). Glomerular filtration rate and creatinine clearance. *Br. J. Clin. Pharm.*, **12**, 7–14

Kleinfelder, H. (1963). Experimentelle Untersuchungen und klinische Erfahrungen mit einem neuen Diureticum. *Dtsch Med. Wochenschr.*, **88**, 1695–702

Kokko, J. P. (1984). Site and mechanism of action of diuretics. *Am. J. Med.*, **77**(SA), 11–17

Lant, A. F. (1981). Modern diuretics and the kidney. *J. Clin. Pathol.*, **34**, 1267–75

Levinsky, N. G. and Levy, M. (1973). Clearance techniques. In Orloff, J., Berliner, R. W. and Geiger, S. R. (Eds.), *Handbook of Physiology: Renal Physiology*. American Physiologic Society, Washington D.C., pp. 103–17

Liedtke, R. R. and Duarte, C. G. (1980). Laboratory protocols and methods for the measurement of glomerular filtration rate and renal plasma flow. In Duarte, C. G. (Ed.), *Renal Function Tests: Clinical Laboratory Procedures and Diagnosis*. Little Brown, Boston, pp. 49–63

Maack, T. (1986). Renal clearance and isolated kidney perfusion techniques. *Kid. Int.*, **30**, 142–51

McEwen, J. (1988). Biochemical pharmacodynamics. *Pharm. Med.*, **3**, 111–20

McEwen, J. (1989). Studies in man with potential therapeutic agents. In Illing, H. P. A. (Ed.), *Xenobiotic Metabolism and Disposition: The Design of Disposition and Metabolism Studies on Novel Compounds*. CRC Press, Boca Raton, pp. 89–97

McMurray, J., Seidelin, P. H. and Struthers, A. D. (1989). Evidence for a proximal and distal nephron action of atrial natriuretic factor in man. *Nephron*, **51**, 39–43

McMurray, J. and Struthers, A. D. (1987). Role of neuroendocrine abnormalities in the enhanced sodium and water retention of chronic heart failure. *Pharm. Toxicol.*, **61**, 209–14

McMurray, J. and Struthers, A. D. (1988). Frusemide pretreatment blunts the inhibition of renal tubular sodium reabsorption by ANF in man. *Eur. J. Clin. Pharm.*, **35**, 333–8

McNabb, W. R., Noormohamed, F. H., Brooks, B. A. and Lant, A. F. (1984). Renal actions of piretanide and three other loop diuretics. *Clin. Pharm. Ther.*, **35**, 328–37

Mejia, G. and Steele, T. H. (1986). Uricosuric diuretics. In Dirks, J. H. and Sutton, R. A. L. (Eds.), *Diuretics: Physiology, Pharmacology and Clinical Use*. W. B Saunders, Philadelphia, pp. 135–48

Navar, L. G. and Schafer, J. A. (1987). Comments on 'Lithium clearance: a new research area'. *N.I.P.S.*, **2**, 34–5

Novello, F. C. and Sprague, J. H. (1957). Benzothiadiazine dioxides as novel diuretics. *J. Am. Chem. Soc.*, **79**, 2028–39

Odlind, B. (1984). Site and mechanism of the action of diuretics. *Acta Pharm. Toxicol.*, **54** (Suppl. 1), 5–15

Puschett, J. B. (1981). Sites and mechanisms of action of diuretics in the kidney. *J. Clin. Pharm.*, **21**, 564–74

Puschett, J. B. (1985). Determination of diuretic sites and mechanisms of action—an outline of the methodology employed. In Puschett, J. B. and Greenberg, A. (Eds.), *The Diuretic Manual*. Elsevier, Amsterdam, pp. 139–52

Puschett, J. B. (1986). Clinical pharmacologic implications in diuretic selection. *Am. J. Cardiol.*, **57** (Suppl. A), 6A–13A

Puschett, J. B. and Rastegar, A. (1974). Comparative study of the effects of metolazone and other diuretics on potassium excretion. *Clin. Pharm. Ther.*, **15**, 397–405

Reyes, A. J. and Leary, W. P. (1987). Natriuretic potency of various drugs. In Andreucci, V. E. and Dal Canton, A. (Eds.), *Diuretics: Basic, Pharmacological and Clinical Aspects*. Martinus Nijhoff, Boston, pp. 506–8

Roberts, C. J. C., Daneshmend, T. K. (1981). Assessment of natriuretic drugs. *Br. J. Clin. Pharm.*, **12**, 465–74

Rose, H. J., O'Malley, K. and Pruitt, A. W. (1977). Depression of renal clearance of furosemide in man by azotemia. *Clin. Pharm. Ther.*, **21**, 141–6

Roy, D. R. and Jamison, R. L. (1985). Countercurrent system and its regulation. In Seldin, D. W. and Giebsch, G. (Eds.), *The Kidney: Physiology and Pathophysiology*. Raven Press, New York, pp. 903–32

Schuster, V. L. and Seldin, D. W. (1985). Renal clearance. In Seldin, D. W. and Giebisch, G. (Eds.), *The Kidney: Physiology and Pathophysiology*. Raven Press, New York, pp. 365–95

Seldin, D. W. and Giebisch, G. (1985). *The Kidney: Physiology and Pathophysiology*. Raven Press, New York

Seldin, D. W. and Rector, F. C. (1973). Evaluation of clearance methods for localisation of site of action of diuretics. In Lant, A. F. and Wilson, G. M. (Eds.), *Modern Diuretic Therapy in the Treatment of Cardiovascular and Renal Disease*. Excerpta Medica, Amsterdam, pp. 97–110

Shackleton, C. R., Wong, N. L. M. and Sutton, R. A. L. (1986). Distal (potassium-sparing) diuretics. In Dirks, J. H. and Sutton, R. A. L. (Eds.), *Diuretics: Physiology, Pharmacology and Clinical Use*. W. B. Saunders, Philadelphia, pp. 117–34

Smith, D. E., Hyneck, M. L., Beradi, R. R. and Port, F. K. (1985). Urinary protein binding, kinetics and dynamics of furosemide in nephrotic patients. *J. Pharm. Sci.*, **74**, 603–7

Smith, H. (1956). *Principles of Renal Physiology*. Oxford University Press, New York

Steinmuller, S. R. and Puschett, J. B. (1972). Effects of metolazone in man: comparison with chlorothiazide. *Kid. Int.*, **1**, 169–81

Teredesai, P. and Puschett, J. B. (1979). Acute effects of piretanide in normal subjects. *Clin. Pharm. Ther.*, **25**, 331–9

Thomsen, K. (1984). Lithium clearance: a new method for determining proximal and distal tubular reabsorption of sodium and water. *Nephron*, **37**, 217–23

van Brummelen, P., Man in 't Veld, A. J. and Schalekamp, M. A. D. H. (1980). Haemodynamic changes during long-term thiazide treatment of essential hypertension in responders and nonresponders. *Clin. Pharm. Ther.*, **27**, 328–36

Weiner, I. M. (1986). General pharmacological aspects of diuretics. In Dirks, J. H. and Sutton, R. A. L. (Eds.), *Diuretics: Physiology, Pharmacology and Clinical Use*. W. B. Saunders, Philadelphia, pp. 3–28

Whelton, A. and Watson, A. J. (1987). The incidence of hypokalaemia and hyperkalaemia associated with diuretic use. In Puschett, J. B. and Greenberg, A. (Eds.), *Diuretics II: Chemistry, Pharmacology and Clinical Applications*. Elsevier, Amsterdam, pp. 677–85

Wilcox, C. S. (1987). Roles of renin angiotensin aldosterone and autonomic nervous systems in the response to diuretic drugs in man. In Puschett, J. B. and Greenberg, A. (Eds.), *Diuretics II: Chemistry, Pharmacology and Clinical Applications*. Elsevier, Amsterdam, pp. 503–9

39
Measurement of Renal Side-effects

Anne Dawnay

Dept of Chemical Pathology, St Bartholomew's Hospital, London EC1A 7BE, UK

INTRODUCTION

Measuring the therapeutic effects of drugs on the kidney has been dealt with elsewhere in this book, and this chapter will concentrate on the methods available for detecting their adverse effects. Space does not permit a detailed critique of each analytical method, but reference has been made to recent reviews.

Conventionally, renal dysfunction is detected by impairment of glomerular filtration rate (GFR), reflected by elevation of the plasma creatinine (cr) or diminution of the creatinine clearance (C_{cr}), and/or proteinuria. These tests alone are not sufficiently sensitive or specific to detect the early stages of drug-induced nephrotoxicity. Impairment of GFR often reflects late, secondary change following a primary insult of sufficient magnitude to the tubules or interstitium. Dipsticks for urine protein are predominantly sensitive to albumin and are only positive at concentrations in excess of 150 mg/l, which is approximately tenfold higher than the normal urine albumin output. Quantitative methods for urine total protein are insensitive and highly imprecise at low (normal) concentrations, and give no indication of the origin of the protein and therefore the possible underlying pathology. The differentiation of glomerular and tubular proteinuria requires the measurement of specific proteins (Peterson *et al.*, 1969).

The heterogeneous nature of the kidney and of the mode of drug toxicity necessitates the use of several tests specific for different aspects of renal integrity. In the last 10 years a bewildering array of new tests for detecting early renal dysfunction have appeared in the literature. Many of these are of unproven value in humans and have assumed, simplistically, that the detection of a drug-associated abnormality equates with toxicity.

In this chapter I have aimed to provide recommendations for screening for adverse effects, taking into account not only what is scientifically most appropriate but also what is feasible, in terms of subject and staff compliance, analytical simplicity, speed and cost. A discussion of what constitutes an adverse effect is outside the scope of this chapter. I believe that persistent and/or consistent abnormalities in screening tests associated with drug administration warrant further investigation to determine whether such changes are innocuous or reflect reversible damage or cell necrosis.

GENERAL CONSIDERATIONS

Urine is a readily accessible fluid but a highly variable and relatively hostile environment. Analytes and their assay methods must be sufficiently robust to withstand the range of urine pH, ionic strength and composition, proteolytic enzymes and contaminating bacteria without elaborate patient preparation or urine collection conditions. Timed urine collections should be avoided whenever possible, because of errors due to incomplete collection of urine passed, incomplete bladder emptying and mistakes in timing.

In most circumstances untimed urine samples are suitable. However, the concentration of most compounds in urine is independent of, and therefore varies inversely with, urine flow rate. This will normally vary between 0.5 and 5 ml/min during the day, depending on fluid intake. Correction for flow rate is achieved most simply by also measuring urine cr, the excretion rate of which is relatively constant (see below), and computing a ratio. Physiologically, urine cr output depends on muscle mass, which in turn varies with age and sex. With some, but not all, analytes this necessitates the use of appropriate reference ranges. The excretion of most compounds in urine does not follow a normal distribution and reference ranges must be derived using non-parametric methods. It is worth noting that most reference ranges are based on the 95th centile of the population and therefore, by definition, 5% will be abnormal. If 20 separate tests are carried out on 100 individuals, 64% will show one or more abnormal results (Rogers and Spector, 1986). The excretion of many proteins is not constant throughout the day, owing to circadian rhythms, posture, exercise, etc. Reference ranges derived from early morning urine samples (i.e. overnight urine) may not be applicable to daytime samples, and vice versa. In general, the type of sample is irrelevant, provided that the same type is consistently used during the study. I have given illustrative reference ranges but these will obviously vary, depending on the method used.

Tests for specific proteins in urine, including enzymes, are notorious for high intraindividual variability and random aberrant results. Fluctuations within the reference range and single abnormal results are probably of little significance. Several samples, to demonstrate consistency within an individual, and/or several subjects, to demonstrate consistency of response, are necessary. This problem has been widely studied in relation to urine albumin (Feldt-Rasmussen and Mathiesen, 1984; Howey *et al.*, 1987; Mogensen, 1987). This does not devalue their use but merits attention when designing protocols and interpreting results.

ASSESSMENT OF GLOMERULAR FILTRATION RATE

The only practicable means of assessing GFR is by C_{cr} and plasma cr and urea. For a full discussion of this subject, I recommend the review by Payne (1986).

Calculation of C_{cr} involves the collection of timed samples, usually over 24 h. Measurement of the volume, and urine and plasma concentrations of cr allow calculation of C_{cr} using the formula uv/p, where u and p are the respective urine and plasma concentrations of cr in identical units and v is the rate of urine flow in ml/min. As a check for inaccurate timing, two consecutive collections should always be made. Plasma cr and urine cr output is not constant over 24 h on a diet containing meat protein (Heymsfield *et al.*, 1983; Mayersohn *et al.*, 1983) and C_{cr} may therefore vary considerably, depending on the timing of the urine collection period and blood sample.

Assessment of GFR is usually for two reasons (Payne, 1986): first, to determine whether it is abnormal and if so to what extent; second, to determine whether it has changed. To detect abnormality demands the use of appropriate reference ranges. C_{cr} steadily declines with age from a mean of 112 ml/min (range 78–146) in the third decade to 78 ml/min (range 52–102) in the eighth decade in men (Rowe *et al.*, 1976a). In contrast, plasma cr measured in the morning in men was unaffected by age (mean 88 μmol/l in the third and 90 μmol/l in the eighth decade) and averaged 10 μmol/l less in women (De Lauture *et al.*, 1973). The constancy of plasma cr with increasing age, in spite of a reduction in C_{cr}, is most likely to be due to a decrease in muscle mass, as reflected by a decreasing urine cr output with age (Rowe *et al.*, 1976b). The detection of change depends on the analytical reproducibility of the measurement and on the biological variability. Day-to-day coefficients of variation for morning plasma cr are some 8% in health (Rosano and Brown, 1982) but may be three times as high (Brochner-Mortensen and Rodbro, 1976) or worse (personal experience) for C_{cr} even after careful instruction. It is a well-known fact that an accurately timed collection of urine is very difficult to obtain.

In nephrotoxicity studies, C_{cr}, plasma cr and urea should be measured on at least two occasions before commencing a study to establish a baseline and to gauge any necessary reduction in drug dose in elderly patients with a naturally reduced GFR if the drug depends on renal clearance. Thereafter, plasma cr measured on samples taken preferably in the morning after a non-meat protein breakfast offers the most precise means of detecting change. Typically, an increase of 30 μmol/l is significant, even if remaining within the reference range. Impairment of GFR due to haemodynamic factors may occur rapidly, e.g. in some forms of nephrotoxicity associated with non-steroidal anti-inflammatory drugs (Garella and Matarese, 1984) or cyclosporine (Walker and Duggin, 1988).

Of all the tests for detecting renal dysfunction, cr is most prone to interference. Ketones, especially acetoacetate, cause positive interference with the assay and prolonged fasting, to an extent that ketones are readily detectable in urine, may be sufficient to cause significant error, especially in a dilute urine sample (Harrison, 1987). Drugs may interfere with cr analysis (e.g. cephalosporin antibiotics) or compete for tubular secretion (e.g. cimeti-dine) (Narayanan and Appleton, 1980; Payne, 1986). In either case this can cause misleading increases in plasma cr and therefore it is advisable to also measure plasma urea. Parent drugs can be tested for analytical interference but their metabolites are not often available. Although comparatively rare, the interference of drugs in laboratory tests should always be borne in mind.

ASSESSMENT OF GLOMERULAR PERMEABILITY

Glomerular proteinuria can only be accurately assessed by specific immunoas-says for proteins of high M_r (>60000). In practice, urine albumin (M_r 66000) is stable, is easy to measure and has been widely studied; there is no evidence that any other protein of high M_r gives more useful information unless an index of selectivity is required.

Urine albumin is readily detected by most types of immunoassay, be they of the unlabelled (e.g. nephelometry, turbidimetry, rocket electrophoresis) or labelled (e.g. isotopic, fluorescent, enzyme) type. The recent recognition that diabetic nephropathy can now be predicted from the early detection of small elevations of albumin (Mogensen, 1987), years in advance of the appearance of clinical proteinuria, has resulted in a proliferation of commercial kits and published in-house assays for urine albumin. Many of these methods are easily automated (Watts *et al.*, 1986; Elving *et al.*, 1989) or are manually so simple (Silver *et al.*, 1986) as to allow the processing of several hundred samples per day. A comprehensive review of the analytical goals and conditions of urine collection and storage is available (Rowe *et al.*, 1989). Normal urine output is <20 mg/24 h (Feldt-Rasmussen and Mathiesen, 1984) or <2.8 mg/mmol cr (Silver *et al.*, 1986) and is typically lower in samples collected while recumbent compared with ambulant and in males compared with females (Silver *et al.*, 1986; Howey *et al.*, 1987). Clinical glomerular proteinuria is known to occur following the use of many drugs, e.g. gold (Hall, 1988), and may be the presenting feature in some forms of non-steroidal anti-inflammatory drug toxicity (Garella and Matarese, 1984). However, there is a dearth of information concerning the use of sensitive urine albumin assays in the early detection of nephrotoxicity.

ASSESSMENT OF TUBULAR DYSFUNCTION

Electrolytes and Water

The measurement of plasma electrolytes (sodium, potassium, calcium, bicar-bonate, chloride) and clinical evaluation of the patient provide the most practicable means of screening for drug-induced abnormalities of water and electrolyte homoeostasis. Magnesium wasting, resulting in hypomagnesaemia, has been reported with aminoglycosides (Davey and Harpur, 1987) and cisplatin (Litterst and Weiss, 1987) but usually occurs in conjunction with hypocalcaemia. The 24 h and fractional excretion of electrolytes, and dynamic tests for urine acidification and concentration, are cumbersome and should only be considered if other evidence suggests that they are necessary.

Low-molecular-weight Proteins (LMWP)

'LMWP' is a term which comprises that group of plasma proteins, generally of M_r less than 35000, which are filtered to a significant extent by the glomerulus. Some 99.95% of the filtered load is absorbed and catabolised in the proximal tubule. Increased excretion of these proteins may be due either to decreased absorption, as a consequence of proximal tubular dysfunction, or to an increase in their serum concentration and therefore a filtered load exceeding the tubular absorptive capacity (Maack *et al.*, 1979; Beetham *et al.*, 1987). This second mechanism is unlikely other than in malignancy, systemic inflammatory processes or renal dysfunction with a plasma cr in excess of some 180 µmol/l (Bernard *et al.*, 1988) and will be apparent from baseline samples. Elevated urine excretion of LMWPs following exposure to drugs, chemicals and heavy metals toxic to the proximal tubule is well proven in healthy volunteers, industrial workers and patients (Weise *et al.*, 1981; Topping *et al.*, 1986; Bernard *et al.*, 1987; Stonard, 1987). Levels may be elevated several hundred-fold in the face of severe proximal tubular damage.

The most widely studied protein in this group is beta-2-microglobulin (b2m) (Schardijn and Statius van Eps, 1987). However, it is rapidly and irreversibly degraded in urine of pH less than 6 (Evrin and Wibell, 1972; Bernard *et al.*, 1982; Davey and Gosling, 1982; Donaldson *et al.*, 1989) and its use is no longer recommended. Retinol-binding protein (RBP) (Peterson and Berggard, 1971) and alpha-1-microglobulin (a1m) (Berggard *et al.*, 1980), both of which are comparatively stable at pH 5 and above (Bernard *et al.*, 1982; Yu *et al.*, 1983; Beetham *et al.*, 1985; Donaldson *et al.*, 1989), are theoretically suitable alternatives and an increasing amount of empirical evidence suggests that this is so (Bernard *et al.*, 1982, 1987; Topping *et al.*, 1986; Beetham *et al.*, 1987). The excretion rate of LMWPs appears to be unaffected by age, sex or water diuresis (Evrin and Wibell, 1972; Wibell and Karlsson, 1976; Beetham *et al.*, 1985; Beetham, 1986). Normal excretion rates are typically <1.7 mg/mmol cr for a1m (Yu *et al.*, 1983) and <13 µg/mmol cr for RBP (Beetham *et al.*, 1985).

Enzymes

The assay of tissue-specific enzymes in serum to detect and monitor tissue damage has a long-established history in clinical chemistry. Such a proven role, together with the cheapness and relative ease of assay, undoubtedly contributed to the application of such assays to urine samples. Urine contains many enzymes whose origin can be located in a particular part of the nephron

(Schmidt and Guder, 1976; Price, 1982). They are generally of high M_r and contamination with their serum counterparts is unlikely, provided that glomerular permeability is normal. Their different distribution not only along the length of the nephron but also to different cellular and subcellular locations in the same part of the nephron suggested that measurement of a panel of enzymes would be a non-invasive means of giving highly specific information concerning the sites affected by nephrotoxins. Such ambitions have generally not been realised, partly because of difficulties experienced with enzyme stability and non-specific effects on activity measurements, often necessitating dialysis or gel filtration of urine samples prior to analysis, and partly because of the difficulties in obtaining corroborative evidence in humans.

The only enzyme to have emerged from an experimental research interest as a serious contender for detecting subclinical toxicity is N-acetyl-beta-D-glucosaminidase (EC 3.2.1.30; NAG). NAG is a lysosomal enzyme found in most parts of the nephron but with toxins affecting the proximal convoluted tubule being the predominant cause of increased excretion in urine. However, in the rat (Stonard, 1987) and dog (Piperno, 1981), experimental papillotoxins also increase NAG excretion. The original assay used a fluorescent substrate (Tucker *et al.*, 1975), necessitating the inclusion of blanks for each urine sample, owing to their highly variable and non-specific endogenous fluorescence. The recent advent of colorimetric substrates, with measurements made at 505 nm (Yuen *et al.*, 1984) or 580 nm (Goren *et al.*, 1986), has obviated the need for blanks, provided that samples are not icteric or blood-stained, and are easily automated. NAG is stable over the pH range 5–8 (Lockwood and Bosmann, 1979) and no inhibitors or activators are known (Piperno, 1981; Mueller *et al.*, 1986). Urine flow rate, age and sex have no appreciable effects on the urine excretion rate (Lockwood and Bosmann, 1979; Houser, 1986; Jung *et al.*, 1986). As with all assays of enzyme activity, reference ranges are highly method-dependent.

A prospective evaluation of NAG excretion compared with plasma cr and urine b2m illustrates its potential use. In a study of 28 patients with normal renal function (plasma cr of <100 μmol/l, no proteinuria and sterile urine) treated with gentamicin, only 1 of 12 patients with an initially normal NAG excretion developed renal failure (increase in plasma cr >50 μmol/l), although 7 showed a marked and persistent increase in the excretion of NAG and, later, of b2m (Gibey *et al.*, 1981). However, 11 of 16 patients with an initially elevated NAG developed renal failure and showed a more rapid increase in NAG and b2m excretion which preceded the increase in plasma cr. Thus, drug-induced abnormalities in the absence of overt renal dysfunction may predict a risk of toxicity which is overt in patients with pre-existing tubular abnormalities. In clinical practice, aminoglycoside use is associated with acute renal failure in 8–26% of patients (Humes, 1988).

Kidney-derived Antigens

The measurement of kidney-derived material to detect renal pathology remains a research tool of promising but, as yet, unproven use (see Dawnay and Cattell, 1987, for review). Only a few of the renal antigens excreted in urine have been isolated and characterised, e.g. ligandin, urine protein-1 and BB-50 from the proximal tubule, Tamm–Horsfall glycoprotein from the thick ascending limb of the loop of Henle and early distal convoluted tubule, and various basement membrane antigens. The past 5 years has seen the development of assays using monoclonal antibodies reactive with specific cellular or subcellular compounds within the nephron. Their reactivity with non-renal antigens is generally unknown and caution should be exercised in the interpretation of results using these assays. Certainly many monoclonal antibodies to B-cells react with kidney antigens which share common epitopes (Fleming *et al.*, 1989).

SUMMARY

Drug-induced nephrotoxicity occurs via numerous mechanisms and may develop acutely or chronically. Sensitive tests to detect subclinical abnormalities may be useful to determine the inherent toxicity of a drug; to compare the relative toxicity of different drugs with a similar therapeutic index; and to select and monitor patients for Phase II trials to minimise the risk of toxicity. Several samples should be obtained from each subject before, during and after drug administration, to determine whether any abnormalities are persistent or random and whether they are reversible.

In the past, nephrotoxicity has often only manifested after widespread clinical use in predisposed patients. Common risk factors include dose and duration of treatment, advancing age, pre-existing renal insufficiency or hepatic disease, hypovolaemia and concurrent nephrotoxic drug administration. Whether the use of sensitive tests to detect subclinical abnormalities during Phase I and Phase II trials will be of useful predictive value merits further evaluation.

REFERENCES

Beetham, R. (1986). The development of immunoassays for retinol-binding protein and their application. PhD Thesis, London University

Beetham, R., Dawnay, A. and Cattell, W. R. (1987). The effect of a synthetic polypeptide on the renal handling of protein in man. *Clin. Sci.*, **72**, 245–9

Beetham, R., Dawnay, A., Landon, J. and Cattell, W. R. (1985). A radioimmunoassay for retinol-binding protein in serum and urine. *Clin. Chem.*, **31**, 1364–7

Berggard, B., Ekstrom, B. and Akerstrom, B. (1980). Alpha-1-microglobulin. *Scand. J. Clin. Lab. Invest.*, **40** (Suppl. 154), 63–71

Bernard, A. M., Moreau, D. and Lauwerys, R. (1982). Comparison of retinol-binding protein and beta-2-microglobulin determination in urine for the early detection of tubular proteinuria. *Clin. Chim. Acta*, **126**, 1–7

Bernard, A. M., Vyskocil, A. A., Mahieu, P. and Lauwerys, R. R. (1987).

Assessment of urinary retinol-binding protein as an index of proximal tubular injury. *Clin. Chem.*, **33**, 775–9

Bernard, A., Vyskocyl, A., Mahieu, P. and Lauwerys, R. (1988). Effect of renal insufficiency on the concentration of free retinol-binding protein in urine and serum. *Clin. Chim. Acta*, **171**, 85–94

Brochner-Mortensen, I. and Rodbro, P. (1976). Selection of routine method for determination of glomerular filtration rate in adult patients. *Scand. J. Clin. Lab. Invest.*, **36**, 35–43

Davey, P. G. and Gosling, P. (1982). Beta-2-microglobulin instability in pathological urine. *Clin. Chem.*, **28**, 1330–3

Davey, P. G. and Harpur, E. S. (1987). In Bach, P. H. and Lock, E. A. (Eds.), *Nephrotoxicity in the Experimental and Clinical Situation* (Part 2). Martinus Nijhoff, Lancaster, pp. 643–58

Dawnay, A. and Cattell, W. R. (1987). In Bach, P. H. and Lock, E. A. (Eds.), *Nephrotoxicity in the Experimental and Clinical Situation* (Part 2). Martinus Nijhoff, Lancaster, pp. 593–612

De Lauture, H., Caces, E., Dubost, P., Tournier, M., Dolle, Y., Weill, J., Boulard, P. and Rossier, J. (1973). In Siest, G. (Ed.), *Reference Values in Human Chemistry*. Karger, Basle, pp. 141–52

Donaldson, M. D. C., Chambers, R. E., Woolridge, M. W. and Whicher, J. T. (1989). Stability of alpha-1-microglobulin, beta-2-microglobulin and retinol binding protein in urine. *Clin. Chim. Acta*, **179**, 73–8

Elving, L. D., Bakkeren, J., Jansen, M., de Kat Angelino, C., de Nobel, E. and van Munster, P. (1989). Screening for microalbuminuria in patients with diabetes mellitus: frozen storage of urine samples decreases their albumin content. *Clin. Chem.*, **35**, 308–10

Evrin, P.-E. and Wibell, L. (1972). The serum levels and urinary excretion of beta-2-microglobulin in apparently healthy subjects. *Scand. J. Clin. Lab. Invest.*, **29**, 69–74

Feldt-Rasmussen, B. and Mathiesen, E. R. (1984). Variability of urinary albumin excretion in incipient diabetic nephropathy. *Diabetic Nephropathy*, **3**, 101–3

Fleming, S., Jones, D. B. and Moore, K. (1989). B-cell markers in the human kidney. *Nephrol. Dial. Transplant.*, **4**, 85–91

Garella, S. and Matarese, R. A. (1984). Renal effects of prostaglandins and clinical adverse effects of nonsteroidal anti-inflammatory agents. *Medicine*, **63**, 165–81

Gibey, R., Dupond, J.-L., Alber, D., Leconte des Floris, R. and Henry, J.-C. (1981). Predictive value of urinary N-acetyl-beta-D-glucosaminidase (NAG), alanine aminopeptidase (AAP) and beta-2-microglobulin (b2m) in evaluating nephrotoxicity of gentamicin. *Clin. Chim. Acta*, **116**, 25–34

Goren, M. P., Wright, R. K. and Osborne, S. (1986). Two automated procedures for N-acetyl-beta-D-glucosaminidase determination evaluated for detection of drug-induced tubular nephrotoxicity. *Clin. Chem.*, **32**, 2052–5

Hall, C. L. (1988). Gold nephropathy. *Nephron*, **50**, 265–72

Harrison, S. P. (1987). More on urinary albumin and creatinine [letter]. *Clin. Chem.*, **33**, 740

Heymsfield, S. B., Arteaga, C. and McManus, C. (1983). Measurement of muscle mass in humans: validity of the 24 hour urinary creatinine method. *Am. J. Clin. Nutr.*, **37**, 478–94

Houser, M. T. (1986). The effects of age and urine concentration on lysozyme and N-acetyl-beta-D-glucosaminidase (NAG) content in urine. *Ann. Clin. Biochem.*, **23**, 297–302

Howey, J. E. A., Browning, M. C. K. and Fraser, C. G. (1987). Selecting the optimum specimen for assessing slight albuminuria, and a strategy for clinical investigation: novel uses of data on biological variation. *Clin. Chem.*, **33**, 2034–8

Humes, H. D. (1988). Aminoglycoside nephrotoxicity. *Kidney Int.*, **33**, 900–11

Jung, K., Schulze, G. and Reinholdt, C. (1986). Different diuresis dependent excretions of urinary enzymes: *N*-acetyl-beta-D-glucosaminidase, alanine aminopeptidase, alkaline phosphatase, and gamma glutamyltransferase. *Clin. Chem.*, **32**, 529–32

Litterst, C. L. and Weiss, R. B. (1987). In Bach, P. H. and Lock, E. A. (Eds.), *Nephrotoxicity in the Experimental and Clinical Situation* (Part 2). Martinus Nijhoff, Lancaster, pp. 771–816

Lockwood, T. D. and Bosmann, H. B. (1979). The use of urinary *N*-acetyl-beta-glucosaminidase in human renal toxicology. *Toxicol. Appl. Pharm.*, **49**, 323–36

Maack, T., Johnson, V., Kau, S. T., Figueiredo, J. and Sigulem, D. (1979). Renal filtration, transport and metabolism of low-molecular-weight proteins: a review. *Kidney Int.*, **16**, 251–70

Mayersohn, M., Conrad, K. A. and Achari, R. (1983). The influence of a cooked meat meal on creatinine plasma concentration and creatinine clearance. *Br. J. Clin. Pharm.*, **15**, 227–30

Mogensen, C. E. (1987). Microalbuminuria as a predictor of clinical diabetic nephropathy. *Kidney Int.*, **31**, 673–89

Mueller, P. W., MacNeil, M. L. and Steinberg, K. K. (1986). Stabilisation of alanine aminopeptidase, gamma glutamyltranspeptidase, and *N*-acetyl-beta-D-glucosaminidase activity in normal urines. *Arch. Environ. Contam. Toxicol.*, **15**, 343–7

Narayanan, S. and Appleton, H. D. (1980). Creatinine: a review. *Clin. Chem.*, **26**, 1119–26

Payne, R. B. (1986). Creatinine clearance: a redundant clinical investigation. *Ann. Clin. Biochem.*, **23**, 243–50

Peterson, P. A. and Berggard, I. (1971). Isolation and properties of a human retinol-transporting protein. *J. Biol. Chem.*, **246**, 25–33

Peterson, P. A., Evrin, P.-E. and Berggard, I. (1969). Differentiation of glomerular, tubular and normal proteinuria: determinations of urinary excretion of beta-2-microglobulin, albumin, and total protein. *J. Clin. Invest.*, **48**, 1189–98

Piperno, E. (1981). In Hook, J. B. (Ed.), *Toxicology of the Kidney*. Raven Press, New York, pp. 31–55

Price, R. G. (1982). Urinary enzymes, nephrotoxicity and renal disease. *Toxicology*, **23**, 99–134

Rogers, H. J. and Spector, R. G. (1986). In Glenny, H. and Nelmes, P. (Eds.), *Handbook of Clinical Drug Research*. Blackwell Scientific, Oxford, pp. 33–58

Rosano, T. G. and Brown, H. H. (1982). Analytical and biological variability of serum creatinine and creatinine clearance: implications for clinical interpretation. *Clin. Chem.*, **28**, 2330–1

Rowe, D. J. F., Dawnay, A. and Watts, G. F. (1989). Microalbuminuria in diabetes mellitus: recommendations for the measurement of albumin in urine. *Ann. Clin. Biochem.* (in press)

Rowe, J. W., Andres, R., Tobin, J. D., Norris, A. H. and Shock, N. (1976a). Age-adjusted standards for creatinine clearance. *Ann. Int. Med.*, **84**, 567–9

Rowe, J. W., Andres, R., Tobin, J. D., Norris, A. H. and Shock, N. W. (1976b). The effect of age on creatinine clearance in men: a cross-sectional and longitudinal study. *J. Gerontol.*, **31**, 155–63

Schardijn, G. H. C. and Statius van Eps, L. W. (1987). Beta-2-microglobulin: its significance in the evaluation of renal function. *Kidney Int.*, **32**, 635–41

Schmidt, U. and Guder, W. G. (1976). Sites of enzyme activity along the nephron. *Kidney Int.*, **9**, 233–42

Silver, A., Dawnay, A., Landon, J. and Cattell, W. R. (1986). Immunoassays for low concentrations of albumin in urine. *Clin. Chem.*, **32**, 1303–6

Stonard, M. D. (1987). In Bach, P. H. and Lock, E. A. (Eds.), *Nephrotoxicity in the Experimental and Clinical Situation* (Part 2). Martinus Nijhoff, Lancaster, pp. 563–92

Topping, M. D., Forster, H. W., Dolman, C., Luczynska, C. M. and Bernard, A. M. (1986). Measurement of urinary retinol-binding protein by enzyme-linked immuno-sorbent assay, and its application to detection of tubular proteinuria. *Clin. Chem.*, **32**, 1863–6

Tucker, S. M., Boyd, P. J. R., Thompson, A. E. and Price, R. G. (1975). Automated assay of *N*-acetyl-beta-glucosaminidase in normal and pathological urine. *Clin. Chim. Acta*, **62**, 333–9

Walker, R. J. and Duggin, G. G. (1988). Drug Nephrotoxicity. *Ann. Rev. Pharm. Toxicol.*, **28**, 331–45

Watts, G. F., Bennett, J. F., Rowe, D. J., Morris, R. W., Gatling, W., Shaw, K. M. and Polak, A. (1986). Assessment of immunochemical methods for determining low concentrations of albumin in urine. *Clin. Chem.*, **32**, 1544–8

Weise, M., Prufer, D., Jaques, G., Keller, M. and Mondorf, A. W. (1981). Beta-2-microglobulin and other proteins as parameter for tubular function. *Contr. Nephrol.*, **24**, 88–98

Wibell, L. and Karlsson, A. (1976). Urinary excretion of beta-2-microglobulin after the induction of a diuresis. *Nephron*, **17**, 343–52

Yu, H., Yanagisawa, Y., Forbes, M. A., Cooper, E. H. and Crockson, R. A. (1983). Alpha-1-microglobulin: an indicator protein for renal tubular function. *J. Clin. Pathol.*, **36**, 253–9

Yuen, C. T., Kind, P. R. N., Price, R. G., Praill, P. F. G. and Richardson, S. C. (1984). Colorimetric assay for *N*-acetyl-beta-D-glucosaminidase (NAG) in patholo-gical urine using the ω-nitrostyryl substrate: the development of a kit and the comparison of manual procedure with the automated fluorimetric method. *Ann. Clin. Biochem.*, **21**, 295–300

X
Assessment of the Effects of Drugs Used in Obstetrics and Gynaecology

40
Abortifacient Drugs

M. Bygdeman

Dept of Obstetrics and Gynaecology, Karolinska Hospital, 104 01 Stockholm, Sweden

INTRODUCTION

Interruption of pregnancy applies to gravidae at less than 28 full weeks' gestation with a quiescent uterus. Practically, in the overwhelming majority of cases, abortion should be performed prior to viability or at less than 22 weeks' gestation.

The global total of legal abortions carried out each year is uncertain, but it is likely to be between 30 and 40 million (Tietze and Henshaw, 1986). Thus, the market for safe and effective abortifacient drugs is considerable. In spite of this fact, the interest among many pharmaceutical companies in developing such drugs has been limited, mainly because of the negative attitude to abortion in general among certain population groups and organisations. While a reduction of the need of legal abortion is desirable, it is more difficult to understand why women for whom a legal termination of an unwanted pregnancy is the only alternative should not be provided with the benefit of scientific progress.

Efficacy and safety of a method for interruption of pregnancy is best assessed by comparison in a double-blind or randomised fashion with an established technique. At present, however, most investigations reported are pilot studies of a single technique and compound, and interpretation is made difficult by the absence of generally accepted working definitions. The significance of key concepts such as successful abortion, complete abortion and induction abortion interval varies according to the author and, occasionally, these concepts are not even explained.

Both surgical and medical methods are of proven value for termination of pregnancy. Abortifacient drugs have an established clinical use for termination of second trimester pregnancy, i.e. natural prostaglandins (PGs), prostaglandin analogues, hypertonic saline, urea and rivanol, and for cervical ripening and dilatation of the cervical canal prior to vacuum aspiration in late first and early second trimester abortions, i.e. prostaglandin analogues. Efforts to develop a medical method as an alternative to vacuum aspiration to terminate early pregnancy have been ongoing for several years. Significant progress has been noted during recent years. Among the drugs used are PG analogues and antiprogestins and combinations of these drugs.

DEFINITION OF STUDY POPULATION

To evaluate the efficacy and safety of abortifacient drugs, it is essential that the study population be strictly defined. For obvious reasons, only patient volunteers can be used. It is preferable, at least initially, to use only healthy subjects with a normal pregnancy. Patients with signs of threatening abortion, i.e. vaginal bleeding or rupture of the membranes, should not be recruited. Otherwise an unrealistic success rate might be obtained. It is not known whether patients with missed abortion are easier or more difficult to induce than viable pregnancies at the same gestational age. However, the risk of complications and side-effects is higher if the intrauterine route of administration is used in these cases, one reason being that after administration the rate of absorption to the general circulation is often significantly increased.

Of major importance is the duration of pregnancy at the time of treatment. In more advanced pregnancies ultrasound examination is recommended to assess the status and the age of the pregnancy. During early pregnancy the daily increase of β-hCG could be used instead when it may not be possible to visualise the pregnancy by ultrasound. During early pregnancy the frequency

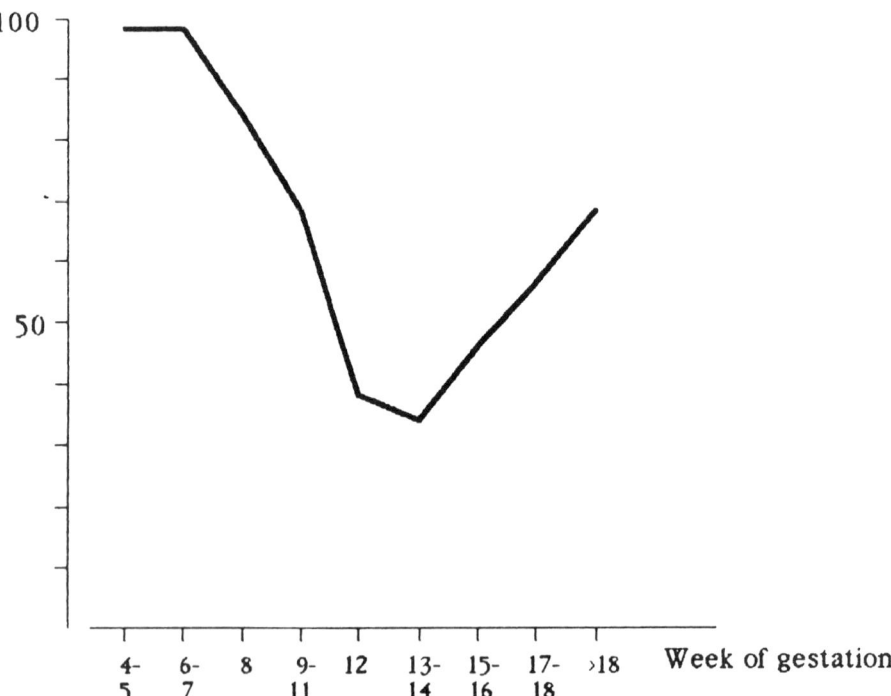

Figure 40.1   Frequency of complete abortion following prostaglandin treatment by various route vs. gestational age. Data from our own studies

of complete abortion following treatment with prostaglandin analogues is directly related to age of gestation. During the first 3 weeks following the first missed menstrual period, a frequency of complete abortions of around 95% could be reached. At later stages of the first trimester the ability of prostaglandins to induce complete abortion declines drastically (Figure 40.1). In the second trimester the incidence of complete abortion increases again (Bygdeman *et al.*, 1976; Bygdeman, 1978). Since the variation in the frequency of complete abortion corresponds to that observed following spontaneous abortion, it is likely that the reason is anatomical rather than dependent on the abortifacient compound used. The frequencies of both minor and major complications are also related to duration of pregnancy. The overall frequency will increase with week of pregnancy (Tietze and Lewit, 1972; Edelman *et al.*, 1974). Certain medical disorders may increase the frequency and the severity of side-effects following treatment with abortifacient drugs. For hypertonic saline, women with pre-existing medical disorders, such as sickle cell disease, moderate to severe anaemia, cardiac or cardiovascular disorders and renal disorders have an increased risk (Brenner, 1972; Kerenyi, 1972; Zuspan *et al.*, 1976). Depending on the prostaglandin used, an increased risk has been reported, for instance, in patients with bronchial asthma, grand-mal seizures and sickle cell anaemia (Brenner, 1975).

MODE OF ACTION

All abortifacient compounds in present use either directly or indirectly result in stimulation of uterine contractility. Hypertonic saline, rivanol and urea all probably act by stimulating endogenous prostaglandin production, probably through induced cellular trauma (Gustavii and Gréen, 1972; Ölund, 1978; Waltman *et al.*, 1973). With hypertonic saline, acute salt poisoning of the products of conception resulting in fetal death is also of importance (Galen *et al.*, 1974). Natural prostaglandins and certain analogues have the unique capacity to stimulate uterine contractility directly during all stages of pregnancy. During early pregnancy and mid-pregnancy intramuscular or intravenous bolus injections of prostaglandins will result in an increase in uterine tonus with irregular contractions superimposed. If the treatment is continued, a regular uterine contractility pattern develops (Toppozada *et al.*, 1972). For both natural PGs and PG analogues used clinically at present, only intrauterine administration allows single administration for termination of second trimester pregnancy (Bygdeman, 1984). Following vaginal administration, intramuscular injections and intravenous injections, the compound will be rapidly metabolised when entering into the circulation (Gréen *et al.*, 1981), while following intra-amniotic administration, the half-life of $PGF_{2\alpha}$ is between 13.5 h and 20 h and of 15-methyl $PGF_{2\alpha}$ between 27 h and 31 h (Gréen *et al.*, 1974, 1976).

As mentioned previously, the response of the mid-pregnant human uterus to single intravenous injections of prostaglandins is characterised by an acute elevation of tonus which gradually returns to a normal level. It has been

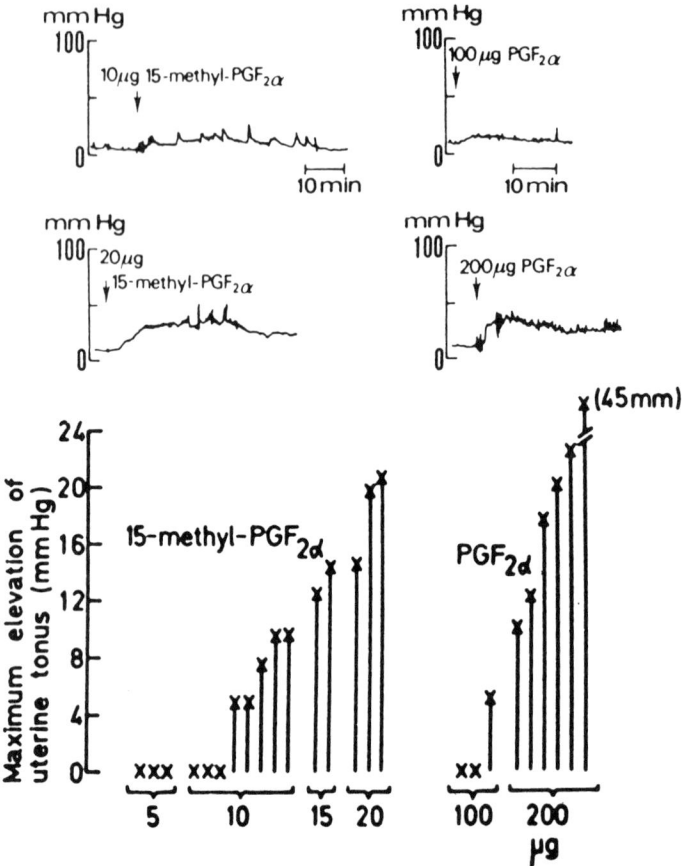

Figure 40.2 Determination of the smallest single intravenous dose of $PGF_{2\alpha}$ and 15-methyl $PGF_{2\alpha}$ that elicits a measurable response at mid-pregnancy in terms of uterine tonus elevation. Upper part of the figure: original tracings. Lower part of the figure: graphic illustration of individual responses obtained from 25 patients. From Newton *et al.* (1977)

shown that the elevation of uterine tonus in mmHg is roughly dose-dependent and can be utilised as a satisfactory measure of evaluating the relative potency of prostaglandins aimed at an abortifacient (Figure 40.2). When threshold doses of 15-methyl $PGF_{2\alpha}$ and $PGF_{2\alpha}$ were compared, the former compound was found to be at least 10 times more potent (Toppozada *et al.*, 1972). This difference corresponds well with the dosages used following, e.g. intra-amniotic administration for termination of pregnancy or 40–50 mg $PGF_{2\alpha}$ and 2.5 mg 15-methyl $PGF_{2\alpha}$ (Bygdeman, 1978). The duration of uterine stimulation is also related to the metabolic turnover of the compound. With 15-methyl $PGF_{2\alpha}$ the duration of the effect was almost double that of $PGF_{2\alpha}$.

Although recording of uterine contractility is a valuable tool in the assessment of new abortifacient drugs, it cannot replace pharmacokinetic studies. It must also be borne in mind that other factors are of importance when the clinical efficacy is evaluated, e.g. the resistance of the cervix.

Antiprogestins, such as RU 486, block the action of progesterone at the receptor level, causing decidual necrosis, bleeding, possibly increased PG production and, eventually, expulsion of the conceptus (Baulieu, 1985; Kelly *et al.*, 1986). The efficacy of the treatment has not been satisfactory. In patients with amenorrhoea of up to 49 days the frequency of complete abortion is reported to be around 60% (Van Look, 1989). Also with respect to antiprogestins, recording of uterine contractility has been found valuable. In early pregnancy the uterus is inactive and the response to the PG analogue sulprostone is characterised by an increase in uterine tonus with superimposed irregular contractions of low amplitude. Treatment with 25 mg RU 486 twice daily resulted in the appearance of regular uterine contractions at 24 h in 2 out of 5 patients, and in all patients at 36, 48 and 72 h after the start of RU 486 treatment. The withdrawal of progesterone influence changed the inactive early pregnant uterus into an active organ. Administration of sulprostone caused an obvious stimulation of both frequency and amplitude in the contractions. In addition, the significantly increased sensitivity to the PG analogue but not to oxytocin was already apparent 24 h after the start of RU 486 treatment (Swahn and Bygdeman, 1988). These experimental findings have been the basis for the highly successful sequential treatment with RU 486 and different prostaglandins for termination of early pregnancy (Bygdeman and Swahn, 1985; Rodger and Baird, 1987).

Cervical tissue has the capacity to form PGE_2, $PGF_{2\alpha}$ and TxA_2 (Christensen *et al.*, 1985) and these compounds probably participate in the physiological progress of cervical ripening at the end of pregnancy. Treatment with, for instance, PGE_2 will induce changes of the cervix similar to those observed at or near term. There are, therefore, good reasons to assume that the softening of the cervix and dilatation of the cervical canal observed after PG treatment prior to vacuum aspiration is due to a stimulating effect of PG on uterine contractility, thereby indirectly affecting the cervix, as well as a direct effect of PGs on the cervix through an increased collagenase activity (Uldbjerg *et al.*, 1987). Also, pretreatment with RU 486 seems to have a similar effect on the cervix but the pretreatment period needed is much longer than for PGs, being 24–48 h (Rådestad *et al.*, 1988). The effect of prostaglandins and antiprogestins on the cervix is best studied in the human by measuring the degree of dilatation by Hegar probes. For biochemical and histological studies of the effect of these compounds, a biopsy from the cervix is needed. For antiprogestins, animal studies can be useful, since these compounds also have a ripening and dilating effect on the cervix in the guinea-pig (Chwalisz *et al.*, 1987).

EVALUATION OF TREATMENT OUTCOME

Efficacy

The primary goal of the treatment depends on the stage of pregnancy at treatment. During early pregnancy, when a non-surgical method to compete with vacuum aspiration is aimed at, only a complete abortion, i.e. passage of the entire conceptus through the cervical canal, is acceptable. Different methods have been used to establish a complete abortion. The best definition of a complete abortion is that curettage has not been necessary from the time of treatment up to the first menstruation (WHO, 1987). Visual assessment, duration and amount of bleeding and gynaecological examinations are helpful in monitoring the abortion process but are not sufficiently precise to be used alone. Since small residues of pregnancy commonly remain in the uterus up to at least the first menstruation (Mandelin, 1978), curettage performed during this period will characterise a significant number of tr··atments as incomplete abortions, although interference would not have been necessary on clinical grounds. Serial ultrasound examinations are useful to establish when the conceptus is expelled, but not reliable for determining whether a complete abortion has occurred. Small residues in the uterus may, as with curettage, be interpreted as an incomplete abortion, although they are of no clinical importance. β-hCG is a valuable tool for following the outcome of the therapy. Experience has shown that a significant and progressive decrease in plasma hCG 1 and 2 weeks after treatment is a reliable sign of clinically complete abortion (Mandelin, 1978; Bygdeman *et al.*, 1984).

In the late first and early part of the second trimester of pregnancy, abortifacient drugs are mainly used to soften the cervix and to dilate the cervical canal prior to vacuum aspiration or dilatation and curettage (Ott, 1977). The degree of cervical dilatation is evaluated subjectively by determining the largest probe which can be introduced without resistance through the cervical canal. It is advantageous to use dilators with a stump end, e.g. Hegar probe. To establish the increase in dilatation there are two possibilities, either measuring the same patient both before start of treatment and at operation or in a randomised, placebo study measuring only at operation. The first alternative, besides being more complicated, has the possible disadvantage that the initial measurement could induce endogenous PG production and, thus, a ripening of the cervix unrelated to the drug treatment. The softness of the cervix may be measured by subjective evaluation of ease of dilatation or objectively by the use of electronic force monitors (Hulka *et al.*, 1974; Rådestad *et al.*, 1988). Of practical importance also is the fact that the treatment period does not exceed 3–4 h and allows outpatient management or, if it is longer, is so uncomplicated that the patient can be at home.

In second trimester abortion the expulsion of the fetus could easily be monitored by vaginal examination. Other factors of importance to be monitored include the induction abortion interval (length of time elapsed between performance of the first step of the procedure and expulsion of the fetus with or without placenta from the uterus), percentage of patients successfully aborted within 12, 24, 36, 48, 60 and 72 h of initiating the termination procedure and, in successfully aborted patients, mean total dose of abortifacient administered (Amy *et al.*, 1976). A complete or incomplete abortion can be visually established, but it is still necessary to follow the patient up to the first menstrual period to ensure that no part of placenta of clinical importance remains. If curettage is performed routinely after expulsion of the fetus and the result of the histopathological examination is used to establish the outcome, practically all patients will be found to have had an incomplete abortion. It is also of importance to describe the allowed time until curettage if the placenta is not expelled spontaneously. The retention rate of the placenta rapidly decreases with time, while the complication rate—for instance, amount of bleeding—increases.

Side-effects and Complications

General complications following termination of pregnancy irrespective of method used include, besides method failure, prolonged duration of bleeding and excessive blood loss, need for recurettage, infection and disturbances in the appearance of the first menstruation. The amount of bleeding should preferably be measured objectively—for instance, by using the procedure described by Newton *et al.* (1977). In many studies, however, especially following treatment during early pregnancy, the patients have subjectively evaluated the bleeding in comparison with their own menstrual bleeding often complemented with measurement of haemoglobin concentration prior to, during and after the bleeding period and with frequency of patients needing blood transfusion recorded (Bygdeman and Van Look, 1988).

Typical prostaglandin side-effects are vomiting and diarrhoea. However, these are transitory, rarely serious and can be treated prophylactically and symptomatically with antiemetics and antidiarrhoeal drugs. Chill, fever and minor episodes of coughing and shortness of breath have occasionally been observed. Although rare, bronchospasm, bradycardia and grand-mal seizures may occur. In second trimester abortion, PG treatment is associated with an increased risk of cervical laceration, especially in primigravidae and when uterine contractility is further augmented with intravenous oxytocin. When a new PG analogue is evaluated as an abortifacient, it is, therefore, advisable to record gastrointestinal side-effects. Different methods have been used, e.g. mean number of episodes per patient, percentage of patients with no such side-effects and percentage of patients with a high frequency of vomiting and diarrhoea, generally more than four episodes. Temperature should be recorded at 4–6 hour intervals, and in second trimester abortion all patients should be examined for status of the cervix following expulsion of the fetus.

Complaints such as nausea, vomiting, dizziness and fatigue are frequent following treatment with antiprogestin with or without the addition of PG analogues (for references see Bygdeman and Van Look, 1988; Van Look, 1989). However, these complaints are pregnancy-related, and since the treatment period has been extended in some studies up to 7 days, it is difficult to know to what extent the side-effects are really drug-related. In this case it is important that the frequency of complaints be recorded both before, daily during treatment and after the end of treatment. If this is done, the increase is found to be only marginal (Swahn *et al.*, 1989).

INTERACTION WITH OTHER DRUGS

Concomitant use of other drugs when testing efficiency and safety of a new compound always involves a risk that the outcome of the trial is affected. This is also true of abortifacient drugs. As mentioned previously, drugs such as hypertonic saline and rivanol act by stimulating the endogenous PG production. Also, following PG treatment the induced uterine contractility will result in an increased PG production from the decidua of importance for the progress of the abortion process. Treatment during the abortion with prostaglandin biosynthesis inhibitors such as salicylic acid or indomethacin will thus result in a significant prolongation of the induction to abortion interval (Waltman *et al.*, 1973; Ölund, 1978). There is no doubt that oxytocin and prostaglandin given in combination result in an additive effect on uterine contractility. However, solid evidence in favour of an enhancement or potentiation of the oxytocic response as influenced by prostaglandin is lacking. Still, combination of the two drugs may increase the risk of overstimulating uterine contractility and, hence, an increased risk of cervical injury and possibly uterine rupture.

ACCEPTABILITY OF TREATMENT

Studies on acceptability of procedures used for termination of pregnancy are few. In some the reaction of the patient is only anticipated, which is not sufficient (Rooks and Cates, 1977). How acceptable a method is to the individual user may eventually become the crucial factor for success of a new method related to fertility regulation if it is implemented into a programme in family planning. The studies published have mainly compared vacuum aspiration with prostaglandin analogues to terminate very early pregnancy. Before being allowed to enter the study, the patient had to accept random allocation to one of the two treatments. Interview schedules with closed and open questions were used to assess the patient's beliefs and evaluations of the procedures before and after treatment, her expectations, experiences and preferences. Sets of rating scales were also answered by each patient (Rosén *et al.*, 1979; 1984). The patients who were treated with prostaglandin remained very positive after the abortion. A majority of these patients intended to use the same procedure in case of a repeated abortion and would also recommend the treatment to a relative or a friend in spite of higher frequency of gastrointestinal side-effects, pain and a longer duration of bleeding than following the surgical procedure. It is not unlikely that most gynaecologists would have anticipated a more negative attitude among the patients.

ACKNOWLEDGEMENT

I am grateful to Astrid Häggblad for typing the manuscript and preparing the figures.

REFERENCES

Amy, J. J., Thiery, M., Bygdeman, M., Kerenyi, T. D., Crawford, J. S. and Karim, S. M. M. (1976). A suggested set of working definitions and criteria applicable to interruption of pregnancy. *Contraception*, **14**, 193–7

Baulieu, E .E. (1985). RU 486: An antiprogestin steroid with contragestive activity in women. In Baulieu, E. E. and Segal, S. J. (Eds.), *The Antiprogestin Steroid RU 486 and Human Fertility Controls*. Plenum Press, New York, pp. 1–25

Brenner, W. E. (1972). Second trimester interruption of pregnancy. In Taymor, M. K. and Green T. H. (Eds.), *Progress in Gynecology*, Vol. 6. Grune and Stratton, New York, pp. 421–44

Brenner, W. E. (1975). The current status of prostaglandins as abortifacients. *Am. J. Obstet. Gynecol.*, **123**, 306–28

Bygdeman, M. (1978). Comparison of prostaglandin and hypertonic saline for termination of pregnancy. *Obstet. Gynecol.*, **52**, 424–9

Bygdeman, M. (1984). The use of prostaglandins and their analogues for abortion. In Newton, J. R. (Ed.), *Clinics in Obstetrics and Gynaecology*, Vol. 11. W. B. Saunders, London, pp. 573–84

Bygdeman, M., Borell, U., Leader, A., Lundström, V., Martin, J. N., Jr., Eneroth, P. and Gréen, K. (1976). Induction of first and second trimester abortion by the vaginal administration of 15-methyl PGF$_{2\alpha}$ methyl ester. In Samuelsson, B. and Paoletti, R. (Eds.), *Advances in Prostaglandin and Thromboxane Research*, Vol. 2. Raven Press, New York, pp. 693–704

Bygdeman, M., Christensen, N. J., Gréen, K. and Vesterqvist, O. (1984). Selfadministration at home of prostaglandin for termination of early pregnancy. In Toppozada, M., Bygdeman, M. and Hafez, E. S. E. (Eds.), *Prostaglandins and Fertility Regulation*. MTP, Lancaster, pp. 83–90

Bygdeman, M. and Swahn, M. L. (1985). Progesterone receptor blockage. Effect on uterine contractility in early pregnancy. *Contraception*, **32**, 45–51

Bygdeman, M. and Van Look, P. F. A. (1988). Antiprogestins for the interruption of pregnancy. In Healy, D. L. (Ed.), *Ballière's Clinical Obstetrics and Gynaecology. Anti-hormones in Clinical Gynaecology*. Ballière Tindall, London, pp. 617–29

Christensen, N. J., Belfrage, P., Bygdeman, M., Floberg, J., Mitzuhashi, N. and Gréen, K. (1985). Bioconversion of arachidonic acid in human pregnant uterine cervix. *Acta Obstet. Gynecol. Scand.*, **64**, 259–65

Chwalisz, K., Qing, S. S., Neef, G. and Elger, W. (1987). The effect of the antigestagen ZK 98,299 on the uterine cervix. *Acta Endocrinol.*, **283** (Suppl.), 113–14

Edelman, D. A., Brenner, W. E. and Berger, G. B. (1974). Effectiveness and complication of abortion by dilatation and vacuum aspiration versus dilatation and rigid metal curettage. *Am. J. Obstet. Gynecol.*, **119**, 473–80

Galen, R. S., Chauhan, P., Wietzner, H. and Navarro, C. (1974). Fetal pathology and mechanism of fetal death in saline induced abortion: a study of 143 gestations and critical review of the literature. *Am. J. Obstet. Gynecol.*, **12**, 347–55

Gréen, K., Bygdeman, M. and Wiqvist, N. (1974). Kinetic and metabolic studies of prostaglandin $F_{2\alpha}$ administered intra-amniotically for induction of abortion. *Life Sci.*, **14**, 2285–97

Gréen, K., Christensen, N. and Bygdeman, M. (1981). The chemistry and pharmacology of prostaglandins with reference to human reproduction. *J. Reprod. Fertil.*, **62**, 269–81

Gréen, K., Granström, E., Bygdeman, M. and Wiqvist, N. (1976). Kinetic and mrtabolic studies of 15-methyl $PF_{2\alpha}$ administered intra-amniotically for induction of abortion. *Prostaglandins*, **11**, 699–711

Gustavii, B. and Gréen, K. (1972). Release of prostaglandin $F_{2\alpha}$ following injection of hypertonic saline for therapeutic abortion. A preliminary study. *Am. J. Obstet. Gynecol.*, **114**, 1099–100

Hulka, J. F., Leffler, H. T., Jr., Anglone, A. and Lachenbruch, P. A. (1974). A new electronic force monitor to measure factors influencing cervical dilatation for vacuum curettage. *Am. J. Obstet. Gynecol.*, **120**, 166–73

Kelly, R. W., Healy, D. L., Cameron, I. and Baird, D. T. (1986). The stimulation of prostaglandin production by two antiprogesterone steroids in human endometrial cells. *J. Clin. Endocrinol. Metab.*, **62**, 1117–23

Kerenyi, T. D. (1972). Technique of late abortion. In Lewit, S. (Ed.), *Abortion Techniques and Services*. Excerpta Medica, Amsterdam, pp. 17–22

Mandelin, M. (1978). Termination of early pregnancy by a single dose 3.0 mg 15-methyl $PGF_{2\alpha}$ methyl ester vaginal suppository. *Prostaglandins*, **16**, 143–51

Newton, J., Barnard, G. and Collons, W. (1977). A rapid method for measuring blood loss using autonomic extraction. *Contraception*, **16**, 269–82

Ölund, A. (1978). The effect of indomethacin on the instillation-abortion interval in Rivanol-induced mid-trimester abortion. *Acta Obstet. Gynecol. Scand.*, **57**, 333–6

Ott, E. R. (1977). Cervical dilatation—A review. *Population Reports*, Series F, No. 6

Rådestad, A., Christensen, N. J. and Strömberg, L. (1988). Cervical ripening with Mifepristone in first trimester abortion. A double-blind randomized biomechanical study. *Contraception*, **38**, 301–12

Rodger, M. W. and Baird, D. T. (1987). Induction of therapeutic abortion in early pregnancy with mifepristone in combination with prostaglandin pessary. *Lancet*, **ii**, 1415–18

Rooks, J. B. and Cates, W., Jr. (1977). Emotional impact of D&E vs. instillation. *Fam. Plann. Perspect.*, **9**, 276–7

Rosén, A.-S., Nystedt, L., Bygdeman, M. and Lundström, V. (1979). Acceptability of a non-surgical method to terminate very early pregnancy in comparison to vacuum aspiration. *Contraception*, **19**, 107–17

Rosén, A.-S., von Knorring, K., Bygdeman, M. and Christensen, N. (1984). Randomized comparison of prostaglandin treatment in hospital or at home with vacuum aspiration for termination of early pregnancy. *Contraception*, **29**, 423–35

Swahn, M. L. and Bygdeman, M. (1988). The effect of the antiprogestin RU 486 on uterine contractility and sensitivity to prostaglandin and oxytocin. *Br. J. Obstet. Gynaecol.*, **95**, 126–34

Swahn, M. L., Ugocsai, G., Bygdeman, M., Kovacs, L., Belsey, E. M. and Van Look, P. F. A. (1989). Effect of oral prostaglandins E_2 on uterine contractility and treatment outcome in women receiving RU 486 (mifepristone) for termination of early pregnancy. *Hum. Reprod.*, **4**, 21

Tietze, C. and Henshaw, S. K. (1986). *Induced Abortion: A World Review 1986*. Alan Guttmacher Institute, New York and Washington

Tietze, C. and Lewit, S. (1972). Joint program for the study of gestation (JPSA). Early medical complications of legal abortion. *Stud. Fam. Plann.*, **3**, 97

Toppozada, M., Beguin, F., Bygdeman, M. and Wiqvist, N. (1972). Response of the midpregnant human uterus to systemic administration of 15(S)15-methyl prostaglandin $F_{2\alpha}$. *Prostaglandins*, **2**, 239–49

Uldbjerg, N., Ulmsten, U. and Ekman, G. (1987). The physiological role of eicosanoids in controlling the form and function of the cervix. In Hillier, K. (Ed.), *Advances in Eicosanoid Research*. MTP, Lancaster, pp. 163–83

Waltman, R., Tricorni, V. and Palay, A. (1973). Aspirin and indomethacin: Effect on instillation/abortion time of mid-trimester hypertonic saline induced abortion. *Prostaglandins*, **3**, 47–58

Van Look, P. F. A. (1989). Antiprogestin: a new era in hormonal regulation of fertility. In *Proceedings of the First Congress of the International Society of Gynecological Endocrinology*. Parthenon Publishing, Carnforth (in press)

WHO Task Force on Post-ovulatory Methods for Fertility Regulation (1987). Menstrual regulation by intramuscular injection of 16-phenoxy-tetranor PGE_2 methyl sulfonylamide or vacuum aspiration. A randomized multicenter study. *Br. J. Obstet. Gynaecol.*, **94**, 949–56

Zuspan, F. P., Ballard, C. A., Bieniarz, J., Brenner, W. E., Corson, S. L., Kaiser, I. H., Kerenyi, T. D., King, T. M. and Tietze, C. (1976). Second trimester abortion—a symposium by correspondence. *J. Reprod. Med.*, **16** (2), 47–64

41
Oxytocic drugs

M. Bamber* and M. G. Elder†

*Rhône-Poulenc Ltd, Rainham Road South, Dagenham, Essex RM10 7XS, UK

†RPMS Institute of Obstetrics and Gynaecology, Hammersmith Hospital,
Ducane Road, London W12 0NN, UK

INTRODUCTION

Oxytocic drugs are those used to stimulate uterine activity. In the past 10–20 years there has been much change in the use of drugs that control uterine activity. Former agents such as 'buccal pitocin' and 'pill ergot' have been overtaken by newer drugs such as the prostaglandins. The assessment of the efficacy and safety of such newer drugs is dependent on measurable observations which reflect uterine activity. This chapter outlines (a) the clinical applications of oxytocic drugs and (b) the methods of evaluation of such agents in each of the above applications.

In current clinical practice there are three groups of oxytocic agents in use: oxytocin, the prostaglandins and their analogues, and ergometrine. These are naturally occurring substances, and are synthesised for therapeutic use. More recently progesterone receptor antagonists have been introduced. These oxytocic agents taken as a group are of benefit in the following clinical applications: (1) induction of labour; (2) augmentation of spontaneous labour; (3) therapeutic abortion; (4) treatment of postpartum haemorrhage; and (5) preoperative cervical softening.

INDUCTION OF LABOUR

Introduction

Prelabour and Labour

Before clinically recognisable labour is established, there is a period of time during which preparation for labour takes place. This preparatory time is called prelabour and lasts approximately 4 weeks. During this time slow but steadily progressive changes occur which enable clinical labour to be completed in a reasonably rapid and safe fashion. These changes are expressed in uterine contractility potential, alterations in the cervix and adaptive changes of the fetal station in the maternal pelvis. Spontaneous uterine contractions, often referred to as Braxton Hicks contractions (Braxton Hicks, 1871), become more frequent and co-ordinated, and the myometrium becomes more sensitive to oxytocin.

Also during the prelabour phase the cervix dilates progressively so that the average cervix already becomes dilated about 2 cm during the last few days prior to the onset of spontaneous labour (Hendricks *et al.*, 1970).

In addition to cervical dilatation, cervical thinning and cervical softening also occur, and by the end of the prelabour phase the internal os is extremely pliable and soft, allowing dilatation to occur readily. Subsequent to these changes the fetal head starts to descend.

Definition/Requirements of Induction

If the concept of prelabour is accepted, it follows that induction of labour must produce enough uterine contractility and associated changes to carry the uterus from whatever state it has achieved during prelabour at the commencement of induction through the completion of the prelabour phase and on into the active phase of clinically evident labour until cervical dilatation is complete (Hendricks, 1983). Therefore, for practical purposes, successful induction of labour implies successful 'completion' of labour. The components of successful completion of labour include the following: completion of cervical ripening and dilatation; effective uterine contractions; duration of labour; mode of delivery; neonatal condition; and other obstetric parameters.

Clinical Evaluation of Oxytocic Drugs in Induction of Labour

Completion of Cervical Ripening and Dilatation

The Use of The Bishop Score

The Bishop (1964) scoring system provides in numerical terms an indicator of the status of a pregnancy and the prospects for its completion. It also provides information on the imminence or otherwise of the spontaneous onset of labour. The score is made up of the following factors: dilatation, effacement, consistency and position of the cervix and the station of the presenting part. The score may range from 0 to 11, and the total score gradually increases as the end of pregnancy approaches. Bishop suggested that elective induction may be successfully and safely performed when the pelvic score totals 9 or more. In a multicentre American study (Friedman *et al.*, 1966) it was demonstrated that the Bishop score was directly related to success of induction of labour and inversely related to the time needed to complete the prelabour phase. Thus, with a Bishop score of 4 or less, at least 4 h was required to complete the prelabour phase, whereas with a score of 11 or 12 only about 1½ h was required to achieve the onset of active phase of labour. Also in this study it was shown that in patients with a very low Bishop score the failure of attempted induction was in excess of 20%, whereas in those patients with a rising score there was a dropping failure rate, a Bishop score of

8 being associated with only 3% failure of induction and that of 10 or more being associated with virtually no induction failures. Studies evaluating the usefulness of prostaglandins (Calder *et al.*, 1975; Mackenzie and Embrey, 1977; Ulmsden *et al.*, 1982) and oxytocin (Calder, 1979) have found the Bishop score to be a helpful indicator of cervical ripening.

During the course of induction of labour it is important to define the actual onset of labour, a point which is often not addressed: O'Driscoll and Meagher (1986) have stated that 'the diagnosis of labour in a case of induction rests solely on dilatation of the cervix'. According to these authors, dilatation is achieved when there has been complete effacement. However, partial dilatation of the cervix can take place without complete effacement.

The Use of The Cervicograph

Once labour has been initiated, the best indicator of progress is the rate of cervical dilatation. This can be measured in the form of a cervicograph. This was pioneered by Friedman (1967) and later made popular by Philpott and Castle (1972) in Southern Africa. In the latter study the authors documented the rate of cervical dilatation from 3 cm dilatation onwards and drew up cervicographs for each patient. They derived an 'Alert Line' to the cervicographs by which they were able to separate efficient from inefficient labour, as reflected in the rate of dilatation of the cervix. The Alert Line joined points representing 1 cm dilatation at zero time (admission) and full dilatation (10 cm) 9 h later, a rate of 1 cm/h. The authors commented that this line was a good guide to the need for intervention and it allowed time for transfer of obstetrically abnormal patients for active management. Furthermore, the Alert Line separated patients with small pelvic size from those of adequate size. The cervicograph provided a graphic record of the rate of cervical dilatation and only essential information was recorded. The effect of oxytocic administration was readily apparent on consulting the cervicograph: if cervical dilatation took place, then the treatment was successful.

Effective Uterine Contractions

Methods for assessment of uterine activity need to measure the parameters of uterine frequency, amplitude and duration. It is also necessary to have a definition for a uterine contraction. The following terminology describes the various characteristics of a uterine contraction waveform.

Contraction interval   The time from the peak of one contraction to the peak of the next. While this unit is often quoted in minutes, the Système Internationale (SI) unit is the second.

Contraction frequency   The number of contractions in a stated time interval. It can be quoted as the inverse of contraction interval (e.g. if the mean contraction interval is 3 min, contraction frequency is said to be '1 in 3' minutes), or as the number of contractions in a standard time-interval (usually 10 min).

Peak contraction pressure   The maximum pressure attained during any particular contraction with reference to atmospheric pressure.

Active contraction pressure The peak pressure minus the 'resting' or 'baseline' tone as measured between contractions.

Onset and offset The beginning and end of each contraction. These are not entirely abrupt and are most conveniently defined as the intersection of regression lines fitted to the ascending and descending slopes of the contractions and an imaginary continuation of the baseline.

Duration The time between contraction onset and offset. This is usually fairly constant for any individual person, despite wide variation in the active contraction pressure (Pontonnier *et al.*, 1975; Seitchik and Chatkoff, 1975).

A number of methods have been used for assessing uterine contractions.

Manual Palpation

This is a relatively inaccurate method and permits only an appreciation of when a uterine contraction has occurred. This method does not evaluate the quality or the exact duration of uterine contractions but gives an indication of their frequency.

External Tocodynamometry

Tocodynamometry is a compound word derived from *toko* meaning 'pertaining to birth' and *dynamometer* meaning 'measurement of force'.

An external method of uterine contraction monitoring was developed and first published by Reynolds in 1948. In this method he introduced the multichannel strain-gauge tocodynamometer: this instrument depended upon the change of electrical resistance which occurred in a thin metal strip when it was bent by an external force. The force was produced by a piston indenting the uterus surrounded by a brass ring attached to the patient's abdomen with adhesive tape. As the uterus contracted, the piston was elevated by the tensing muscle. The increased force was transmitted by the piston to the end of the thin metal strip. The change in resistance was measured and recorded with a spark galvanometer. The records obtained could be analysed for (a) frequency of contractions; (b) regularity of contractions; (c) total relative work per unit period of time; (d) characteristics of contractions—e.g. intensity of contractions, contraction time, contraction duration and relaxation time, and contraction and relaxation rates.

The disadvantges of this system included (a) the inability to accurately measure intrauterine pressure, since this consists of the two components intra-amniotic pressure and local uterine muscle tension, the latter of which may not be representative of the uterus as a whole; (b) the large size and fragility of the apparatus.

Continuation of these studies using a multiple tocodynamometer technique showed that a normal contraction wave originates at the fundus of the uterus and passes down towards the cervix (Hellman *et al.*, 1950).

At about this period another method was developed, which was based on the principle that a weight laid on a muscle is raised when the muscle contracts and sinks back again when the muscle relaxes (Bell, 1952). This method was cumbersome and impractical.

The next attempt to develop an acceptable external method for recording intrauterine pressure was devised by Smyth and published in 1957. The principles of Smyth's method were as follows. If a small area of the abdominal and underlying uterine wall is turned into a flat diaphragm by pressing upon the external surface with a flat plate, the pressures upon each side of the body wall will be equal; by measuring the force upon the plate the internal pressure can be measured if the area of contact is known. To define the area of contact exactly and also to eliminate any pressure arising from bending of the body wall at the edges of the flattened area, the pressure plate is surrounded by a guard-plate which is held exactly level with the measuring area and flattens an additional 'surround' of body tissues. The force on the 'surround' or guard-ring is not measured. Although theoretically effective, there were several practical drawbacks to this method. The instrument needed to be applied to the patient over a fluid-filled part of the uterus, thus restricting the patient's choice of posture. In addition, the instrument needed to be held in position by a stiff elastic belt passed around the patient. Absence of adequate application of the belt could result in loss of contact and an inability to maintain continuous measurements.

Although Smyth claimed that his external method was an accurate reflection of intrauterine pressure, subsequent comparisons of records using his method and direct recordings of intrauterine pressure showed similarity in 70–100% of cases (Wood *et al.*, 1965).

For the above reasons, external methods of monitoring uterine activity have not continued to be used for scientific evaluation but have proved to be useful tools when used as an adjunct to continuous fetal heart monitoring (Steer, 1977).

The Measurement of Intrauterine Pressure

Interest in the measurement of intrauterine pressure began as early as 1872 (Miller, 1981), but the development of modern intrauterine measurement techniques began in the late 1940s and early 1950s (Alvarez and Caldeyro-Barcia, 1950; Caldeyro-Barcia and Alvarez, 1952).

In the earlier paper Alvarez and Caldeyro-Barcia introduced a method of measurement of intrauterine pressure by means of a catheter introduced into the uterine cavity. Recording of amniotic fluid pressure was achieved by connecting the catheter tubing to a water or mercury manometer, depending on whether the measurements were being taken during pregnancy or labour. The manometer was connected to an ink recording system. These workers noted that the intensity of uterine contractions during the first and second stages of labour varied between 25 and 70 cm of water. The average value of the 'tonus' (defined as a 'more or less straight and horizontal line between two contractions') varied between 8 and 17 cm of water and the frequency of contractions was between 2 and 6 contractions per 10 min.

In another publication in 1952 the same authors described further characteristics of uterine contractility, using a modification of their earlier technique. The *intensity* of each contraction was measured by the increase it causes in intrauterine pressure (over tonus pressure). In normal labours the average intensity of each contraction ranged between 30 and 50 mmHg, in some cases reaching up to 60 mmHg. The *value* of the uterine contractility in a given period of time was roughly proportional to the product of the intensity and the frequency of the contractions. In the tracing of the amniotic (intrauterine) pressure this value was accurately measured by the area included within the elevations caused by the contractions. The authors commented that the higher the value of this area the more rapidly labour progresses, provided that no other factors such as incoordination of the contractions intervene. This value of intensity × frequency was further defined by Caldeyro-Barcia and other colleagues in a paper in 1957. They again stated that (a) the intensity of each contraction is measured by the *rise* in pressure it produces in the amniotic fluid; (b) the frequency of the contractions is expressed by the number of contractions per 10 min; (c) the product (intensity × frequency) of the contractions was called 'uterine activity' and was expressed in Montevideo Units (MU). Thus, MUs can be derived by summing all the individual active pressures in a given 10 min period or by multiplying mean active pressure by the mean frequency per 10 min over the same period. Since its introduction the MU has attained greater world-wide acceptance than any other method of quantifying uterine activity. The normal range of MUs during labour was 150–250. The MU measurement had two deficiencies: it did not measure the duration of contractions and it was difficult to quantify electronically. In 1967, in an attempt to take the parameter of duration of uterine contractions into account, Samir *et al.* in Egypt introduced The Alexandria Unit—average amplitude (intrauterine pressure, mmHg × average duration (min) × average frequency per 10 min).

Developments in microelectronics in the 1970s allowed rapid online quantification of uterine activity to become possible. A number of methods have been described utilising computers.

In 1971 Braaksma and colleagues compared values obtained from quantification of uterine activity by manual and computer (digital) methods in non-pregnant women, and found most parameters to be comparable. In 1972 Jilek and his colleagues described an instrument which used a voltage-controlled oscillator to convert pressure (expressed as a voltage) into a train of pulses that could be accumulated into a counter. The counter was set with a time base of 2, 5 or 10 min, as required. The number of pulses accumulated in an interval of time was then representative of the area under the contraction curve. This technique measured total contraction area. Making use of this method, Hon and Paul in the following year (1973) described the quantitation of uterine activity and defined a uterine activity unit (UAU) as a unit of evaluation. They proposed that 1 UAU be defined as 1 Torr-min, which in turn was equivalent to a rectangle 1 mmHg high which lasts for 1 min. The authors commented that, in their view, the total area under the intrauterine pressure curve seemed to be meaningful in clinical terms as measured by cervical dilatation and duration of labour. Their technique has been utilised in a number of studies reported since (Huey *et al.*, 1976; Miller *et al.*, 1976). A method of expressing UAU every 10 min by a bar graph printout on the uterine activity channel of the fetal monitoring trace has been made commercially available as part of a fetal monitoring system (Miller *et al.*, 1980).

In 1978 Steer *et al.*, in order to overcome the disadvantages met with fluid-filled polythene catheters which had been in use hitherto (Csapo, 1970; Chan *et al.*, 1973; Tutera and Newman, 1975), designed a catheter with a pressure transducer at the tip. The transducer was mounted on the end of a 900 mm catheter and was situated so that it measured lateral pressure and not impact or head-on pressure. The catheter and transducer were sealed with a silicone rubber sleeve, giving the catheter a diameter of 2.7 mm. The transducer was connected by a plug at the distal end of the catheter to a 2 m flexible extension cable which was in turn connected to the contraction socket of the fetal monitor.

The same group of workers went on to develop an infusion system which automatically adjusted oxytocin infusion to suit the individual requirement of the patient—termed a Closed Loop Oxytocin Infusion System (Carter and Steer, 1980). At the same time this group introduced a new parameter, the Uterine Activity Integral (UAI)—this unit measured the active contraction area above basal pressure over a period of 15 min and was defined as $UAI = P^{900}p\,dt$ kPa s. The upper limit of safe induced activity was determined to be 1500 kPa s/15 min, since, above this level, fetal hypoxia as shown by fetal heart rate changes became unacceptably common, occurring in greater than 50% of cases. Adequate progress in labour only occurred above 500 kPa s/15 min, and therefore the authors suggested this as the lower limit.

The techniques and units described above are useful in measuring the work required to dilate the cervix and can be used for monitoring both the induction and the augmentation of labour. While these units may provide a scientific means of evaluating the effect of oxytocic agents, in a clinical context cervical dilatation is the more relevant clinical measurement. However, a continuous record of uterine contraction is essential for better interpretation of fetal heart rate traces. Because of the possible (although uncommon) risks (Chan *et al.*, 1973; Fernandez-Rocha and Oullette, 1976; Amato, 1977) associated with intrauterine pressure transducers, external tocodynamometry is the preferred clinical method.

Duration of Labour

There is often difficulty in defining the exact onset of labour (Jeffcoate, 1961). The differentiation between painful contractions which lead to dilatation of the cervix and eventual delivery of the baby, and those which do not, is sometimes only possible in retrospect. O'Driscoll insisted that onset of labour can only be diagnosed if the cervix is fully effaced, but this has been questioned by other workers (Bidgood, 1988). In practice, various arbitrary limits have been set, with specific dilatation of the cervix being required before a diagnosis of labour and active-phase progress can be accepted. The artificial rupture of membranes may be taken as a commencement point in those labours which are induced. The end of labour is usually defined as the end of the second stage—i.e. delivery of the baby. The duration of labour is usually recorded in completed hours and fractions of an hour to the nearest 10 min.

Mode of Delivery

Five types of delivery can be categorised:

(i) Spontaneous vertex vaginal delivery without mechanical assistance.
(ii) Delivery assisted by the use of 'straight' (non-rotational) forceps such as Simpson's, Neville Barnes or Milne-Murray's.
(iii) Delivery assisted by 'rotational' forceps such as Kielland's or Moolgusker's.
(iv) Vacuum delivery (Ventouse).
(v) Caesarean section.

Fetal/Neonatal Condition

The fetal heart rate pattern is an important measure of fetal well-being and abnormalities in this pattern often reflect fetal hypoxia (Studd *et al.*, 1982). The condition of the newborn infant may be measured by means of Apgar Score as in Table 41.1, the range being 0–10.

Table 41.1

	Apgar score		
	0	*1*	*2*
Heart rate	absent	<100	>100
Respiratory effort	none	slow irregular	good
Muscle tone	limp	flexion	active
Reflex irritability	none	grimace	cough/sneeze
Colour	pale	blue	pink extremities

Other Obstetric Variables

Other important variables which may be taken into consideration are: age; height; gestation; parity; reason for induction; weight of the newborn; analgesia of the mother; and oxytocic dosage.

AUGMENTATION OF SPONTANEOUS LABOUR

Oxytocin is the oxytocic of choice for improving the efficiency of dysfunctional labour. It is also indicated when the membranes have spontaneously ruptured and have not been followed by onset of uterine contractions.

For practical purposes, the methods used to evaluate oxytocic therapy in the augmentation of spontaneous labour are similar to those described for the induction of labour.

THERAPEUTIC ABORTION

Prostaglandins administered by various routes, including intravenous and intravaginal, have been used successfully for the termination of first- and second-trimester pregnancies. In contrast, the early- and mid-pregnant uterus is relatively unresponsive to oxytocin, which makes this drug unsuitable as the sole agent for inducing abortion. However, oxytocin can be used to enhance the abortifacient effects of other oxytocic agents.

Menstrual Regulation

Primary prostaglandins have been used with some effect for menstrual regulation—i.e. within 6 weeks of the last menstrual period, when administered into the uterus or intravaginally (Csapo *et al.*, 1973; Karim, 1976; Takagi *et al.*, 1977). More recently, steroids with antiprogestogen activity have also been introduced as abortifacients in early pregnancy (Cameron and Baird, 1988; Iqbal, *et al.*, 1988; Swahn and Bygdeman, 1988).

The means of evaluation of efficacy in these studies were:

(1) Onset of uterine contractions, in minutes from administration of prostaglandin.
(2) Onset of uterine bleeding, in hours and minutes from time of administration of prostaglandin.
(3) Duration of uterine bleeding, in days.
(4) Quantity of uterine bleeding, in ml.
(5) Nature of expulsion of uterine contents:
   (a) complete evacuation was termed 'complete abortion';
   (b) incomplete evacuation was termed 'incomplete abortion';
   (c) non-expulsion of contents of uterus was termed a 'failed abortion'.
(6) Measurement of plasma progesterone, oestradiol and HCG levels.
(7) Dose of prostaglandin used.
(8) Measurement of pulse, BP and temperature.

In the study carried out by Swahn and Bygdeman (1988), the effect of the antiprogestogen on uterine contractility was also recorded. Intrauterine pressure recordings took place at 24 h, 36 h, 48 h and 72 h after administration of the antiprogestogen. These measurements were recorded with a Grass Polygraph connected to a pressure transducer, which was inserted extra-amniotically through the cervical canal into the upper part of the uterus with its tip 1–2 cm from the fundus. The degree of uterine contractility was quantified by planimetric measurement of the total pressure area per 10 min period and by calculating Montevideo Units (see page 537).

First-trimester Abortions

Although prostaglandins have been used for inducing abortion in first trimester, a major drawback associated with their use was the high prevalence of side-effects, the commonest being vomiting, diarrhoea, pyrexia, headaches and local phlebitis at the infusion site.

The parameters used to monitor prostaglandin activity in this indication were similar to those used for menstrual induction. The need or otherwise of surgical evacuation and analgesia type and quantity may also be documented.

Second-trimester Abortions

Prostaglandins E_2 and F_2 have been in use for the induction of second-trimester abortions for several years (Beazley and Gillespie, 1971; Wiqvist *et al.*, 1971; Cameron and Baird, 1984).

The sensitivity of the uterus to oxytocic drugs increases with increasing gestation, and in this respect the prostaglandins have been found to be clinically effective and, in most cases, to have an acceptable incidence of side-effects. The routes of administration have been intravenous, intra-amniotic and vaginal. Similar to the indication of termination of early first-trimester pregnancies, the important parameters to evaluate in second trimester included:

(1) The time of onset and severity of lower abdominal pain.

(2) The time of onset of vaginal bleeding.

(3) The time of expulsion of the products of conception.

(4) The nature of expulsion of uterine contents, complete or incomplete.

(5) The time of commencement of oxytocic administration, and the time of abortion. These values can be used to calculate the induction–abortion interval, expressed in hours and minutes. The total dose required to effect abortion can also be measured.

(6) In the case where extra-amniotic catheters were used, the time of their expulsion was recorded.

(7) A record of the need or otherwise of surgical evacuation of the uterus and the time this took place.

(8) Pulse, blood pressure and temperature were measured for a period before, throughout and for several hours after the treatment procedure.

(9) Details of any operative and additional medical treatment were recorded.

(10) Following discharge from hospital, follow-up took place where a record could be made of any further vaginal bleeding, abdominal pain or vaginal discharge. A vaginal examination was conducted at this visit.

In an attempt to reduce the induction–abortion interval as well as the dose of prostaglandin used, the concurrent use of intravenous oxytocin has been tried (Coltart and Coe, 1975). In these situations the timing of administration of oxytocin and the dose used would require to be documented.

Prostaglandins are usually contraindicated in patients with severe cardiovascular disease and hypertension and those with asthma. Hypersensitivity to prostaglandins is another contraindication. For those patients who have undergone previous extensive abdominal surgery, and/or who may have uterine abnormalities such as fibroids, intra-amniotic injections are also contraindicated.

TREATMENT OF POSTPARTUM HAEMORRHAGE

The oxytocic effect of ergometrine is used in the management of the third stage of labour—i.e. from the time of delivery of the baby to the expulsion of the placenta. Ergometrine is used to enhance contraction of the uterus and placental separation and to prevent atonic postpartum haemorrhage. It is also extremely useful in cases of established obstetric haemorrhage. Oxytocin may also be used on its own in the management of the third stage of labour.

Prostaglandins have been advocated by some workers as useful in the treatment of postpartum haemorrhage (Tagaki *et al.*, 1976; Hayashi *et al.*, 1981; Thiery, 1986), but this type of management has not been widely adopted.

The first to investigate systemically the value of prostaglandin administration for primary postpartum uterine hypotony was a Japanese research group in Tokyo (Tagaki *et al.*, 1976). These workers defined postpartum haemorrhage as haemorrhage exceeding 400 ml in primiparas and 300 ml in multiparas, and set these parameters for treatment with prostaglandin by various routes. Further, to assess the effectiveness of their various methods, they measured (a) the total blood loss during the 2 h period following intramuscular or intramyometrial injection, or after the start of an intravenous infusion, and (b) the interval between treatment of and the onset of uterine contraction.

In 1981 Hayashi and co-workers reported preliminary results of a multicentre trial which were later updated. As did the previously quoted Japanese workers, this group examined the usefulness of prostaglandin F_2 in severe postpartum haemorrhage. However, their treatment criteria included the following: (1) an episode of hypotension (a systolic or diastolic pressure drop of 30 mmHg or more); (2) a decrease in haemoglobin concentration of 3 g or more without transfusion; (3) a decrease in haemoglobin concentration of 2 g with 500 ml blood transfusion; or (4) estimated blood loss of 1000 ml or more. Patients were entered into the study if they were haemorrhaging secondary to uterine atony and did not respond to conventional treatment with oxytocin, methylergonovine and uterine massage. The possibility of genital tract lacerations and retained placental fragments was ruled out before the patient was entered into the study. Success was defined as 'satisfactory management of the bleeding without surgical intervention'. Vital signs were recorded at 15 min intervals and side-effects were noted. Estimated blood loss was noted before and after prostaglandin administration. Haematocrit and haemoglobin concentrations were noted at 24 h and 48 h after therapy began, and the effect on uterine muscular tone was noted periodically. Other investigators have used similar treatment entry and efficacy criteria (Henson *et al.*, 1983; Thiery, 1986).

PREINDUCTION CERVICAL RIPENING AND PREOPERATIVE CERVICAL SOFTENING

The prostaglandins have been found to be of great benefit in softening and dilating the cervix before interruption of pregnancy, whether at term, in the second trimester or before suction curettage during early pregnancy. They have been most widely applied at term to ripen the cervix in the course of inducing labour. This topic has been addressed above (pages 533–534).

Cervical incompetence and subsequent spontaneous abortions can occur following vacuum aspiration for termination of first-trimester pregnancy (Wright *et al.*, 1972). Preoperative softening may reduce this risk. The prostaglandins have been shown to lower the resistance of the cervix to mechanical dilatation (Dingfelder *et al.*, 1975) and to allow cervical dilatation to occur prior to vacuum aspiration (Prasad *et al.*, 1978; Welch and Elder, 1982).

In 1974 Hulka and co-workers reported the development of an instrument which enabled the measurement and recording of the force exerted on the internal os during dilatation. The instrument consisted of a series of dilators designed to be fitted to a force transducer in a dilator 'handle', a strip-chart system to record the force exerted on one channel and a recording of total force exerted over time on a second channel. In addition, there was a digital readout to indicate the cumulative force exerted over time, or total force–time integral (TFTI). The transducer chosen was a linear variable differential transformer (LVDT), which translated the displacement of an iron slug into a proportional output voltage. To make the output voltage read force rather than displacement, the LVDT was arranged in a handle with a spring load at one end and a mechanical coupling and latching mechanism at the other end, which was open to accept the specially shaped ends of the dilators. The force of dilatation was transmitted mechanically to the spring load, displacing the iron slug from its zero-force position in the magnetic coupling circuit of the LVDT. The slug displacement was directly proportional to the force exerted, thus yielding a voltage which was an exact linear function of the axial force exerted. The voltage output was amplified, scaled and displaced on one channel of a strip-chart recorder. As each separate dilator was inserted, a display of the force–time integral was recorded. A continuous summation of the individual force–time integrals was provided by a numerical integration which yielded a number displayed as the cumulative force–time integral (cumulative FTI). These investigators demonstrated that Hegar dilators required more force than Pratt dilators, that the cervix was most resistant at 9 mm diameter and that less force was required with more advanced weeks of gestation. The instrument described above was successfully utilised in a cervical dilatation study conducted by Dingfelder and co-workers in California (1975).

The development of another instrument was reported in 1981 in Glasgow (Fisher *et al.*, 1981). This instrument consisted of a cylindrical stainless steel casing which contained a linear displacement transducer, a compression spring and a stainless steel piston. The transducer sensor was attached to the inner end of the piston and the dilators were, in turn, screwed into the outer end. An axial force on the dilator displaced the piston against the spring and the displacement was monitored by the transducer. The spring gave a displacement of 1 mm for a 5 kg force. The output signal was processed by an electronic converter giving an output of 0.1 V DC for a 0.45 kg force. For each patient the peak force applied to each dilator for sizes 3–8 mm inclusive was noted and summed to give an expression of total force. This value was then taken to represent the cervical resistance for each patient: as an example, in a group of 22 nulliparous pregnant women the mean + standard error of the mean total resistance was 4.5 + 0.5 kg. One year later these workers examined cervical resistance in a group of pregnant and non-pregnant women and found that the highest recordings were in postmenopausal women (Anthony *et al.*, 1982).

Similarly, Welch and Elder (1982) described a cervical resistance evaluating system in pregnant patients who were administered prostaglandin prior to termination of their pregnancy. The force (in kilograms) needed to fully insert individual Hegar dilators was measured by means of a spring gauge attached to its handle. Pressure between the operator's hand, principally the thenar eminence, and the butt of the spring gauge caused compression of the spring, the force being registered directly on a scale (0.3–1.5 kg) by a pointer which did not return when the force ceased to be applied. The reduction in the cervical resistance to the passage of a dilator was assessed by determining the maximum diameter of Hegar dilator that could be passed with a force of less than 0.3 kg.

Aside from cervical resistance, another measurable component of cervical softening is the cervical canal diameter (in millimetres). This can be measured after the treatment period as the largest dilator which can be inserted without force. In addition, the need or otherwise of further dilatation can be recorded (Prasad *et al.*, 1978). If further dilatation is necessary, the ease of further dilatation can be recorded by means of a four-point scale (none, easy, moderate, difficult).

SIDE-EFFECTS OF OXYTOCIC DRUGS

As part of the evaluation of oxytocic drugs, documentation of the nature and extent of side-effects is necessary. Below are listed side-effects which have been described for the oxytocic agents in clinical practice.

Oxytocin

Oxytocin has antidiuretic properties and in high doses may lead to fluid retention and, at worst, water intoxication (Liggins, 1962). Thus, caution should be exercised in cases of cardiac disease and pre-eclampsia. Some workers have suggested an association between oxytocin and neonatal jaundice (Ghosh and Hudson, 1972; Calder *et al.*, 1974). Buchan (1979) has reported decreased erythocyte deformability and increased haemolysis in umbilical cord blood following oxytocin infusion. Rupture of the uterus may occur in rare circumstances (Daw, 1972).

Prostaglandins

Because of their pharmacological properties, prostaglandins may cause gastrointestinal stimulation (nausea, vomiting and diarrhoea), a rise in temperature and a rise in blood pressure, and may induce bronchospasm. Thus, they should be avoided in patients with cardiovascular disease and those with asthma.

Ergometrine

Ergometrine rarely causes side-effects, apart from occasional vomiting. Peripheral vascular spasm may occur after overdosage, and a transient rise in blood pressure may be observed.

Antiprogestogens

Apart from their antiprogestational activity, antiprogestogens have antiglucocorticoid effects through their high binding affinity for the glucocorticoid receptors. As a result, plasma levels of cortisol rise during antiprotestogen treatment of pregnant women (Kovacs *et al.*, 1984). One group of workers has reported a subjective increase in bleeding associated with a fall in haemoglobin concentration (Couzinet *et al.*, 1986), and acute haemorrhage necessitating emergency curettage has also been reported (Kovacs *et al.*, 1984; Cameron and Baird, 1988).

SUMMARY

The development of sophisticated technology, along with better understanding of physiological processes have enabled recently introduced oxytocic agents to be more scientifically and accurately evaluated. This allows for more effective and safe use of these agents in patients.

ACKNOWLEDGEMENTS

I should like to thank Dr P. J. Steer for allowing me to read and consult his MD thesis, 1986, and Mrs Hazel Gunn for her excellent secretarial help.

REFERENCES

Alvarez, H. and Caldeyro-Barcia, R. (1950). Contractility of human uterus recorded by new methods. *Surg. Gynaecol. Obstet.*, **91**, 1–13

Amato, J. C. (1977). Fetal monitoring in a community hospital. A statistical analysis. *Obstet. Gynecol.*, **50**, 269–74

Anthony, G. S., Fisher, J., Coutts, J. R. T. and Calder, A. A. (1982). Forces required for surgical dilatation of the pregnant and non-pregnant human cervix. *Br. J. Obstet. Gynaecol.*, **89**, 913–16

Beazley, J. M. and Gillespie, A. (1971). Double-blind trial of prostaglandin E₂ and oxytocin in induction of labour. *Lancet*, **1**, 152–5

Bell, G. H. (1952). Abnormal uterine action in labour. *J. Obst. Gynaecol. Br. Emp.*, **59**, 617–23

Bidgood, K. A. (1988). Oxytocin augmentation of labour. In Chamberlain, G. (Ed.), *Contemporary Obstetrics and Gynaecology*. Butterworths, London, pp. 225–42

Bishop, E. H. (1964). Pelvic scoring for elective induction. *Obstet. Gynecol.*, **24**, 266–8

Braaksma, J. T., Veth, A. F. L., Janssens, J., Stolte, L. A. M., Eskers, T. K. A. B., Hein, P. R. and Van Der Weide, H. (1971). A comparison of digital and non-digital analysis of contraction records obtained from the non-pregnant uterus *in vivo. Am. J. Obstet. Gynecol.*, **110**, 1075–82

Buchan, P. C. (1979). Pathogenesis of neonatal hyperbilirubinaemia after induction of labour with oxytocin. *Br. Med. J.*, **ii**, 1255–7

Calder, A. A. (1979). In Kierse, M. J. N. C., Anderson, A. B. M. and Bennebroek Gravenhoist, J. (Eds.), *Human Parturition*. University Press, Leiden, pp. 201–17

Calder, A. A., Moar, V. A., Ounsted, M. K. and Turnbull, A. C. (1974). Increased bilirubin levels in neonates after induction of labour by intravenous prostaglandin E₂ or oxytocin. *Lancet*, **ii**, 1339–42

Caldeyro-Barcia, R. and Alvarez, H. (1952). Abnormal uterine action in labour. *J. Obstet. Gynaecol. Br. Commonw.*, **59**, 646–54

Cameron, I. T. and Baird, D. T. (1984). The use of 16, 16-dimethyl *trans* delta 2 prostaglandin E1 methyl ester (gemeprost) vaginal pessaries for the termination of pregnancy in the early second trimester. A comparison with extra-amniotic prostaglandin E₂. *Br. J. Obstet. Gynaecol.*, **91**, 1136–40

Cameron, I. T. and Baird, D. T. (1988). Early pregnancy termination: a comparison between vacuum aspiration and medical abortion using prostaglandin (16, 16 dimethyl-*trans*-D₂-PGE, methyl ester) or the antiprogestogen RU 486. *Br. J. Obstet. Gynaecol.*, **95**, 271–6

Carter, M. C. and Steer, P. J. (1980). A closed-loop oxytocin infusion system: preliminary results of clinical trials. In Rolfe, P. (Ed.), *Fetal and Neonatal Physiological Measurements*. Pitman Press, Bath, pp. 165–76

Chan, W. H., Paul, R. H. and Toews, J. (1973). Intrapartum fetal monitoring— maternal and fetal morbidity and perinatal mortality. *Obstet. Gynecol.*, **41**, 7–13

Coltart, T. M. and Coe, M. J. (1975). Intravenous prostaglandins and oxytocin for mid-trimester abortion. *Lancet*, **1**, 174–5

Couzinet, B., Lestrat, N., Ulmann, A., Baulieu, E. E. and Schaison, G. (1986). Termination of early pregnancy by progesterone antagonist RU 486 (Mifepristone). *New Engl. J. Med.*, **315**, 1565–70

Csapo, A. I. (1970). The diagnostic significance of intrauterine pressure—I. *Obstet. Gynaecol. Surv.*, **25**, 403–35

Csapo, A. I., Mocsary, P. and Nagy, T. (1973). The efficacy and acceptability of the 'prostaglandin impact' in inducing complete abortion during the second week after the missed menstrual period. *Prostaglandins*, **3**, 125–39

Daw, E. (1973). Oxytocin-induced rupture of the primigravid uterus. *J. Obstet. Gynaecol. Br. Commonw.*, **80**, 374–5

Dingfelder, J. R., Brenner, W. E. and Hendricks, C. H. (1975). Reduced cervical resistance by prostaglandin suppositories prior to dilatation for induced abortion. *Am. J. Obstet. Gynecol.*, **122**, 25–30

Fernandez-Rocha, L. and Oulette, R. (1976). Fetal bleeding; an unusual complication of fetal monitoring. *Am. J. Obstet. Gynecol.*, **125**, 1153–4

Fisher, J., Anthony, G. S., McManus, T. J., Coults, J. R. T. and Calder, A. A. (1981). Use of a force measuring instrument during cervical dilatation. *J. Med. Eng. Tech.*, **5**, 194–5

Friedman, E. A., Niswander, K. R., Bayonet-Rivera, N. P. and Sachtleben, M. R. (1966). Relation of prelabour evaluation in inducibility and the course of labour. *Obstet. Gynecol.*, **28**, 495–501

Ghosh, A. and Hudson, F. P. (1972). Oxytocic agents and neonatal hyperbilirubinaemia. *Lancet*, **ii**, 823–5

Hayashi, R. H., Castillo, M. S. and Noah, M. L. (1981). Management of severe postpartum haemorrhage due to uterine atony using an analogue of Prostaglandin F_2. *Obstet. Gynecol.*, **58**, 426–9

Hellman, L. M., Harris, J. and Reynolds, S. R. M. (1950). Characteristics of the gradients of uterine contractility during the first stage of true labour. *Bull. Johns Hopkins Hosp.*, **86**, 234–48

Hendricks, C. H. (1983). Second thoughts on induction of labour. In Studd, J. (Ed.), *Progress in Obstetrics and Gynaecology*, Vol. 3. Churchill Livingstone, London, pp. 101–12

Hendricks, C. H., Brenner, W. E. and Kraus, G. (1970). Normal cervical dilatation pattern in late pregnancy and labour. *Am. J. Obstet. Gynecol.*, **106**, 1065–82

Henson, G., Gough, J. D. and Gillmer, M. D. G. (1983). Control of persistent primary postpartum haemorrhage due to uterine atony with intravenous prostaglandin E_2. *Br. J. Obstet. Gynaecol.*, **90**, 280–2

Hicks, J. B. (1871). On the contractions of the uterus throughout pregnancy: their physiological effects and their value in the diagnosis of pregnancy. *Trans. Obstet. Soc., London*, 216

Hon, E. H. and Paul, R. H. (1973). Quantitation of uterine activity. *Obstet. Gynecol.*, **42**, 368–70

Huey, J. R., Al-Hadjer, A. and Paul, R. W. (1976). Uterine activity in the multiparous patient. *Am. J. Obstet. Gynecol.*, **126**, 682–6

Hulka, J. F., Lefler, H. T., Anglone, A. and Lachenbruch, P. A. (1974). A new electronic force monitor to measure factors influencing cervical dilatation for vacuum curettage. *Am. J. Obstet. Gynecol.*, **120** (2), 166

Iqbal, P. K., Hopkins, R. E., Stevenson, T. C., Mayers, F. N. and Gartside, M. W. (1988). *Br. J. Obstet. Gynaecol.*, **95**, 827–8

Jeffcoate, T. N. A. (1961). Prolonged labour. *Lancet*, **ii**, 61–7

Jilek, J., Hon, E. H. and Yeh, S. Y. (1972). A technique for the measurement of uterine activity. *Med. Res. Eng.*, **11**, 4–5

Karim, S. M. M. and Ratnam, S. S. (1976). Termination of pregnancy with prostaglandin analogues. In Sammulsson, B. and Paoletti, R. (Eds.), *Advances in Prostaglandin and Thromboxane Research*. Raven Press, New York, p. 727

Kovacs, L., Sas, M., Resch, B. A., Ugoscai, G., Swahn, M. L., Bygdeman, M. and Rowe, P. J. (1984). Termination of very early pregnancy by RU 486—an antiprogestational compound. *Contraception*, **29**, 399–410

Liggins, G. C. (1962). The treatment of missed abortion by high dosage syntocinon intravenous infusion. *J. Obstet. Gynaecol. Br. Commonw.*, **69**, 277–81

Mackenzie, I. L. and Embrey, M. P. (1977). Cervical ripening with intravaginal prostaglandin E₂ gel. *Br. Mr. J.*, **2**, 1381–4

Miller, F. C. (1981). Quantitation of uterine activity. *Clin. Perinatol.*, **8**, 27–34

Miller, F. C., Mueller, E. and Vellick, K. (1976). Quantitation of uterine activity in 100 primiparous patients. *Am. J. Obstet. Gynecol.*, **124**, 398–405

O'Driscoll, K. and Meagher, D. (1986). In O'Driscoll, K. and Meagher, D. (Eds.), *Active Management of Labour*. Baillière Tindall, London, pp. 24–31

Philpott, R. H. and Castle, W. M. (1972). Cervicographs in the management of labour in primigravidae. The alert line for detecting abnormal labour. *J. Obstet. Gynaecol. Brit. Commonw.*, **79**, 592–8

Pontonnier, G., Puech, F., Granjean, H. and Holland, M. (1975). Some physical and biochemical parameters during normal labour. *Biol. Neonate*, **26**, 159

Prasad, R. N. V., Lim, C. and Wong, Y. C. (1978). Vaginal administration of 16, 16-dimethyl-*trans*-D²-PGE, methyl ester (ONO 802) for pre-operative cervical dilatation in first trimester nulliparous pregnancy. *Singapore J. Obstet. Gynaecol.*, **9**, 69–71

Reynolds, J. R. M., Heard, O. O., Bruns, P. and Hellman, L. M. (1948). A multichannel straingage tokodynamometer—an instrument for studying patterns of uterine contractions in pregnant women. *Bull. Johns Hopkins Hosp.*, **82**, 449–69

Samir, E. S., Gaafar, A. A. and Toppozada, H. K. (1967). A new unit for evaluation of uterine activity. *Am. J. Obstet. Gynecol.*, **98**, 900–3

Seitchik, J. and Chatkoff, M. L. (1975). Intrauterine pressure waveform characteristics in hypocontractile labor before and after oxytocin administration. *Am. J. Obstet. Gynecol.*, **123**, 426–34

Smyth, C. N. (1957). The guardring tocodynamometer—an absolute measurement of intra-amniotic pressure by a new instrument. *J. Obstet. Gynaecol. Br. Commonw.*, **64**, 59–66

Steer, P. J. (1977). Monitoring of labour. *Br. J. Hosp. Med.*, **17**, 219–25

Studd, J. W. W., Cardozo, L. D. and Gibb. D. M. F. (1982). The management of spontaneous labour. In Studd, J. (Ed.), *Progress in Obstetrics and Gynaecology*, Vol. 2. Churchill Livingstone, London, pp. 60–72

Swahn, M. L.and Bygdeman, M. (1988). The effect of the antiprogestin RU 486 on uterine contractility and sensitivity to prostaglandin oxytocin. *Br. J. Obstet. Gynaecol.*, **95**, 126–34

Takagi, S., Sakata, H., Yoshida, T., Nakazawa, S., Fujii, K. T., Tominaga, Y., Iwasa, Y., Ninagawa, T., Hiroshima, T., Tomida, Y., Itoh, K. and Matsukawa, R. (1977). Termination of early pregnancy by ONO-802 (16, 16-Dimethyl-*trans*-D²-PGE, methyl ester). *Prostaglandins*, **14**, 791–8

Thiery, M. (1986). Prostaglandins for the treatment of hypotonic postpartum haemorrhage. *Prostaglandins Perspectives*, **2** (3), 11–12

Tutera, G. and Newman, R. L. (1975). Fetal monitoring; its effect on the perinatal mortality and caesarean section rates and its complications. *Am. J. Obstet. Gynecol.*, **122**, 750–4

Ulmsden, U., Wingerup, L., Belfrage, P., Ekman, G. and Wiqvist, N. (1982). Intracervical application of prostaglandin gel for induction of term labour. *Obstet. Gynecol.*, **56**, 336–9

Welch, C. and Elder, M. G. (1982). Cervical dilatation with 16,16-dimethyl-*trans*-D²-PGE, methyl ester vaginal pessaries before surgical termination of first trimester pregnancies. *Br. J. Obstet. Gynaecol.*, **89**, 849–52

Wiqvist, N., Bygdeman, M. and Toppozada, M. (1971). Induction of abortion by the intravenous administration of prostaglandin F_2. A critical evaluation. *Acta Obstet. Gynecol. Scand.*, **50**, 381–9

Wood, C., Bannerman, R. H. O., Booth, R. T. and Ankerton, J. H. M. (1965). The prediction of premature labour by observation of the cervix and external tocography. *Am. J. Obstet. Gynecol.*, **91**, 396–402

Wright, C., Campbell, S. and Beazley, J. (1972). Second trimester abortion after vaginal termination of pregnancy. *Lancet*, **1**, 1278–9

XI
Assessment of Drug Activity in the Skin

42
Measurement of Skin Response to Drugs

Sam Shuster, P. M. Farr and C. M. Lawrence

University Dept of Dermatology, Royal Victoria Infirmary,
Newcastle upon Tyne NE1 4LP, UK

INTRODUCTION

The increasing use of drugs for the treatment of skin disease has exposed the poverty of traditional methods for assessing therapeutic response. The wider employment of good clinical trial practice has, of course helped, but however good the design, the limits of detection are dictated by sensitivity of the measures of response. There are a number of objective methods available which could be more generally used, as well as several which would be better avoided. In this chapter we give a brief account of some of the more important methods and their uses and limitations. Our problem in presenting this briefly is the very nature of skin as an organ, the bland appearance of which conceals a riot of different tissues and functions. Thus, our account will mostly be a series of discrete structural and functional attributes which are affected by drugs, with a few examples of the response of specific reactions which can to some extent be used as models of disease. For a fuller account, see Greaves and Shuster (1989a,b).

SKIN STRUCTURES, FUNCTIONS AND CONSTITUENTS

Epidermal Cell Replication

Some indication of epidermal cell replication can be obtained by the time to disappearance of dye applied to the stratum corneum (Baker and Blair, 1968; Roberts and Marks, 1980), but the method has never been properly validated and there are problems of avidity, penetration and loss. Great differences are seen likewise with the various methods for measuring cell cycle events, and the mitotic index is too variable for reliability (Dover and Wright, 1989). The stathmokinetic method measures the birth rate of cells by counting mitoses in sequential biopsies at timed intervals after the local injection of vinblastine to ensure mitotic arrest (Duffill *et al.*, 1976, 1977); it is very time-consuming but it is doubtful that the other less rigorous procedures are worth doing.

Stratum Corneum

Structural

The number and size of scales can be measured, and their ease of removal gives a measure of adhesion (Nicholls and Marks, 1977; Roberts and Marks, 1980). The surface pattern of scale can be studied by a skin-surface recording device or photography, but numerical analysis is complex. These methods are now well established but are little used in the study of drug action.

Functional

The simplest way to study the stratum corneum barrier function is by measuring evaporative loss of water. With such methods the magnitude of water loss is dependent on rate of flow of the collecting gas (Johnson and Shuster, 1969a), and a simpler if less informative method uses an electrical sensing device (the Servomed Evaporimeter) to measure water vapour pressure differences, on and above the skin surface (Blickmann and Serup, 1987). Percutaneous absorption is studied *in vivo* by measurement of drug or metabolites in the blood, urine or faeces or a radiolabelled tracer, but analysis of concentration in successive Cellophane-tape-stripped layers of stratum corneum provides an interesting and simple way of predicting steady state absorption (Tojo and Lee, 1989).

Skin Constituents

Direct Analysis

Changes in a variety of skin constituents have been measured as an index of drug action and it has proved important (1) to dissociate epidermis from dermis because of their grossly different composition; (2) to use an appropriate unit of reference—in the epidermis this is usually DNA, and in the dermis the simplest unit is surface area, using a rotary punch biopsy (Shuster and Bottoms, 1963). The importance of the point of reference first became apparent when the effect of ageing and corticosteroids on skin collagen was studied (Shuster and Bottoms, 1963; Shuster *et al.*, 1967) and serious errors of interpretation were made until collagen content was related to skin surface area and not unit mass (see below, and Kohn and Schider, 1989). The former is an *absolute* quantity per unit of skin, the latter *relative* to the base unit chosen.

Tissue Fluids

Needle perfusion of the skin is neither pleasant nor satisfactory, and suction blisters are now used (Kistala, 1968) for analysis of tissue constituents and the kinetics of drugs in the skin.

Skin and Lesion Thickness

Measurement of skin and lesion thickness is a simple and important method of studying the cutaneous response to drugs. The normal epidermis contributes only about 5%, and variation in skin thickness with site, age and sex is due principally to differences in the dermal collagen layer (Shuster *et al.*, 1975).

The Harpenden Skinfold Caliper

The Harpenden Skinfold Caliper was designed to measure subcutaneous fat (Tanner and Whitehouse, 1955) but can be used to measure skin thickness at sites where the skin can be picked up separately from the underlying tissue. The caliper gives a resolution of 0.1 mm and measurements are reproducible with little observer bias (Cook and Shuster, 1980; Lawrence and Shuster, 1985a); it has been used to measure normal and atrophic skin (McConkey *et al.*, 1963), skin lesions and the response to inflammation and drugs (Moss *et al.*, 1981; Friedmann *et al.*, 1983; Marsden *et al.*, 1983; Lawrence and Shuster, 1985b, 1987). It is inexpensive, portable, easy to use and robust, but it can only be used where a fold of skin can be lifted separate from the underlying fat (Lawrence and Shuster, 1985a).

The Radiographic Method

In the radiographic method (Meema *et al.*, 1964) an X-ray beam is directed tangentially through skin flattened by a wooden block, using metal plates to facilitate focusing and alignment (Black, 1969). Skin thickness is measured from the radiographic image. The technique has been used in endocrine disease and to measure corticosteroid-induced dermal thinning (Black *et al.*, 1973; Tan *et al.*, 1981). Disadvantages are the use of ionising radiation, the equipment and the limitation to certain skin sites.

Ultrasound

In the ultrasound method (Alexander and Miller, 1979; Kirsch *et al.*, 1984) a transducer, offset from the skin by a water-bath, detects the pulse transit time, oscillograph peaks representing the water–skin, dermis–fat and fat–muscle interfaces. Skin thickness is calculated from the distance between the first and second peaks, using a constant for the speed of sound in skin (Tan *et al.*, 1981). Ultrasound is used to measure normal and atrophic skin thickness, and it tends to underestimate somewhat (Tan *et al.*, 1982; Lawrence and Shuster, 1985a). The equipment is portable and the method is quick, harmless and capable of being used at any skin site, but it gives poor results in inflamed skin (Lawrence and Shuster, 1985a) because it fails to detect the lower limit of the dermis and because inflammation may extend beyond that interface.

Histology

Histology has a limited use, because it is invasive and because of distortion by elastic recoil of the tissue after removal and subsequent shrinkage during fixation (Dykes and Marks, 1977; Tan *et al.*, 1982).

Physical Properties of Dermis

A variety of devices are now available to measure the extensile response to a linear, shear, rotational or suctional force, and can demonstrate the effects on connective tissue of drugs such as corticosteroids. It is surprising that these methods have not been used more often in the study of drug action (see Cook, 1989, for review).

Blood Vessels

Increased skin blood flow is a feature of inflammatory dermatoses, and the response to ultraviolet radiation and chemical irritants. Measurement of vascular changes in skin may, therefore, be used to monitor disease severity and response to treatment, and, as in the case of topical corticosteroid-induced vasoconstriction (Barry and Woodford, 1977), as a bioassay of potency.

Cutaneous blood flow can be measured by thermal (Forrest and Williams, 1989) or radioactive isotope clearance (Tsuchida, 1979). These techniques are time-consuming, and the data they produce may be difficult to interpret. Consequently, they have not found wide clinical application. Laser Doppler flowmetry has been used increasingly (Tur *et al.*, 1983; Farr and Diffey, 1986a). In this technique a low-intensity laser beam of red light is shone onto the skin surface and the Doppler frequency shift of the remitted light is used to calculate the blood flux, a value related to the product of the number of red blood cells in the field of view and their average velocity (Nilsson *et al.*, 1980): absolute flow cannot be calculated.

Increased cutaneous blood flow is usually accompanied by dilatation of superficial vessels and several methods are used to quantify this (see Forrest and Williams, 1989).

Visual Grading

Small differences in erythemal intensity can be detected but the eye is poor at estimating their magnitude.

Colour Comparison Charts and Optical Filters

The intensity of erythema can be graded, using known colour standards, and although it is subjective, the method has advantages over visual grading, because the eye performs well in the null system used in the matching of two colours. A series of filters with high transmittance for red light and decreasing transmittance for blue/green light has been used to quantify erythema by observing which of the filters just causes the erythema to disappear.

Reflectance Spectrophotometry

The methods are objective and quantitative. Haemoglobin in the vessels of the superficial dermis is the main cutaneous chromophore of green light. The consequent reduction in reflectance of green light re-emitted from inflamed skin has been used to quantify erythema (Farr and Diffey, 1985), and computer-controlled spectrophotometers allow reliable *in vivo* measurement of the spectral reflectance (Wan *et al.*, 1983).

Hair

The effect of drugs on hair is complex and the main features to be measured are: (1) density (number/cm^2), (2) diameter (microscopy), (3) growth rate, (4) cycle, (5) colour, (6) physical properties and (7) surface appearance.

Growth Rate

Growth rate is measured after marking the hair, light hair with black dye and dark hair with bleach, and remeasuring after a timed period, the rate being 0.3–0.4 mm/day.

Hair Cycle

Hair cycle duration can usually be inferred by rate of hair growth and mean hair length and is the main determinant of the regional differences in hair appearance. Further information is obtained by examining plucked follicles: normally 5–15% of the scalp hairs are in the resting phase (anagen) and cytostatic drugs produce atrophic follicles.

Nail

The rate of nail growth (about 0.1 mm/day) is easily measured and will, for example, demonstrate the effect of cytostatic drugs such as methotrexate (Dawber, 1970). The nail is marked with a file at the apex of the lunula, and the distance the scratch has travelled over a fixed period of time is measured from the proximal nail fold cuticle or the lunula; these two measurements should be the same. There is a small difference in rate of growth of different fingernails and sequential measurements should, therefore, be done on the same fingers.

The Sebaceous Gland

The effects of drugs such as 13-*cis*-retinoic acid and various hormones used for treatment of acne can be assayed by their effect on the sebaceous glands. The simplest method is to measure sebum output, most often on the forehead, over a timed period. The sebum is either collected onto absorbent paper and measured gravimetrically or else onto ground glass and measured by light transmission. Gland function can also be studied by measuring sebaceous lipogenesis, using [^{14}C]-glucose or acetate as substrate. This has been done in isolated glands but it is simpler to measure total dermal lipogenesis and express in relationship to surface area (see Thody and Shuster, 1989a,b for a review of methods and the effect of drugs).

Sweat Gland Function

The effect of drugs on sweat rate or sweat constituents is best measured using chemically induced sweating either by intradermal injection of a cholinergic drug or more often by iontophoresis of 0.1% pilocarpine with 4 mA for 5 min (see Johnson and Shuster, 1969b; Collins, 1989). Sweat is collected onto filter papers, in capsules stuck on to the skin or under plastics held in place with strapping, over a 15–20 min period and measured gravimetrically. Sweat, Na, K, Cl and urea are the most frequently assayed constituents.

Skin Sensation

Pain

Pain is an uncommon manifestation of skin disease and is discussed elsewhere (see Lynn, 1989).

Itch

Itch can be measured subjectively by simple grading or by marking on a 10 cm scale. The most reproducible and probably the best method is to use scratch as a measure of itch (Shuster, 1981). Scratch can be measured by needle electrodes, or by amplifying discharges along nerve fibres, but is most easily measured by limb movement meters or by monitoring bed movement at night (Felix and Shuster, 1975). Both arm and leg movement are measured because itch-provoked scratch is done mostly by the arms, arm movement mostly being due to scratch, whereas leg movement represents restlessness. Because of the variation from night to night, measurements are made over two consecutive nights.

Self-image

The depressing effect of skin disease on self-image has been assessed subjectively by psychological questionnaires and psychometrically, e.g. after topical treatment of acne (Shuster, 1981), but methodological and clinical details have not been published in full.

SPECIFIC DISEASES AND DRUGS

Psoriasis

Clinical Assessment

Erythema, scale, palpability and area of involvement are scored clinically. Area is seriously overestimated by most observers, e.g. using the rule of nines (Ramsay and Lawrence, 1989), and the addition of the component scores to make a single overall score (as in the now widely used PASI method; Friedrickson and Pettersson, 1978) is unacceptable, as it presumes a numerically equivalent relationship of those components to response.

Objective Measurements

Change in lesion thickness measured by calipers and transepidermal water loss correspond well to therapeutic response (Shuster *et al.*, 1980) and allow calculation of a $T_{\frac{1}{2}}$ for plaque regression (Farr *et al.*, 1987). There are no published studies of the use of X-ray and ultrasound techniques but our own (unpublished) evidence is that ultrasound gives variable and unsatisfactory recordings.

Adolescent Acne

Drugs act either by reducing the rate of sebum production or by antibiotic activity. Despite claims to the contrary, there is no evidence of a primary effect on duct keratinisation or that duct blockage plays any part in the disease (Shuster, 1989).

Clinical Response

Clinical response is usually estimated by a global clinical grading or by separate grades for the different components of the disease in specific areas (Burke and Cunliffe, 1984). Less often, individual lesions are counted but it is not clear whether this offers much advantage over clinical grading. Antibiotic effect is usually studied by the clinical response.

Measurement of Sebum Excretion Rate

See above. This is a simple assay of the effect of drugs which improve acne by a sebostatic effect.

Dermatitis and Eczema

Dermatitis and eczema constitute the largest group of diseases requiring study and one of the least susceptible to existing methods of measurement. The symptom of itch can be measured indirectly as scratch, but the extent and degree of dermatitis is still assessed by simple clinical grading, although lesion thickness, transepidermal water penetration and skin blood flow could be used.

Corticosteroids

Potency

The vasoconstrictor assay (Barry and Woodford, 1977) is still widely used to rank topical corticosteroids. This is surprising, as the inhibitory effect on induced inflammation (e.g. anthralin inflammation or contact sensitivity) should give greater sensitivity (Lawrence and Shuster, 1985b).

Atrophy

Since the study of Black *et al.* (1973) skin thickness measurements have been widely used to assess collagen loss after corticosteroids. However, there are serious reservations, because changes in skin thickness are only an indirect measure of dermal collagen content (Shuster *et al.*, 1975). More importantly, most studies of the atrophic potency of corticosteroids are concerned with the small changes which occur in the first weeks of treatment and there is no evidence that these changes are due to collagen loss. Thus, most of the published measurements of the atrophic potency of topical corticosteroids are of dubious relevance.

Other Drugs

Effects are usually assayed clinically on the disease process, occasionally on related models (e.g. histamine wealing and antihistamines; see below) or pharmacological properties (e.g. cytostatic drugs on nail growth).

THE RESPONSE OF INFLAMMATION TO THERAPY

There are few good models of skin disease, and of these the response to inflammatory agents and its modification by drugs is the most often used to study the effect of drugs. (For a review of the pharmacological agents associated with different types of inflammation, see Greaves and Lawlor, 1989).

Ultraviolet Erythema

Minimal Erythema Dose (MED)

Adjacent areas of skin are exposed to geometrically increasing doses of radiation and the lowest dose required to achieve erythema is noted, usually at 24 h. The difficulty in judging this threshold point is compounded by the varying definitions, which range from a faint erythema (Epstein, 1962) to a uniform redness with sharp borders (Willis and Kligman, 1970). More importantly, the minimal erythema dose is a single point at the foot of the dose–response curve and therefore cannot characterise the biological event.

Erythema Dose–Response Curves

For these reasons full erythema dose–response curves are better than the frequently used MED. Inhibition of the early erythemal response to UVB can be used to measure the effect of cyclo-oxygenase inhibition in skin (Farr and Diffey, 1986b).

Weal Reactions

Measurement of Weals

The response to spontaneous wealing and to vasoactive agents such as histamine and its antagonists can be measured as weal area, weal thickness and calculated volume (Cook and Shuster, 1980). Weal area is measured at the time of maximum definition by transferring the inked outline on Cellophane-tape-stripped stratum corneum and computing the area on a digitising pad (Humphreys and Shuster, 1987) or planimeter (Krause and Shuster, 1985b). Weal thickness is measured by calipers and dose–response curves can be used to study the effect of disease and drugs. Rate constants of weal formation and disappearance can also be used to analyse the effect of drugs and different wealing agents (Cook and Shuster, 1980; Humphreys *et al.*, 1987).

Dermographic Wealing

A spring-loaded stylus is used to produce shear distortion as the stylus is moved across the skin, and weal diameter is used to construct weal force–response curves using a series of different forces. Site and skin frictional resistance are important (Krause and Shuster, 1985). The response to H_1 receptor antagonists can be demonstrated by a shift in the force–response curve and in dermographic threshold (Krause and Shuster, 1984, 1985a).

Irritant Inflammation

The effect of drugs can be studied by their action on inflammation induced by various chemicals, e.g. detergents (Berardesea and Maibach, 1988), weak acids or anthralin. Although the response is measured as erythema, skin blood flow, oedema and transepidermal water loss, their mechanisms and response to drugs differ, and this can be used for therapeutic assay, e.g. the response to anthralin (Lawrence and Shuster, 1985b, 1987; Lawrence *et al.*, 1986).

Immune Reactions

The Immediate (Antigen–IgE) Response)

This response is usually measured by the weal and flare reaction to antigen introduced by pricking, but this is less satisfactory than intradermal injection, which allows construction of dose–response curves and measurement of weal kinetics (Humphreys *et al.*, 1987). This response has been used to study the effect of antihistamines, corticosteroids, cromoglycates, cyclo-oxygenase inhibitors, cyclosporin and other agents. The delayed response to antigens such as house-dust mite which occurs in patients with atopy remains semi-quantitative, and dose–response curves have not yet been established.

The Delayed (Lymphocyte-borne) Response

This response is measured by sensitisation, e.g. with dinitrochlorobenzene (DNCB) (Moss *et al.*, 1981). The capacity of a particular population to become sensitised is measured by using different sensitising doses and the degree of sensitisation is measured 3–4 weeks later by the magnitude of the 48 h response to increasing concentrations of DNCB, measured as thickness by calipers (area does not change linearly with response). Erythema blood flow and transepidermal water loss have been used less extensively. These measurements have been used to study the effects of drugs such as corticosteroids and cyclosporin.

REFERENCES

Alexander, H. and Miller, D. L. (1979). Determining skin thickness with pulsed ultrasound. *J. Invest. Derm.*, **72**, 17–19
Baker, H. and Blair, C. P. (1968). Cell replacement in the stratum corneum in old age. *Br. J. Derm.*, **80**, 367–72
Barry, B. W. and Woodford, R. (1977). Vasoconstructor activities and bioavailabilities of proprietary corticosteroids assessed using a non-occluded multiple dosage regimen. *Br. J. Derm.*, **97**, 555–60
Berardesea, A. and Maibach, H. I. (1988). Racial differences in sodium lauryl sulphate induced cutaneous irritation. *Contact Derm.*, **18**, 65–70
Black, M. M. (1969). A modified radiographic method of measuring skin thickness. *Br. J. Derm.*, **81**, 661–8
Black, M. M., Shuster, S. and Bottoms, E. (1973). Skin collagen and thickness in Cushing's syndrome. *Arch. Derm. Forsch.*, **246**, 365–8

Blickmann, C. W. and Serup, J. (1987). Reproducibility and variability of trans-epidermal water loss measurement. Studies on the Servo Med evaporimeter. *Acta Derm. Ven. (Stockholm)*, **678**, 206–10

Burke, B. M. and Cunliffe, W. J. (1984). The assessment of acne vulgaris—the Leeds technique. *Br. J. Derm.*, **111**, 83–92

Collins, K. J. (1989). Measurement of sweating and sweat-gland function. In Greaves, M. W. and Shuster, S. (Eds.), *Handbook of Experimental Pharmacology*, Vol. II. Springer Verlag, Heidelberg, pp. 19–22

Cook, T. H. (1989). Mechanical properties of human skin. In Balin, A. K. and Kligman, A. M. (Eds.), *Aging and the Skin*. Raven Press, New York, pp. 205–25

Cook, L. J. and Shuster, S. (1980). Histamine formation and absorption in man. *Br. J. Pharm.*, **69**, 579–86

Dawber, R. P. R. (1970). The effect of methotrexate, corticosteroids and azathioprine on fingernail growth in psoriasis. *Br. J. Derm.*, **83**, 680–3

Dover, E. and Wright, N. A. (1989). Methods for the study of proliferative rates in epidermis. In Greaves, M. W. and Shuster, S. (Eds.), *Handbook of Experimental Pharmacology*, Vol. II. Springer-Verlag, Heidelberg, pp. 3–11

Duffill, M., Appleton, D., Dyson, P., Shuster, S. and Wright, N. A. (1977). The measurement of cell cycle time in squamous epithelium using the metaphase arrest technique with vincristine. *Br. J. Derm.*, **96**, 493–502

Duffill, M., Wright, N. A. and Shuster, S. (1976). The cell proliferation kinetics of psoriasis examined by three *in vivo* techniques. *Br. J. Derm.*, **94**, 355–62

Dykes, R. J. and Marks, R. (1977). Measurement of skin thickness; a comparison of in vivo techniques and conventional histometric methods. *J. Invest. Derm.*, **69**, 275–8

Epstein, J. H. (1962). Polymorphous light eruptions. Wavelength dependency and energy studies. *Arch. Derm.*, **85**, 82–8

Farr, P. M. and Diffey, B. L. (1985). The erythemal response of human skin to ultraviolet radiation. *Br. J. Derm.*, **113**, 65–76

Farr, P. M. and Diffey, B. L. (1986a). The vascular response of human skin to ultraviolet radiation. *Photochem. Photobiol.*, **44**, 501–7

Farr, P. M. and Diffey, B. L. (1986b). A quantitative study of the effect of topical indomethacin on cutaneous erythema induced by UVB and UVC erythema. *Br. J. Derm.*, **115**, 453–90

Farr, P. M., Diffey, B. L. and Marks, J. M. (1987). Phototherapy and dithranol treatment of psoriasis: new lamps for old. *Br. Med. J.*, **294**, 205–7

Felix, R. H. and Shuster, S. (1975). A new method for the measurement of itch and the response to treatment. *Br. J. Derm.*, **93**, 303–12

Forrest, M. J. and Williams, T. J. (1989). Blood flow—including microcirculation. In Greaves, M. W. and Shuster, S. (Eds.), *Pharmacology of the Skin*, Vol. I. Springer-Verlag, Heidelberg, pp. 117–27

Friedmann, P. S., Moss, C., Shuster, S. and Simpson, J. M. (1983). Quantitative relationships between sensitising dose of DNCB and reactivity in normal subjects. *Clin. Exp. Immunol.*, **53**, 709–15

Friedrickson, T. and Pettersson, N. (1978). Severe psoriasis—oral therapy with a new retinoid. *Dermatologica*, **157**, 238–44

Greaves, M. W. and Lawlor, F. (1989). Specific acute inflammatory responses. In Greaves, M. W. and Shuster, S. (Eds.), *Handbook of Experimental Pharmacology*, Vol. I. Springer-Verlag, Heidelberg, pp. 479–90

Greaves, M. W. and Shuster, S. (1989a). *Handbook of Experimental Pharmacology*, Vol. I. Springer-Verlag, Heidelberg

Greaves, M. W. and Shuster, S. (1989b). *Handbook of Experimental Pharmacology*, Vol. II. Springer-Verlag, Heidelberg

Humphreys, F., Krause, L. B. and Shuster, S. (1987). The effects of astemizole and indomethacin on weal and flare reactions to histamine 48/80 and house dust mite antigen. *Br. J. Derm.*, **116**, 435

Humphreys, F. and Shuster, S. (1987). The effect of nedocromil on weal reactions in human skin. *Br. J. Clin. Pharm.*, **24**, 405–8

Johnson, C. and Shuster, S. (1969a). The measurement of transepidermal water loss. *Br. J. Derm.*, **81** (Suppl. 4), 40–5

Johnson, C. and Shuster, S. (1969b). Eccrine sweating in psoriasis. *Br. J. Derm.*, **81**, 119–24

Kirsch, J. M., Hanson, M. E. and Gibson, J. R. (1984). The determination of skin thickness using conventional diagnostic ultrasound equipment. *Clin. Exp. Derm.*, **9**, 280–5

Kistala, W. (1968). Suction blister device for separation of viable epidermis from dermis. *J. Invest. Derm.*, **50**, 128–37

Kohn, R. R. and Schnider, S. L. (1989). Collagen changes in aging skin. In Balin, A. K. and Kligman, A. M. (Eds.), *Aging and the Skin*. Raven Press, New York, pp. 131–2

Krause, L. B. and Shuster, S. (1984). The effect of terfenadine on dermographic wealing. *Br. J. Derm.*, **110**, 73–80

Krause, L. B. and Shuster, S. (1985a). A comparison of astemizole and chlorpheniramine in dermographic urticaria. *Br. J. Derm.*, **112**, 447–53

Krause, L. B. and Shuster, S. (1985b). Enhanced weal and flare response to histamine in chronic idiopathic urticaria. *Br. J. Clin. Pharm.*, **20**, 486–8

Lawrence, C. M., Howel, D. and Shuster, S. (1986). Site variations in anthralin inflammation of forearm skin. *Br. J. Derm.*, **114**, 609–13

Lawrence, C. M. and Shuster, S. (1985a). Comparison of ultrasound and caliper measurement of normal and inflamed skin thickness. *Br. J. Derm.*, **112**, 195–200

Lawrence, C. M. and Shuster, S. (1985b). Mechanism of anthralin inflammation: 1. Dissociation of response to clobetasol and indomethacin. *Br. J. Derm.*, **113**, 107–15

Lawrence, C. M. and Shuster, S. (1987). Effect of arachidonic acid on anthralin inflammation. *Br. J. Clin. Pharm.*, **24**, 125–31

Lynn, B. (1989). Structure, function and control: afferent nerve endings in the skin. In Greaves, M. W. and Shuster, S. (Eds.), *Handbook of Experimental Pharmacology*, Vol. I. Springer-Verlag, Heidelberg, pp. 117–24

McConkey, B., Fraser, G. M., Bligh, A. S. and Whiteley, H. (1963). Transparent skin and osteoporosis. *Lancet*, **i**, 693–5

Marsden, J. R., Coburn, P. R., Marks, J. M. and Shuster, S. (1983). Measurement of the response of psoriasis to short term application of anthralin. *Br. J. Derm.*, **109**, 209–18

Meema, H. E., Sheppard, R. H. and Rappoport, A. (1964). Roentgenographic visualisation and masurement of skin thickness and its diagnostic application in acromegaly. *Radiology*, **82**, 411

Moss, C., Friedman, P. S. and Shuster, S. (1981). Impaired contact hypersensitivity in untreated psoriasis and the effects of photochemotherapy and dithranol/UV-B. *Br. J. Derm.*, **105**, 503–8

Nicholls, S. and Marks, R. (1977). Novel techniques for the estimation of intracorneal adhesion *in vivo*. *Br. J. Derm.*, **96**, 595–602

Nilsson, G. E., Tenland, T. and Oberg, P. A. (1980). Evaluation of a laser Doppler flowmeter for measurement of tissue blood flow. *IEEE Trans. Biomed. Engng*, **BME-27**, 597–604

Ramsay, B. and Lawrence, C. M. (1989). Comparison of subjective and objective methods of assessment of psoriasis plaque area. *Br. J. Derm.*, **120**, 293

Roberts, D. and Marks, R. (1980). The determination of regional and age variations in the rate of desquamation: a comparison of four techniques. *J. Invest. Derm.*, **74**, 13–16

Shuster, S. (1981). Reason and the rash. *Proc. Roy. Inst. Gr. Brit.*, **53**, 136–63

Shuster, S. (1989). The blocked duct and the dying mythology of acne. *Proceedings of Conference on Acne, Cardiff, March 1988.* In Marks, R. and Plowig, G. (Eds.), *Acne and Related Disorders*, Ch. 16, pp. 81–6

Shuster, S., Black, M. M. and MacVitie, E. (1975). The influence of age and sex on skin thickness, skin collagen and density. *Br. J. Derm..*, **93**, 639–43

Shuster, S. and Bottoms, E. (1963). Senile degeneration of skin collagen. *Clin. Sci.*, **25**, 487–91

Shuster, S., Raffle, E. J. and Bottoms, E. (1967). Skin collagen in rheumatoid arthritis and the effects of corticosteroids. *Lancet*, **i**, 525–7

Shuster, S., Rawlins, M. D., Rogers, S., Chadirk, W., Marks, J. M. and Comaish, S. (1980). Objective comparison of the response of psoriasis to treatment with PUVA and dithranol. In Turner, P. (Ed.), *Proceedings of First World Conference on Clinical Pharmacology and Therapeutics.* Macmillan, London, pp. 421–3

Tan, C. Y., Marks, R. and Payne, P. (1981). Comparison of xeroradiographic and ultrasound detection of corticosteroid induced dermal thinning. *J. Invest. Derm.*, **76**, 657–67

Tan, C. Y., Statham, B., Marks, R. and Payne, P. A. (1982). Skin thickness measurement by pulsed ultrasound: its reproducibility, validation and variability. *Br. J. Derm.*, **106**, 657–67

Tanner, J. M. and Whitehouse, R. H. (1955). The Harpenden Skinfold Caliper. *Am. J. Phys. Anthrop.*, **13**, 743–6

Thody, A. J. and Shuster, S. (1989a). The sebaceous gland. *Phys. Rev.* (in press)

Thody, A. J. and Shuster, S. (1989b). The sebaceous glands. In Greaves, M. W. and Shuster, S. (Eds.), *Handbook of Experimental Pharmacology*, Vol. I. Springer-Verlag, Heidelberg, pp. 233–46

Tojo, K. and Lee, A. R. C. (1989). A method for predicting steady-state rate of skin penetration *in vivo. J. Invest. Derm.*, **92**, 105–8

Tsuchida, Y. (1979). Rate of skin blood flow in various regions of the body. *Plastic Reconstruct. Surg.*, **64**, 505–8

Tur, E. *et al.* (1983). Basal perfusion of the cutaneous microcirculation: measurement as a function of anatomic position. *J. Invest. Derm.*, **81**, 442–6

Wan, S., Parrish, J. A. and Jaenicke, K. F. (1983). Quantitative evaluation of ultraviolet induced erythema. *Photochem. Photobiol.*, **37**, 643–8

Willis, I. and Kligman, A. M. (1970). Aminobenzoic acid and its esters. *Arch. Derm.*, **102**, 405–17

43
Drugs for Eczema

John R. Gibson and Vasant K. Manna†*

*Dermatology Section, †Dept of Clinical Investigation, The Wellcome Research Laboratories, Langley Court, Beckenham, Kent BR3 3BS, UK

INTRODUCTION

The majority of drugs used in dermatology were not initially developed for the skin but are spin-offs from drug development in other fields, e.g. corticosteroids, antibiotics. At the time of writing, the concept of developing an agent specifically for the treatment of eczema is somewhat underworked. Thus, the approach that has been taken here is to present a brief overview of the issues which need to be considered rather than a finely detailed commentary on research methodologies. The latter would be premature in the case of drug development for eczema, in view of the poor definition of pathogenesis and the relatively unrefined status of most volunteer models that could be relevant to the drug development process. However, a range of measurement techniques that may be applicable to eczema research are mentioned and referenced below, and are described in detail in the chapter 'Measurement of Skin Responses to Drugs'. A selection of volunteer models is also briefly presented and commented upon. The major aim is to provide the reader with an overall plan for the drug development process in eczema and to stimulate him/her to further develop the range of available techniques and models in a critical and logical manner, thus helping to bring dermatopharmacology into line with the more advanced areas of drug research and development. It is hoped that, in the future, problem-orientated drug development for skin diseases will result in the production of a new generation of agents with optimised dermatological benefits.

Before considering the process of human drug evaluation in eczema, it is important to clarify a few basic issues such as the definition of the disease and the possible targets for therapeutic intervention. These points will be briefly dealt with in the first two sections of this chapter.

Although, in its stricter sense, dermatitis refers to any inflammation of the skin, it is commonly used interchangeably with eczema to denote a pruritic, papulovesicular or lichenified condition occurring as a result of the interaction of the skin with a variety of endogenous and/or exogenous factors (Burton *et al.*, 1986). For the purpose of this chapter these terms will be used synonymously. Eczema occurs in acute, subacute and chronic stages, each with a wide range of severity, with corresponding clinical and histological features. In addition, eczema embraces several distinct clinical subtypes

(Table 43.1), each being associated with various predisposing and triggering factors. While it is easy to identify certain of these (e.g. a genetic predisposition in atopic eczema, a specific allergen or irritant in contact dermatitis), in other cases such associations may be unclear and/or controversial. Broadly speaking, however, it is likely that in many situations a given genetic background predisposes to the blend of immunological, pharmacological and anatomical features needed to prime the subject to respond to triggering factors (internal and/or external) leading to a pathway of inflammatory events which initiate and interweave with a range of secondary reactions to create the spectrum of clinical features known as eczema.

Table 43.1   Examples of eczema sub-types

Atopic
Contact allergic
Contact irritant
Discoid/nummular
Infective
Pompholyx
Seborrhoeic
Venous stasis

TARGETING DRUGS IN ECZEMA

The currently available therapeutic armamentarium for eczema consists of:

(1) Emollient applications and soap substitutes.
(2) Topical, and occasionally systemic, corticosteroids.
(3) Topical and systemic antimicrobial agents, including antibiotics, antifungals and antivirals.
(4) Systemic antihistamines.
(5) Sedatives and tranquillisers.
(6) Orally administered essential fatty acids, e.g. gamma-linolenic acid.
(7) Orally administered immunosuppressants such as azathioprine and cyclosporin.
(8) Psoralens plus ultraviolet light (PUVA).

Possible targets for new agents in eczema are outlined in Figure 43.1. It is clear that this diagram represents an oversimplification of highly complex interrelated events in the pathogenesis of the disease. One relatively straightforward example of this is the role of *Staphylococcus aureus* in both exacerbating atopic eczema via a series of inflammatory events, possibly based on an immunological trigger (Dahl, 1983), and further complicating the process by causing frank superinfection of the diseased skin.

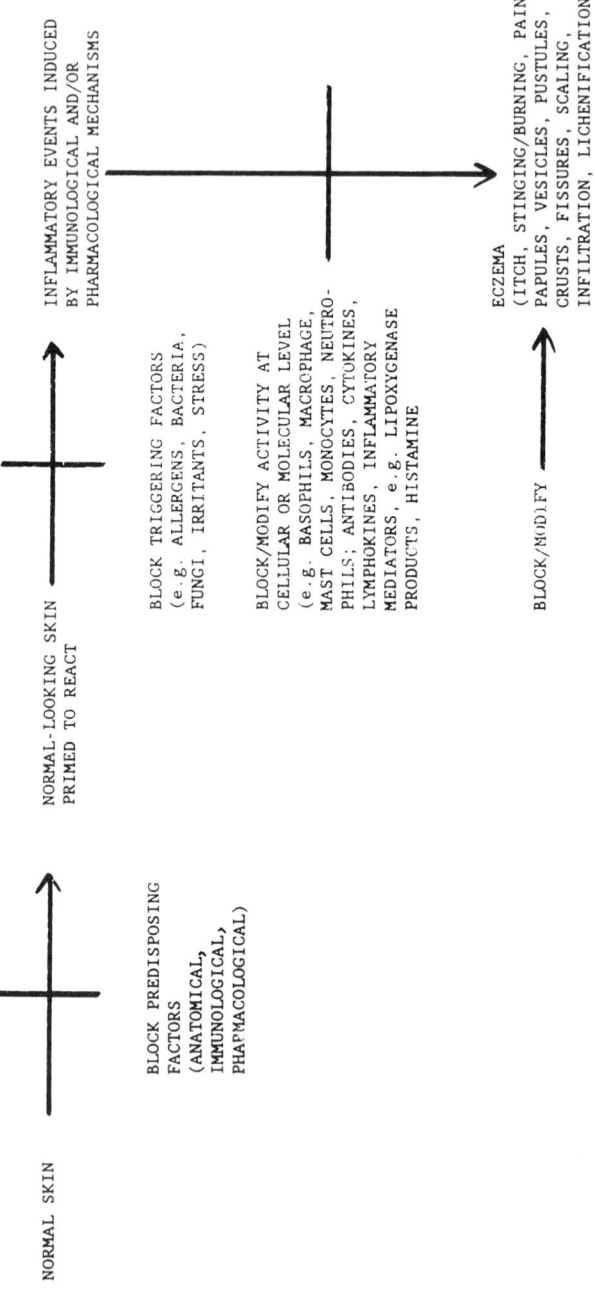

Figure 43.1 Drug targets in eczema (Ring and Dorsch, 1985; Burton *et al.*, 1986; Hanifin, 1986; Leung and Geha, 1986)

There are several important, interrelated aspects to be considered when targeting drugs for eczema. They are:

(1) The specific pathophysiological process(es) to be modified and the optimum stage (timing) for intervention.
(2) The choice of a broad- versus a narrow-spectrum approach.
(3) The route of administration for the agent (systemic or topical).

In addition, consideration needs to be given to whether the target represents a fundamental, primary event or a secondary complication.

At one end lies a broad-spectrum, systemically administered attack on inflammatory and/or immunological events occurring early in the pathogenesis of the disease. This approach is likely to strike one or more of the important targets and be highly effective, e.g. systemic corticosteroids, but may carry with it the risk of an unacceptable level of adverse effects. Conversely, a topically administered, specifically targeted, narrow-spectrum agent given after the onset of the disease is less likely to be highly effective in the full range of eczema subtypes and may miss several key targets, but has a greater chance of avoiding unwanted effects. The ideal drug is clearly one that could be used safely, effectively and conveniently to intervene at the earliest possible stage in the disease process. When more than 10% of the surface area of the skin is involved, and particularly if the distribution of the disease is patchy, oral therapy may be the preferred mode of administration.

THE EVALUATION OF DRUGS FOR ECZEMA

When developing a drug for the treatment of 'eczema', it is likely that the condition to be focused on will be that associated with the atopic state (Champion and Parish, 1986). Indeed, from a therapeutic viewpoint, all the general headings for targets normally considered in the management of eczema are relevant to this form of the disease, although the exact details concerning pathogenesis may vary from one subtype of eczema to another. These headings include psychosomatic aspects; irritant, allergic and microbial triggers; immunological and inflammatory disturbances; anatomical and microanatomical derangement (Hanifin, 1986; Leung and Geha, 1986). However, it should be remembered that differences in pathogenesis may yield one approach to therapy, a viable proposition in one eczema subtype, but not in another. Conversely, other approaches may be more broadly relevant. Compare, for example, the successful specific treatment of seborrhoeic dermatitis with an imidazole antifungal agent (Green *et al.*, 1987) with the use of topical corticosteroid therapy for all forms of eczema. Thus, it may be appropriate to evaluate drug effects in a range of eczema subtypes, and the extent to which such exploration will be necessary in the early phases of clinical development will depend on the pharmacological profile of the agent and, in particular, the nature and specificity of its therapeutic attack. Data from such studies must be interpreted against a background of genuine understanding of important pathophysiological (Hanifin, 1986; Leung and Geha, 1986) and clinical (Burton *et al.*, 1986; Champion and Parish, 1986) aspects of the various eczema subtypes and of exactly what one is trying to achieve.

With suitable modification and a creative, flexible approach, the general plan and specific techniques described below can be used, as appropriate, to evaluate all subtypes of eczema and the effects of all potentially useful drugs, regardless of the proposed mechanism of action. Clearly, some techniques will be more suitable than others in any given situation. It is appreciated that when applying a drug either topically or systemically for the treatment of skin diseases, it is important to gather information on all aspects of its effects in humans. However, for the purposes of this chapter, the focus will be on the skin. The depth to which early human exploratory work is taken will depend, in part, on what is known about the therapeutic class to which the test substance belongs. For example, in the case of a topical corticosteroid, the key questions would relate to speed and degree of efficacy versus the risk of well-known adverse effects, e.g. skin thinning. On the other hand, the question asked of a drug based on an unproven concept would be: does it work? and if so, is the mechanism of action that which was proposed? or did the agent perform as predicted pharmacodynamically at a molecular or cellular level and yet fail to benefit the disease process?

Essentially, what needs to be done in the early phase human evaluation of both topical and systemic agents is to:

(1) Establish that the test substance has the potential to be effective in eczema.

(2) Define the optimal dosage regimen.

(3) Define the pharmacokinetic and pharmacodynamic profile of the drug in human skin, as well as systemically.

(4) Determine the likely relative efficacy of the agent as compared with standard therapies, allowing preliminary judgements to be made regarding commercial viability.

(5) Estimate the risk/benefit profile of the agent.

In the case of topical therapy, the vehicle and concentration of active agent in the formulation need to be optimised. These aims may appear logical and obvious, but it is surprising how often fundamental principles are ignored in dermatological drug development—e.g. failure to determine, at an early stage, optimal dosing regimes for topical corticosteroid therapy, or failure to determine with reasonable precision the changes in corticosteroid concentration in a given vehicle needed to achieve definite changes in clinical efficacy (Gibson *et al.*, 1984, 1987).

The early clinical development plans for both topical and systemic drugs are summarised in Figures 43.2 and 43.3. The exact timing of the 'important associated activities' may vary from project to project, but attention should be paid to each of them at an appropriate time. It is worth recalling that some of the advantages of dermatological drug development are that clinical changes are readily visible and usually occur quickly, and, in the case of topical

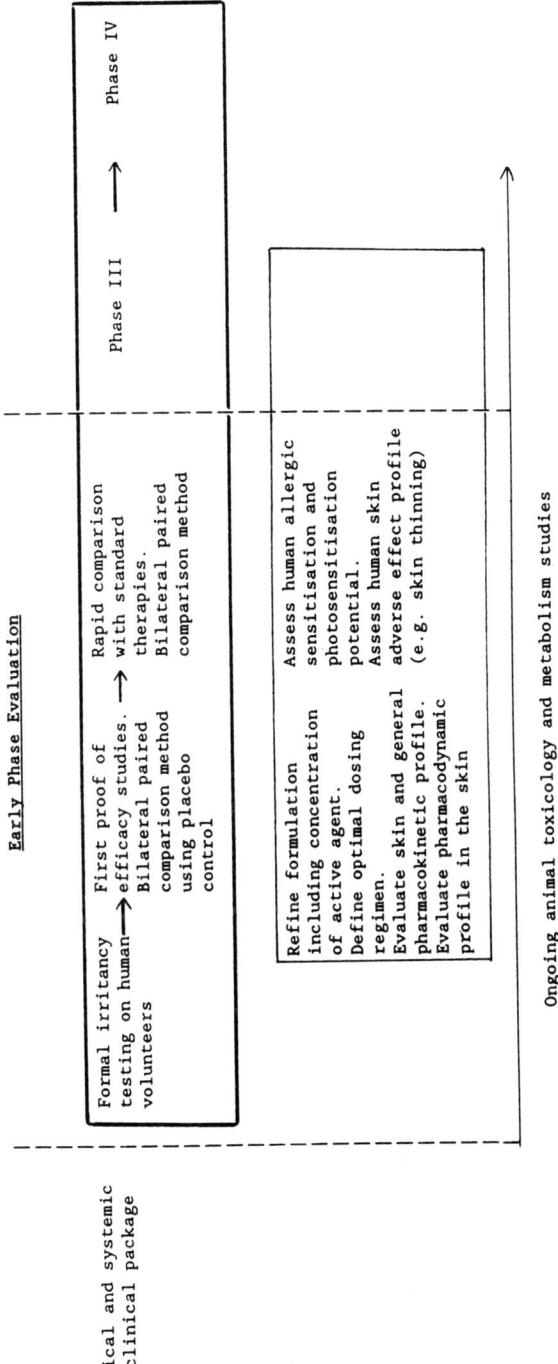

Figure 43.2 The clinical development plan for topical eczema drugs: thick box, primary pathway; thin box, important associated activities

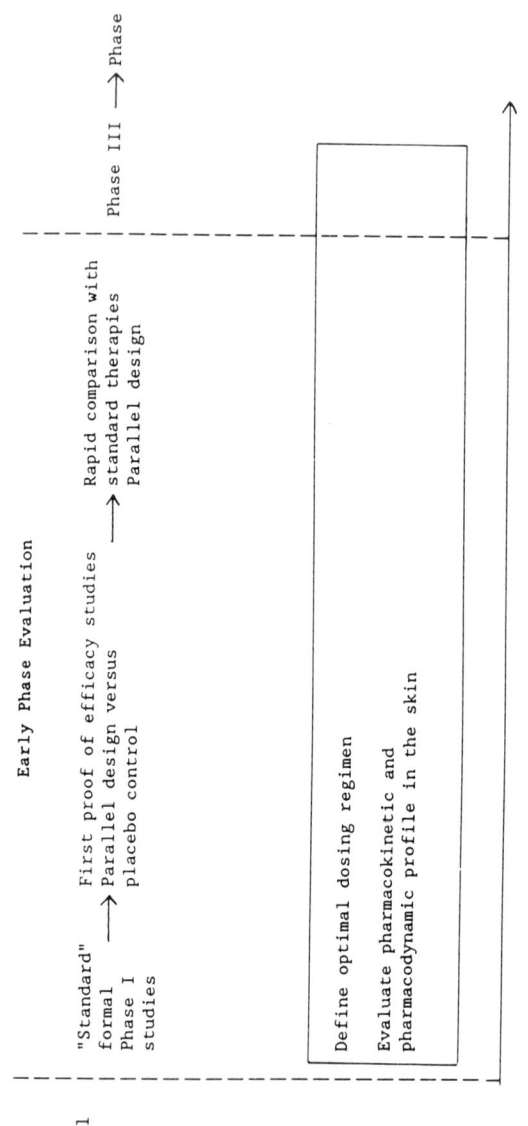

Figure 43.3   The clinical development plan for systemic eczema drugs

therapy, the safety margin is generally good. In addition, the skin represents the ideal organ for exploring human *tissue* pharmacology in a relatively low-invasive manner and this should be exploited as fully as possible (Camp and Greaves, 1987).

With regard to drugs for topical application, it is sensible to gain some experience of use in normal human skin before proceeding to patients, owing to the inflammatory nature of the eczema process and its propensity for exacerbation following irritation. This can be most simply done in normal human volunteers using an occlusive technique involving Finn chambers and a simple double-blind assessment evaluating epidermal and dermal changes ('dryness'/scaling, erythema, papules, vesiculation, infiltration/induration, erosion/ulceration), much like the method used in allergic contact dermatitis patch test clinics (Bronaugh and Maibach, 1982; Wilkinson and Rycroft, 1986). Alternatively, repeated application techniques, with or without occlusion, can be used (Bronaugh and Maibach, 1982). With regard to systemic drugs, 'standard' Phase I studies evaluating safety and general human pharmacology will be needed.

Table 43.2 details the established and potential uses of volunteer models and studies in patients. The backbone of the exercise is the treatment of

Table 43.2 The real and/or potential uses of volunteer models and patient studies

Volunteer models	Patient studies
Irritancy, allergenicity, photosensitising and skin thinning potential in normal skin (Epstein, 1977; Hjorth, 1977; Maibach and Marzulli, 1977; Marzulli and Maibach, 1977; Bronaugh and Maibach, 1982; Frosch, 1982; Jordan and King, 1982; Kaidbey, 1982; Buehler and Ritz, 1985; Frosch and Wendt, 1985)	Efficacy, safety and acceptability in various eczema sub-types (Akers, 1982; Allen, 1982)
Drug pharmacokinetics and pharmacodynamics in normal and experimentally challenged/damaged skin (Fowle *et al.*, 1971; Malone *et al.*, 1974; Plummer *et al.*, 1977; Barry and Woodford, 1978; Sussman *et al.*, 1983; Hensby *et al.*, 1984; Gibson *et al.*, 1987; Guy *et al.*, 1987)	Drug pharmacokinetics and pharmacodynamics in diseased skin (Kobza Black *et al.*, 1982)
Refinement of topical formulation, including concentration of active agent (Malone *et al.*, 1974; Gibson *et al.*, 1987)	Refinement of topical formulation, including concentration of active agent (Gibson *et al.*, 1984, 1987)
Definition of treatment regimen (Woodford *et al.*, 1983)	Definition of treatment regimen (Sudilovsky *et al.*, 1981; Harst *et al.*, 1982)

patients with eczema to establish efficacy. However, experimental volunteer models can be of value if they are used judiciously and if it is recognised that few, if any, of them have been fully refined and that in some instances their exact roles have yet to be unequivocally established.

The important issues in any given study in the early evaluation of eczema drugs are:

(1) The population to use—patients or volunteers?
(2) The model/eczema subtype to study and the experimental design.
(3) What to measure?—clinical symptoms and signs; pharmacological, immunological and anatomical/structural parameters.
(4) How to perform measurements?

The best overall assessment will probably be obtained using data generated from creatively designed and rigorously conducted studies in both patients and volunteers. Some of the references given below relate to the evaluation of psoriasis, as this disease tends to have been studied more extensively, and as some lessons learned from that field are relevant to eczema.

The Population to be Studied

The most fundamental question to be answered is: does the drug work in eczema? This obviously requires to be tested in patients. In assessing irritancy potential prior to use in eczema, one may choose to use normal volunteers, volunteers with a 'normal' skin but with a personal and/or family history of atopy, or the 'normal' skin of patients with eczema. In practice, a screening study as discussed above in normal volunteers should suffice, with the majority of data concerning irritancy being collected during the clinical phase of development.

The Model/Eczema Subtype to Study and the Experimental Design

Study design, with the possible exception of early dose determination work, should be double-blind and pay due regard to the need for proper controls, full randomisation and other statistically important considerations. Whenever possible, the bilateral, symmetrical, paired-comparison method should be used, as this permits the asking of the highly discriminating questions—which side is better and to what degree? (Akers, 1982; Allen, 1982; Gibson *et al.*, 1987), and utilises the valuable resource of the study population in the most efficient manner, with the subject acting as his own control (Allen, 1982). The theoretical objection that drug administered to one site may affect another is unlikely to be of practical significance (except in the case of antimicrobial therapy) if small amounts of drug are applied to limited areas of diseased/experimentally damaged skin.

Table 43.3 lists a range of models that could be considered in the evaluation and development of drugs for eczema. In many cases, further refinement

Table 43.3 Patient/volunteer models of real and/or potential use

Challenge system/inducer	Model category	References
Dinitrochlorobenzene (DNCB)	Eczema/dermatitis	Friedmann et al. (1983)
Rhus	Eczema/dermatitis	Kaidbey and Kligman (1976)
Sodium lauryl sulphate (SLS)	Inflammation/dermatitis	Van Neste et al. (1986)
Croton oil	Inflammation	Kaidbey and Kligman (1974)
Dithranol	Inflammation	Lawrence and Shuster (1985, b)
Kerosene	Inflammation	Kaidbey and Kligman (1974)
LTB$_4$	Inflammation	Camp et al. (1984)
Tetrahydrofurfuryl nicotinate	Inflammation	Hensby et al. (1984)
UVB	Inflammation	Rupp et al. (1983); Tan et al. (1986); Torrent et al. (1988)
Intradermal antigen, compound 48/80, histamine	Weal and flare mimicking Type I allergy/inflammation	Fowle et al. (1971); Gibson (1989) Stahle and Hagermark (1984)
Skin stripping (Sellotape)	Epidermal disruption/inflammation/ hyperaemia	Wells (1957)
Intradermal histamine/trypsin	Itch	Rajka (1969); Woodward et al. (1985)
Atopic eczema	Itch	Wahlgren et al. (1988)
Topical corticosteroids	Human vasoconstriction assay	Barry (1983); Gibson et al. (1984, 1987); Cornell and Stoughton (1985)
Topical corticosteroids	Skin thinning	Wendt and Frosch (1982); Gibson et al. (1984); Thomas and Black (1985)

would be needed to optimise their value. In some instances, e.g. presensitisation and rechallenge with dinitrochlorobenzene (DNCB), the ethical status of the test system is open to question. For a variety of reasons, which include the lack of definitive knowledge concerning critical aspects of the pathogenesis of various eczema sub-types, it is most likely that the best use of models is not as a predictor of efficacy in eczema *per se* (that is best left to studies in patients), but rather as a set of methods for refining topical formulations (Malone *et al.*, 1974; Gibson *et al.*, 1987) and dosing regimens (Woodford *et al.*, 1983) and for acquiring further knowledge of the agent's human dermatopharmacology (Hensby *et al.*, 1984; Stahle and Hagermark, 1984; Gibson, 1989). Thus, if it has been established in a screening programme that an agent has a 'therapeutic' effect in a given human model system, it could be utilised for the purposes specified above with greater ease, efficiency and accuracy than in a typical clinical trial setting, owing to the higher level of standardisation and speed of subject recruitment possible when performing volunteer studies. Models need not be assumed to be mechanistically relevant to the eczema process in order to be of value, provided that they are shown to be relevant to the test agent in question. However, it is of great importance not to attempt extrapolation of results gained from model systems to the clinical situation until it has been unequivocally established that this is scientifically valid.

The ideal model would be ethical, simple to use, reliable in response both to the challenge modality and the test therapies, non-invasive and non-scarring, reproducible and clinically relevant. Of the models listed in Table 43.3 the following would appear to represent a reasonable range of potentially useful methods: croton oil, tetrahydrofurfuryl nicotinate, sodium lauryl sulphate (SLS) and LTB_4-induced inflammation; Sellotape stripping; weal and flare reactions following histamine, compound 48/80 and antigen challenge; the human vasoconstriction assay (for corticosteroids only); and itch assessment; and ultrasound for examining skin thinning. Rapid screening using small numbers of volunteers should be used to fine-tune the choice of models used to assess any given agent.

The four 'inflammation' models simply represent a range of methods for inducing various types of inflammatory changes in the skin which may respond to certain anti-inflammatory agents. They would be considered when a novel agent with a suitable anti-inflammatory profile was being evaluated. They utilise a range of insults from both the chemical and biological ends of the spectrum.

Sellotape stripping may be used as an entity in itself to produce epidermal derangement (Frodin and Skogh, 1984) accompanied by hyperaemia, as an adjunct to the human vasoconstriction assay for corticosteroid assessment (Wells, 1957) and as a method for ensuring greater penetration of drug into skin challenged by various modalities.

Weal and flare reactions may be usefully employed in the evaluation of both systemic (Fowle *et al.*, 1971) and topical (Gibson, 1989) agents with antihistamine effects, as well as those with an ability to modify mast cell (Stahle and Hagermark, 1984; Gibson, 1989) and/or basophil behaviour. This model could readily be extended to assess drug effects on various other vasoactive substances besides histamine (Hagermark *et al.*, 1978; Soter *et al.*, 1983).

The human vasoconstriction assay has been used with great success to screen topical corticosteroids for clinical activity (Barry, 1983), for determining the bioavailability of corticosteroids from their vehicles (Barry and Woodford, 1978) and for predicting the relative clinical potencies of topical corticosteroid preparations (Gibson *et al.*, 1984, 1987; Cornell and Stoughton, 1985). An excellent review of this model has been prepared by Barry (1983). It is probably the most used and refined of all the methods outlined in Table 43.3, but unfortunately its use is currently limited to the evaluation of topical corticosteroids.

Volunteer models for the assessment of itching usually utilise intracutaneous injections of histamine or various proteases, e.g. trypsin, papain, or the epicutaneous application of cowhage extract (Rajka, 1969; Hagermark, 1973; Woodward *et al.*, 1985; Spilker, 1987). Parameters which are usually measured are itch threshold, duration and intensity (Hagermark, 1973; Woodward *et al.*, 1985). It should be noted that the sensation induced by pruritogenic agents varies qualitatively, depending on the depth to which the injection is given (Woodward *et al.*, 1985). The role of available models of experimentally induced itch in predicting with accuracy that a drug will act as an antipruritic agent in eczema remains to be clarified.

Measurement of itching in patients may be performed by subjective evaluation with or without the added sophistication of the use of data loggers (Wahlgren *et al.*, 1988; Doherty *et al.*, 1989) or by limb meters (Krause and Shuster, 1983; Savin *et al.*, 1986) which evaluate scratching as a direct correlate of itching. Several important weaknesses have recently been stressed concerning the use of the latter method (Gibson, 1987). A simple, subjective evaluation currently appears to be the method of choice in terms of both practicality and clinical relevance.

For studies in patients, preference should be given in the early stages to evaluating subtypes of eczema which lend themselves to assessment by the bilateral paired-comparison method. Thus, atopic eczema, venous stasis eczema and contact dermatitis would be appropriately selected in circumstances where a broad-spectrum anti-inflammatory effect is anticipated.

What to Measure and How to Measure It

Techniques for evaluating drug effects on eczema and experimentally challenged skin are summarised in Table 43.4. These are described in detail in the chapter 'Measurement of Skin Responses to Drugs'. They may be usefully applied in a range of models and clinical conditions.

In all clinical and volunteer studies, characteristic symptoms and signs (e.g. itching, stinging/burning, pain, erythema, blanching, papules, vesicles, pustules, infiltration/induration, scaling) produced by the challenge modality or clinical condition, and modification of these by the test agent, can be readily evaluated using carefully constructed scoring systems performed under blinded conditions (Allen, 1982; Wendt and Frosch, 1982). The most important aspects of such evaluations are summarised in Table 43.5. Despite the subjective nature of these assessments, they remain of central importance in dermatological studies, they are surprisingly accurate and reproducible

Table 43.4 Measurement techniques of real and/or potential value

Technique	Useful in	References
Blinded, carefully constructed, subjective scoring systems based on clinical symptoms and signs	Patient studies and volunteer models	Allen (1982); Wendt and Frosch (1982); Cornell and Stoughton (1985); Gibson et al. (1987)
Measurement of area and/or volume	Weal and flare studies	Fowle et al. (1971)
Laser Doppler velocimetry/flowmetry	Volunteer models with a sufficient inflammatory component to increase skin blood flow, including weal and flare studies	Holloway and Watkins (1977); Engelhart and Kristensen 1983); Holloway (1983); Bisgaard and Kristensen (1984); Drouard et al. (1984); Stevensen et al. (1987)
	Specially adapted forms of the human vasoconstriction assay	Bisgaard et al. (1986)
Measurement of transepidermal water loss (TEWL) by evaporimetry	Patient studies and volunteer models which involve functional disturbance of the epidermis	Nilsson (1977); Scott et al. (1982); Frodin and Skogh (1984); Werner and Lindberg (1985); Blichmann and Serup (1987)
Skin thickness determination, using calipers, ultrasound or radiographically	Volunteer studies to determine the skin-thinning potential of topical agents	Black (1969); Dykes and Marks (1977); Tan et al; (1982)
Skin absorption of radiolabelled drug	Studies to determine drug pharmacokinetics where the use of pharmacodynamic endpoints is not feasible	Guy et al. (1987); Rougier and Lotte (1987)
Suction blisters and skin windows	Patient studies and volunteer models of eczema/inflammation to determine skin drug levels and effects at a molecular and cellular level	Kobza Black et al. (1977, 1985); Michel and Dubertret (1985); Cunningham and Camp (1987)

Table 43.5 Points to consider in performing subjective skin evaluations

Experience and training is invaluable.

Use a double-blind, fully randomised study design with adequate controls.

Use the bilateral, paired comparison method or multiple lesions/challenge sites within the same subject where possible. This allows use of highly discriminating questions—which side is better? and to what degree (slightly better, better, very much better)?—or ranking of treatment effects.

Scoring systems for individual symptoms and signs should include the full range of possibilities, e.g. no response—intense response, using a 5–10-point scale with clinically meaningful and evenly separated spacing between descriptive terms. An overall 'severity' score incorporating grouped signs should also be included.

Progress in the condition should be scored with a similarly constructed scale, e.g. very much worse–completely cleared.

when performed by a trained, experienced investigator, and their value should not be underestimated. Suitable methods of eliciting the subject's opinion should be used to add to the database. Properly 'educated' patients and volunteers often agree with the investigator's evaluation.

Measurement of the area of weals and flares produced by various intradermally injected challenge substances, e.g. histamine, is a simple, reliable and reproducible method of objectively evaluating drug effects on these parameters (Fowle *et al.*, 1971; Gibson, 1989) and has been extensively used to determine the time of onset, intensity and duration of drug activity in man. The theoretically more appropriate measurement of weal volume is technically more difficult and does not add significantly to the usefulness of the data obtained.

Laser Doppler velocimetry/flowmetry is useful as an objective measure of cutaneous blood flow and has been utilised to study the pharmacodynamic response following application of topical vasodilators (Guy *et al.*, 1985). It may be used to provide objective data to supplement and expand upon subjective evaluation when assessing drug effects in skin inflammatory disease/models where the drug under test directly or indirectly has an effect on cutaneous blood flow. To date, it has been of no value in situations where blood flow is reduced below normal baseline values, e.g. corticosteroid-induced vasoconstriction (Bisgaard *et al.*, 1986).

The measurement of transepidermal water loss (TEWL) by evaporimetry (Blichmann and Serup, 1987) provides a practical and objective method for determining the effect of treatment on the return to full functional integrity of the epidermis, particularly the stratum corneum. Normal functioning of the stratum corneum, as determined by its ability to restrict TEWL to a baseline level, may occur several days after the skin has returned to normal, as judged by the naked eye (Grice, 1980).

Several methods have been used to determine the thickness of skin. They include the use of calipers, histometric techniques, X-rays and ultrasound (Dykes and Marks, 1977; Tan *et al.*, 1982; Thomas and Black, 1985; Kingston and Lowe, 1987). Currently, with regard to dermatological drug development, the key purpose of such work is to determine the relative skin-thinning effects of topical corticosteroid preparations and future competitors to such agents. This is probably best done using subjective assessment (Wendt and Frosch, 1982) and ultrasound (Tan *et al.*, 1982; Gibson *et al.*, 1984).

Methods involving the use of radiolabelled agents (Guy *et al.*, 1987; Rougier and Lotte, 1987) to evaluate and/or predict the rate, depth and degree of penetration of drugs into and through the skin are currently under development and may prove to be of value in the future evaluation of topically applied agents.

Suction blister (Kobza Black *et al.*, 1977) and skin window (Cunningham and Camp, 1987) techniques permit the sampling of biological fluids derived from the deeper epidermis/upper dermis and allow the determination of skin drug levels at or near the target site following systemic administration, as well as the study of the effects of drugs (topical and systemic) on mediators of inflammation and other parameters at a molecular or cellular level. For example, they could be used to verify whether an agent with a particular pharmacological profile, e.g. lipoxygenase blockade, does actually perform that role in human skin *in vivo*. However, owing to lack of hard pathophysiological data, such work would not necessarily accurately predict that the test agent would be effective in the treatment of eczema.

CONCLUSIONS

The key element in the early phase evaluation of drugs for eczema is proof of efficacy in a clinical setting, as determined by the eyes and palpating fingers of a skilled clinician. However, much could be gained in terms of clarification of pathogenesis, definition of an agent's pharmacological profile and refinement of dose and treatment schedules by more detailed study involving the use of a range of techniques in volunteer models and patients. Before this ideal can be attained, a great deal of work will be needed to refine, validate and standardise the currently available methods. Human skin has the supreme advantage of accessibility. The development of new purpose-orientated means by which dermatopharmacology may be advanced to a stage where the skin takes its place as an ideal organ for the study of human tissue pharmacology must remain the goal of those who work in this area.

REFERENCES

Akers, W. A. (1982). Topical corticosteroids: proof of efficacy in skin diseases. In Kligman, A. M. and Leyden, J. J. (Eds.), *Safety and Efficacy of Topical Drugs and Cosmetics*. Grune and Stratton, New York, pp. 1–23

Allen, A. M. (1982). Design methodology in trials of topical drugs. In Kligman, A. M. and Leyden, J. J. (Eds.), *Safety and Efficacy of Topical Drugs and Cosmetics*. Grune and Stratton, New York, pp. 25–49

Barry, B. W. (1983). Dermatological formulations: percutaneous absorption. In Swarbrick, J. (Ed.), *Drugs and the Pharmaceutical Sciences*, Vol. 18. Marcel Dekker, New York, Basle, pp. 264–95

Barry, B. W. and Woodford, R. (1978). Activity and bioavailability of topical steroids. *In vivo/in vitro* correlations for the vasoconstrictor test. *Journal of Clinical Pharmacy*, **3**, 43–65

Bisgaard, H. and Kristensen, J. K. (1984). Quantitation of microcirculatory blood flow changes in human cutaneous tissue induced by inflammatory mediators. *Journal of Investigative Dermatology*, **83**, 184–7

Bisgaard, H., Kristensen, J. K. and Sondergaard, J. (1986). A new technique for ranking vascular corticosteroid effects in humans using laser-Doppler velocimetry. *Journal of Investigative Dermatology*, **86**, 275–8

Black, M. M. (1969). A modified radiographic method for measuring skin thickness. *British Journal of Dermatology*, **81**, 661–6

Blichman, C. W. and Serup, J. (1987). Reproducibility and variability of trans-epidermal water loss measurement. Studies on the Servo Med evaporimeter. *Acta Dermato-Venereologica*, **67**, 206–10

Bronaugh, R. L. and Maibach, H. I. (1982). Evaluation of skin irritation: correlations between animals and humans. In Kligman, A. M. and Leyden, J. J. (Eds.), *Safety and Efficacy of Topical Drugs and Cosmetics*. Grune and Stratton, New York, pp. 51–62

Buehler, E. V. and Ritz, H. L. (1985). Patch testing techniques for risk assessment of allergic contact dermatitis. In Maibach, H. I. and Lowe, N. J. (Eds.), *Models in Dermatology*, Vol. 2. Karger, Basle, pp. 251–63

Burton, J. L., Rook, A. and Wilkinson, D. S. (1986). Eczema, lichen simplex, erythroderma and prurigo. In Rook, A., Wilkinson, D. S., Ebling, F. J. G., Champion, R. H. and Burton, J. L. (Eds.), *Textbook of Dermatology*, Vol. 1, 4th edn. Blackwell Scientific, Oxford, pp. 367–418

Camp, R. D. R. and Greaves, M. W. (1987). Inflammatory mediators in the skin. *British Medical Bulletin*, **43**, 401–14

Camp, R., Jones, R. R., Brain, S., Woollard, P. and Greaves, M. (1984). Production of intraepidermal microabscesses by topical application of leukotriene B_4. *Journal of Investigative Dermatology*, **82**, 202–4

Champion, R. H. and Parish, W. E. (1986). Atopic dermatitis. In Rook, A., Wilkinson, D. S., Ebling, F. J. G., Champion, R. H. and Burton, J. L. (Eds.), *Textbook of Dermatology*, Vol. 1, 4th edn. Blackwell Scientific, Oxford, pp. 419–34

Cornell, R. C. and Stoughton, R. B. (1985). Correlation of the vasoconstriction assay and clinical activity in psoriasis. *Archives of Dermatology*, **121**, 63–7

Cunningham, F. M. and Camp, R. D. R. (1987). New assays for inflammatory mediators in skin diseases. In Maibach, H. I. and Lowe, N. J., *Models in Dermatology*, Vol. 3. Karger, Basle, pp. 39–45

Dahl, M. V. (1983). *Staphylococcus aureus* and atopic dermatitis. *Archives of Dermatology*, **119**, 840–6

Doherty, V., Sylvester, D. G. H., Kennedy, C. T. C., Harvey, S. G., Calthrop, J. G. and Gibson, J. R. (1989). Treatment of itching in atopic eczema with antihistamines with a low sedative profile. *British Medical Journal*, **298**, 96

Drouard, V., Wilson, D. R., Maibach, H. I. and Guy, R. H. (1984). Quantitative assessment of UV-induced changes in microcirculatory flow by laser Doppler velocimetry. *Journal of Investigative Dermatology*, **83**, 188–92

Dykes, P. J. and Marks, R. (1977). Measurement of skin thickness: a comparison of two *in vivo* techniques with a conventional histometric method. *Journal of Investigative Dermatology*, **69**, 275–8

Engelhart, M. and Kristensen, J. K. (1983). Evaluation of cutaneous blood flow responses by ^{133}Xe washout and a laser-Doppler flowmeter. *Journal of Investigative Dermatology*, **80**, 12–15

Epstein, J. H. (1977). Photocontact allergy in humans. In Marzulli, F. N. and Maibach, H. I. (Eds.), *Advances in Modern Toxicology*, Vol. 4 *(Dermatotoxicology and Pharmacology)*. Halsted Press, New York, pp. 413–26

Fowle, A. S. E., Hughes, D. T. D. and Knight, G. J. (1971). The evaluation of histamine antagonists in man. *European Journal of Clinical Pharmacology*, **3**, 215–20

Friedman, P. S., Moss, C., Shuster, S. and Simpson, J. M. (1983). Quantitative relationships between sensitizing dose of DNCB and reactivity in normal subjects. *Clinical and Experimental Immunology*, **53**, 709–15

Frodin, T. and Skogh, M. (1984). Measurement of transepidermal water loss using an evaporimeter to follow the restitution of the barrier layer of human epidermis after stripping the stratum corneum. *Acta Dermato-Venereologica*, **64**, 537–40

Frosch, P. J. (1982). Methods for quantifying the cutaneous adverse effects of topical corticosteroids. In Kligman, A. M. and Leyden, J. J. (Eds.), *Safety and Efficacy of Topical Drugs and Cosmetics*. Grune and Stratton, New York, pp. 119–34

Frosch, P. J. and Wendt, H. (1985). Human models for quantification of corticosteroid adverse effects. In Maibach, H. I. and Lowe, N. J. (Eds.), *Models in Dermatology*, Vol. 2. Karger, Basle, pp. 5–15

Gibson, J. R. (1987). The use of antihistamines with a low sedative potential in the treatment of the itching of atopic eczema. *Clinical and Experimental Dermatology*, **12**, 469–70

Gibson, J. R. (1989). Topically applied drugs in type I allergic reactions. In Maibach, H. I. and Lowe, N. J. (Eds.), *Models in Dermatology*, Vol. 4. Karger, Basle (in press)

Gibson, J. R., Hough, J. E., Marks, P. and Webster, A. (1987). Effect of concentration on the clinical potency of corticosteroid ointment formulations. In Shroot, B. and Schaefer, H. (Eds.), *Pharmacology and the Skin*, Vol. 1. Karger, Basle, pp. 214–22

Gibson, J. R., Kirsch, J. M., Darley, C. R., Harvey, S. G., Burke, C. A. and Hanson, M. E. (1984). An assessment of the relationship between vasoconstrictor assay findings, clinical efficacy and skin thinning effects of a variety of undiluted and diluted corticosteroid preparations. *British Journal of Dermatology*, **111** (Suppl. 27), 204–12

Green, C. A., Farr, P. M. and Shuster, S. (1987). Treatment of seborrhoeic dermatitis with ketoconazole. II. Response of seborrhoeic dermatitis of the face, scalp and trunk to topical ketoconazole. *British Journal of Dematology*, **116**, 217–21

Grice, K. A. (1980). Transepidermal water loss in pathological skin. In Jarret, A. (Ed.), *The Physiology and Pathophysiology of the Skin*, Vol. 6. Academic Press, London, pp. 2147–55

Guy, R. H., Bucks, D. A. W., McMaster, J. R., Villaflor, D. A., Roskos, K. V., Hinz, R. S. and Maibach, H. I. (1987). Kinetics of drug absorption across human skin *in vivo*. In Shroot, B. and Schaefer, H. (Eds.), *Pharmacology and the Skin*, Vol. 1. Karger, Basle, pp. 70–76

Guy, R. H., Tur, E. and Maibach, H. I. (1985). Optical techniques for monitoring cutaneous microcirculation. Recent applications. *International Journal of Dermatology*, **24**, 88–94

Hagermark, O. (1973). Influence of antihistamines, sedatives and aspirin on experimental itch. *Acta Dermato-Venereologica*, **53**, 363–8

Hagermark, O., Hokfelt, T. and Pernow, B. (1978). Flare and itch induced by substance P in human skin. *Journal of Investigative Dermatology*, **71**, 233–5

Hanifin, J. M. (1986). Pharmacophysiology of atopic dermatitis. *Clinical Reviews in Allergy*, **4**, 43–65

Harst, L. C. A. v. d., de Jonge, H., Pot, F. and Polano, M. K. (1982). Comparison of two application schedules for clobetasol 17 proprionate. *Acta Dermato-Venereologica*, **62**, 270–3

Hensby, C. N., Maloubier, A., Civier, A., Shroot, B. and Ortonne, J. P. (1984). A model for studying the anti-prostaglandin activity of drugs in human skin. *British Journal of Dermatology*, **111** (Suppl. 27), 147–51

Hjorth, N. (1977). Diagnostic patch testing. In Marzulli, F. N. and Maibach, H. I. (Eds.), *Advances in Modern Toxicology*, Vol. 4 *(Dermatotoxicology and Pharmacology)*. Halsted Press, New York, pp. 341–51

Holloway, G. A. (1983). Laser Doppler measurement of cutaneous blood flow. In Rolfe, P. (Ed.), *Non-invasive Measurements: 2*. Academic Press, London, pp. 219–49

Holloway, G. A. and Watkins, D. W. (1977). Laser Doppler measurement of cutaneous blood flow. *Journal of Investigative Dermatology*, **69**, 306–9

Jordan, W. P. and King, S. E. (1982). Human experimental contact dermatitis. In Kligman, A. M. and Leyden, J. J. (Eds.), *Safety and Efficacy of Topical Drugs and Cosmetics*. Grune and Stratton, New York, pp. 193–205

Kaidbey, K. (1982). Assessment of topical photosensitizers in humans. In Kligman, A. M. and Leyden, J. J. (Eds.), *Safety and Efficacy of Topical Drugs and Cosmetics*. Grune and Stratton, New York, pp. 213–19

Kaidbey, K. H. and Kligman, A. M. (1974). Assay of topical corticosteroids by suppression of experimental inflammation in humans. *Journal of Investigative Dermatology*, **63**, 292–7

Kaidbey, K. H. and Kligman, A. M. (1976). Assay of topical corticosteroids. Efficacy of suppression of experimental Rhus dermatitis in humans. *Archives of Dermatology*, **112**, 808–10

Kingston, T. P. and Lowe, N. J. (1987). Experimental assessment of human cutaneous irritant reactions using anthralin. In Maibach, H. I. and Lowe, N. J. (Eds.), *Models in Dermatology*, Vol. 3. Karger, Basle, pp. 74–83

Kobza Black, A., Barr, R. M., Wong, E., Brain, S., Greaves, M. W., Dickinson, R., Shroot, B. and Hensby, C. N. (1985). Lipoxygenase products of arachidonic acid in human inflamed skin. *British Journal of Clinical Pharmacology*, **20**, 185–90

Kobza Black, A., Greaves, M. W. and Hensby, C. N. (1982). The effect of systemic prednisolone on arachidonic acid, and prostaglandin E_2 and $F_{2\alpha}$ levels in human cutaneous inflammation. *British Journal of Clinical Pharmacology*, **14**, 391–4

Kobza Black, A., Greaves, M. W., Hensby, C. N., Plummer, N. A. and Eady, R. A. J. (1977). A new method for recovery of exudates from normal and inflamed human skin. *Clinical and Experimental Dermatology*, **2**, 209–16

Krause, L. and Shuster, S. (1983). Mechanism of action of antipruritic drugs. *British Medical Journal*, **287**, 1199–200

Lawrence, C. M. and Shuster, S. (1985a). Mechanism of anthralin inflammation. I. Dissociation of response to clobetasol and indomethacin. *British Journal of Dermatology*, **113**, 107–15

Lawrence, C. M. and Shuster, S. (1985b). Mechanism of anthralin inflammation. II. Effect of pretreatment with glucocorticoids, anthralin and removal of stratum corneum. *British Journal of Dermatology*, **113**, 117–22

Leung, D. Y. M. and Geha, R. S. (1986). Immunoregulatory abnormalities in atopic dermatitis. *Clinical Reviews in Allergy*, **4**, 67–86

Maibach, H. I. and Marzulli, F. N. (1977). Phototoxicity (photoirritation) of topical and systemic agents. In Marzulli, F. N. and Maibach, H. I. (Eds.), *Advances in*

Modern Toxicology, Vol. 4 *(Dermatotoxicology and Pharmacology)*. Halsted Press, New York, pp. 211–23

Malone, T., Haleblian, J. K., Poulsen, B. J. and Burdick, K. G. (1974). Development and evaluation of ointment and cream vehicles for a new topical steroid, fluclorolone acetonide. *British Journal of Dermatology*, **90**, 187–95

Marzulli, F. N. and Maibach, H. I. (1977). Contact allergy: predictive testing in humans. In Marzulli, F. N. and Maibach, H. I. (Eds.), *Advances in Modern Toxicology*, Vol. 4 *(Dermatotoxicology and Pharmacology)*. Halsted Press, New York, pp. 353–72

Michel, L. and Dubertret, L. (1985). A simple method for studying chemotaxis, vascular permeability and histological modifications induced by mediators of inflammation *in vivo* in man. *British Journal of Dermatology*, **113** (Suppl. 28), 61–6

Nilsson, G. E. (1977). Measurement of water exchange through skin. *Medical and Biological Engineering and Computing*, **15**, 209–18

Plummer, N. A., Hensby, C. N., Kobza Black, A. and Greaves, M. W. (1977). Prostaglandin activity in sustained inflammation of human skin before and after aspirin. *Clinical Science and Molecular Medicine*, **52**, 615–20

Rajka, G. (1969). A method for evaluation on the influence of experimental itch of topically applied drugs. *Acta Dermato-Venereologica*, **49**, 163–6

Ring, J. and Dorsch, W. (1985). Altered releasability of vasoactive mediator secreting cells in atopic eczema. *Acta Dermato-Venereologica*, Suppl. 114, 9–23

Rougier, A. and Lotte, C. (1987). Correlations between horny layer concentration and percutaneous absorption. In Shroot, B. and Schaefer, H. (Eds.), *Pharmacology and the Skin*, Vol. 1. Karger, Basle, pp. 81–102

Rupp, W., Badian, M., Dagrosa, E., Ganshorn, F., Lucena, M., Petri, W. and Sittig, W. (1983). Kinetics of UV-erythema in normal subjects. *British Journal of Dermatology*, **109** (Suppl. 25), 111–13

Savin, J. A., Dow, R., Harlow, B. J., Massey, H. and Yee, K. F. (1986). The effect of a new non-sedative H_1-receptor antagonist (LN2974) on the itching and scratching of patients with atopic eczema. *Clinical and Experimental Dermatology*, **11**, 600–2

Scott, R. C., Oliver, G. J. A., Dugard, P. H. and Singh, H. J. (1982). A comparison of techniques for the measurement of transepidermal water loss. *Archives of Dermatology*, **274**, 57–64

Soter, N. A., Lewis, R. A., Corey, E. J. and Austen, K. F. (1983). Local effects of synthetic leukotrienes (LTC_4, LTD_4, LTE_4 and LTB_4) in human skin. *Journal of Investigative Dermatology*, **80**, 115–19

Spilker, B. (1987). Clinical evaluation of topical antipruritics and antihistamines. In Maibach, I. H. and Lowe, N. J. *Models in Dermatology*, Vol. 3. Karger, Basle, pp. 55–61

Stahle, M. and Hagermark, O. (1984). Effects of topically applied clobetasol-17-propionate on histamine release in human skin. *Acta Dermato-Venereologica*, **64**, 239–42

Stevenson, J. M., Maibach, H. I. and Guy, R. H. (1987). Laser Doppler and photoplethysmographic assessment of cutaneous microvasculature. In Maibach, H. I. and Lowe, N. J., *Models in Dermatology*, Vol. 3. Karger, Basle, pp. 121–40

Sudilovsky, A., Muir, J. G. and Bocobo, F. C. (1981). A comparison of single and multiple applications of halcinonide cream. *International Journal of Dermatology*, **20**, 609–13

Sussman, G. L., Petillo, J. J., Zisblatt, M., Vukovich, R. A., Neiss, E. S. and Shocket, A. L. (1983). Inhibition of compound 48/80 induced mediator release following oral administration of tiaramide hydrochloride in normal subjects. *Annals of Allergy*, **51**, 367–70

Tan, C. Y., Statham, B., Marks, R. and Payne, P. A. (1982). Skin thickness measurement by pulsed ultrasound: its reproducibility, validation and variability. *British Journal of Dermatology*, **106**, 657–67

Tan, P., Flowers, F. P., Araujo, O. E. and Doering, P. (1986). Effect of topically applied flurbiprofen on ultraviolet-induced erythema. *Drug Intelligence and Clinical Pharmacy*, **20**, 496–9

Thomas, R. H. M. and Black, M. M. (1985). Corticosteroids: cutaneous atrophy. In Maibach, H. I. and Lowe, N. J. (Eds.), *Models in Dermatology*, Vol. 2. Karger, Basle, pp. 30–4

Torrent, J., Izquierdo, I., Barbanoj, M. J., Moreno, J., Lauroba, J. and Jane, F. (1988). UV-induced erythema model: a tool in dermatopharmacology for testing the topical activity of non-steroidal anti-inflammatory agents in man. *Methods and Findings in Experimental and Clinical Pharmacology*, **10**, 341–5

Van Neste, D., Masmoudi, M., Leroy, B., Mahmoud, G. and Lachapelle, J. M. (1986). Regression patterns of transepidermal water loss and of cutaneous blood flow values in sodium lauryl sulfate induced irritation: a human model of rough dermatitic skin. *Bioengineering and the Skin*, **2**, 103–18

Wahlgren, C.-F., Hagermark, O., Bergstrom, R. and Hedin, B. (1988). Evaluation of a new method of assessing pruritus and antipruritic drugs. *Skin Pharmacology*, **1**, 3–13

Wells, G. C. (1957). The effect of hydrocortisone on standardized skin-surface trauma. *British Journal of Dermatology*, **69**, 11–18

Wendt, H. and Frosch, P. J. (1982). *Clinco-pharmacological Models for the Assay of Topical Corticoids*. Karger, Basle

Werner, Y. and Lindberg, M. (1985). Transepidermal water loss in dry and clinically normal skin in patients with atopic dermatitis. *Acta Dermato-Venereologica*, **65**, 102–5

Wilkinson, J. D. and Rycroft, R. J. G. (1986). Contact dermatitis. In Rook, A., Wilkinson, D. S., Ebling, F. J. G., Champion, R. H. and Burton, J. L. (Eds.), *Textbook of Dermatology*, Vol. 1, 4th edn. Blackwell Scientific, Oxford, pp. 435–532

Woodford, R., Haigh, J. M. and Barry, B. W. (1983). Possible dosage regimens for topical steroids, assessed by vasoconstrictor assays using multiple applications. *Dermatologica*, **166**, 136–40

Woodward, D. F., Conway, J. L. and Wheeler, L. A. (1985). Cutaneous itching models. In Maibach, H. I. and Lowe, N. J. (Eds.), *Models in Dermatology*, Vol. 1. Karger, Basle, pp. 187–95

44
Drugs Affecting Hair Growth

Ervin Novak

Clinical Development 2, The Upjohn Company, 700 Portage Road, Kalamazoo, MI 49001, USA

INTRODUCTION

The greatest impact on the study of hair was the discovery of the hair growth cycles[1] and their characterisation.[2] Hair follicles undergo periods of growth (anagen), quiescence (telogen) and transition (catagen). The cycle can be determined by examination of plucked hairs and by trichograms which give the percentage of growing versus quiescent follicles.[3] Hair follicles in anagen and telogen phases differ in their response to X-ray irradiation, illustrating the importance of controlled hair growth studies.[4] Cohens[5] and Oliver[6] showed that follicular growth depends on the interaction between the dermal papilla and the epidermal position of the follicle. Hamilton[7] proved that the stimulating factor for common baldness is androgen and that hair follicles are active target organs of testosterone (incorporation and metabolism). Testosterone in the hair follicle is converted to two major metabolites: dihydrotestosterone and androstenedione. The enzyme 5-alpha-reductase converts testosterone to dihydrotestosterone. The activity of this enzyme is 3–8 times higher in anagen than in telogen follicles.[8] The formation of dihydrotestosterone is also higher in hair follicles from the frontal scalp than from the occipital scalp.[9] Price[10] observed that in hair follicles predisposed to baldness increased dihydrotestosterone production played an important role in androgenic alopecia. Many theories have been offered trying to explain baldness: stress, lack of vascularity, lack of innervation, overinnervation, insufficiency of vitamins and hormones, mental disturbances and bad eating habits. However, hair transplantation demonstrated conclusively that the scalp which produces hairs abundantly in some areas but not in others can support hair growth when hairs are grafted onto the bald areas.[11]

Baldness is still widely misunderstood. The process of balding is slow—not a general destruction, but a systematic involution of hair follicles culminating in follicles similar to those of the fetus, but there is no diminution in their absolute numbers. Regardless of how totally bald the scalp of a young person is, a seeding of quiescent terminal hair follicles can always be found. During balding, the scalp follicles progressively diminish in size over successive generations of hair cycles, eventually resembling growing vellus follicles. Baldness thus proceeds with exquisite order and uniformity over a long period of time.[12]

In every normal scalp there are 80–85% of hairs in anagen (80000–85000 hairs), 1–2% in catagen (1000–2000 hairs) and 10–20% in telogen (10000–20000 hairs). Practically all the hairs in a normal scalp biopsy are in anagen. Catagen is a rare finding, and an occasional follicle may be in telogen. Human scalp hairs, if more than 100 μm in diameter, have a medulla with a thick, more or less pigmented cortex, surrounded by the cuticle and encased in the three layers of internal root sheath. All this material forms on the hair matrix and moves upward at the rather uniform speed of 0.3–0.4 mm per day (about 1 cm per month). In catagen the entire lower part of the follicle, the cyclic or transient portion, undergoes complicated involuntary changes.

Hair diseases can be divided into those that lead to *deformed hairs*, with possible loss through breakage; and the *true alopecia*, in which hair is lost completely, either temporarily or permanently. In either case microscopic changes of the hair follicle may be expected.[13] Hair formation depends on a delicately balanced interaction between the dermal papilla and the hair matrix, and any major disturbance will lead to loss of hair. The initial assessment of alopecia should determine whether the hair follicles remain (non-cicatricial alopecia) with the potential for hair regrowth, or have been permanently lost (cicatricial alopecia).[13–18]

COMPONENTS OF A PHASE I AND PHASE II CLINICAL PROGRAMME (Establishing Safety and Efficacy)

There is an absence of published or approved guidelines for the evaluation of drugs affecting hair growth. It is, therefore, desirable that any clinical programme for a hair growth claim be discussed with the regulatory officials in the early stages of the clinical development programme. The following hair growth evaluation programme pertains to the development of a treatment for male pattern baldness (alopecia androgenetica, androgenic alopecia). Almost all adult males have some degree of thinning hair during their ageing process. It usually starts with the recession of the frontal hair line and can progress to the vertex and to the top of the scalp, with the hair intact at the sides and the occiput.[18,19] It is considered a hereditary condition and a polygenic or multifactorial mode of inheritance is suggested. The complexity of pattern baldness, lack of animal models, difficulties of interpretation and evaluation and lack of positive controls (comparators) mandates placebo-controlled studies in Phase II. Only one hair growth stimulating agent (topical minoxidil solution) so far has been approved in the US for male pattern baldness, which is a testimony to the difficulties and complexities we face in developing drugs affecting hair growth.

Accordingly, most of the published data are based on the experience obtained with the development of minoxidil (topical). For this reason the safety evaluations included a large battery of cardiovascular testing called for by the antihypertensive-vasodilator properties of minoxidil. For new agents with different mechanism(s) of action appropriate modifications in the investigative approach dictated by the characteristics of the test drug must be taken into consideration and be employed.

It should be emphasised that male pattern baldness should not be considered a pathological condition, and consequently both Phase I and Phase II studies deal with otherwise healthy individuals. However, male volunteers have to be selected with caution during enrolment into these studies. The investigator has to be familiarised with the pharmacology and the kinetics of the study drug obtained from *in vitro* and animal (*in vivo*) data (e.g. effects on vasodilation-hypertensive patients) and to select (and/or exclude) the right patient population for the study.

PHASE I STUDIES

Before broader Phase I safety studies are undertaken, the irritation, sensitisation and photoirritation properties of the topically applied test drug are established.

The Draize (Modified) Skin Sensitisation Study

The purpose of this double-blind, randomised, complete block-design study is to determine and compare the potential for irritation and sensitisation of the topically applied test drug (solution, gel or ointment) of different concentrations (e.g. 3% and 5%) and the vehicle (placebo) in a repeated insult patch test.[20] All healthy screened subjects simultaneously receive all treatments. Each subject has a series of patches, each containing one test solution, applied to their backs or upper arms three times weekly for 3 consecutive weeks. Each patch remains in place for 48–72 h.

Each patch size is evaluated for irritation prior to replacement patch application. Approximately 2 weeks after the sensitisation phase, challenge applications are made by applying test patches to a previously unpatched site. An evaluation of irritation and sensitisation is made for each test preparation at 48 h and 96 h post challenge. In addition, delayed-sensitisation readings are made to demonstrate delayed sensitivity.[20]

The Modified Photo-Draize Skin Sensitisation Study

This study determines and compares the irritation and photosensitisation potentials of topically applied solutions and the vehicle in a randomised, double-blind, complete block design trial in healthy screened subjects. The screened subjects are given applications of each test solution three times (3 successive days) weekly for 3 successive weeks on the back or arms. Each test area is irradiated with visible light each time a patch is changed. Two weeks later, challenge applications (two of each test solution) are made to two previously unpatched test sites. After 24 h patches are removed from one test area, the area is irradiated with visible light, and patches are reapplied. Ninety-six hours post challenge, both test sites are evaluated for irritation and for induction of photoallergic or allergic contact sensitisation to the solutions tested.[21]

Photoirritation (Phototoxicity) Study

This randomised, double-blind, complete block design trial is conducted to determine and compare the photoirritation (phototoxicity) potential of the test drug and the vehicle. All screened subjects simultaneously receive all treatments. Solution-soaked patches, two for each test solution, are applied for 1 h to test areas on the arms of each subject. Solutions (approximately 0.2 ml) are applied to Cellophane-stripped glistening skin. Test areas are separated so that one could be irradiated while the other is not. At 1 h one test site is irradiated, the other site serving as a control. Irritancy readings are made at 48 h post patch application.[22]

21 Day Cumulative Irritancy Potential

This randomised, double-blind, complete block design trial attempts to determine the relative irritancy potential of topically applied test solutions (two or more concentrations) as compared with that of the vehicle alone and with that of a hair tonic. Subjects (healthy males and females) simultaneously receive all treatments. Saturated patches with 0.2 ml of the test solutions (one test solution per patch) are secured to each subject's back with occlusive bandages. Fresh patches are applied each weekday and patch sites undergo evaluation each time the patch is removed. That provides the investigator with 15 irritancy scores over the 21 day course of study. Pairwise comparisons of test solutions are then made.[23]

PHARMACODYNAMIC STUDIES

Measuring Percutaneous Absorption of Test/Drug in Man

The percutaneous absorption and excretion of test drug solutions labelled with ^{14}C are measured in healthy bald adult male subjects.[24] These subjects are randomly assigned to the testing groups, and all receive nine topical applications of their assigned solution concentration to a bald area on the scalp, on study days 1 and 9. Urine and faeces are collected to measure excretion of radioactivity. Radioactivity from the skin surface and pillowcase washes is also recovered and measured.

On the morning of study day 1, the subjects report to the laboratory and each has 1 ml of radioactive test solution applied to 200 cm^2 on the bald scalp by a pipette. The material is spread evenly over the outlined area with a glass rod, which is saved and subsequently assayed for retained radioactivity. The subjects are instructed to avoid touching the treated area with their hands, or allowing hats or other objects to come into contact with the scalp. In addition, no washing of the application site is allowed until the subjects report back to the laboratory 24 h later. On days 2–8, the subjects themselves apply 1 ml of non-radioactive test formulation to the scalp each morning and evening. On the morning of day 9, the subjects report again to the laboratory and another 1 ml of radioactive test solution is applied. A 4 mm punch biopsy of the test site is performed immediately following the 24 h wash of the second application. The specimen is separated into epidermis and dermis by the technique of heat separation, and each is analysed for radioactive content.

The data from this study allow one to estimate the magnitude of absorption of the test drug of different concentrations under various clinical conditions.

Measuring Cutaneous Blood Flow in Man after Test Drug Application

If the assumed mechanism of action of the test drug is vasodilation, cutaneous blood flow post application of test drug is measured.

In this double-blind study the screened healthy, balding, male volunteers are randomly assigned to receive test drug applied topically to the scalp twice on successive days. The treatments used are different concentrations of test drug and a placebo control (vehicle). In all treatment groups cutaneous blood flow is measured by the following two non-invasive techniques: (1) the laser Doppler velocimetry (LDV) operating on the Doppler principle; (2) the Photopulse plethysmography (PPG) using a diode that emits infrared light and determines changes in blood volume passing through the microcirculation by the percentage of incident radiation absorbed. On study days 1 and 2 blood pressure and pulse rates are obtained before the drug is applied. Baseline measurement of blood flow in the scalp skin at the intended site of drug application is made with both techniques, LDV on one half of the scalp and PPG on the other half.

On day 1 the total 0.25 ml contents of the pipette containing the randomly assigned test drug is distributed uniformly over 100 cm^2 on each side of the bald scalp area. The solution is released slowly from the pipette, to avoid run-off and the need to rub it into the bald scalp with the fingers. A 15 min drying period is allowed after drug application before the recording begins. The LDV and PPG probes are then positioned on the scalp at the site of drug application. Cutaneous blood flow is recorded continuously for 40–60 min, and then intermittently for 4 h. Blood pressure and pulse rates are taken after the 4 h recording. Volunteers are asked not to wash their scalp prior to day 2. On day 2 vital signs and a baseline blood flow measurement are again obtained. This measurement serves as both the 24 h measurement for day 1 and the predrug measurement for day 2. The same randomly assigned formulation as on day 1 is applied to the same scalp site, and cutaneous blood flow is recorded as on day 1. Vital signs are again obtained after the 4 h session.[25]

Histologic Study of Male Pattern Baldness

The screened, bald, healthy male subjects are assigned at random to receive the test drug or the vehicle (placebo). A technician applies 1 ml of the assigned solution to the bald area of the subject's scalp in the morning and evening each day for 16 consecutive weeks. The medication is allowed to dry completely before the subject leaves the clinic. Evaluations are made through week 24.[26]

At the pretreatment examination all subjects should have normal blood chemistries, CBC, urinalysis, EKG, pulse rate and blood pressure. Blood and urinalysis specimens are taken again at weeks 4, 20 and 24; and an EKG is taken monthly. Blood pressure, pulse rate and body weight are checked daily for the first 2 weeks and then weekly. Blood levels for test drug are assayed pretrial and at weeks 2, 4, 8, 16 and 24.

A few hairs are plucked from the balding scalp of each subject pretrial and at weeks 12 and 16, or more often, and are examined under magnification for changes in shaft diameter and length, depth of hair roots and degree of pigmentation. A punch biopsy from the vertex or the parietal areas of the scalp is obtained with a No. 4 Baker disposable punch pretrial and at weeks 12 and 25 (9 weeks after the last application of medication). Ten normal control (also bald) subjects from the same population are also biopsied in this manner.

The punch-biopsied tissue cores are divided in a transverse plan at the approximate junction of dermis and subcutis. Cut surfaces are stained with aqueous eosin to ensure proper orientation during embedding and sectioning. Continuous serial sections are cut from all paraffin blocks. Microscopy is done with an American Optical Series Ten microscope. Quantitative measurements are done with an American Optical ocular micrometer specifically calibrated. Hair shaft diameters were measured to 0.001 mm.

Qualitatively, the presence or absence of follicular dysplasia, epidermal changes, sebaceous epithelial changes and vascular changes are followed and inflammation is evaluated as slight, moderate or marked. Hair shaft diameters are usually measured at the level of the sebaceous ducts or higher. Quantitative determinations include: (1) hair shaft diameter; (2) density or total follicular structures, total anagen follicles, total vellus follicles and total telogen germinal units (per mm^2) and; (3) percentage of telogen and vellus follicles. Detailed micrometric *in situ* measurements of transverse sections of human scalp hair have been reported,[27] and other different histopathological techniques of biopsied scalp tissue can be employed.[13,14]

Systemic Safety and Local Tolerance

To evaluate the systemic safety and local tolerance of the test drug, up to four times the usual dosage is applied for 14 days up to eight times daily to the scalps and chests of healthy bald male subjects in a randomised, double-blind trial. For the scalp evaluation, males in good health with early, progressive, premature thinning of the scalp hair (male pattern baldness Type III,

Hamilton's Scale[19]) are selected; for the chest evaluation, healthy, adult male volunteers with non-hairy chests are selected.

A pioneer step-up design is employed, and no new group is started until safety is shown for the previous study group. Subjects are randomised within each group and test drug application times are as follows:

two times/day: 8 a.m., 8 p.m.
four times/day: 8 a.m., 12 noon, 4 p.m., 8 p.m.
six times/day: 8 a.m., 10.25 a.m., 12.50 p.m., 3.15 p.m., 5.35 p.m., 8 p.m.
eight times/day: 8 a.m., 9.45 a.m., 11.25 a.m., 1.05 p.m., 2.50 p.m., 4.35 p.m., 6.20 p.m., 8 p.m.

All volunteers must not have had prior allergy or intolerance to the test drug. There are no restrictions placed on dietary intake except when fasting is required for laboratory tests. In addition, all subjects receive fluids ad lib and smoking is permitted if it was the normal custom of the volunteer. If the test drug has vasodilatory properties, the exclusion criteria should include hypertension (with sitting blood pressure above 140/90); major medical and mental illnesses; and concomitant dermatological disorders of the scalp. The volunteer should not be on any form of medication for 1 week prior to the study or during the study.

Extensive sampling for bioavailability of absorbed and excreted test drug is also carried out. Standard laboratory parameters are measured on days −1 and 14 (haematology, serum chemistries, urinalysis, vital signs, body weight). If the drug under investigation has vasodilatory properties, cardiac function is measured before and after applications of drug on day 14 by echocardiograms, electrocardiographic analysis and chest X-rays, and frequent vital-signs measurements and body-weight monitoring are performed.

The biopharmaceutical serum and urine data are compared with the safety (tolerance) data. The accumulation of the test drug in the skin and absorption of the test drug through the skin from the two different areas (scalp and chest) are assessed and compared.

PHASE II STUDIES

Dose–Response Study in Male Pattern Baldness

Healthy men with either pattern III vertex or pattern IV male pattern baldness are selected. A history, physical examination, electrocardiogram, chest X-ray, M-mode electrocardiogram (for vasodilatory agents) and laboratory evaluations (haematology, serum chemistries including thyroid function test and urinalysis) are obtained prior to inclusion and repeated at 2 and 6 months post study start. Test drug blood levels are assessed at 2 and 6 weeks post study start. The age of the subject is about 18–49 years, with the duration of baldness from 12 months to 30 years and the vertex balding area (elliptic or circular shape) size varying from 15 to 120 cm.[28]

In this double-blind study, the subjects are randomly assigned to one of the treatment groups, and the test drugs of different concentrations or the placebo vehicle are applied to the bald area of the scalp using a Dab-o-matic calibrated or bottle or calibrated dropper. Treatments are applied twice daily for 6 months.

Efficacy is determined by four methods.

(1) Counting the vellus hair, non-vellus hair and total hairs always by the same evaluator within a target 1 inch diameter on the mid-vertex area at baseline and at each subsequent visit.

(2) The two longest diameters (X and Y) of the vertex balding area are measured at baseline and at 6 months post study start.

(3) At completion of the study (6 months) the subject and the investigator assess the amount of hair growth, using the scale: no growth, minimal hair growth (apparent hair growth over baseline), moderate hair growth (obvious new hair growth) or dense hair growth.

(4) Shedding is assessed on a monthly basis by the subjects and standardised photographs are taken monthly to corroborate the subjective assessments.

Safety assessment (systemic and local) are done at or closely before enrolment and repeated at 2 and 6 month intervals as listed in the first paragraph of this section. In addition, a correlation between the efficacy data (stimulation of hair growth) and pharmacokinetic data is assessed.

Among the concentrations of test drug studied, one concentration is chosen for use in later trials. That concentration is based on a statistically significant increase in the evaluated efficacy parameters (in total and non-vellus target area hair counts) at study completion time (6 months) with acceptable safety.

Safety and Efficacy of Test Drug versus Placebo

The purpose of this study is to determine efficacy and safety of the test drug in the treatment of male pattern baldness as compared with placebo (vehicle). Duration of the study is 8 months and the test drug and placebo are randomly assigned.[28-31]

Inclusion criteria: Male subjects with Type III or Type IV vertex alopecia (by Hamilton's Scale),[19] with non-vellus hair present throughout the bald area (Type IV must have a band of hair growth across the entire bridge of the scalp). The balding vertex area should be 3–10 cm in transverse diameter and 4 cm in vertical diameter. Further inclusion criteria are: good health, dark hair and normal electrocardiogram.

Exclusion criteria: In addition to those specified under 'Systemic Safety and Local Tolerance' known hypersensitivity to test drug or class of similar drugs; non-compliant subjects; female patients; concomitant therapy with drugs with pharmacological activity similar to that of the test drug, steroids, cytotoxic agents, hair-growth remedies; subjects who participated previously in a similar study or are participating currently in an investigational drug study.

Efficacy is measured by the following methods: the mean change of non-vellus hair counts from week 1 to week 32 (8 months); investigators' and patients' subjective evaluations of visible hair growth; standardised photographs; results of the pull test. A 1.0 cm square area is permanently marked (tattooed in) and the non-vellus hair in that designated area is clipped and counted at weeks 0, 16 and 32. Also, the degree of hair shading is assessed by the hair pull test, grasping 15–40 hairs at three distinct areas adjacent to the test area on the scalp and gently tugging at every visit, and counted. If hair growth is noticed by the patient or investigator during the study period on other parts of the subject's body than the scalp, this should also be recorded.

Safety measurements: Monitoring of blood pressure (seated) and pulse rate, body weight, and electrocardiographic evaluation obtained at 0, 8, 16, 24 and 32 weeks. Clinical assessment (complete physical examination before and after week 32, including a detailed evaluation of the scalp), laboratory evaluations (haematology, blood chemistries, urinalysis at weeks 0, 8, 16 and 32) and serum drug level evaluations at weeks 8, 16 and 32.

The subjects at week 0 are instructed about the frequency and method of test drug applications (one or more times daily); about the amount of application with a calibrated dropper (1 ml or more); about the defined area of application; and about the spread of the medication on the applied area (centrifugally with one fingertip). The medication should be applied 60–90 min after washing the hair.

Other study designs use evaluation procedures similar to those above with the subjects applying the vehicle (placebo) for 4 months and then crossing over to the test drug for the full 12 months medication period.[31]

SUMMARY

Phase I studies for the evaluation of drugs affecting hair growth should establish the systemic safety and local tolerance in healthy bald male volunteers (male pattern baldness, androgenic alopecia). Special evaluations can be included in these studies if the character of the test drug warrants it (e.g. scalp blood flow studies if the test drug is a vasodilator). In Phase II studies the efficacy, dose response, pharmacokinetic parameters, and systemic and local safety are evaluated.

The studies described here are 'tailored' for male pattern baldness, but with modifications they could be employed in the evaluation of drugs for female pattern baldness and also for alopecia areata when taking into consideration the different aetiology, course, prognosis and some other specific characteristics of these alopecias. In all of these studies co-operation with statisticians, regulatory agencies, pathologists, dermatopathologists, experienced clinical investigators, pharmacologists and pharmacokineticists is necessary in the early stage of planning of these studies. This team approach is imperative, because of lack of experience with drugs affecting hair growth, because of inexperience and difficulties of interpretation of the results of these studies and also because of the difficulties in quantifying hair growth. Different methods can now be used to evaluate these results, and with the 'explosion' of hair growth research in the last decade, there are now available better and more sophisticated approaches[26-45] used by a large pool of experienced clinical investigators.

REFERENCES

1. Dry, F. W. (1926). The coat of the mouse (*Mus musculus*). *J. Genet.*, **16**, 287–340
2. Chase, H. B. (1954). Growth of the hair. *Physiol. Rev.*, **34**, 113–26
3. Binet, D., Dompmartin-Pernot, D. and Aron-Brunetiere, R. (1981). An objective approach of the diagnosis of diffuse alopecia: The trichogram. In *Hair Research—Status and Future Aspects*, Ed. Orfanos, Montagna, Stuttgen; Springer-Verlag, Berlin, Heidelberg, New York, pp. 277–82
4. Chase, H. B. (1949). Greying of hair. I. Effects produced by single doses of X-rays on mice. *J. Morphol.*, **84**, 57–80
5. Cohen, J. (1965). The dermal papilla. In Lyne, A. G. and Short, B. F. (Eds.), *Biology of the Skin and Hair Growth*. Angus and Robertson, Sydney, pp. 183–99
6. Oliver, R. F. (1966). Whisker growth after removal of the dermal papilla and lengths of follicle in the hooded rat. *J. Embryol. Exp. Morphol.*, **15**, 331–47
7. Hamilton, J. B. (1942). Male hormone is prerequisite and incitant in common baldness. *Am. J. Anat.*, **71**, 451–80
8. Takayasu, S. and Adachi, K. (1972). The conversion of testosterone to 17-β-hydroxy-5a-androstan-3-one(dihydrotestosterone) by human hair follicles. *J. Clin. Endocrinol. Metab.*, **34**, 1098–101
9. Takashima, I. and Montagna, W. (1971). Studies of common baldness of the stump-tailed macaque (*Macaca speciosa*). VI. The effect of testosterone on common baldness. *Arch. Dermatol.*, **103**, 537–44
10. Price, V. H. (1975). Testosterone metabolism in the skin. *Arch. Dermatol.*, **111**, 1496–502
11. Orentreich, N. (1959). Autographs in alopecias and other selected dermatological conditions. *Ann. N.Y. Acad. Sci.*, **83**, 463–79
12. Montagna, W. and Carlissle, X. (1981). Consideration on hair research and hair growth. In *Hair Research—Status and Future Aspects*. Eds. Orfanos, Montagna and Stuttgen; Springer-Verlag, Berlin, Heidelberg, New York, pp. 3–11
13. Pinkus, H. (1980). Alopecia. Clinicopathologic correlations. *Int. J. Dermatol.*, **19**, 245–53
14. Abell, E. and Carry, M. M. (1986). The pathologic effect of minoxidil in male pattern alopecia. *J. Invest Dermatol.*, **86**, 459 (abstract)
15. Burton, J. L. *et al.* (1979). Male pattern alopecia and masculinity. *Br. J. Dermatol.*, **100**, 567–71
16. Kligman, A. M. (1961). Pathologic dynamics of human hair loss. *Arch. Dermatol.*, **83**, 175–98
17. Landow, R. K. (1983). *Handbook of Dermatology Treatment*. Jones Medical Publications, Greenbrae, California, pp. 159–60
18. Smith, M. A. and Wells, R. S. (1964). Male type alopecia, alopecia areata and normal hair in women. *Arch. Dermatol.*, **89**, 95–8
19. Hamilton, J. B. (1951). Patterned loss of hair in man: types and incidence. *Ann. N.Y. Acad. Sci.*, **53**, 708–11
20. Marzulli, F. N. and Maibach, H. I. (1977). Predictions of contact dermatology in man. In *Dermatology and Pharmacology*. Halsted Press, New York

21. Draize, J. H., Woodards, G. and Calvary, H. D. (1944). Methods for the study of irritation and toxicity of substances applied topically to the skin and mucous membranes. *J. Pharmacol. Exp. Ther.*, **83**, 377–90
22. Marzulli, F. N. and Maibach, H. I. (1970). Perfume phototoxicity. *J. Soc. Cosmet. Chem.*, **21**, 695–715
23. Philips, L. 2nd, Sainberg, J., Maibach, H. I. and Akers, W. A. (1972). A comparison of rabbit and human skin response to certain irritants. *Toxicol. Appl. Pharm.*, **21**, 369–82
24. Franz, T. J. (1985). Percutaneous absorption of minoxidil in man. *Arch. Dermatol.*, **121**, 203–6
25. Wester, R. C., Maibach, H. I., Guy, R. H. and Novak, E. (1984). Minoxidil stimulates cutaneous blood flow in human balding scalps: pharmacodynamic measured by laser Doppler velocimetry and photopulse plethysmography. *J. Invest. Dermatol.*, **82**, 515–17
26. Headington, J. T. and Novak, E. (1984). Clinical and histologic studies of male pattern baldness treated with topical minoxidil. *Curr. Ther. Res.*, **36**, 1098–106
27. Headington, J. T. (1984). Transverse microscopic anatomy of the human scalp: a basis for a morphometric approach to disorders of the hair follicle. *Arch. Dermatol.*, **120**, 449–56
28. Olsen, E. A., DeLong, E. R. and Weiner, M. S. (1986). Dose-response study of topical minoxidil in male pattern baldness. *J. Am. Acad. Dermatol.*, **15**, 30–37
29. Storer, J. S., Brzuskiewicz, J., Floyd, H. and Rice, J. C. (1986). Topical minoxidil for male pattern baldness. *Am. J. Med. Sci.*, **291**, 328–33
30. DeVillez, R. L. (1985). Topical minoxidil therapy in hereditary androgenic alopecia. *Arch. Dermatol.*, **121**, 197–202
31. Olsen, E. A., Weiner, M. S., DeLong, E. R. and Pinnell, S. R. (1985). Topical minoxidil in early male pattern baldness. *J. Am. Acad. Dermatol.*, **13**, 185–92
32. Kvedar, J. C. and Baden, H. P. (1987). Topical minoxidil in the treatment of male pattern alopecia. *Pharmacotherapy*, **7**, 191–7
33. Vanderveen, E. E., Ellis, C. N., Kang, S. *et al.* (1984). Topical minoxidil for hair regrowth. *J. Am. Acad. Dermatol.*, **11**, 416–21
34. Novak, E., Franz, T. J., Headington, J. T. *et al.* (1985). Topically applied minoxidil in baldness. *Int. J. Dermatol.*, **24**, 82–7
35. Weiss, V. C., West, D. P. and Muller, C. E. (1981). Topical minoxidil in alopecia areata. *J. Am. Acad. Dermatol.*, **5**, 224–6
36. Baden, H. P. and Kubilus, J. (1983). Effect of minoxidil on cultured keratinocytes. *J. Invest. Dermatol.*, **81**, 558–60
37. Kubilus, J., Kvedar, J. C. and Baden, H. P. (1987). Effect of minoxidil on pre- and postconfluent keratinocytes. *J. Am. Acad. Dermatol.*, **16**, 648–52
38. Cohen, R. L., Alves, M. E. A. F., Weiss, V. C., West, D. P. and Chambers, D. A. (1984). Direct effect of minoxidil on erpidermal cells in culture. *J. Invest Dermatol.*, **82**, 90–3
39. Galbraith, G. M. P. and Thiers, B. H. (1985). *In vitro* suppression of human lymphocyte activity by minoxidil. *Int. J. Dermatol.*, **24**, 249–51
40. Murad, S., Clayton, J. and Pinnell, S. R. (1986). Selective depression of lysyl hydroxylase activity in human skin fibroblasts by minoxidil [abstract]. *J. Invest. Dermatol.*, **86**, 496
41. Uno, H., Cappas, A. and Schlagel, C. (1985). Cyclic dynamics of hair follicles and the effects of minoxidil on the bald scalps of stumptailed macaques. *Am. J. Dermatopathol.*, **7** (3), 283–97
42. Uno, H., Cappas, A. and Brigham, P. (1987). Action of topical minoxidil in the bald stump-tailed macaque. *J. Am. Acad. Dermatol.*, **16**, 657–68

43. Roenigk, H. H. and Kuruvilla, S. (1987). Topical minoxidil for male pattern alopecia in two sets of twins. *Cutis*, **39**, 329–32
44. Rietschel, R. L. and Duncan, S. H. (1987). Safety and efficacy of topical minoxidil in the management of androgenetic alopecia. *J. Am. Acad. Dermatol.*, **16**, 677–85
45. Shupack, J. L., Kassimir, J. J., Thirumoorthy, T. *et al.* (1987). Dose-response study of topical minoxidil in male pattern alopecia. *J. Am. Acad. Dermatol.*, **16**, 673–6

XII
Assessment of Drugs Used for the Treatment of Metabolic Disorders

45
Hypolipidaemic Drugs

R. H. Jay and D. J. Betteridge

Dept of Medicine, University College and Middlesex School of Medicine, The Rayne Institute, London WC1E 6JJ, UK

INTRODUCTION

Coronary heart disease (CHD) is the principal cause of death in the Western world, accounting for about one-third of the total mortality. The probability of developing CHD is increased in the presence of certain risk factors. A large number of these are statistical associations, and better termed 'risk markers', but the major factors thought to play a causal role in the underlying processes of atherogenesis and thrombosis include hypercoagulability, diabetes, hyperinsulinaemia, smoking, hypertension and hyperlipidaemia. These factors are interrelated and often coexist.

The role of hyperlipidaemia in coronary atherosclerosis may be better defined by considering the separate lipoprotein classes, the properties of which are summarised for reference in Table 45.1. Low-density lipoprotein (LDL) is the major carrier of plasma cholesterol and is responsible for its atherogenic effect. Conversely high-density lipoprotein (HDL), which normally carries 20–30% of plasma cholesterol, is inversely related to atherosclerotic risk in epidemiological studies and is thought to protect against atheroma. The role of triglyceride is more controversial, since its major carrier, very-low-density lipoprotein (VLDL), varies in concentration inversely with HDL, a factor not always taken into account in studies showing an association between triglycerides and CHD. However, it has been implicated as an independent coronary risk factor in some studies (Castelli, 1986).

Chylomicrons, the carriers of dietary triglyceride, are not associated with atherosclerosis, even when present in great excess. The most important complication of severe hypertriglyceridaemia is acute pancreatitis, which is associated with levels above about 11 mmol/l. Intermediate-density lipoproteins (IDL), the remnants of catabolism of chylomicrons and VLDL, are normally cleared efficiently from plasma and therefore present only at low concentration, but they build up in the rare type III hyperlipoproteinaemia which is associated with premature atherosclerosis, especially of the cerebral and peripheral vessels.

Apolipoprotein (apo) B100 is the structural apoprotein associated with the VLDL–IDL–LDL series of lipoproteins and may be a better predictor of CHD than plasma cholesterol (Anon., 1988). Apo A1, the structural apoprotein of the HDL series, correlates inversely with CHD risk. More

Table 45.1 Lipoprotein classification

Property	Chylomicrons	VLDL	IDL	LDL	HDL
Diameter (nm)	80–500	30–80	25–35	20	10
Electrophoresis	Origin	Pre-beta	Broad beta	Beta	Alpha
Density	<0.95	0.95–1.006	1.006–1.019	1.019–1.063	1.063–1.21
Principal core lipid	Exogenous triglyceride	Triglyceride, cholesterol esters	Cholesterol esters, triglyceride	Cholesterol esters, triglyceride	Cholesterol esters
Major apoproteins	AI, AII, B48, CII, CIII	B100, CII, CIII	B, CIII, E	B100	AI, AII, CIII
Effect on atheroma	Nil	+	+++	+++	Protects
Drug treatment	Diet: drugs ineffective	Fibrates, nicotinic acid, omega-3 fish oils	Fibrates, nicotinic acid	Resins, nicotinic acid, fibrates, probucol	Fibrates, nicotinic acid, omega-3 fish oils and resins raise. Probucol lowers

recently Lp(a), a variant of LDL with an additional apoprotein, apo(a), attached to the apo B via a disulphide bridge, has been shown to correlate with CHD (Rhoads *et al.*, 1986) and interest in this particle is growing. The effects of lipid-lowering therapy on Lp(a) have been little studied.

The potential for reduction of coronary risk by lipid lowering has been demonstrated by a number of interventional studies which have been recently reviewed (Thompson, 1986), but none of the currently available lipid-lowering drugs is ideal.

LIPID-LOWERING DRUGS

Since the aim of lipid-lowering therapy is to reduce the risk of CHD, or to delay its onset, any potential drug must be convenient, well-tolerated, effective and safe over long periods of treatment. In addition, it must not interact with drugs used in the treatment of CHD, other conditions predisposing to atherosclerosis or causes of secondary hyperlipidaemia (Table 45.2), and must not adversely affect other factors in the patient's risk profile. The latter has been a problem with antihypertensive drugs. Thiazide diuretics and beta blockers have theoretical disadvantages due to their adverse effects on lipid and glucose metabolism, and this may account to some extent for the failure of many blood-pressure-lowering trials to demonstrate a beneficial effect on the rate of CHD. Conversely, lipid-lowering drugs affecting adipose tissue lipolysis may increase insulin sensitivity and have beneficial effects on blood coagulation and fibrinolysis.

PLASMA LIPOPROTEIN ESTIMATION

Blood for lipoprotein analysis is obtained after an overnight fast of 14 h to ensure that triglyceride levels are not elevated by postprandial chylomicronaemia. During this period water may be taken, but caffeine-containing drinks are forbidden, since these can affect the lipoprotein profile. Assessment should be based on at least two separate measurements in view of the fluctuation in levels from day to day. Plasma protein changes associated with posture and venous occlusion can significantly affect lipoprotein levels, and therefore the circumstances of venepuncture must be standardised, as should

Table 45.2 Causes of secondary hyperlipidaemia

Dietary	Alcohol
Diabetes	Drugs
Hypothyroidism	thiazide diuretics
Obesity	beta blockers
Chronic renal failure	oral contraceptives
Nephrotic syndrome	isotretinoin
Dysglobulinaemia	

the choice between serum and EDTA-anticoagulated plasma. Samples are usually obtained after sitting for 10 min and venous occlusion released after the vein is entered and before withdrawing the blood.

Clinical laboratories without facilities for ultracentrifugation commonly measure total cholesterol, triglyceride and HDL cholesterol after precipitation of the apo-B-containing lipoproteins with heparin and manganese (Warnick and Albers, 1978). A similar precipitation method using phosphotungstate had to be modified to avoid precipitating part of the HDL fraction, and comparison of several precipitation procedures reveals the importance of details of technique (Warnick *et al.*, 1985). LDL cholesterol can be calculated by the Friedewald formula (Friedewald *et al.*, 1972):

$$\text{LDL cholesterol} = \text{total cholesterol} - \text{HDL cholesterol} - \frac{\text{triglyceride}}{K}$$

K is 2.19 when the units are mmol/l and 5 when the units are mg/dl. The formula assumes a constant ratio of cholesterol and triglyceride in VLDL, and becomes inaccurate when triglyceride concentration exceeds 5 mmol/l.

HDL_2 and HDL_3 subfractions may be separated by a double-precipitation technique (Warnick *et al.*, 1982), but further analysis involves complete separation of lipoproteins by ultracentrifugation (Lindgren *et al.*, 1972). Measurement of apoproteins A1, B and Lp(a) in whole serum gives additional measures of atherosclerotic risk.

Detailed analysis of lipoprotein subclasses may be performed by rate-zonal ultracentrifugation (Patsch *et al.*, 1974). Since there is a continuum of lipoprotein densities, this technique gives more detailed information on the distribution of lipoproteins within each class. Complementary information may be obtained by use of apoprotein analysis to allow a distinction to be made between a change in particle size and particle numbers. Apoprotein B100, the main structural lipoprotein of the VLDL–IDL–LDL series, remains constant during the metabolism of a particle. Therefore, a change in the apo B content of a fraction obtained by ultracentrifugation implies a change in particle numbers.

CHOICE OF SUBJECTS

The effects of drugs on the lipoprotein profile vary according to the abnormality present. For example, the percentage reduction in triglyceride levels achieved by fibrates increases with higher initial levels. These drugs lower the LDL cholesterol in hypercholesterolaemia; but when used for hypertriglyceridaemia, the LDL cholesterol may actually rise. Therefore, early studies in normal volunteers may not reflect the response of hyperlipidaemic patients. When the latter are employed, they must represent a homogeneous diagnostic group, and should be screened for causes of secondary hyperlipidaemia (Table 45.2), especially diabetes and hypothyroidism, which are common and often unsuspected.

Hyperlipidaemic subjects may be selected in terms of either the lipoprotein pattern or the underlying diagnostic group (Table 45.3). The latter is preferable in the early phase of drug evaluation, since similar lipoprotein profiles may result from differing mechanisms and therefore respond differently to treatment. 'Common' or 'polygenic' hyperlipidaemias, representing the upper end of the population lipoprotein distribution, make up a heterogeneous group, and some patients with specific inherited disorders may be included in error if family screening has not revealed a characteristic pattern.

The commonest inherited disorder is familial combined hyperlipidaemia. These subjects vary in their lipoprotein pattern, both within families and within individuals over time, and the diagnosis depends on family screening. It is, therefore, difficult to establish strict diagnostic criteria suitable for use in clinical trials.

A more easily defined diagnostic group is familial hypercholesterolaemia, which may be characterised by the finding of a total cholesterol above 7.5 mmol/l, due to raised LDL cholesterol, and the presence of tendon xanthomas in the patient or affected family member. This condition occurs with a frequency of 1 in 500, and represents a significant proportion of attenders at lipid clinics.

Hypertriglyceridaemia is more variable in extent than hypercholesterolaemia, with levels ranging from 2.3 mmol/l to 75 mmol/l or more in some cases. It is more dependent on environmental influences such as diet and alcohol intake, and a high proportion of cases of moderate hypertriglyceridaemia (2.3–5.6 mmol/l) have an underlying cause such as diabetes, alcohol excess or obesity. Wider variations in both pretreatment levels and response to treatment will be seen in this group than in hypercholesterolaemia.

DIET

Diet is the major environmental factor influencing plasma lipoprotein levels and its modification is the first line of treatment in all types of hyperlipidaemia (Ad Hoc Committee, 1984). The major dietary determinants of plasma cholesterol are the amount and fatty acid type of dietary triglyceride. The effect of individual fatty acids on plasma cholesterol still remains to be fully delineated. The conventional wisdom that saturated fats raise cholesterol and polyunsaturates lower it has been challenged by recent studies of monounsaturates and individual saturated fatty acids (Bonanome and Grundy, 1988).

Dietary cholesterol intake may also affect plasma cholesterol, and cholesterol restriction represents part of the lipid-lowering diet (Table 45.4). Dietary treatment is usually pursued alone for 3–6 months before adding drugs, and it is important that patients be on a stable diet before entry into a trial.

Therefore, during treatment the diet should be assessed to ensure a constant food energy intake, total fat intake, ratio between fatty acid types (saturates/polyunsaturates/mono-unsaturates), and cholesterol intake. The

Table 45.3 Primary hyperlipidaemias

Condition	Prevalence	Lipoproteins	Typical lipid levels (mmol/l)	Atherosclerosis	Remarks
Familial hypercholesterolaemia (heterozygous)	1:500	LDL ↑ VLDL→ or ↑ HDL→ or ↓	Cholesterol 7.5–15 Triglyceride <5	+++	Tendon xanthomas, corneal arcus
Familial combined hyperlipidaemia	1:200	VLDL and LDL ↑ or → HDL→ or ↓	Cholesterol 6.5–10 Triglyceride 2.5–12	++	Lipoprotein pattern varies within family
Remnant (type III) hyperlipidaemia	1:10,000	IDL ↑ HDL→ or ↓	Cholesterol 9–14 Triglyceride 9–14	+++	Palmar and tuberous xanthomas, cerebral and peripheral atheroma
Familial hypertriglyceridaemias	Unknown	VLDL ↑ Chylomicrons→ or ← HDL→ or ↓	Cholesterol <12 Triglyceride 6–250	±	Several types: eruptive xanthomas, lipaemia retinalis, pancreatitis
'Polygenic' hypercholesterolaemia		LDL ↑ HDL→ or ↓	Cholesterol 6.5–9 Triglyceride normal	+	Frequency depends on population and definition
'Polygenic' hypertriglyceridaemia		VLDL ↑ HDL→ or ↓	Cholesterol normal Triglyceride 5–10	?+	As above

Table 45.4   American Heart Association dietary phases

Phase I	30% calories as fat; equal proportions of saturated, mono-unsaturated and polyunsaturated; under 300 mg cholesterol
Phase II	25% calories as fat; equal proportions of fatty acid types; 200–250 mg cholesterol
Phase III	20% calories as fat; equal proportions of fatty acid types; 100–150 mg cholesterol

latter varies widely from day to day, and therefore accurate assessment requires analysis of several days' weighed dietary inventory. In practice a 3 day estimated record is commonly used, since the aim is to ensure consistency rather than analyse dietary composition in detail.

DURATION OF TREATMENT

Since lipid-lowering therapy is a long-term preventative treatment, the speed of the fall in plasma lipids is seldom of practical concern. The action of fibrates on triglyceride levels takes only a few days, while probucol may take several months to reach its full activity in reducing plasma cholesterol. In clinical practice it is usual to monitor response after 1–3 months. Therefore, the length of a trial period must depend upon the mechanism of action and the results of animal studies. A suggested minimum is 4 weeks, to allow repeated lipoprotein assessments and to allow a stable plateau of response to be achieved.

Similar considerations apply to the washout phase between treatments in a crossover study and the initial period of withdrawal of previous therapy. For resins and fibrates a month is adequate, but probucol accumulates in body fat and requires at least 3 months' washout.

ETHICAL CONSIDERATIONS

Current lipid-lowering drugs have been shown to reduce the incidence of coronary events over as little as 5 years (Thompson, 1986; Frick *et al.*, 1987) in populations with moderate hyperlipidaemia. The benefit is presumed to be correspondingly higher in more severe disorders such as familial hyper-cholesterolaemia, and the use of placebo over periods of several months cannot be justified. Although the risk of physical harm is probably small, the psychological effect on the patient's perception of the importance of treatment may be considerable. Treatment withdrawal should, therefore, be kept to the minimum necessary to obtain baseline data, and comparisons should be made with baseline levels and existing therapy rather than placebo when studying subjects with severe lipid abnormalities.

ADVERSE EFFECTS

Table 45.5 lists the principal side-effects of lipid-lowering drugs in current use. Many of these are troublesome and reduce compliance in long-term treatment, while some are potentially dangerous. Prolongation of the Q–T interval on the ECG may predispose to ventricular arrhythmias in patients with pre-existing heart disease. Although this has not been reported in humans taking probucol, cases have been reported in non-human primates. Q–T prolongation is easily missed on routine reading of an ECG and specific measurements should be made if this possible side-effect is suspected. Similarly, post-dose hypotension is potentially hazardous in patients with heart disease and should be specifically assessed when drugs cause vasodilation.

Muscle pains or elevations of plasma levels of muscle enzymes may occur in patients taking fibrates or HMG CoA reductase inhibitors, both of which inhibit cholesterol synthesis. Severe rhabdomyolysis resulting in renal failure has been reported in patients taking lovastatin in conjunction with immuno-suppressive treatment following heart transplantation. Raised plasma levels of liver enzymes also occur with several drugs, and therefore monitoring of both liver and muscle enzymes is important.

Cholelithiasis is common in hypertriglyceridaemia, and an increased rate of cholecystectomy was seen in patients on active treatment in one long-term trial of clofibrate (Committee of Principal Investigators, 1978). The potential effect of a drug on gallstone formation may be assessed by measurement of the cholesterol saturation of bile obtained from the intubated duodenum after stimulation with cholecystokinin. Cholesterol, phospholipids and bile acid concentrations are measured and saturation is derived from tables (Carey, 1978).

Another potentially serious long-term side-effect is cataract. This was originally noted with triparanol (Laughlin and Carey, 1962), which inhibited cholesterol synthesis at a late stage in the pathway and led to accumulation of desmosterol and other intermediates in the lens. More recently a small,

Table 45.5   Adverse effects

Drug	Effect
Resins	Gastrointestinal
HMG CoA reductase inhibitors	Gastrointestinal, raised liver enzymes, myositis, rashes, headache
Nicotinic acid	Gastrointestinal, raised liver enzymes, flushing, rashes, hypotension, glucose intolerance
Fibrates	Gastrointestinal, raised liver enzymes, gallstones, myositis, impotence, hair loss, rashes
Probucol	Gastrointestinal, impotence, rashes, headache, Q–T interval prolongation on ECG

non-significant excess of cataract surgery was seen in the group treated with gemfibrozil in the Helsinki heart study (Frick *et al.*, 1987), and very high doses of lovastatin have been associated with cataract formation in dogs (Illingworth, 1986). It may be that any drug affecting cholesterol synthesis adversely affects metabolism in the lens, which is isolated from plasma as a source of cholesterol. Drug licensing authorities will therefore require evidence that this has been sought in trials of new agents. Routine ophthalmoscopy is inadequate for early detection of this problem, and the pattern of any lens opacities should be carefully recorded by an ophthalmologist before treatment and again periodically on therapy.

Finally, drugs interfering with cholesterol synthesis may theoretically affect steroid hormone production by reducing the supply of cholesterol to the synthetic pathway. This should become apparent during maximal stimulation of hormone production, an approach used to assess the safety of lovastatin (Illingworth and Corbin, 1985).

MECHANISMS OF ACTION

With early lipid-lowering drugs empirical use was followed later by elucidation of mechanisms of action. With increased understanding of lipoprotein metabolism, modern drug development is targeted at specific steps in the metabolic pathways. Some regulatory steps which are targets for present or future agents are listed in Table 45.6. This final section outlines some of the methods used for studying mechanisms of currently available agents in humans.

Table 45.6 Sites of action

Process	Targets
1. ↓ Cholesterol synthesis	HMG CoA reductase
	Mevalonate pyrophosphate dehydrogenase
2. ↑ Bile salt production	Enterohepatic recirculation
	Cholesterol 7α-hydroxylase
3. ↓ Cholesterol absorption	Pancreatic lipase
	Micelle formation
	Uptake into mucosal cell
	Acyl CoA: acyltransferase
4. ↑ LDL clearance	LDL receptor (direct action or secondary to 1 and 2 above)
5. ↓ VLDL secretion	Phosphotidate phosphohydrolase
	NEFA release from adipose tissue lipolysis
6. ↑ VLDL catabolism	Lipoprotein lipase
7. ↑ HDL maturation	Lecithin: cholesterol acyltransferase

Clearly, changes in both production and removal of a lipoprotein may alter its plasma concentration and these may be assessed by use of radioactive tracers. In the case of HDL this distinction is especially important, since one possible mechanism for its protective effect is its role in reverse cholesterol transport, and raising plasma levels by inhibiting its catabolism may theoretically be counterproductive. Saku *et al.* (1985) demonstrated that gemfibrozil increased apo AI and apo AII turnover by labelling patient's own HDL and measuring the levels and specific activity of the apoproteins.

Grundy *et al.* (1981), in their studies of the metabolic effects of nicotinic acid, used ^{3}H-labelled glycerol as a substrate for triglyceride synthesis and incorporation into VLDL. In order to eliminate effects of dietary carbohydrate and fat intake on VLDL production, subjects were given a fat-free, mildly hypocaloric liquid diet for 36 h before the [^{3}H]-glycerol injection and during the 48 h period of blood sampling. VLDL was separated by ultracentrifugation and its activity and lipid composition were assayed.

VLDL production is stimulated by an increase in levels of non-esterified fatty acids (NEFA), in blood entering the liver. Plasma levels of NEFA vary according to the nutritional state, and release from adipose tissue may be stimulated by adrenaline. Therefore, conditions of measurement must be standardised as in the study of Rifkind (1966), in which both fasting and adrenaline-stimulated levels were measured in relation to clofibrate therapy.

Adams *et al.* (1974) and Kissebah *et al.* (1974) have used an infusion of ^{14}C-labelled palmitate to assess the metabolism of triglycerides and NEFA. This allows calculation of the rate of clearance of NEFA from the plasma concentration and activity at equilibrium during a 2 h infusion. After discontinuing the infusion, the clearance of label from lipoproteins containing endogenous triglyceride could be followed. Clearance of infused intralipid may be similarly used as a measure of catabolism of lipoproteins containing exogenous triglyceride.

Both chylomicrons and VLDL are catabolised by the endothelial enzymes lipoprotein lipase and hepatic lipase. These may be detached from their endothelial binding sites by injection of heparin 40 u/kg intravenously and the lipolytic activity of plasma obtained 10 min after the injection may be assayed. The activity of the two enzymes may be distinguished by inactivating one with a specific antibody or after separation by affinity chromatography (Eisenberg *et al.*, 1984).

The uptake of LDL into cells occurs via both a high-affinity receptor and an independent scavenger mechanism. The two pathways may be distinguished by examining the clearance rates of both the native particle and LDL which has been chemically modified to block recognition of lysine or arginine residues by the LDL receptor. The difference in clearance rates gives an index of LDL receptor activity (Packard and Shepherd, 1983).

The predominant target organ for HMG CoA reductase inhibitors is the liver. Percutaneous liver biopsy is a potentially hazardous procedure, but patients undergoing elective cholecystectomy have been used to study the acute effects of drugs on wedge biopsies obtained at operation. Changes in HMG CoA reductase activity of peripheral blood monocytes in response to drugs have been measured (Schneider *et al.*, 1984), and plasma mevalonate levels may be used as a measure of cholesterol synthesis (Parker *et al.*, 1984).

As physicians undertaking later-phase trials of new agents increasingly expect details of drug mechanisms, verification in humans of animal data on underlying mechanisms is desirable at an early stage of development.

REFERENCES

Adams, P. W., Kissebah, A. H., Harrigan, P., Stokes, T. and Wynn, V. (1974). The kinetics of plasma free fatty acid and triglyceride transport in patients with idiopathic hypertriglyceridaemia and their relation to carbohydrate metabolism. *Eur. J. Clin. Invest.*, **4**, 149–61

Ad Hoc Committee to design a dietary treatment for hyperlipoproteinaemia (1984). Recommendations for treatment of hyperlipidaemia in adults. A joint statement of the nutrition committee and the council on arteriosclerosis. *Circulation*, **69**, 1065A–1090A

Anon. (1988). Apolipoprotein B and atherogenesis (leader). *Lancet* , **i**, 1141–2

Bonanome, A. and Grundy, S. M. (1988). Effect of dietary stearic acid on plasma cholesterol and lipoprotein levels. *New Engl. J. Med.*, **318**, 1244–8

Carey, M. C. (1978). Critical tables for calculating the cholesterol saturation of native bile. *J. Lipid Res.*, **19**, 945–55

Castelli, W. P. (1986). The triglyceride issue, a view from Framingham. *Am. Heart J.*, **112**, 432–7

Committee of Principal Investigators (1978). A cooperative trial in the primary prevention of ischaemic heart disease using clofibrate. *Br. Heart J.*, **40**, 1069–118

Eisenberg, S., Gavish, D., Oschry, Y., Fainaru, M. and Deckelbaum, R. J. (1984). Abnormalities in very low, low and high density lipoproteins in hypertriglyceridaemia. Reversal towards normal with bezafibrate treatment. *J. Clin. Invest.*, **74**, 470–82

Frick, M. H., Elo, O., Haapa, K., Heinonen, O. P., Heinsalmi, P., Helo, P., Huttunen, J. K., Kaitaniemi, P., Koskinen, P., Manninen, V., Mäenpää, H., Mälkönën, M., Mänttäri, M., Norola, S., Pasternak, A., Pikkarainen, J., Romo, M., Sjöblom, T. and Nikkilä, E. K. (1987). Helsinki Heart Study: primary-prevention trial with gemfibrozil in middle-aged men with dyslipidaemia. Safety of treatment, changes in risk factors, and incidence of coronary heart disease. *New Engl. J. Med.*, **317**, 1237–45

Friedewald, W. T., Levy, R. I. and Fredrickson, D. S. (1972). Estimation of the concentration of low-density lipoprotein cholesterol in plasma without the use of the preparative ultracentrifuge. *Clin. Chem.*, **18**, 499–502

Grundy, S. M., Mok, H. Y. I., Zech, L. and Berman, M. (1981). Influence of nicotinic acid on metabolism of cholesterol and triglycerides in man. *J. Lipid Res.*, **22**, 24–36

Illingworth, D. R. (1986). Specific inhibitors of cholesterol biosynthesis as hypocholesterolaemic agents in humans: mevinolin and compactin. In Fears, R., Levy, R. I., Shepherd, J. *et al.* (Eds.), *Pharmacological Control of Hyperlipidaemia*. Prous, Barcelona, pp. 231–49

Illingworth, D. R. and Corbin, D. (1985). The influence of mevinolin on the adrenal response to corticotropin in patients with heterozygous familial hypercholesterolaemia. *Proc. Natl Acad. Sci. USA*, **82**, 6291–4

Kissebah, A. H., Adams, P. W., Harrigan, P. and Wynn, V. (1974). The mechanism of clofibrate and tetranicotinylfuranose (Bradilan) on the kinetics of plasma free fatty acids and triglyceride transport in type IV and type V hypertriglyceridaemia. *Eur. J. Clin. Invest.*, **4**, 163–74

Laughlin, R. C. and Carey, T. F. (1962). Cataracts in patients treated with triparanol. *J. Am. Med. Assoc.*, **181**, 339–40

Lindgren, F. T., Jensen, L. C. and Hatch, F. T. (1972). The isolation and quantitative analysis of serum lipoproteins. In Nelson, G. J. (Ed.), *Blood Lipids and Lipoproteins*. Wiley-Interscience, New York, pp. 181–274

Packard, C. J. and Shepherd, J. (1983). Low-density lipoprotein receptor pathway in man. Its role in regulating plasma low-density lipoprotein. *Atherosclerosis Rev.*, **11**, 29–63

Parker, T. S., McNamara, D. J., Brown, C. D., Kolb, R., Ahrens, E. H. Jr., Alberts, A., Tobert, J., Chen, J. and DeSchepper, P. J. (1984). Plasma mevalonate as a measure of cholesterol synthesis in man. *J. Clin. Invest.*, **75**, 795–804

Patsch, J. R., Sailer, S., Kostner, G., Sandhofer, F., Halasek, A. and Braunsteiner, H. (1974). Separation of the main lipoprotein density classes from plasma by rate-zonal ultracentrifugation. *J. Lipid Res.*, **15**, 356–66

Rhoads, G. G., Dahlen, G., Berk, K., Morton, N. E. and Dannenberg, A. L. (1986). Lp(a) lipoprotein as a risk factor for myocardial infarction. *J. Am. Med. Assoc.*, **256**, 2540–4

Rifkind, B. M. (1966). Effects of CPIB ester on plasma free fatty acid levels in man. *Metabolism*, **15**, 673–5

Saku, K., Gartside, P. S., Hynd, B. A., Mendoza, S. G. and Kashyap, M. L. (1985). Apolipoprotein AI and AII metabolism in patients with primary high density lipoprotein deficiency associated with familial hypertriglycerinaemia. *Metabolism*, **34**, 754–64

Schneider, A. G., Ditschuneit, H. H., Stange, E. F. and Ditschuneit, H. (1984). Regulation of 3-hydroxy-3-methylglutaryl coenzyme A reductase in freshly isolated human mononuclear cells by fenofibrate. In Carlson, L. A. and Olsson, A. G. (Eds.), *Treatment of Hyperlipoproteinaemia*. Raven Press, New York, pp. 181–4

Thompson, G. R. (1986). Evidence that lowering serum lipids favourably influences coronary heart disease. *Quart. J. Med.*, **238**, 87–95

Warnick, G. R. and Albers, J. J. (1978). A comprehensive evaluation of the heparin-manganese precipitation procedure for estimating high density lipoprotein cholesterol. *J. Lipid Res.*, **19**, 65–76

Warnick, G. R., Benderson, J. and Albers, J. J. (1982). Quantitation of high-density-lipoprotein subclasses after separation by dextran sulphate and Mg^{2+} precipitation. *Clin. Chem.*, **28**, 1574

Warnick, G. R., Nguyen, T. and Albers, A. A. (1985). Comparison of improved precipitation methods for quantification of high density lipoprotein cholesterol. *Clin. Chem.*, **31**, 217–22

46
Antidiabetic Drugs

Daniel C. Howey

Eli Lilly and Company, William N. Wishard Memorial Hospital,
1001 West Tenth St, Indianapolis, IN 46202, USA

INTRODUCTION

The safe and cost-effective development of new drugs has never been more dependent on well-designed early studies. There are a large number of potential sites of drug action and there are no templates for early phase human drug trials in diabetes. Thus, success will demand an understanding of the disease, its pathophysiology and the tools available to study it. As always, studies in normal volunteers will be crucial to the design and safe conduct of clinical trials. However, if the pharmacology of new drugs is directed at specific abnormalities, the expected pharmacology may not be manifest in normal people. Therefore, early studies of drug action in patients with diabetes will be of great importance to clinical trials design and product decision-making.

THE CLASSIFICATION OF DIABETES MELLITUS

The NDDG (National Diabetes Data Group, 1979) and WHO (World Health Organization Study Group, 1985) devised simple classification systems for diabetes mellitus to aid the collection of epidemiological and investigational data. The classifications include insulin-dependent diabetes, non-insulin dependent diabetes, malnutrition-induced diabetes, impaired glucose tolerance, gestational diabetes, secondary diabetes mellitus and statistical risk categories.

INVESTIGATIONAL AGENTS

Currently cyclosporin, aldose reductase inhibitors and peptides are under investigation as treatments for diabetes. In addition, there are a few metabolic agents in various stages of development.

The recognition that insulin-dependent diabetes mellitus (IDDM) may have immunological underpinnings stimulated a number of clinical trials over the years with a variety of agents used to inhibit immune function. Most of these trials met with mixed results (Skyler, 1987). However, recent attempts to inhibit autoimmune destruction of islet cells in IDDM with cyclosporin (Cohen *et al.*, 1984) have met with promising results (Canadian-European Randomized Control Trial Group, 1988).

Over the last 10 years, several investigators have proposed a theory of glucotoxicity which places aldose reductase prominently in the chain of events leading to the development of diabetic retinopathy, cataracts and neuropathy (Kinoshita and Nishimura, 1988). The discovery of an important interrelation between aldose reductase, sorbitol dehydrogenase, myoinositol metabolism and (Na^+, K^+)-ATPase activity promises to explain the mechanism underlying diabetic complications (Greene *et al.*, 1988). Clinical studies of several inhibitors of aldose reductase currently under way are providing keys to the epidemiological relationships between glucose control and complications (Larson, 1988).

Recombinant DNA technology is ushering in the age of genetically engineered peptides. Cholecystokinin, somatostatin, pancreatic polypeptide, insulin-like growth factors I and II, glucagon and gastrointestinal polypeptide are several of the polypeptides which affect carbohydrate metabolism. The manufacture and modification of these peptides is within the reach of this technology. Even recombinant human insulin can be modified to introduce desirable characteristics. For instance, Brange and Markussen have recently created analogues of insulin with increased solubility for rapid absorption (Brange *et al.*, 1988) and decreased solubility for delayed absorption and longer action (Markussen *et al.*, 1987).

The few new drugs designed to affect hyperglycaemia focus on disparate physiological and biochemical processes in diabetes. The approaches include inhibition of glucagon secretion with somatostatin analogues, enhancing insulin secretion with alpha-2 antagonists, metabolic intervention with fatty acid oxidation inhibitors and inhibition of carbohydrate absorption from the gastrointestinal tract with glucosidase inhibitors (Mohrbacher *et al.*, 1987).

THE CONTROL OF CARBOHYDRATE METABOLISM

Blood glucose concentration is the result of a balance between glucose production, absorption from meals and uptake by tissues. Perturbations of this balance may result in disease. The complexity of the systems determining this balance offers opportunities for both success and failure in drug development. There are a number of points in the control of these systems where a new drug might act. To get the most from their studies, the designers of early trials must be familiar with the biochemistry and pathophysiology of diabetes.

PHARMACOLOGICAL METHODS

Assessment of Antidiabetic Drug Action

Carbohydrate, Amino Acid and Lipid Metabolism

Assessing the effects of a drug on glucose control will be a major concern for any trial of an antidiabetic agent. Average glycaemia over a period of several months can be assessed with haemoglobin Alc levels (Peacock, 1984). Over the short term, blood glucose control can be evaluated by use of assays performed in a clinical laboratory or at home by the patient. Clinical laboratories should use an enzymatic assay for glucose and pursue rigorous analytical goals (Fraser, 1986). Under appropriate circumstances home glucose monitoring will produce reliable data (Pohl *et al.*, 1985). The reliability of blood glucose records obtained from patients can be substantially improved with the use of glucose meters capable of storing data (Mazze *et al.*, 1984). Blood glucose data may be represented in a variety of useful ways to reflect the dynamic nature of this variable (Service *et al.*, 1987). The best measures for assessing overall glycaemic control are the average fasting glucose level and haemoglobin Alc (Shamoon *et al.*, 1986).

The glucose clamp (Andres *et al.*, 1966) is an extremely useful pharmacodynamic tool. The objective is to maintain a subject's glucose level constant in the face of a hypoglycaemic stimulus with an intravenous glucose infusion. The 'clamp' can be performed manually or under computer control (Verdonk *et al.*, 1980). Hypoglycaemic drugs can be evaluated safely and pharmacodynamic data can be obtained without interference from counterregulatory hormones.

Hetenyi has extensively reviewed radiotracer techniques used to measure the metabolic clearance of glucose, lactate, pyruvate, glycerol, alanine and other amino acids (Hetenyi *et al.*, 1983). These techniques are particularly useful in determining the effects of drugs on the 'flow' of metabolites between the liver and the peripheral tissues. Unfortunately, the data from these popular techniques are often rendered by 'mathematical models' which are difficult, if not impossible, to validate. One must keep in mind that radiotracer studies simply measure the metabolic clearance rate of the metabolite under study (Radziuk and Lickley, 1985). These studies are best performed by investigators with experience in the use of radiotracers. Studies should be kept simple and must have sound designs.

Respiratory or indirect calorimetry is a time-honoured technique developed around the turn of the century which estimates the metabolic rate by measuring the consumption of oxygen and production of carbon dioxide (Ferrannini, 1988). This non-invasive technique can be used to determine the rates of carbohydrate and lipid consumption; i.e. carbohydrate and lipid 'burned' to CO_2 and H_2O. Although of somewhat limited availability, indirect calorimetry may provide information complementary to metabolic clearance of glucose determined with radioactive tracers.

Insulin Secretion

Insulin secretory capacity can be assessed by measuring insulin levels following a standardised stimulus. Area-under-the-insulin-curve can be calculated and followed over time. The stimulus can be as time-worn as an oral (Bagdade, 1967) or intravenous glucose tolerance test (Melani *et al.*, 1967). Mixed meals, such as liquid dietary supplements, may be substituted for glucose for a more 'physiological' stimulus. Sampling for insulin and glucose should be similar to literature sources to aid in interpretation. Tolbutamide, glucagon, arginine and leucine have been used to stimulate insulin secretion. These secretagogues are only rarely used.

C-peptide has been used for many years as an index of insulin secretion (Faber and Binder, 1986). Its most useful application lies in determining secretory capacity in people with insulin antibodies. C-peptide is a by-product of the synthesis of insulin and is secreted in a molar ratio with insulin. C-peptide probably does not undergo significant first-pass hepatic metabolism after secretion. The kidney metabolises and excretes C-peptide (Zavaroni *et al.*, 1987), making the use of urinary C-peptide a simple index of insulin secretion (Meistas *et al.*, 1981).

Insulin Sensitivity

Insulin resistance is an important pathophysiological feature of both non-insulin-dependent diabetes mellitus (NIDDM) and IDDM. By definition, insulin resistance occurs when an increment of serum insulin produces a less-than-normal response in glucose uptake. From the point of view of insulin receptors, insulin resistance can be categorised as being caused by prereceptor (insulin or insulin-receptor antibodies), receptor-mediated (reduced insulin-receptor affinity or number) and postreceptor abnormalities. Unfortunately, insulin-receptor assays have declined in popularity and availability, owing to several limitations and other problems. These assays require large blood sample volumes and are generally limited to studies of monocytes or red blood cells. The widespread application to human liver, fat and muscle cells has been hindered by the invasive nature of the sampling techniques. In addition, there is confusion over the interpretation of the results of these assays (Nattrass and Dodds, 1987).

Postreceptor defects in insulin action cannot be measured with receptor-binding assays. By their very nature postreceptor defects are only observed during *in vivo* or *in vitro* studies of insulin action. Bergman has extensively reviewed the theoretical background and the methods of measuring these defects in insulin action discussed below (Bergman *et al.*, 1985; Ader and Bergman, 1987).

Himsworth and Kerr developed the first practical and standardised protocol to evaluate insulin sensitivity (Himsworth, 1936; Himsworth and Kerr, 1939). The protocol required two oral glucose tolerance tests: one with and one without an intravenous insulin injection. Before the development of insulin radioimmunoassays, these investigations discovered much of what we hold true regarding insulin resistance in diabetes mellitus, obesity and ageing.

IVGTT and OGTT coupled with serum insulin assays have, in general, supported these concepts over the years.

Reaven and colleagues pioneered the insulin suppression test as a measure of insulin sensitivity. This technique involves infusing adrenaline and propranolol (Shen *et al.*, 1970) or somatostatin (Harano *et al.*, 1978) to inhibit endogenous insulin secretion. The subjects are also given an infusion of glucose and insulin. After 90 min the plasma glucose reaches a new steady state (SSPG). The higher the SSPG, the greater the resistance to the effects of insulin. The SSPG correlates well with results obtained from the euglycaemic glucose clamp described next (Greenfield *et al.*, 1981). This test is simple to perform but the use of adrenaline and propranolol may be associated with hypertension, bradycardia and other cardiac arrhythmias (Lampman *et al.*, 1981).

Insulin dose–response studies are the 'gold standard' for evaluating insulin sensitivity (Rizza *et al.*, 1981). These studies require the glucose clamp. The dose–response study can be used to differentiate decreased insulin sensitivity (a shift to the right of the half-maximal effect) from decreased responsiveness (reduced maximal effect). Combinations of defects are not unusual in NIDDM and they can be readily detected with this procedure. The glucose clamp requires a large investment in staff, time and equipment.

Bergman and colleagues have developed an insulin sensitivity index called the frequently sampled intravenous glucose tolerance test (FSIGT) (Beard *et al.*, 1986). The FSIGT requires sequential intravenous injections of glucose and tolbutamide followed by an analysis of glucose data using 'minimal modeling' techniques. The FSIGT correlates well with insulin sensitivity measured by glucose clamp studies (Bergman *et al.*, 1987). This technique seems to be developing into a standardised protocol that may require a small number of samples and a simple analysis. If this is the case, the FSIGT could be easily integrated into clinical trials of NIDDM that require repeated measurement of insulin sensitivity over time.

Counterregulatory Mechanisms in Defence of Hypoglycaemia

The central nervous system depends predominantly on glucose as a fuel and is exquisitely sensitive to acute hypoglycaemia (Siesjö, 1988). Neuroglycopenia is the limiting toxicity of insulin and the sulphonylureas. A drug may produce hypoglycaemia by decreasing production, decreasing absorption or increasing uptake. If compensation does not occur, hypoglycaemia will result. Neuroglycopenia follows and brain damage or death will result.

Glycogenolysis and gluconeogenesis are the primary metabolic events called on to correct hypoglycaemia. Glycogenolysis is prompt but short-lived. Gluconeogenesis is the major contributor to the recovery of blood glucose. Glucagon is the primary stimulus for increased glucose production and adrenaline is of secondary importance. Cortisol and growth hormone have minimal effects on the acute response. Unfortunately, the secretion of glucagon and adrenaline decrease with time in most people with IDDM and in many with NIDDM (Gerich, 1988). Although the ability to modulate glucose production will be a desirable feature of any new drug for diabetes, complete inhibition of gluconeogenesis would be anathema.

A GENERIC APPROACH TO THE EARLY EVALUATION OF A DRUG FOR DIABETES

Given the plethora of opportunities to affect insulin secretion, gluconeogenesis and carbohydrate metabolism, it is impossible to design a single 'generic' approach to early drug studies in humans. However, if we assume that a drug is developed for NIDDM and that it works by increasing glucose utilisation, suppressing glucose production or by *directly* improving insulin resistance, some general principles can be invented. We must accept two caveats. First, if there is sufficient reason to enter Phase I studies, the lack of pharmacology in normals should not be the sole reason for not proceeding into patients. Second, the 'shotgun' approach to the selection of 'things-to-measure' will not work in human studies, owing to ethical restrictions on blood loss, among other considerations. A sensible and efficient approach demands that a specific or, at the very least, a proposed mechanism of action be at hand. For the discussion that follows, space dictates a Spartan approach to selecting 'things-to-measure'.

Phase I

Normal volunteers are traditionally used for Phase I studies. However, drugs that ameliorate insulin resistance may not produce demonstrable effects in normal subjects. Attempts to evaluate the effects of drugs on insulin resistance in normals are fruitless. Drugs that affect gluconeogenesis may work in normals but the effects in NIDDM may be considerably greater. In these situations, confirmation of activity must be performed in patients with diabetes. The activity of drugs that stimulate glucose utilisation either directly or by stimulating insulin secretion may be confirmed promptly in normal subjects.

In addition to the standard safety measures used during Phase I for any drug, serum glucose should be measured during all volunteer studies. Frequent measurements during the expected period of drug action and careful monitoring for symptoms and signs of hypoglycaemia should suffice. Multiple-dose studies should be performed in diabetic volunteers, unless hypoglycaemia poses no threat to normals.

First Study: *Absorption, Bioavailability and Metabolism*

This is typically a normal volunteer study. There is little need to include patients unless the peculiarities of diabetes or obesity are expected to significantly affect drug disposition.

For all drugs that affect glucose levels, a fall from fasting glucose of 20% should be sufficient to confirm activity. If the initial doses are expected to drop serum glucose by greater than 20%, the study should be performed under the glucose clamp or at the very least with an infusion of glucose to prevent serious hypoglycaemia. The glucose clamp will produce useful pharmacodynamic data.

For drugs expected to increase glucose utilisation, serum insulin and glucose levels at intervals determined during animal studies should suffice for the first pharmacodynamic evaluation. Respiratory calorimetry may be quite useful for these drugs.

For a drug working by affecting gluconeogenesis, tritiated glucose should be used at this time to attempt to measure effects on glucose production. The use of the glucose clamp, i.e. any infusion of a large quantity of 'cold' glucose, may complicate the analysis of radiotracer studies (Finegood *et al.*, 1988).

Second Study: *Dose-ranging to Initial Toxicity or Efficacy*

If toxic effects are encountered with a drug expected to stimulate glucose utilisation before any effects on glucose, the drug may not be viable. This may not hold true for drugs affecting insulin resistance. It may not be wise to make a recommendation regarding drugs affecting gluconeogenesis without knowing their mechanism of action and the differential effects on diabetic and normal animal models.

If pharmacological action is reached prior to toxic effects, dose-ranging to toxicity may be performed in normals or diabetics with the glucose clamp. This technique will provide adequate protection from hypoglycaemia and excellent dose–response data. However, the maximum duration of glucose clamp studies is usually less than 24 h. Thus, only single-dose escalations on a weekly basis are practical.

Third Study: *Counterregulatory Response to Hypoglycaemia*

This evaluation is critical for drugs affecting glucose utilisation or gluconeogenesis; however, this study may not be relevant for an agent that directly affects insulin resistance. The results of these studies form the basis of the recommendations for treatment of hypoglycaemia or overdose. Drugs stimulating glucose utilisation should produce responses similar to insulin-induced hypoglycaemia. Measure serum insulin, adrenaline, glucagon, growth hormone and cortisol and use insulin as a control. If counterregulation is similar to insulin-induced hypoglycaemia, then oral or intravenous glucose or injectable glucagon is the treatment of choice.

For a drug affecting gluconeogenesis, glucagon and adrenaline may not reverse the hypoglycaemia. In this case it may not be wise to continue. Dosing with drug to produce hypoglycaemia should be performed with extreme caution. As an alternative, the drug can be given at a dose expected to fall short of hypoglycaemia while infusions of glucagon or epinephrine are given to reverse effects. These studies will require radiotracers to measure glucose production.

Fourth Study: *Bioavailability and Drug Action with Food*

There is nothing about the diets recommended for diabetes that would suggest the use of other than normal volunteers for this mundane study. However, if appropriately controlled and compared with placebo, an evaluation of a drug's effects on meal-time glucose concentrations could make patient studies particularly interesting.

Phase II

It is virtually impossible to make sensible recommendations for the design of Phase II trials. However, several guidelines might be useful.

Selection of Patients

Early studies should avoid patients with complications of diabetes or concomitant diseases, or those taking drugs other than sulphonylureas (or a biguanide). Patients requiring insulin may be in an advanced stage of their disease and less responsive. Patients with NIDDM must have abnormal glucose tolerance, hyperinsulinaemia and insulin resistance off drug therapy

Selection of Drugs for Comparison

Choose a sulphonylurea with pharmacokinetic and pharmacodynamic profiles similar to the drug under study. Hold insulin and biguanides until later.

Study Design

Randomised crossover studies are highly recommended. Blinding the volunteers is imperative. A person with diabetes will usually experience an improvement in blood glucose control following enrolment into a study. This will hold true for those on placebo. A period of up to 3–6 weeks may be required to obviate this effect.

Monitoring Techniques

Targets for glucose control are difficult to provide. Normalisation of glucose control is the ideal. In general, a new agent that does not meet or exceed the effects of a sulphonylurea will probably not be successful. Blood glucose control is best determined by performing daily blood glucose measurements from one fasting level up to eight throughout the day. Home glucose monitoring with meters capable of storing the results will be a boon to data collection and determination of compliance levels. An intensive monitoring day on a research unit during which blood glucose is measured hourly might be included at regular intervals. Intensive monitoring days are only practical during short trials. Even the best volunteers will rebel after three or four sessions. Haemoglobin Alc levels take at least 6–12 weeks to change appreciably and are of limited value during short studies.

Any drug which effectively lowers blood glucose might be expected to improve insulin sensitivity. The selection of the technique used to measure insulin sensitivity will depend primarily on availability. Using the technique correctly and obtaining repeated measures over time are of paramount importance.

REFERENCES

Abernethy, D. R. and Greenblatt, D. J. (1986). Drug disposition in obese humans. An update. *Clinical Pharmacokinetics*, **11**, 199–213

Ader, M. and Bergman, R. N. (1987). Insulin sensitivity in the intact organism. *Baillière's Clinical Endocrinology and Metabolism*, Vol. 1. Ballière Tindall, pp. 879–910

Andres, R., Swerdloff, L., Pozefsky, D. and Coleman, D. (1966). Manual feedback technique for the control of blood glucose concentration. In Skeggs, L. T. (Ed.), *Automation in Analytical Chemistry, Technician Symposia 1965*. Mediad Incorporated, New York, pp. 486–91

Bagdade, J. D., Bierman, E. L. and Porte, D. (1967). The significance of basal insulin levels in the evaluation of the insulin response to glucose in diabetic and nondiabetic subjects. *Journal of Clinical Investigation*, **46**, 1549–57

Beard, J. C., Bergman, R. N., Ward, W. K. and Porte, D. (1986). The insulin sensitivity index in nondiabetic man: correlation between clamp-derived and IVGTT-derived values. *Diabetes*, **35**, 362–9

Bergman, R. N., Finegood, D. T. and Ader, M. (1985). Assessment of insulin sensitivity *in vivo*. *Endocrine Reviews*, **6**, 45–86

Bergman, R. N., Prager, R., Volund, A. and Olefsky, J. (1987). Equivalence of the insulin sensitivity index in man derived by the minimal model method and the euglycemic glucose clamp. *Journal of Clinical Investigation*, **79**, 790–800

Bloudin, R. A., Kolpek, J. H. and Mann, H. J. (1987). Influence of obesity on drug disposition. *Clinical Pharmacy*, **6**, 706–14

Brange, J., Ribel, U., Hansen, J. F., Dodson, G., Hansen, H. T., Havelund, S., Melberg, S. G., Norris, F., Norris, K., Snael, L., Sorensen, A. R. and Voigt, H. O. (1988). Monomeric insulins obtained by protein engineering and their medical implications. *Nature*, **333**, 679–82

Brownlee, M., Cerami, A. and Vlassara, H. (1988). Advanced products of nonenzymatic glycosylation and the pathogenesis of diabetic vascular disease. *Diabetes/Metabolism Reviews*, **4**, 437–51

Canadian-European Randomized Control Trial Group (1988). Cyclosporin-induced remission of IDDM after early intervention. *Diabetes*, **37**, 1574–82

Cohen, D. J., Loertscher, R., Rubin, M. F., Tilney, N. L., Carpenter, C. B. and Strom, T. B. (1984). Cyclosporin: a new immunosuppressive agent for organ transplantation. *Annals of Internal Medicine*, **101**, 667–82

Faber, O. K. and Binder, C. (1986). C-peptide: an index of insulin secretion. *Diabetes/Metabolism Reviews*, **2**, 331–45

Feldman, M. and Schiller, L. R. (1983). Disorders of gastrointestinal motility associated with diabetes mellitus. *Annals of Internal Medicine*, **98**, 378–84

Ferrannini, E. (1988). The theoretical bases of indirect calorimetry: a review. *Metabolism*, **37**, 287–301

Finegood, D. T., Bergman, R. N. and Vranic, M. (1988). Modeling error and apparent isotope discrimination confound estimation or endogenous glucose production during euglycemic glucose clamps. *Diabetes*, **37**, 1025–34

Fraser, C. (1986). Analytical goals for glucose analyses. *Annals of Clinical Biochemistry*, **23**, 379–89

Gerich, J. E. (1988). Glucose counterregulation and its impact on diabetes mellitus. *Diabetes*, **37**, 1608–17

Greene, D. A., Lattimer, S. A. and Sima, A. A. F. (1988). Pathogenesis and prevention of diabetic neuropathy. *Diabetes/Metabolism Reviews*, **4**, 201–21

Greenfield, M. S., Doberne, L., Kraemer, T. and Reaven, G. (1981). Assessment of insulin resistance with the insulin suppression test and the euglycemic clamp. *Diabetes*, **30**, 387–92

Harano, Y., Hidaka, H., Takatsuki, K., Ohgaku, S., Haneda, M., Motoi, S., Kawgoe, K., Shigeta, Y. and Abe, H. (1978). Glucose, insulin and somatostatin infusion for the determination of insulin sensitivity *in vivo*. *Metabolism*, **27**, 1449–52

Hetenyi, G., Perez, G. and Vranic, M. (1983). Turnover and precursor-product relationships of nonlipid metabolites. *Physiological Reviews*, **63**, 606–67

Himsworth, H. P. (1936). Diabetes mellitus. Its differentiation into insulin-sensitive and insulin-insensitive types. *Lancet*, **1**, 127–30

Himsworth, H. P. and Kerr, R. B. (1939). Insulin-sensitive and insulin-insensitive types of diabetes mellitus. *Clinical Science*, **4**, 119–52

Isacson, D. and Stålhammar, J. (1987). Prescription drug use among diabetics—a population study. *Journal of Chronic Diseases*, **49**, 651–60

Kinoshita, J. H. and Nishimura, C. (1988). The involvement of aldose reductase in diabetes complications. *Diabetes/Metabolism Reviews*, **4**, 323–38

Lampman, R. M., Santinga, J. T., Bassett, D. R. and Savage, P. J. (1981). Cardiac arrhythmias during epinephrine-propranolol infusions for measurement of *in vivo* insulin resistance. *Diabetes*, **30**, 618–20

Larson, E. R., Lipinski, C. A. and Sarges, R. (1988). Medicinal chemistry of aldose reductase inhibitors. *Medicinal Research Reviews*, **8**, 159–86

Lebovitz, H. E. and Feinglos, M. N. (1983). The oral hypoglycemic agents. In Ellenberg, M. and Rifkin, H. (Eds.), *Diabetes Mellitus: Theory and Practice*. Medical Examination Publishing Company, New Hyde Park, pp. 591–609

Markussen, J., Hougaard, P., Ribel, U., Sorensen, A. R. and Sorensen, E. (1987). Soluble prolonged-acting insulin derivatives. I. Degree of protraction and crystallizability of insulins substituted in the termini of the B-chain. *Protein Engineering*, **1**, 205–13

Mazze, R. S., Shamoon, H., Pasmantier, R., Lucido, D., Murphy, J., Hartmenn, K., Kuykendall, V. and Lopatin, W. (1984). Reliability of blood glucose monitoring by patients with diabetes mellitus. *American Journal of Medicine*, **77**, 211–17

Meistas, M. T., Zadik, Z., Margolis, S. and Kowarski, A. A. (1981). Correlation of urinary excretion of C-peptide with the integrated concentration and secretion rate of insulin. *Diabetes*, **30**, 639–43

Melani, F., Lawecki, J., Bartelt, K. M. and Pfeiffer, E. F. (1967). Serum insulin levels in subjects with normal metabolism, obese patients and diabetics after intravenous administration of glucose, tolbutamide and glucagon. *Diabetologia*, **3**, 422–6

Mohrbacher, R. J., Kiorpes, T. C. and Bowden, C. R. (1987). Pharmacologic intervention in diabetes mellitus. *Annual Reports in Medicinal Chemistry*, **22**, 213–22

Morgensen, C. E., Schmitz, A. and Christensen, C. K. (1988). Comparative renal physiology relevant to IDDM and NIDDM patients. *Diabetes/Metabolism Reviews*, **4**, 453–83

National Diabetes Data Group (1979). Classification and diagnosis of diabetes mellitus and other categories of glucose intolerance. *Diabetes*, **28**, 1039–57

Nattrass, M. and Dodds, K. E. (1987). Interpretation of radioreceptor assays. *Annals of Clinical Biochemistry*, **24**, 13–21

Peacock, I. (1984). Glycosylated haemoglobin: measurement and clinical use. *Journal of Clinical Pathology*, **37**, 841–51

Pohl, S. L., Gonder-Frederick, L., Cox, D. J. and Evans, W. S. (1985). Self-measurement of blood glucose concentration: clinical significance of patient-generated measurements. *Diabetes Care*, **8**, 617–19

Polonsky, K. S. and Rubenstein, A. H. (1986). Current approaches to measurement of insulin secretion. *Diabetes/Metabolism Reviews*, **2**, 315–29

Radziuk, J. and Lickley, H. L. A. (1985). The metabolic clearance of glucose: measurement and meaning. *Diabetologia*, **28**, 315–22

Rendel, M., Lassek, W. D., Ross, D. A., Smith, C., Kernek, S., Williams, J., Brown, M., Willingmyre, L. and Yamamoto, L. (1983). A pharmaceutical profile of diabetic patients. *Journal of Chronic Diseases*, **36**, 193–202

Rendel, M., Rasbold, K., Nierenberg, J., Krohn, R., Hermanson, G., Klenk, D. and Smith, P. K. (1986). Comparison and contrast of affinity chromatographic determinations of plasma glycated albumin and total glycated plasma protein. *Clinical Biochemistry*, **19**, 216–20

Rizza, R. A., Mandarino, L. J. and Gerich, J. E. (1981). Mechanisms of insulin resistance in man: assessment using insulin dose-response curve in conjunction with insulin-receptor binding. *The American Journal of Medicine*, **70**, 169–76

Ruiz-Cabello, F. and Erill, S. (1984). Abnormal serum protein binding of acidic drugs in diabetes mellitus. *Clinical Pharmacology and Therapeutics*, **36**, 691–5

Service, F. J., O'Brien, P. C. and Rizza, R. A. (1987). Measures of glucose control. *Diabetes Care*, **10**, 225–37

Shamoon, H., Mazze, R., Pasmantier, R., Lucido, D. and Murphy, J. A. (1986). Assessment of long-term glycemia in type I diabetes using multiple blood glucose values stored in a memory-containing reflectometer. *American Journal of Medicine*, **80**, 1086–92

Shen, S. W., Reaven, G. M. and Farquhar, J. W. (1970). Comparison of impedance to insulin-mediated glucose uptake in normal subjects and in subjects with latent diabetes. *Journal of Clinical Investigation*, **49**, 2151–60

Siesjö, B. K. (1988). Hypoglycemia, brain metabolism, and brain damage. *Diabetes/Metabolism Reviews*, **4**, 113–44

Skyler, J. S. (1987). Immune intervention studies in insulin-dependent diabetes mellitus. *Diabetes/Metabolism Reviews*, **4**, 1017–35

Tsuchiya, S., Sakurai, T. and Sekiguchi, S. (1984). Nonenzymatic glycosylation of human serum albumin and its influence on binding capacity of sulfonylureas. *Biochemical Pharmacology*, **33**, 2967–71

Verdonk, C. A., Rizza, R., Westland, R. E., Nelson, R. L., Gerich, J. E. and Service, F. J. (1980). Glucose clamping using the Biostator GCIIS. *Hormone and Metabolic Research*, **12**, 133–5

World Health Organization Study Group (1985). *Diabetes Mellitus*. Technical Report Series No. 727, Geneva

Zavaroni, I., Deferrari, G., Lugari, R., Bonora, E., Garibotto, G., Dall'aglio, E., Robaudo, C. and Gnudi, A. (1987). Renal metabolism of C-peptide in man. *Journal of Clinical Endocrinology and Metabolism*, **65**, 494–8

Zysset, T. and Wietholtz, H. (1988). Differential effect of type I and type II diabetes on antipyrine disposition in man. *European Journal of Clinical Pharmacology*, **34**, 369–75

XIII
Assessment of the Effects of Chemotherapeutic Agents

47
Antibacterial Drugs

A. Pickup

Abbott Laboratories Ltd, Abbott House, Moorbridge Road, Maidenhead, Berkshire SL6 8JG, UK

INTRODUCTION

Phase II trials of antibacterial therapy are inherently different from those with most other pharmacological agents. Principally this is because the aim is to achieve a cure rather than palliation of symptoms, but also because one is attempting to have an effect on an agent which has invaded the body and not produce a response from the body itself.

It is important to take into account more than simply the mechanics of clinical trials. This is, therefore, intended to be a guide to approaching some of the problems and questions which may be encountered during the Phase II investigation of a unique class of drugs.

AIM

The aim of early trials is to establish a risk:benefit ratio, the dosage regimen and serious ADR profile, to enable Phase III studies to be properly designed. It is important, during these early trials, some of which may be open, that as much pharmacokinetic data is collected as possible. The kinetics of a drug may be very different in the very sick patient compared with the healthy volunteer. For example, erythromycin readily crosses the blood–brain barrier in meningitis, but only very poorly in the healthy state. Clearly, classical single and/or rising dose studies cannot be included in the evaluation of an antibiotic. The initial Phase II studies in patients may also be preceded by a serum bactericidal activity (SBA) test. In this test the serum of volunteers in Phase I studies is used as a culture medium for the study of pathogens. The test determines the dilution of a serum sample from a subject taking the antibiotic which will still kill $\geq 99.9\%$ of the test pathogen *in vitro* over 18–24 h. It is well described in the literature (Washington, 1981). The data acquired will not provide an answer to the clinical question of which dose to use first, but compared with results *in vitro* and HPLC assays of serum concentrations from volunteers, it can be very useful in early identification of unexpected lack of, or enhancement of, activity; the former may be due to an interaction in the case of a combination, and the latter to an active metabolite with a long half-life or higher potency than the parent compound.

PATIENT SELECTION

As the efficacy in man is unknown initially, the temptation is to choose patients who are not particularly unwell, and this may lead to under assessment of the dosage regimen to be used in Phase III trials; patients with mild infections may improve spontaneously and thus consideration should always be given to a control group, even in very early studies.

Open or controlled studies in patients who are not seriously ill may also lead to overenthusiastic reporting of the efficacy of a new drug. Conversely, use in very ill patients may not be ethically justified at this early stage, unless all else has failed, or may give an overly pessimistic view of the compound's efficacy.

There is much controversy surrounding the inclusion and exclusion criteria for clinical trials of antibiotics. In early trials, patients should not have been treated with a plethora of agents immediately prior to entering the study. It is often felt that it is unnecessary to ensure that the organism(s) being treated should be sensitive to both agents in a comparative study, as this does not parallel the clinical situation; in fact, this is very important for two reasons.

Firstly, in the case of an open study, including organisms resistant to one of the agents results in treating infections inherently 'more difficult' to eradicate; also, it is not difficult to imagine resistance rates *in vitro* for an old established agent being somewhat higher than for a new agent with a novel mode of action. Excluding patients randomised to the older agent because organisms are resistant to it, but not those randomised to the new agent, will result in unbalanced groups favouring the older antibiotic.

Secondly, if the study is double blind there is no way of knowing which treatment the patient is taking in the event of there being resistance *in vitro* to one of the agents. The blind may not be broken and thus the patient should be withdrawn from the study. The patient may continue to be treated blindly, if the clinician wishes, with study medication, assuming they are improving, but the result must be assessed quite separately from those patients meeting all the entry criteria.

ASSESSMENT

In all clinical trials of antibiotics there will be two basic criteria for the assessment of success, namely, bacteriological eradication and clinical outcome; also there may be additional secondary criteria such as change in colour of sputum or appearance of the urine. These criteria allow an early assessment of response, and generally a decision to continue the patient in early Phase II studies may be made by the third day, or even earlier. In the event of lack of efficacy, the patient may then be either discontinued from the study or transferred to the comparative compound if the study is controlled by the presence of a group taking a standard reference therapy. This has the benefit of the inclusion, in early trials, of patients who are relatively well but who do have clinically significant infections.

The two methods of assessing 'cure' in antibacterial trials, namely symptomatic and bacteriological, are quite different and must be analysed and interpreted entirely separately, the bacteriological assessment being the 'gold standard'. Examples of non-concurrence of the two criteria are well known; asymptomatic significant bacteriuria is not uncommon and yet frequently it is impossible to culture bacteria in the presence of acute dysuria and frequency. It is not unusual to find pathogens in the sputum of clinically cured, acute or chronic bronchitis; equally, symptoms of acute bronchitis may persist for some time despite apparent eradication of the causative organisms.

Mistakes in this area are all too easily made because the final assessment of efficacy at the end of the course of therapy is not performed correctly. It is worth mentioning at this point that *all* patients should, if possible, undergo a 'final assessment' even if it has been decided to withdraw him/her from the study in order to prescribe another antibiotic. In this respect in particular one should be aware of the care needed in obtaining/handling the final specimen. Principally the sample is often taken too soon after cessation of treatment; the urine especially, for example, may have inhibitory concentrations of the antibiotic present for several days after the last dose. Samples taken too early lead to the false impression that the antibiotic has been effective unless a late follow up is carried out after 5 days or more.

There are at least two further important pitfalls to avoid.

Firstly, it is well recognised that disappearance of bacteria and/or symptoms may occur in 50% of urinary-tract infections treated without an antibiotic; so these parameters of efficacy should not be blindly regarded as indicators of success. Secondly, differentiating between relapse and reinfection in the event of bacteria occurring in the 'final specimen' should pose no problems, but often does. It is likely that patients involved in these early trials will be those who attend relatively frequently with, for example, urinary-tract infections or acute exacerbations of chronic bronchitis. It is often helpful to use such patients in early Phase II studies but it must be remembered that not only will they tend to be, as a group, more difficult to treat, but also they are by definition more prone to reinfection; it is essential, therefore, to take meticulous care in typing the organism(s). The reappearance of the original organism is a treatment regimen failure, but the appearance of a new organism should not be considered as such.

DOSE RANGING

A good estimate of the appropriate dose must be achieved before starting Phase II studies, and in contra-distinction to other classes of drug, this will generally be possible by assessing the absorption, distribution, metabolism and excretion in Phase I trials together with MIC and MBC data from studies *in vitro*. This assessment will be further enhanced by assessing efficacy in some animal models.

Dose-escalation or dose-ranging studies, in which a number of different dosages are given to the same patient randomly on several different occasions, are clearly not feasible. It is, however, important to obtain some dosage regimen data in parallel group studies. Doses employed should generally be different by multiples of two (e.g. 200 mg b.d. vs 400 mg b.d.); the lowest dose must be expected to have some clinical efficacy based upon the preclinical data, but this may be exceeded in the higher dose group. Apparent toxicity must be carefully monitored in these studies, as the decision to opt for the higher dosage in Phase III studies will be predicated to some extent upon the apparent risk/benefit ratio. It may be that the lower dose is 100% effective in eradicating bacteria and producing clinical cure or that there is no difference between the two dosage regimens tested; in this case it may be prudent to try a still lower dose although the plasma/tissue concentrations achieved in these initial studies must be borne in mind together with the data on known MICs/MBCs. Gaining information about tissue distribution reasonably early in Phase II studies is of great value in assisting with these calculations. Single or multiple doses may be given to patients about to undergo surgery, e.g. tonsillectomy or nephrectomy. This can yield vital information to assist in choosing the correct dosage for Phase III studies. It should not be forgotten, however, that some tissue distribution characteristics change in the presence of infection, e.g. erythromycin and meningitis.

Despite careful consideration of these points, it may still appear that a lower dose than that predicted from the preclinical programme is effective. This may relate to the presence of a metabolite which also has activity against the bacteria under study. It is likely, under these circumstances, that discrepancies will be seen between HPLC and microbiological methods of measuring plasma concentrations—both should be done at this stage, if at all possible.

Paying careful attention to all these issues will enable an assessment to be made at the end of the Phase III programme as to how many patients could be offered the new drug with hope of success in a busy clinical setting. It will also help to ensure that the agent is launched at the correct dosage, an absolutely vital aspect from both the commercial, as well as the medical, points of view.

REFERENCE

Washington, J. A. (II) (1981). *Laboratory Procedures in Clinical Microbiology*, Springer-Verlag, New York, pp. 715–28

48
Antiviral Drugs

Whaijen Soo

Dept of Clinical Virology, Hoffman–La Roche Inc., 340 Kingsland St, Nutley, NJ 07110–1199, USA

INTRODUCTION

Viral infections lead to a spectrum of diseases of varying severity and duration. Infections caused by many respiratory and enteric viruses, for example, usually lead to acute illnesses without much chronicity. The aims of antiviral therapy for these acute viral infections should be early resolution of signs and symptoms associated with the disease as well as prevention of secondary complications. This strategy can also be applied to therapy for recurrent episodes of acute illness caused by some of the herpes virus infections such as herpes simplex and varicella zoster. Most known antiviral agents are only effective when given early during an acute infection. To maximise the clinical benefits of these drugs, use during a prodromal phase or even for postexposure prophylaxis should be considered, if the safety and tolerance of a particular drug have been well established.

Infections by papillomaviruses, hepatitis viruses and immunodeficiency viruses, on the other hand, might not cause obvious acute illnesses but can cause chronic diseases leading to serious clinical sequelae. The aims of antiviral therapy for these chronic viral infections, therefore, should be to arrest the progression of the disease and reduce the chance of late adverse consequences. Since drugs for chronic viral illnesses will probably be used for an extended period of time, tolerance can be a difficult issue. Risk-to-benefit ratio has to be determined for each drug with regard to the viral illness to be treated.

Immunisation should remain the primary approach to the prevention of viral infections. When effective vaccines are not available for use in a particular target population, chemoprophylaxis should be considered. These circumstances include use in immunodeficient individuals and individuals with hypersensitivity to a particular vaccine, as well as in conjunction with late vaccination. For seasonal chemoprophylaxis against diseases such as influenza, drug therapy should be initiated as soon as an outbreak is recognised. For other prophylactic use, the duration and the timing of initiation of prophylaxis will depend on knowledge of the natural history of the disease to be treated.

DRUG CLASSES

Attempts to develop antiviral therapy in the past 50 years have met with only very limited success. This is because animal viruses are obligatory, intracellular parasites carrying genes that programme only a limited number of virus-specific functions while taking advantage of a large number of normal human biochemical mechanisms to survive. Therefore, targets for antiviral therapy are very limited and frequently difficult to identify. Up to now, most successful antiviral drugs, such as idoxuridine, vidarabine and zidovudine, are nucleoside analogues that selectively interfere with viral nucleic acid synthesis by inhibiting viral polymerases. This selection can be made more specific if the activation of the drug can only be achieved by a virus-specific process, as with acyclovir (Balfour, 1984). Other successful targetings include drugs such as amatadine and rimatadine, which interfere with the entry of the influenza virus (Koff and Knight, 1979). Recent advances in molecular virology and recombinant technology, however, have enabled us to better understand the virus life cycle, and thus recognise additional virus-specific functions to be targeted for potential therapeutic intervention. These new target sites include, for example, virus-specific integrase, protease and regulatory enzymes responsible for amplification of viral replication (Mitsuya and Broder, 1987). Simple screening procedures suitable for high-flux random screening can now be developed to identify drug candidates which inhibit these target sites.

A different approach to antiviral therapy is the use of immunomodulators. This is a relatively new class of compounds, many of which have non-specific immunomodulatory effects. The primary objective for the use of an immunomodulator is to enhance the cytotoxic killing of infected cells which serve as reservoirs for further spread of the virus. One particular immunomodulator, alpha-interferon, has been extensively studied. Alpha-interferon, however, has independent immunomodulatory and antiviral effects, probably through different mechanisms of action (Clemens and McNurlan, 1985). It is possible that the efficacy of alpha-interferon against viral hepatitis and papilloma viral infection, for example, is due to both the antiviral and the immunomodulatory effects of this compound. Other immunomodulators such as gamma-interferon and interleukin-2 have also been studied for their potential use against various viral diseases. These immunomodulators clearly do not have a direct antiviral effect. Although there is preliminary evidence suggesting that these immunomodulators can indeed enhance immune functions in patients with viral illnesses (Weinhold *et al.*, 1988), it is too early to predict whether the observed immunomodulatory effects can be translated into clinical efficacy.

PROPHYLAXIS

Aims of Therapy

The aim of chemoprophylaxis is to prevent the infection and/or clinical manifestation of disease caused by a particular virus. For viral infections leading to significant chronic sequelae, prevention of infection is critical. For viral infections causing only acute illnesses, prevention of clinical disease should be adequate. In the latter case, the development of an immune response to subclinical infections could be a potentially desirable feature of prophylaxis, since immunity may be established against reinfection.

Study Design

To demonstrate efficacy of chemoprophylaxis in a natural setting usually requires a large number of patients, because of low infection rates. This problem can be circumvented in early phase evaluation by the selection of a subpopulation with higher infection rates, such as prison inmates, nursing home residents and other institutionalised populations (Atkinson *et al.*, 1986), as well as individuals who are less immunocompetent because of medications, transplantations or lack of vaccination. If such a subpopulation is not available, the use of an artificial challenge model can be considered (Dawkins *et al.*, 1968). The extrapolation of data from challenge to natural studies, however, is not always successful. This is because the viral load, the infection rate and the strains of virus used in a challenge study might be very different from those occurring in the natural setting.

Owing to the unpredictability of the outbreak and the variability of the immune status of each individual against a particular viral infection, efficacy data from uncontrolled, open studies are not reliable. Phase II pilot efficacy studies, therefore, should be double-blind and controlled, while Phase I single and multiple ascending-dose pharmacokinetic and tolerance studies can remain open and uncontrolled.

CLINICAL ASSESSMENTS

The primary efficacy end-point is prevention of laboratory-documented viral illness during chemoprophylaxis. Laboratory documentation is especially critical in respiratory viral infections, because many different respiratory viruses cause diseases with similar signs and symptoms. For example, in a prophylaxis study comparing rimantadine with placebo in young volunteers, 14% of those who took drug had clinical diagnosis of influenza A illness, yet only 3% had true influenza A illness documented by the laboratory (Dolin *et al.*, 1982). On the other hand, laboratory documentation might not be required for study on suppression of recurrence, since in this case patients are usually familiar with the specific clinical signs and symptoms associated with the disease, so that accurate diagnosis can be made clinically.

The severity of viral illness that develops during chemoprophylaxis should also be monitored. Illness developing during chemoprophylaxis could be less severe or with fewer complications, which supports further the activity of the drug.

Laboratory Assessments

Many methods are now available to confirm virus infection. Antibody tests are available for the detection of either seroconversion or increases in antibody titres (Van Voris *et al.*, 1985). Other tests such as antigen-capture assays detect the presence of the virus or its components in the infected individuals. Viral culture, if positive, is a useful indication for the infectivity of the patients. Negative culture results, however, may not always indicate the absence of the virus, and could be due to the difficulty in standardising the culture technology itself, especially if virus is sensitive to exposure outside the host or is present in very low titres.

ACUTE INFECTIONS

The aims of treatment for acute infection include some or all of the following: relief of signs and symptoms of acute viral illnesses, early resolution of viral lesions, reduction in viral shedding and prevention of secondary complications. Usually similar study designs and efficacy parameters can be used for initial infection as well as recurrent episodes of illness. In some viral diseases, however, the signs and symptoms may be different between initial infection and subsequent recurrences.

Study Design

The timing of initiation of therapy and the frequency of efficacy measurements are two elements critical to a successful treatment study on acute viral infections. The earlier drug treatment can be started, the more likely benefits of the drug can be shown. Results from studies on influenza A and herpes simplex showed that, to have significant efficacy against these acute illnesses, drugs must be given within 48 h after signs and symptoms of diseases are first noted. Ideally, drug therapy should not be initiated until laboratory diagnosis is made. However, when a rapid diagnostic test is not available, treatment may be started without laboratory diagnosis if the disease is life-threatening or the drug under study is relatively non-toxic. Under these circumstances, a retrospective laboratory diagnosis should be made. Drug therapy can be commenced even earlier with self-initiation of therapy by patients, provided that pretherapy baseline information can be accurately recorded by patients themselves or through other types of arrangements.

Many acute infections are self-limited and patients usually recover without therapy in a few days. Therefore, efficacy of drug can be demonstrated only during a narrow window of time. Demonstration of more rapid improvement with therapy might require that patients be monitored frequently with more than one observation per day. This close monitoring may require housing patients with diseases that otherwise would not require hospitalisation, a procedure bound to increase the cost of a study and present additional management problems.

Since there is much variation in the clinical course of acute disease among infected individuals, drug efficacy for symptomatic relief can only be evaluated in double-blind, controlled studies. Although early phase tolerance studies can still be open and uncontrolled, it should be emphasised that toxicities of a drug can sometimes be confused with symptoms and signs of the disease to be treated. In this case, further clarification of drug toxicity can only be obtained from a controlled study.

Clinical Assessments

Clinical Signs and Symptoms

The most important efficacy parameters in clinical assessments are measurements of signs and symptoms. Since clinical manifestations of an acute infection include many signs and symptoms, analysis of change in each sign and symptom individually can be cumbersome and often uninterpretable. One approach to simplify this analytical nightmare is to establish a simple scoring system for signs and symptoms, as was used in studies with rimantadine for the treatment of influenza A illness (Hall *et al.*, 1987). Another approach is to select only key symptoms as primary parameters for analysis. For example, only pain and itching were evaluated in most studies with acyclovir and interferons for the treatment of herpes simplex (Sacks, 1988) and herpes zoster (Winston *et al.*, 1988). A third approach employs 'transformed' parameters that provide general measurement of the rate of recovery from illness. Examples of 'transformed' parameters include 'time to 50% improvement' and 'time to last fever', which were effectively used in data analysis of rimantadine studies (Wingfield *et al.*, 1969). These parameters help to eliminate repeated analysis at each time-point.

Quality of Life

Improvement of quality of life in acute viral illnesses can provide supportive evidence for the activity of the drug. Simple evaluation of productivity such as return to work, class attendance, etc., can sometimes provide useful evidence for practical benefits of the drug. For example, in a study in college students who had acute influenza illness, those who were treated with rimantadine were able to return to classes earlier than those who were treated with placebo (Van Voris *et al.*, 1981).

More sophisticated instruments are now available to help evaluate changes in overall behaviour or perceptions such as psychosocial functioning and general well-being. These methods will be discussed later in this chapter.

Resolution of Viral Lesions

This clinical assessment is primarily restricted to herpetic lesions. Resolution of viral lesions is usually measured by time to healing, time to crusting and duration of vesicle/ulcer. Some of these parameters are more appropriate than others for a particular type of herpetic lesion, depending on the natural course of the disease. For example, time to crusting is probably more reliable than time to healing for herpes zoster lesions, since crust in this disease may persist for variable periods of time. It should be emphasised that a precise definition of these parameters might not be as critical as a simple one that is strictly followed, especially among different study centres in a multicentre trial. In addition, consistent observations of lesions by one or only a very limited number of observers are required, since the assessment of lesions can be subjective.

Prevention of Complications

The particular viral disease under study determines the difficulty with which this parameter can be adequately assessed. Prevention of dissemination of lesions in herpes zoster in immunocompromised patients, for example, is easy to demonstrate, since dissemination can be clearly defined and the incidence of dissemination without drug therapy is high. In a study to evaluate alpha-interferon for the treatment of zoster in immunosuppressed patients with cancer, dissemination of zoster occurred in 58% of patients who received placebo, but only in 17% of those who received interferon (Winston *et al.*, 1988). On the other hand, to demonstrate prevention of secondary complications such as pneumonia or death from influenza infection requires a large number of patients, since the incidence of complications is low. In some viral diseases, a clear-cut causal relationship between the primary infection and secondary complications can be difficult to establish.

Laboratory Assessments

Viral culture data provide key measurements of an antiviral effect. Presence of viruses from either herpetic lesions or nasal wash of patients with influenza illness, for example, can be identified by culture. The sensitivity of culture techniques depends on the particular viral disease under study. For influenza virus, quantitative techniques for viral isolation have been well established, and data on viral shedding are fairly reliable. These culture assays were effectively used to demonstrate that significantly fewer patients with influenza illness were shedding virus after 2 day therapy with rimantadine as compared with those who received placebo. In addition, those who continued to shed virus despite rimantadine therapy had significantly lower viral titres as compared with placebo recipients (Van Voris *et al.*, 1981). On the other hand, interpretation of viral culture data from studies with herpes simplex is not as straightforward. Positive culture cannot be obtained from herpetic lesions in up to 50% of recurrent episodes, so that culture-negative and culture-positive lesions might have to be evaluated separately (Sacks, 1988).

CHRONIC INFECTION

The primary aims of therapy for chronic viral illnesses should be to arrest disease progression and reduce the chance of late adverse sequelae of infection. The ultimate goal is to completely eliminate pre-existing viral infection, but is probably not realistic at the present time. Owing to viral-gene integration and the development of latency, active viral replication does not take place in many infected cells. Phenotypically and functionally, these cells closely resemble their non-infected counterparts, leaving few targeting opportunities for drug therapy.

Study Design

The evaluation of antiviral agents for chronic viral illness frequently follows a two-step process. Virological markers are usually used as end-points for drug activity during early phase studies so that a long study period can be avoided. Activity of a drug can also be supported by positive data from measurements of immune functions and quality of life, although it is usually difficult to interpret results of these latter measurements in early phase open studies. Once drug activity is demonstrated and therapeutic index determined, long-term studies will be needed to evaluate efficacy on the basis of clinical end-points which can be rare and might require months or even years to reach.

The response of patients with chronic viral illnesses to therapy frequently depends on the length of the disease at the time of therapy. In diseases such as chronic hepatitis B and human papilloma virus infection, it has been shown that the longer patients have had the disease the less likely it is that they will respond. To ensure a balanced study population, stratification of patients based on the length of their disease should be considered.

Since measurements of virological markers and immune functions are fairly standardised and objective, early phase efficacy and tolerance studies can be open and uncontrolled in design. However, Phase III studies should always be double-blind and controlled. Dose-range and the frequency of dosing to be used in early phase studies should be determined on the basis of effective *in vitro* antiviral concentrations and single-dose pharmacokinetics of the drug in humans.

Clinical Assessments

Death or Life-threatening Events

When possible, death or life-threatening events should be used as clinical end-points. These parameters provide the most impressive and often dramatic results for the efficacy of a drug. For example, in a placebo-controlled Phase II study on zidovudine in patients with Acquired Immunodeficiency Syndrome (AIDS) or advanced AIDS-Related Complex (ARC), only 1 of 145 patients taking the drug but 16 of 137 patients taking placebo died after 3–6 months of treatments (Fischl *et al.*, 1987). This convincing evidence for efficacy resulted in an early termination of the study, leading to the registration approval of the drug. Death or life-threatening events due to other chronic viral illnesses could take a lifetime to develop or occur with very low incidence. In these diseases clinical assessments would have to focus on quality of life and other measurements discussed below.

Quality of Life Measurements

Methodology to measure quality of life has been developed over the past decade. Some of these methods, such as the General Health Rating Index (Ware, 1984) and the Sickness Impact Profile (Bergner, 1984), have been developed to assess the sense of well-being and satisfaction with life, intellectual functioning, overall physical condition, overall emotional state and ability to perform in social roles. Other more specific instruments, such as the Psychological General Well-being Schedule (Dupuy, 1984), have been designed primarily to measure general psychological status. It should be emphasised that there is no single method that is sensitive, specific and yet able to cover the breadth of all aspects of quality of life. A composite index, based on all available instruments, should be developed for each chronic viral illness under study.

Other Assessments

Depending on the disease, other assessments may be appropriate. For example, patients with human immunodeficiency virus (HIV) infection also develop neurological abnormalities and cognitive function impairment. Thus, demonstration of improvement in neurological and cognitive functions can be supportive evidence for efficacy (Schmitt *et al.*, 1988). In patients with chronic hepatitides, specific measurements are also available for the evaluation of signs and symptoms associated with compromised liver functions.

Laboratory Assessments

Virological Measurements

Commercial assays are now available for quantitative measurements of components associated with various viruses such as hepatitis B virus (HBV) and HIV. In HBV infection, the plasma levels of both HBV-DNA and HBV-DNA polymerase seem to correlate well with the amount of viral particles. A significant decrease in these parameters with therapy should therefore reflect antiviral activity of the drug. Moreover, continuous suppression of these HBV viral markers has been associated with reversion of serological status of patients and improvement in liver histology (Alexander *et al.*, 1987). In HIV infection, suppression of the viral core antigen (P24) plasma level correlates well with survival (Jackson *et al.*, 1988).

Viral cultures so far are not reliable efficacy parameters for chronic viral illnesses due to problems with reproducibility. Once available, viral culture data may provide useful additional information. For example, the culturing procedures for HIV often use co-culturing of peripheral blood lymphocytes with target cells. Negative culture results could therefore suggest elimination of both circulating viruses and infected peripheral T-cells.

Another method to evaluate the reduction and elimination of infected cells is a DNA probe assay. This method has been successfully used to demonstrate that alpha-interferon treatment is effective in the elimination of HBV in liver biopsies of patients with chronic active hepatitis B, as well as in the elimination of subclinical infection by human papillomavirus in patients with genital warts. With the availability of 'polymerase chain-reaction' technology to increase its sensitivity, the DNA probe assay can now be expanded for use in other viral diseases such as HIV.

Antibodies against specific viral antigens represent another important class of markers for virological assessments. The presence of these antibodies is commonly correlated with a less active phase of viral replication. Appearance of these antibodies during drug therapy, therefore, strongly suggests that the activity of the disease has been slowed down or arrested. For example, appearances of antibodies to HBV core antigen and surface antigen have been established as major milestones for efficacy in the therapy of chronic active hepatitis B (Perrillo *et al.*, 1988).

Immunological Measurements

When the immune system serves as the direct target of a virus, as with HIV infection, normalisation or improvement of immune function will be key evidence for efficacy. In other viral illnesses improvement in immune functions can only be used as supportive evidence.

Several immunological tests have been widely used for the evaluation of various immune functions. Routine cell counts of total and various subtypes of white blood cells provide a quick glimpse of overall status of the immune system. Specific measurements of subsets of T lymphocytes, such as helper population (T4) and suppressor population (T8), are critical for the evaluation of drug therapy for HIV diseases but are not generally useful for other viral illnesses. Other measurements of immune functions are now possible for testing both *in vitro* and *in vivo*. The most commonly used *in vitro* assay is the lymphocytic response to mitogenic and antigenic stimulation, a general assay to assess the overall functional status of cellular immunity (Yarchoan and Nelson, 1983). More specific assays such as antibody-dependent cell-mediated cytotoxicity should be used only when infected cells can serve directly as target cells for cytotoxic killing in the *in vitro* assay (Weinhold *et al.*, 1988). Cutaneous delayed-type hypersensitivity (DTH) tests have been widely used to evaluate the T-cell functionality *in vivo* (Yarchoan *et al.*, 1986). However, the DTH test has not been standardised so far, and cannot be considered a validated efficacy parameter at the present time.

Other Assessments

Additional efficacy parameters may be used when their association with the disease under study is clearly established. For example, improvement in liver function tests during therapy is supportive evidence for the efficacy of drugs for chronic hepatitis B and chronic non-A, non-B hepatitis, while improvement in liver histology is considered key evidence for efficacy for both chronic hepatitides. Any new parameter being explored as a potential efficacy end-point should preferably be tested first with established drugs.

DEVELOPMENT OF RESISTANT STRAINS

The emergence of drug-resistant strains of poliovirus was reported in laboratories as early as 1961 (Melnick *et al.*, 1961), but the clinical significance of drug-resistance has not been adequately evaluated, because of limited clinical use of antiviral drugs. Drug-resistant strains of various viruses have, however, clearly been isolated from man. These resistant strains may have either existed in the environment before drug therapy and were selected during drug treatment, or have arisen by mutation from sensitive progenitor strains during therapy.

Early detection of resistant strains depends on the availability of sensitive laboratory methods and the careful study design of clinical trials. In studies on acute infections, for example, symptoms and signs of the illness as well as viral shedding should be followed during the entire length of the study, so that any rebound in illness and/or viral shedding late in drug therapy can be recognised and potential emergence of resistant strains of virus evaluated. Virulence and infectivity of drug-resistant strains of virus can best be studied in a postcontact study. In chronic infections the emergence of resistant strains should always be considered a possible cause for the loss of response to drug therapy.

SAFETY EVALUATION

Standard evaluations of adverse reactions are discussed elsewhere in this book. However, it is important to emphasise that in early phase studies when a control arm is not used, the toxicities of a drug may be exaggerated because of difficulty in separating toxicities associated with the drug from symptoms and signs of the illness. For example, the gastrointestinal toxicities seen in patients who received rimantadine or amantadine for acute influenza illness could be due to either drug or the illness (Hall *et al.*, 1987). Similarly, haematological and neurological toxicities from HIV infection have made evaluation of toxicities of zidovudine (Richman *et al.*, 1987) and dideoxycytidine (Yarchoan *et al.*, 1988) difficult. When no control arm is included in a trial for comparison, careful attention should be given to the temporal relationship of the observed toxicity and drug therapy, as well as the reversibility of side-effects after termination of therapy. If possible, rechallenge with drug should be considered to provide direct evidence for the causal relationship. In life-threatening diseases such as AIDS, one should caution not to drop the development of a drug candidate until it is clearly demonstrated that the limiting toxicity is due to the agent under study.

CONCLUSIONS

The search for new antiviral drugs has shifted in recent years from limited nucleoside research and opportunism to rational drug design, including the establishment of target sites and development of screening procedures to identify lead compounds targeted at these sites. Antiviral research has been accelerated tremendously by the mobilisation of the scientific research community to discover treatment for AIDS. It is expected that, through this research effort, many new classes of drugs will be developed in the next few decades, not only for HIV infection but for other viral illnesses as well.

Methodologies for the evaluation of antiviral drugs have been developed for many viral illnesses. For prophylaxis, a small early phase study with the artificial challenge model should provide useful information on the activity of the drug, but a large study in a natural setting is ultimately required to establish the efficacy of the drug. For acute infections, drug therapy should be initiated early, and the signs and symptoms of illness should be monitored frequently during drug therapy to demonstrate early improvement. Reduction of viral shedding should be demonstrated, and the potential development of resistant strains should be followed closely. For chronic viral infections, viral markers, quality of life measurements and, if appropriate, immunological parameters should be evaluated for drug activity in early phase trials. Since correlation between reduction in viral markers, improvement in immune functions and efficacy in clinical end-points, such as survival or prevention of disease progression, has not been established, arbitrary end-points for these laboratory parameters frequently have to be defined for determination of drug activity, followed by long-term trials to evaluate efficacy in clinical end-points.

For many viral illnesses, treatments are either available or under development for control of the disease, but no cure is on the horizon. With the availability of new biotechnologies such as recombinant DNA technology, monoclonal antibody methodology, and better drug delivery systems, however, there could be no boundary for future antiviral therapy. For the first time, these technologies can provide us with opportunities to consider cure instead of control of the disease. Laboratory assessments for cure of viral diseases will require more sensitive diagnostic tests to verify eradication of infection. Clinical evaluation for cure will require studies with a much longer follow-up and a larger number of patients on a scale similar to that used for vaccine studies.

REFERENCES

Alexander, G. J. M., Brahm, J., Fagan, E. A., Smith, H. M., Daniels, H. M., Eddleston, A. L. W. F. and Williams, R. (1987). Loss of HBsAg with interferon therapy in chronic hepatitis B virus infection. *Lancet*, **ii**, 66–8

Atkinson, W. L., Arden, A. H., Patriarca, P. A., Leslie, N., Lui, K.-J. and Gohd, R. (1986). Amantadine prophylaxis during an institutional outbreak of type A (H1N1) Influenza. *Arch. Int. Med.*, **146**, 1751–6

Balfour, H. H. (1984). Acyclovir and other chemotherapy for herpes group viral infections. *Ann. Rev. Med.*, **35**, 279–91

Bergner, M. (1984). The sickness impact scale. In Wenger, N. K., Mattson, M. E., Furgerg, C. D. and Elinson, J. (Eds.), *Assessment of Quality of Life in Clinical Trials of Cardiovascular Therapies*. Le Jacq Publishing, New York, pp. 152–9

Clemens, M. J. and McNurlan, M. A. (1985). Regulation of cell proliferation and differentiation by interferons. *Biochem. J.*, **226**, 345–60

Dawkins, A. T., Gallager, L. R., Togo, Y., Hornick, R. B. and Harris, B. A. (1968). Studies on induced influenza in man. *J. Am. Med. Assoc.*, **203**, 1095–9

Dolin, R., Reichman, R. C., Madore, H. P., Maynard, R., Linton, P. N. and Weber-Jones, J. (1982). A controlled trial of amantadine and rimantadine in the prophylaxis of influenza A infection. *New Engl. J. Med.*, **307**, 580–4

Dupuy, H. J. (1984). The psychological general well-being index. In Wenger, N. K., Mattson, M. E., Furberg, C. D. and Elinson, J. (Eds.), *Assessment of Quality of Life in Clinical Trials of Cardiovascular Therapies*. Le Jacq Publishing, New York, pp. 170–83

Fischl, M. A. D. A., Richman, D. D., Grieco, M. H., Gottlieb, M. S., Volberding, P. A., Laskin, O. L., Leedom, J. M., Groopman, J. E., Mildvan, D., Schooley, R. T., Jackson, G. G., Durack, D. T., King, D. and the AZT Collaborative Working Group (1987). The efficacy of azidothymidine (AZT) in the treatment of patients with AIDS and AIDS-related complex. *New Engl. J. Med.*, **317**, 185–91

Hall, C. B., Dolin, R., Gala, C. L., Markovitz, D. M., Zhang, Y. Q., Madore, P. H., Disney, F. A., Talpey, W. B., Green, J. L., Francis, A. B. and Pichichero, M. E. (1987). Children with influenza A infection: treatment with rimantadine. *Pediatrics*, **80**, 275–82

Jackson, G. G., Paul, D. A., Falk, L. A., Rubenis, M., Despotes, J. C., Mack, D., Knigge, M. and Emeson, E. E. (1988). Human immunodeficiency virus antigenemia (p24) in the Acquired Immunodeficiency Syndrome (AIDS) and the effect of treatment with zidovudine. *Ann. Int. Med.*, **108**, 175–80

Koff, W. C. and Knight, V. (1979). Effect of rimantadine on influenza virus replication. *Proc. Soc. Exp. Biol. Med.*, **160**, 246–53

Melnick, J. L., Crowther, D. and Barrera-Oro, J. (1961). Rapid development of drug-resistant mutants of poliovirus. *Science, N.Y.*, **134**, 551–3

Mitsuya, H. and Broder, S. (1987). Strategies for antiviral therapy in AIDS. *Nature*, **325**, 773–8

Perrillo, R. P., Regenstein, F. G., Peter, M. G., DeeSchryver-Kecskemeti, K., Bodicky, C. J., Campbell, C. R. and Kuhns, M. C. (1988). Prednisone withdrawal followed by recombinant alpha interferon in the treatment of chronic type B hepatitis. *Ann. Int. Med.*, **108**, 95–100

Richman, D. D., Fischl, M. A., Grieco, M. H., Gottlieb, M. S., Volberding, P. L., Laskin, O. L., Leedom, J. M., Groopman, J. E., Mildvan, D., Hirsch, M. S., Jackson, G. G., Durack, D. T., Nusinoff-Lehrman, S. and the AZT Collaborative Working Group (1987). The toxicity of azidothymidine in the treatment of patients with AIDS and AIDS-related complex. *New Engl. J. Med.*, **317**, 192–7

Sacks, S. L. (1988). Treatment of genital herpes. In DeClercq, E. (Ed.), *Clinical Use of Antiviral Drugs*. Martinus Nijhoff, Boston, pp. 87–114

Schmitt, F. A., Bigley, J. B., McKinnis, R., Logue, P. E., Evans, R. W., Drucker, J. L. and the AZT Collaborative Working Group (1988). Neurophysiological outcome of zidovudine treatment of patients with AIDS and AIDS-related complex. *New Engl. J. Med.*, **319**, 1573–8

Van Voris, L. P., Betts, R. F., Hayden, F. G., Christmas, W. A. and Douglas, G., Jr. (1981). Successful treatment of naturally occurring influenza A/USSR/77 H1N1. *J. Am. Med. Assoc.*, **245**, 1128–31

Van Voris, L. P., Betts, R. F., Menegus, M. A., Murphy, B. R., Roth, F. K. and Douglas, G., Jr. (1985). Serological diagnosis of influenza A/USSR/77 H1N1 infection: value of ELISA compared to other antibody techniques. *J. Med. Virol.*, **16**, 315–20

Ware, J. (1984). General health rating index. In Wenger, N. K., Mattson, M. E., Furberg, C. D. and Elinson, J. (Eds.), *Assessment of Quality of Life in Clinical Trials of Cardiovascular Therapies*. Le Jacq Publishing, New York, pp. 184–8

Weinhold, K. J., Lyerly, H. K., Matthews, T. J., Tyler, D. S., Ahearne, P. M., Stine, K. C., Langlois, A. J., Durack, D. T. and Bolognesi, D. P. (1988). Cellular anti-gp120 cytolytic reactivities in HIV-1 seropositive individuals. *Lancet*, **i**, 902–4

Wingfield, W. L., Pollack, D. and Grunert, R. R. (1969). Therapeutic efficacy of amantadine HCl and rimantadine HCl in naturally occurring influenza A2 respiratory illness in man. *New Engl. J. Med.*, **281**, 579–84

Winston, D. J., Eron, L. J., Ho, M., Pazin, G., Kessler, H., Pottage, J. C., Jr., Gallagher, J., Sartiano, G., Ho, W. G., Champlin, R. E. and the Hoffman–La Roche Zoster Study Group (1988). Recombinant interferon alpha-2a for treatment of herpes zoster in immunosuppressed patients with cancer. *Am. J. Med.*, **85**, 147–51

Yarchoan, R., Klecker, R. W., Weinhold, K. J., Markham, P. D., Lyerly, H. K., Durack, D. T., Gelmann, E., Nusinoff-Lehrman, S., Blum, R. M., Barry, D. W., Shearer, G. M., Fischl, M. A., Mitsuya, H., Gallo, R. C., Collins, J. M., Bolognesi, D. P., Myers, C. E. and Broder, S. (1986). Administration of 3'-azido-3'-deoxythymidine, an inhibitor of HTLV-III/LAV replication, to patients with AIDS or AIDS-related complex. *Lancet*, **i**, 575–80

Yarchoan, R. and Nelson, D. L. (1983). A study of the functional capabilities of human neonatal lymphocytes for *in vitro* specific antibody production. *J. Immunol.*, **131**, 1222–8

Yarchoan, R., Perno, C. F., Thomas, R. V., Klecker, R. W., Allain, J.-P., Wills, R. J., McAtee, N., Fischl, M. A., Dubinsky, R., McNeely, M. C., Mitsuya, H., Pluda, J. M., Lawley, T. J., Leuther, M., Safai, B., Collins, J. M., Myers, C. E. and Broder, S. (1988). Phase I studies of 2',3'-dideoxycytidine in severe human immunodeficiency virus infection as a single agent and alternating with zidovudine(AZT). *Lancet*, **i**, 76–80

49
Anticancer Drugs

Lee Schacter, Marcel Rozencweig, Claude Nicaise, Renzo Canetta, Susan Kelley and Laurie Smaldone

Pharmaceutical R&D Division, Bristol-Myers Co., 5 Research Parkway, Wallingford, CT 06492, USA

INTRODUCTION

The assessment of anticancer agents represents a unique combination of problems in drug development. The treatment of cancer requires compounds which can kill neoplastic human cells with minimum toxicity to normal cells and tissues. Since, at the present time, no drugs are available which are truly selective for cancer cells, collateral damage is an expected, if unwanted, consequence of cancer chemotherapy. The vast majority of active anticancer agents are cytotoxic compounds which have significant side-effects and a very small therapeutic index. Therefore, such agents are commonly given at the highest doses possible, despite the routine occurrence of toxicities which would be considered unacceptable in drugs used for other diseases.

The goal of any treatment must be to benefit the individual being treated. When testing Phase I cancer agents, the hope, however remote, is that the patient may benefit from the new therapy. Clinical trials of anticancer agents are predicated on this objective. Within this constraint three critical items of information must be obtained as the result of Phase I trials of cytotoxics for cancer chemotherapy. One is to determine how much of the new agent can be given safely. This is the maximum tolerated dose (MTD) of the new agent. Second, the dose-limiting toxicity(ies) (DLT) and other side-effects of the agent must be identified so that additional patients can be treated more safely. At this point the evaluation of the new agent is a largely qualitative one and, as a practical matter, restricted to the analysis of acute events or cumulative toxicities which appear fairly quickly. Finally, information about the effects of schedule on toxicity is sought.

The recent interest in so-called 'biological response modifiers' (BRMs) such as interferon, tumour necrosis factor and monoclonal antibodies poses a new set of challenges to the development of agents for the treatment of malignant diseases. End-points in addition to or other than toxicity or tumour shrinkage need to be defined for the early testing of such materials.

The design of clinical trials of new oncological drugs has recently been discussed at length (Begg, 1988; Levinthal, 1988; Piantadosi, 1988). This review will first consider the testing of traditional cytotoxic compounds for the therapy of cancer and then discuss approaches to the evaluation of the new 'biological' substances.

PHASE I—CYTOTOXIC AGENTS

Selection of Patients for Early Clinical Trials of Antineoplastic Agents

Because of the toxicity associated with traditional cytotoxic agents (Table 49.1), these compounds are *not* tested in normal human subjects. Such studies are performed in seriously ill individuals with malignancy.

Table 49.1 Common toxicities of cytotoxic agents

Myelosuppression	Renal dysfunction
Immune suppression	Hepatic dysfunction
Nausea, vomiting	Pulmonary dysfunction
Anorexia	Mucositis
Alopecia	

Cancer patients selected for Phase I trials must meet two kinds of criteria; the first designed to protect them from unnecessary risks while maximising the chance of benefit, and the second to allow adequate testing of the agent. To protect the patient, only individuals for whom no effective treatment of their malignancy is available are entered into Phase I trials. This usually means progressive disease following surgery, radiation therapy and/or chemotherapy. Because the toxicity of the new agent is uncertain, it is important that those receiving the drug be able to metabolise and excrete it normally. Thus, they need to have adequate hepatic and renal function. In addition, most cytotoxics affect the bone marrow. Patients receiving these agents in Phase I studies must have adequate marrow function as demonstrated by normal numbers of circulating white blood cells and platelets.

If there is to be any opportunity for the patient to benefit from the new agent, those treated cannot have very advanced, preterminal disease. Subjects must be well enough to be able to be followed so that any response or delayed toxicity can be observed. Patients must, therefore, have a life expectancy of at least 8–12 weeks following drug administration (Table 49.2).

Table 49.2 Commonly used inclusion and exclusion criteria for Phase I trials

Inclusion	*Exclusion*
Histologically confirmed cancer	Pregnancy or lactation
Age >18 and <75	Brain metastases
Performance status WHO ≤3	Active infection
Life expectancy >9 weeks	Major organ dysfunction
No cytotoxic within 4 weeks (6 weeks for nitrosoureas)	Any medical or psychiatric condition which would put patient at risk
$WBC > 4000/mm^3$, platelets $> 100\,000/mm^3$	
Serum creatinine ≤1.5 mg/dl	
Normal hepatic function	
Ability to give informed consent	

The type of patient entered when the MTD is approached may differ from those treated at the lowest dose of drug. At the beginning of the Phase I trial, heavily pretreated patients of poor performance status are usually entered. Since no toxicity is expected at the starting dose, such patients can be safely treated. As experience with the drug accumulates, better-risk individuals are given the drug.

It is important to determine the MTD in patients with both good and poor performance characteristics. When toxic events are first observed, patients with fewer risk factors for toxicity, such as prior therapy or poor performance status, must be included. If this is not done, the dose chosen for Phase II and Phase III trials may be significantly lower than appropriate for patients with less advanced disease.

Conduct of Phase I Trials

Adverse events can reasonably be expected to occur in at least some patients treated with new cytotoxic agents. Trials with these compounds should only be conducted by experienced investigators and at institutions with the facilities to provide adequate care regardless of the toxicity encountered.

Determination of Starting Dose

A primary goal of Phase I cytotoxic drug testing is to determine the maximally tolerated dose (MTD) of the new agent. It is important to detect the earliest indications of toxicity so that no patient is placed at unwarranted risk for serious complications. The first human subjects should be exposed to doses which can reasonably be expected to cause little or no toxicity. In addition, the starting dose should not be too remote from efficacious levels.

The starting dose in man is based on data from animals. Retrospective analyses in a large series of cytotoxic drugs of the relationship between doses causing toxicity in animals and dose-causing toxic events in humans makes it possible to predict a safe starting dose for a new agent in humans from animal studies (Penta *et al.*, 1979; Rozencweig *et al.*, 1981, 1982). A safe starting dose in man for the vast majority of cytotoxic drugs has been empirically found to be either one-tenth of the LD_{10} in rodents or one-third of the lowest dose causing toxicity (toxic dose low: TDL) in a larger mammal such as the dog. In many cases these two doses are very close and either can be used. If, however, there is a large discrepancy between one-tenth of the LD_{10} in rodents and the TDL in dogs, the lower starting dose should be chosen to reduce the risk to patients.

Dose Calculation

Many drugs are dosed on a mg/kg basis or a fixed dose regardless of the patient's size. Because of the narrow margin between therapeutic and toxic doses for cytotoxic drugs, the amount administered must be more carefully determined. A number of studies (Crawford *et al.*, 1950; Pinkel, 1958; Freireich *et al.*, 1966) have demonstrated that dosing based on surface area is the most accurate method for administering comparable doses of cytotoxic drugs to patients. In addition, comparison of toxic and therapeutic effects between species is most accurate when body surface area is used as the denominator. Nomograms have been developed to convert height and weight into surface area (m^2) for both adults and children as well as conversion factors from mg/kg to mg/m^2 for various species (Freireich *et al.*, 1966). Almost all cytotoxic drugs are administered on a m^2 basis whether in early clinical trials or routine clinical use.

Dose Escalation

Traditional cytotoxic drugs rarely show activity at doses completely devoid of side-effects. Because the starting dose in Phase I is chosen to be non-toxic, it is important to make the transition from an inactive non-toxic starting dose to an active dose as rapidly as possible, to minimise the number of patients treated at inactive levels. There are two general approaches to dose escalation regardless of schedule.

The first is an empiric approach in which doses are increased according to a predetermined numerical formula. One such formula is referred to as the Fibonacci escalation, named for an Italian mathematician who described this type of numerical sequence (Geller, 1984). The pattern described by Fibonacci is 1, 1, 2, 3, 5, ... If this scheme is followed, the first dose is n, the second $2n$, the third $3n$, and so on. In practice a modification of the Fibonacci progression is used. Other formulas can be used such as doubling the dose until the first signs of toxicity are observed and then increasing it at a slower rate (e.g. 20% or 33%) until the MTD has been identified. As the MTD is approached, the dose may have to be increased *or* decreased to clearly define the MTD, depending on the pattern of toxicity observed.

The second general approach to dose escalation is based on drug pharmacokinetics. The human MTD for many cytotoxics occurs when the area under the plasma drug concentration–time curve (AUC or $C \times T$) is the same as the AUC in mice at the mouse LD_{10} (EORTC Group, 1984). While it may be possible to use the AUC to determine dosing, this approach remains unproven.

Retreatment Interval

The time between treatments with a new agent is determined by toxicology data from animals, the nature of the agent being studied and preliminary observations in treated patients. For example, a new chemotype demonstrating delayed hepatotoxicity in animals will require prolonged careful monitoring of liver function prior to retreatment, while an analogue of an existing drug such as doxorubicin, which is known to cause early cytopenia as the first manifestation of its toxicity, may be dosed more frequently in Phase I. To ensure the safety of patients, frequent (twice/week) laboratory studies are needed. It is critical not to miss the first signs of adverse effects on the marrow, liver or kidneys. In addition, a weekly history and physical is done, to disclose the presence of symptoms or signs of side-effects.

In many trials a patient started at a particular dose level can be retreated at the next higher dose level *if* he/she has shown no toxicity at that level *and* if other patients administered the drug at the higher level have been followed for a long enough period to determine its safety.

Number of Patients at Each Dose Level

In the vast majority of Phase I trials of cytotoxic agents, three patients are entered at each dose level. The number of patients at each dose level is kept small, to allow the most rapid possible increase in dose from a non-toxic inactive level to an active, albeit a toxic, one. *Assuming* that there is a probability of achieving toxicity in 50% of the patients at a given dose level, the chance of toxicity occurring in three patients is $0.5 \times 0.5 \times 0.5 = 0.125$. This number of patients gives an 87.5% confidence (1.0–0.125) that the dose is non-toxic if no adverse events are seen. If four patients are entered, the confidence becomes 93.75% and with five patients it becomes 96.875% (Geller, 1984). Many, if not most, trials enter additional patients if one or more of three patients at any given dose level exhibit toxicity, to ensure the validity of the observation and to be able to give a probability of such an event occurring. At the suspected MTD, experience is expanded in a larger number of patients to more clearly identify the optimal dose and the toxicities which may be expected in Phase II trials enroling patients with various risk factors.

End-point of Phase I Trials for Cytotoxics

The objectives of Phase I trials for cytotoxic agents are to: (1) identify the most common toxicities; (2) define the dose (MTD) at which these toxicities become a significant risk to the patient. Achievement of these goals allows the design of Phase II efficacy trials.

Cytotoxic agents can cause a wide variety of toxicities. Prominent targets of these drugs are the bone marrow, oral mucosa, hair follicles and gastrointestinal mucosa. These organs must be monitored closely for toxic effects. Toxicities are generally rated by use of the scales promulgated by the World Health Organization (WHO publication No. 48, WHO Publications Centre USA, 49 Sheridan Ave., Albany, N.Y. 12210). The MTD is defined as the highest dose which can be safely administered. For haematological parameters, reversible WHO grade IV toxicity is usually considered dose-limiting.

Determination of Route and Schedule

Cytotoxic drugs can be given by various routes and schedules. Preclinical studies often provide some information on whether or not the new agent's activity is route- or schedule-dependent. Unless preclinical trials unambiguously point to superior activity via a particular route or schedule, most drugs are tested by intravenous administration using more than one schedule. Patient and physician convenience are an important factor in determining schedules.

For cytotoxic drugs the interval between dosing is a function of the time it takes to recover from drug-induced toxicity. The higher the dose, the longer recovery usually takes. For most new cytotoxic agents the MTD and DLT are determined using three different schedules: a single dose given at intervals determined by the time to full recovery (usually every 3 or 4 weeks); daily doses for 5 days, with retreatment when there is full recovery; and once weekly for 4 weeks, again with retreatment when there is full recovery. Testing of prolonged daily treatment is not routinely performed until the toxicity of the drug in man has been evaluated and the possibility of a cumulative effect determined.

Most cytotoxics are given intravenously in Phase I, but if oral absorption in animals has been good and GI toxicity mild, the oral route might be chosen.

EARLY PHASE II—CYTOTOXIC AGENTS

In Phase I the critical issue addressed is the determination of the MTD of the new agent and the identification of the toxic effects of the compound. In Phase II the emphasis is the identification of antitumour activity.

There are two goals in early Phase II trials of cancer drugs. First, to avoid treating large numbers of patients with ineffective agents. Second, to avoid false-negative results. It is more important not to mistakenly label as inactive an agent which has activity than to label as active one which is not. An error in identifying as active an agent which is not will be corrected as trials continue. If an active agent is erroneously labelled as ineffective, its development may be abandoned.

Response and Survival

The ultimate goal of cancer chemotherapy is cure. However, to date, few cytotoxic drugs have had an obvious and dramatic impact on survival in Phase II studies. Trials designed to detect increased survival with non-curative agents require large numbers of patients and prolonged follow-up. It is generally accepted that tumour shrinkage is required for improved survival, and that the higher the response rate, the more likely it is that these responses will result in prolonged life expectancy. Therefore, response is used in Phase II as a surrogate for survival. Response *per se* can also be clinically important, reducing tumour burden, relieving symptoms and improving quality of life.

Response Criteria

For the purpose of these trials, activity is defined as the ability to induce complete and/or partial responses. A complete response is defined as the complete disappearance of all signs and symptoms of the disease for at least 4 weeks. A partial response is the reduction by 50% or more in the volume of all measurable disease for 4 weeks or more. Other types of responses have been defined (mixed, less than partial and stabilisation), but these are generally considered of little clinical or biological significance. Measurable is generally defined as any mass which can be palpated or seen by an imaging technique and whose size can be determined. Pleural effusions or lep-tomeningeal disease would not be considered measurable. To measure the mass, the two largest perpendicular diameters are multiplied. If more than one measurable mass is present, the size of each is determined and summed. An overall response rate, the sum of the complete and partial rates, is usually reported.

Spectrum of Activity

In addition to determining the ability of the new agent to induce complete and partial responses, the spectrum of activity is also determined. New agents are usually tested in malignancies which are common and/or have lesions which can be followed for response. Typically, Phase II studies will be conducted in breast cancer, non-small-cell lung cancer, small-cell lung cancer, colorectal cancer, hypernephroma, melanoma and squamous cell carcinoma of the head and neck. In addition, if preclinical trials suggested activity against a specific cell type, such as lymphocytes, the agent will also be tried in the treatment of malignancies derived from that tissue.

Patient Selection

A key issue in the design of Phase II trials is the type of patients entered. For the majority of cancers, the response to any therapy is reduced following relapse from prior treatment. Patients who have been exposed to a number of cytotoxic drugs before receiving a new agent are far less likely to respond to the new agent than previously untreated individuals. A good example of this phenomenon is the response of small-cell lung cancer patients to the cytotoxic drug etoposide. Previously untreated patients with this disease have a 40+% response rate, while previously treated individuals rarely respond. In Phase II trials the best interests of the patients and the need to test the new agent in an advantageous setting must be considered. It is generally considered ethical to use a new agent in previously untreated patients who cannot be cured by surgery or radiotherapy, if there is no effective chemotherapy for that malignancy (Table 49.3). For cancers which respond to existing drugs it may still be ethical to use a new agent as first-line chemotherapy if the natural history of the disease is such that a delay in therapy will not reduce the efficacy of standard drug treatment.

Table 49.3 Response of cancer to existing chemotherapy

Unresponsive to existing chemotherapy	Minor response to existing chemotherapy	Response to chemotherapy
Melanoma	Colorectal cancer	Breast cancer
Hypernephroma (renal cell carcinoma)	Hepatoma	Small-cell lung cancer
	Squamous cell carcinoma of the head and neck	Lymphoma (Hodgkin's and non-Hodgkin's)
Pancreatic carcinoma	Non-small-cell lung cancer	Leukaemia (all forms)
		Germ cell tumours

While investigators differ in their opinions on when to test a Phase II agent for each human cancer, the goal is always to test the new agent in patients with the best possible chance of responding.

Duration of Treatment

Few tumours respond to a single cycle of any chemotherapeutic agent. Unless there is clear-cut progression, two cycles of therapy are given before response is assessed.

Statistical Considerations

The statistical goal of a Phase II trial is to estimate the response rate (defined above) to the new agent. This goal must be pursued in the light of the ethical mandate to treat the smallest number of patients possible with an ineffective agent. If no responses are seen in 14 consecutive patients, there is a 95% probability that the response rate is <20%. If 19 consecutive patients show no response, it is possible to be 95% sure that the response rate is <15% (Geller, 1984). If no responses are seen in 14 or 19 patients, the drug is generally considered to be of little value as a single agent in that disease.

As more patients are entered, the accuracy with which the response rate can be predicted increases. To estimate the response to within ±15% of its true value with 95% confidence, 45 patients must be entered. Most trial designs call for the entry of a fixed number of *evaluable* patients, usually 24 or 30 (Gehan and Schniederman, 1973). Once activity has been observed, expanded Phase II trials allow for more careful definition of activity in a specific patient population.

Response data should be based on evaluable patients. Evaluable patients are all individuals entered into the study who met the entry criteria and for whom sufficient data are available to allow evaluation of response. Very sick patients are not entered into such studies. Patients must be expected to live long enough to receive two courses of treatments and long enough beyond that time-point so that an effective agent can exert its antitumour activity.

The end-point of the early Phase II trial of a new cytotoxic is the identification of sufficient activity to warrant further development. The end-point of late Phase II trials is the more accurate definition of the degree and spectrum of activity, as well as further quantitative determination of acute and chronic side-effects.

PHASE I—'BIOLOGICAL RESPONSE MODIFIERS' (BRMs)

Cytotoxics vs BRMs

Cytotoxic drugs are obtained by synthesis, by extraction of plants or as fermentation products of bacteria and fungi. They are identified by their ability to kill human cancer cells. BRMs, in contrast, are mammalian cell products which may be expected to influence cell growth and division on the basis of their known or suspected roles *in vivo*. Included under this rubric are entities such as monoclonal antibodies, tumour necrosis factor, assorted growth factors, and interleukins. The rationale for using cytotoxics is their ability to act directly on malignant cells. In contrast, BRMs are used with the expectation that they will augment, supplement, activate or initiate a process in which tumour cells are killed via naturally occurring anti-tumour mechanisms.

Phase I End-points for BRMs

Phase I trials of these agents should attempt to determine the dose, route and schedule for the agent which will maximise the biological response sought. While it is critical to note any toxicities encountered, the amount of a biological agent administered need not be escalated to the MTD once the dose required to achieve the optimal biological response is identified. The dose–effect curve for a BRM may demonstrate an optimal concentration, making the use of a BRM at higher or lower doses counterproductive.

The Phase I end-point is, therefore, a function of the agent's biological activity and the way it is expected to be used in the treatment of malignancy. For a biological material designed to elicit an immune response to a tumour, that end-point would be some measure of tumour immunity. If a monoclonal antibody is being tested, optimal localisation at the tumour site relative to other parts of the body as well as the ability to elicit an immune response to the tumour might be used as end-points. Unfortunately, these biological end-points are not always known with certainty at the start of clinical trials with BRMs.

Because some BRMs are extremely expensive, cost can become a factor and an undesirable end-point in testing these agents.

Selection of Patients

In addition to the criteria applicable to patients being treated with cytotoxics, patients entered on Phase I trials of biological agents must be able to mount an appropriate response to such agents. For example, if the new agent is designed to stimulate an immune response to tumour, patients entered in the trial must be able to mount such an immune response. The criteria for selection will depend on the nature of the agent being tested and the end-point defined. Patients who would be eligible for Phase I studies of cytotoxic agents may not be eligible for similar trials of BRMs.

Starting Dose

If toxicity is observed in animal models, the starting dose for a biological agent can be based in part on those observations. However, many BRMs show little if any acute toxicity (e.g. monoclonal antibodies), so that the starting dose must be based either on endogenous levels of naturally occurring compounds or another rational extrapolation from animal trials.

Dose Escalation

In Phase I trials of BRMs a specific response end-point, e.g. tumour immunity or immune response, is sought. Therefore, dose may need to be increased or decreased from the starting dose to define this end-point. Doses must be modified on the basis of experience gained during the trial.

Statistical Considerations

Statistical end-points for BRMs must be individualised, depending on the parameter being followed.

EARLY PHASE II—BRMs

As with cytotoxics, the primary objective of Phase II testing of BRMs is to treat cancer. Response criteria may differ from those applied to cytotoxics, depending on what activity is being sought in the BRM.

SUMMARY

Early clinical trials for anticancer drugs represent a unique set of challenges. For traditional drugs, the need to treat at doses close to the MTD places an emphasis on the careful identification and monitoring of the pattern of toxicities. Testing the newer biological agents presents an even greater challenge, as appropriate end-point(s) for each must be individually determined and appropriately measured.

REFERENCES

Begg, C. B. (1988). Selection of patients for clinical trials. *Semin. Oncol.*, **15**, 434–40

Crawford, J. D., Terry, M. E. and Rourke, G. M. (1950). Simplification of drug dosage calculation by application of the surface area principle. *Pediatrics*, **5**, 783–90

EORTC Pharmacokinetics and Metabolism Group. (1987). Pharmacokinetically guided dose escalation in phase I clinical trials. Commentary and proposed guidelines. *Eur. J. Cancer Clin. Oncol.*, **23**, 1083–7

Freireich, E. J., Gehan, E. A., Rall, D. P., Schmidt, L. H. and Sipeer, H. E. (1966). Quantitative comparison of toxicity of anticancer agents in mouse, rat, hamster, dog, monkey and man. *Cancer Chemother. Rep.*, **50**, 219–44

Gehan, E. A. and Schniederman, M. A. (1973). Experimental design of clinical trials. In Holland, J. F. and Frei, E. (Eds.), *Cancer Medicine*. Lea and Febiger, Philadelphia, pp. 531–53

Geller, N. L. (1984). Design of phase I and II clinical trials in cancer: a statistician's view. *Cancer Invest.*, **2**, 483–91

Levinthal, B. G. (1988). An overview of clinical trials in oncology. *Semin. Oncol.*, **15**, 414–22

Penta, J. S., Rozencweig, M., Guarino, A. M. and Muggia, F. M. (1979). Mouse and large-animal toxicology studies of twelve antitumour agents: Relevance to starting dose for phase I clinical trials. *Cancer Chemother. Pharm.*, **3**, 97–101

Piantadosi, S. (1988). Principles of clinical trial design. *Semin. Oncol.*, **15**, 423–33

Pinkel, D. (1958). The use of body surface area as a criterion of drug dosage in cancer chemotherapy. *Cancer Res.*, **18**, 853–6

Rozencweig, M., Dodion, P., Nicaise, C., Piccart, M. and Kenis, Y. (1982). Approach to phase I trials in cancer patients. In Cortes-Funes, J. H. and Rozencweig, M. (Eds.), *New Approaches in Cancer Therapy*. Raven Press, New York, pp. 1–13

Rozencweig, M., Von Hoff, D. D., Staquet, M. J., Schein, P. S., Penta, J. S., Goldin, A., Muggia, F. M., Freireich, E. J. and DeVita, V. T. Jr. (1981). Animal toxicology for early clinical trials with anticancer agents. *Cancer Clin. Trials*, **4**, 21–8

XIV
Assessment of Drugs Affecting the Inflammatory Process and Pain

50
Drugs Affecting the Immune Response

M. Rooney and G. W. Duff

University of Edinburgh, Dept of Medicine, University of Edinburgh, Rheumatic Diseases Unit, Northern General Hospital, Ferry Road, Edinburgh EH5 2DQ, UK

INTRODUCTION

This chapter is concerned with the investigation of drug-induced changes in immune function. Before discussing specific investigative techniques, a few general points should be made. Many tests for evaluation of the immune system are complex, time-consuming and expensive. The tests chosen should, therefore, be informative, discriminating and, most important, clinically relevant. More than in most other areas of therapeutic evaluation, immunological assays require scrupulous technique in sample collection, cell separation and culture methods. All systems of evaluation must be rigorously standardised with normal values obtained for each laboratory. The complex cellular events that are measured as immune function give rise to large interassay and interindividual variations. Therefore, controls must be included with each batch. Finally, discrepancies in results from *in vitro* and *in vivo* studies of the same immunological phenomenon are common; the former must therefore be interpreted with caution and should not be viewed in isolation.

THE IMMUNE SYSTEM

Cells and cellular interactions involved in the adaptive immune response are outlined in Figure 50.1. Following the processing and presentation of antigen by cells expressing MHC class II, T cells (primarily T helper cells) are stimulated via their antigen receptor to express growth factor genes, leading to clonal proliferation. This process is augmented by cytokines from the antigen-presenting cells. Activated T helper cells are necessary for B cell proliferation and differentiation in the presence of antigen, and induce cytotoxic T cells that bind antigen on target cells with subsequent cell death. Following T cell activation, T cell-mediated suppression occurs which down-regulates the immune response. As well as cell-to-cell interactions via surface receptors, cellular responses of mature immunocytes are modulated by soluble peptide cytokines. Thus, analysis of the cell populations involved and

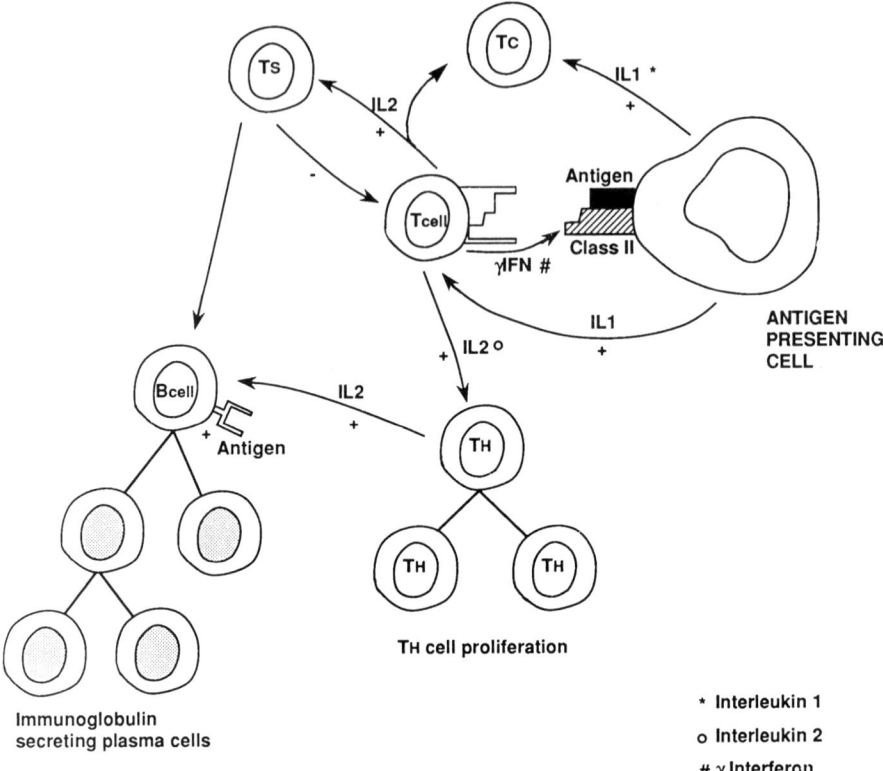

Figure 50.1 Diagrammatic representation of the adaptive immune response. The division of T cells into helper (Th), suppressor (Ts) and cytotoxic (Tc) subsets is based on functional activity. Differences in expression of surface markers may be related to ontogenic progression of cells of similar lineage

evaluation of their functional capacity are an important aspect of assessing immunomodulation.

Investigation of immune regulation can broadly be divided into the following categories: assessment of (1) T cell function; (2) B cell function; (3) accessory cell function; (4) complement function; (5) reactive oxygen production; (6) cytokine function; and (7) intercellular adherence function.

The reader is also referred to Chapter 49 on anticancer therapy, where areas of immune regulation are also considered.

T LYMPHOCYTE EVALUATION

T lymphocyte evaluation can be divided into numerical and functional assays. The latter are more informative but the former are often complementary and a necessary initial step for the functional assays.

Total lymphocyte numbers can be derived from peripheral blood films and total peripheral blood white cell counts. Two tests are in common use to distinguish T from B lymphocytes, which are morphologically identical: (1) spontaneous sheep red cell rosetting;[1] (2) recognition of lineage-specific surface markers by antibodies.

The first method is based on the principle that lymphocytes with surface receptors for sheep red cells are thymus-derived, i.e. T cells. Lymphocytes with these receptors will bind clusters of sheep cells and form E (erythrocyte) rosettes. Using the method described by Wilson *et al.*,[2] optimal identification of T cells can be achieved. This method is economical and fast, though somewhat insensitive.

The second method involves identification of T cells using T-cell-specific monoclonal antibodies. All T cells express the CD3 complex on their surface.[3] An arrangement of three polypeptides, it is usually related to the T cell antigen receptor and appears to modulate the cellular response to antigen, although its definitive functions remain unclear. Monoclonal antibodies (Mab) directed against various epitopes on this structure enable detection of all classes of T cell. This method is probably the most sensitive but is relatively expensive. Lymphocyte subset-specific monoclonal reagents are now commercially available in kits with detailed protocols. The method of choice is indirect immunofluorescence where the second antibody is fluorochrome-labelled. Fab_2 fragment is preferable, to avoid non-specific adherence to cells bearing Fc receptors.

Reductions in the absolute numbers of total white cells (leucopenia) or of lymphocytes (lymphopenia) are a common feature of immunosuppressive drugs, reflecting suppression of proliferation and maturation of bone marrow progenitor cells. For example, Hanly and Bresnihan[4] have shown a fall in total lymphocyte numbers in the peripheral blood of patients with rheumatoid arthritis treated with gold salts. We have obtained similar results (Figure 50.2). However, it is important to remember that reduction in circulating T cells can simply indicate sequestration elsewhere. Thus, only direct evaluation of progenitor cell production by bone marrow aspirate can address this question definitively.

Identification of Changes in T Lymphocyte Subpopulations

A number of cell markers have been described which divide the total T cell population into distinct maturational and functional subsets. These include variation in E-receptor expression, receptors for different Ig classes, differential binding of lectins and, more recently, expression of differentiation antigens using T cell subset-specific monoclonal antibodies.

The two methods most commonly used are:

(1) Identification of T cells bearing receptors for IgG (T suppressor/cytotoxic cells, Ts/Tc).[5] Identification of T cells bearing receptors for IgM (T helper cells, Th).[5] This older technique is still used in some studies.

(2) Identification of T cell subsets using monoclonal antibodies primarily

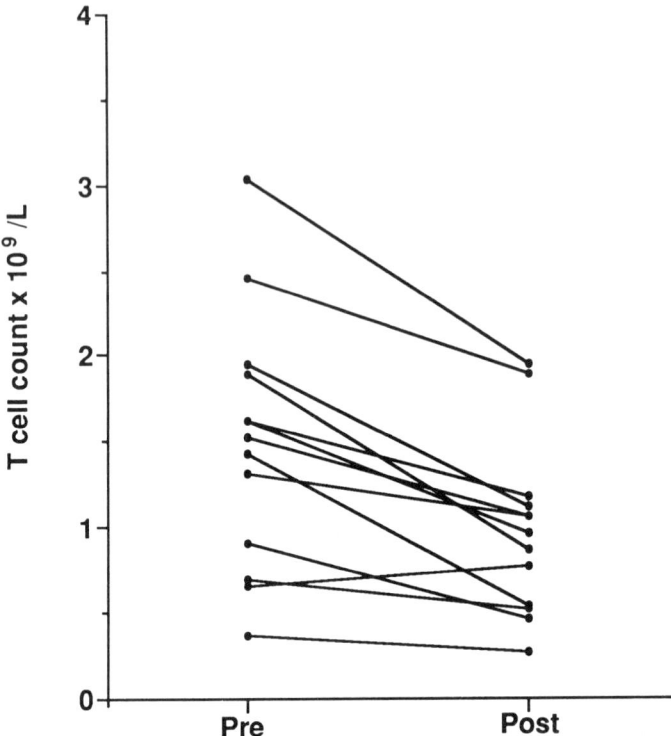

Figure 50.2 Change in T lymphocyte count of patients with rheumatoid arthritis before and after treatment with gold salts

distinguishing functional Th and Ts population.[6,7] This is now the conventional method and is most widely used.

As well as expressing the CD3 complex, T cells express surface proteins that divide the population into three functionally distinct groups: the helper (Th), suppressor (Ts) and cytotoxic (Tc) cells. T helper cells are characterised by the surface marker CD4 (T4). They are important (Figure 50.1) in T cell maturation, B cell activation and Tc maturation by the generation of cytokines following interactions with macrophages.

Ts and Tc cells express the antigen CD8 (T8). Functionally they are involved in down-regulation of the immune response (Ts) and cytotoxicity of target cells (virally infected or tumour cells). Initially there was considerable interest in the discovery of this functional division of cell populations that were thought to be ontogenetically distinct. Alterations in the normal Th/Ts ratio have been recorded in a number of diseases, including rheumatoid arthritis, and more recently in acquired immunodeficiency syndrome (AIDS).[8] Reduction in the Th population is a recognised feature of drugs with immunomodulating properties. For example, Veys *et al.*[9] showed not only an increase in the Th/Ts ratio in patients with acute RA, but also that the ratio reverted towards normal following antirheumatic therapy. More recently, the T helper population has been divided into two functionally distinct populations according to the presence of additional surface markers. T helper cells bearing the 4B4 marker appear to be true helper-inducers, while those with low 4B4 expression but high 2H4 expression are inducers of suppression. However, there is increasing evidence that, rather than distinct populations, the latter are simply immature forms which, when appropriately stimulated, express the 4B4 molecule on their surface.[10]

The CD4 and CD8 surface glycoproteins exist in soluble form in plasma and can be detected by ELISA (see pp. 665–6). Preliminary work suggests that measurement of these soluble forms in plasma may be useful in monitoring immunological disease activity[11] and they are of potential use in monitoring immunomodulation.

Fluorescein-activated Cell-sorting Techniques (FACS)

In recent years cell-sorting techniques have advanced considerably. With fluorescein-activated cell-sorting techniques, cells labelled with monoclonal antibodies tagged with fluorescein can be sorted and quantified in a fraction of the time required when manual methods are used. Here individual cells are incorporated in tiny droplets and electrically charged, depending on whether they are fluorescein-labelled or not. Subsequently, labelled and unlabelled cells are separated by passing them through a strong electric field. With the widespread availability of automated cell sorters, this technique has become a basic routine in immunology laboratories.

T Cell Functional Assays

Transformation

On exposure to antigen, specific T cells are activated by signals transduced by the T cell antigen receptor. This results in cell cycle initiation. Some agents, acting non-specifically on T cells, also generate a stimulating signal and induce T cell blastogenesis with *de novo* synthesis of DNA. In addition to specific antigens (e.g. tetanus toxoid), a range of mitogenic stimuli are commonly used to evaluate lymphocyte proliferative function. These include: (1) plant-derived lectins, e.g. phytohaemagglutinin, concanavalin A, pokeweed mitogen; (2) antigenic preparations with non-specific mitogenic effects—purified protein derivative, *Candida albicans*, streptokinase, streptodornase; (3) allogenic cells (usually lymphocytes).

Synthesis of DNA requires the nucleotide thymidine. By measuring incorporation into DNA of tritium-labelled thymidine, lymphocyte proliferation can be estimated. The DNA from cell lysates is deposited on a paper filter and beta emission is measured by scintillation counting.[12]

T cell mitogenesis requires not only the appropriate antigen/mitogen, but also growth factors from antigen presenting (accessory) cells (which do not, themselves, proliferate). In transformation experiments it is usual to supplement culture with serum or other growth-supporting medium. Autologous serum should not be used, as this often contains inhibitors of lymphocyte transformation. The same standard 'batch' of medium should be used throughout a series of experiments. This *in vitro* method is widely used to evaluate the effect of immunomodulatory drugs on both T lymphocyte and accessory cell function. For example, Lipsky and Ziff[13] have shown that incubation of normal peripheral blood mononuclear cells (PBMNC) with therapeutic concentrations of gold salts resulted in inhibition of mitogen- and antigen-induced cellular proliferation. Such results show functional inhibition but do not indicate whether the agent (gold) interferes with the antigen presenting cells in the culture or with the responding T cells. However, by separating adherent and non-adherent cell populations and treating them separately, Lipsky and Ziff showed that T cell mitogenesis could be restored with untreated adherent cells, indicating that the immunomodulatory properties of gold primarily involved a reduction in the ability of monocytes to present antigen.

Antigen-specific stimulation can also be used to assess modulatory drugs, especially in cell-mediated immunity by skin testing for delayed-type hypersensitivity responses. Skin testing evaluates both the afferent and efferent limbs of the cell-mediated immune response (CMI) *in vivo* and is therefore a useful technique for drug evaluation.[14] However, since responses to previously encountered antigens vary widely in the population, results can be difficult to interpret.

When immunomodulation results in suppression of the afferent limb of the CMI response, established immunity, such as a positive tuberculin reaction, will often remain unchanged but the capacity of cells *in vivo* to respond to a novel antigen (such as keyhole limpet haemocyanin) will be impaired. In contrast, when immunomodulation affects the effector limb of the CMI response pre-existing responses are also diminished. For example, corticosteroids mainly suppress the effector limb of the CMI response.[15]

T Lymphocyte Cytotoxicity

Sensitised T lymphocytes kill antigen-bearing target cells *in vitro*.[16] A number of target cells have been used, including tumour cell lines, virally infected cells and allogenic lymphocytes. This immune function is an important component of graft rejection. Cyclosporin A has been shown to affect both T lymphocyte transformation and the generation of effector cytotoxic T cells in a mixed lymphocyte reaction (MLR).[17,18] By varying the time at which the drug is added to the culture system, e.g. pre- or post-mitogen/antigen stimulation, it is possible to resolve the mechanisms that are affected. For example, Klaus has shown that cyclosporin does not directly influence priming of T helper cells to antigen but inhibits early events in the generation of cytotoxic function when cells are primed in the presence of cyclosporin. However, if cyclosporin is added post priming, effector, i.e. cytotoxic, function is not inhibited.[19]

B CELLS

B cells mediate the humoral immune response following their maturation into immunoglobulin-producing plasma cells. Since the majority of plasma cells are found in the lymphoid organs, changes in the number of circulating B cells are probably of limited value as an indicator of immune modulation. Further, since these cells (unlike plasma cells) are morphologically indistinguishable from T cells, their detection relies on the presence of surface immunoglobulin or other cell-specific markers. Methods of detection have a number of inherent technical problems.[20] Three methods commonly used are identification by:

(1) *Complement rosette formation* B cells, unlike most T cells, bear complement receptors (CR1, 2 and 3). Using red cells coated with complement component C3b, the rosetting cells can be enumerated.[21]

(2) *Surface immunoglobulin detection* B cells can be demonstrated directly using fluorescein-labelled anti-human immunoglobulin antibodies.[22]

(3) *Anti-surface immunoglobulin rosette formation* The surface IgG can also be demonstrated by rosette formation with anti-IgG conjugated red cells.[23]

B Cell Function

B cell activation leads to immunoglobulin production. Measurement of immunoglobulin levels is probably a more meaningful indicator of immunomodulation than is cell enumeration (Figure 50.3). For example, gold salts have been shown to reduce raised serum Ig levels in patients with RA.[24] Further, the magnitude of this fall appears to correlate with clinical improvement. In studies of immunomodulation, quantitative as well as qualitative assays are necessary. Using subclass-specific antisera and WHO standards, accurate immunoglobulin quantification can be obtained by: (1) single radial immunodiffusion;[25] (2) immunoelectrophoresis;[26] (3) immunoassay;[27] and (4) nephelometry.[28]

Methods (2)–(4) are more sensitive but more complex, and the choice probably depends on the size of the project and available resources. It should be noted that immunoglobulin levels vary with age, sex and even from day to day in an individual and therefore should be carefully controlled. Although a useful screening technique, changes in immunoglobulin levels are a relatively non-specific indicator of immune function. Thus, suppression of immunoglobulin levels should indicate interference with antigen processing and presentation by accessory cells, the generation and delivery of T cell help, and B cell function. Immunoglobulins and Ig complexes are often sequestered in body tissues, and there can be a considerable delay in detecting significant changes in serum Ig following drug exposure. However, measurement of immunoglobulin production by B cells *in vitro* is very quantitative and gives results relatively quickly.[29]

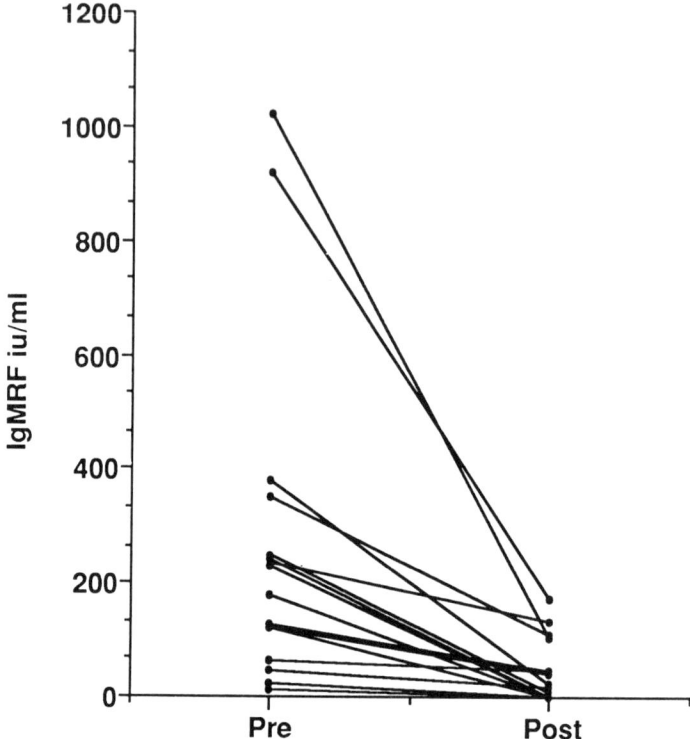

Figure 50.3 Change in serum IGM rheumatoid factor (IgMRF) measured by ELISA in patients with rheumatoid arthritis before and after treatment with gold salts for 1 year

Immunoglobulin Production by B Cells

Peripheral blood mononuclear cells (which include monocytes), and T and B cells, can be cultured for about 7 days and release immunoglobulins spontaneously or with polyclonal B cell activators such as pokeweed mitogen (PWM). The effects of putative immunomodulators can be easily assessed by addition to the cultures. However, *ex vivo* experiments are more relevant physiologically. The agent is given *in vivo* by different protocols and at different dosages and cells are subsequently removed for *in vitro* testing of Ig production. For example, Rooney *et al.*[30] noted that peripheral blood mononuclear cells (PBMC) from patients with rheumatoid arthritis showed highly significant falls in immunoglobulin production following treatment of the patients with gold salts (Figure 50.4). Using an *in vitro* model, Rosenberg and Lipsky[31] obtained similar results, but, by addition of untreated monocytes, Olsen and Jasin[32] showed that immunoglobulin production could not be wholly restored, indicating that the treatment was not simply affecting accessory cell function but also inhibited B cell function. For the detection of low levels of immunoglobulin, laser nephelometry and immunodiffusion

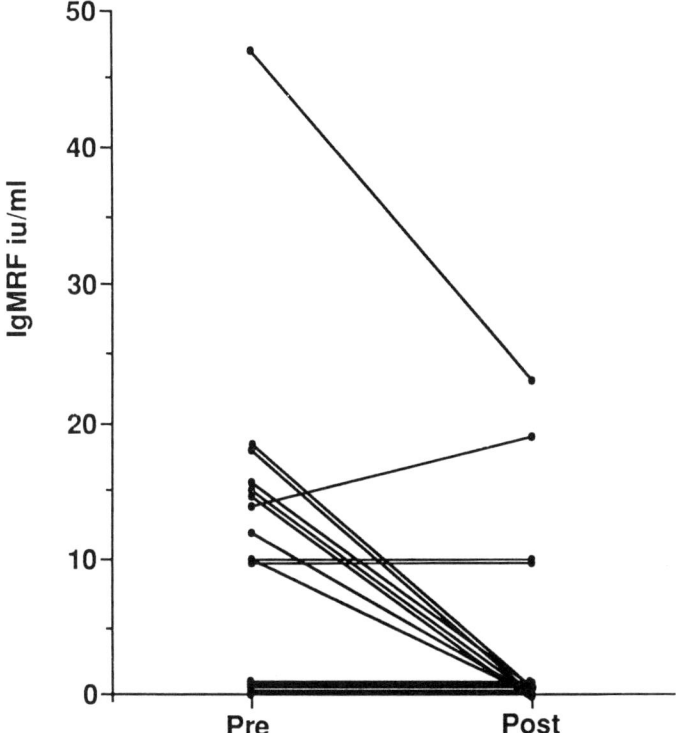

Figure 50.4   Change in spontaneous IgM rheumatoid factor (IgMRF) production by peripheral blood mononuclear cells following gold therapy.

techniques are unsuitable. Here a radioimmunoassay or an enzyme-linked immunosorbent assay (ELISA) should be used.

Enzyme-linked Immunosorbent Assays

This sensitive, reproducible and safe method for quantifying antigens or antibodies is very valuable in studies of immunomodulation. The principle of the method is to link an enzyme to either antigen or antibody, and, following complex formation in the solid phase, the amount of unknown antigen or antibody can be calculated from the enzyme action on added chromogenic substrate. Introduced by Engvell and Perlman,[33] three methods are now commercially available.

   (1) *Competitive assay*   The antigen to be assayed competes with the adsorbed antigen for the enzyme-labelled antibody.
   (2) *Sandwich technique (I)*   Unlabelled antibody binds the antigen to be

assayed, the latter being detected by subsequent addition of an enzyme-labelled specific antibody.

(3) *Sandwich technique (II)*   Adsorbed antigen is bound by the antibody to be assayed, the latter being detected by enzyme-labelled anti-immunoglobulin.

The third method is probably the most useful, as it allows quantitative differentiation of immunoglobulin subclasses. A detailed review of this topic is provided by O'Sullivan *et al.*[34]

CHEMOTAXIS AND RANDOM MIGRATION

Assessment of the biological events involved in microbial killing is also used to assess immune function. Cells of neutrophil or monocyte lineage respond by chemotaxis or random migration to chemoattractants *in vitro*. Particulate stimuli can be opsonised by antibody and/or complement. Immunoadherence, phagocytosis and metabolic responses, including intracellular killing of pathogens, can all be measured *in vitro*.

Methods of analysing chemotaxis and migration include:

(1) *The Boyden microscope technique*   The passage of leucocytes through a filter paper in response to a chemoattractant (e.g. casein) is measured.[35]

(2) *Rebuck skin window*   This is an *in vivo* assessment of leucocyte migration to the site of induced inflammation. Following superficial dermal abrasion, cells adhering to a coverslip applied to the lesion are counted after different periods of time.[36] For example, Jessop *et al.*[37] have shown, using the skin window technique, that gold salts inhibit monocyte migration.

These two simple methods, though measuring the end result of complex processes, are useful indicators of interference with early monocyte/macrophage function and neutrophil chemotaxis.

COMPLEMENT

Investigation of the complement system is of limited value in Phase II studies of immunomodulators. Reductions in complement components are almost always associated with disease or primary deficiency and only rarely follow drug-induced immunomodulation in the absence of a hypersensitivity reaction. However, in assessing therapeutic effects in disease states characterised by hypocomplementaemia, e.g. systemic lupus erythematosus,[38] measurement of the total haemolytic complement[39] or components C3 and C4[25,40] is useful.

SUPEROXIDE PRODUCTION

The superoxide radical (O_2^-) is a highly reactive intermediate produced in biological systems when one electron is removed from oxygen during the respiratory burst in phagocytes. These and similar radicals may participate in bacterial killing and damage macromolecules. They are toxic to cells and overproduction has been found in a number of immunologically mediated diseases, including RA.[41] For example, Roisman *et al.* have shown that gold salts inhibit superoxide production by phagocytic cells.[42] Detection of the O_2^- radical is based on its ability to reduce cytochrome C when incubated with isolated granulocytes.[43] This reaction is inhibited by superoxide dismutase, an enzyme that destroys O_2^- activity.

CYTOKINES

The immune response is based on the selective growth and differentiation of one or a small number of lymphocyte clones. The binding of antigen to lymphocyte receptors stimulates the expression of genes that encode lymphocyte growth factors. Additionally, growth factors are produced by antigen presenting cells (mainly macrophages but also endothelial cells) and in many cases they have proinflammatory effects in addition to their activities on lymphocytes. These soluble mediators of immunity are also called cytokines.

Cytokines may be defined as inducible peptides with receptor-mediated effects on the proliferation, maturation and functional activities of many cell types, including those of the immune system. At present five families of cytokines are recognised: the interleukins; the interferons; the cytotoxins (tumour necrosis and lymphotoxin); haematopoietic factors (colony stimulating factors); and transforming growth factors. Interleukins, one of the families of cytokines, are involved in many stages of the immune response.[44] The three criteria that define an interleukin are (1) production of leukocytes (though not necessarily exclusively); (2) production during inflammation or immune response; (3) a known primary sequence. There are, at present, eight defined interleukins (see Table 50.1) but it is certain that many others will be characterised in future. Other cytokines, such as interferons, tumour necrosis factor and colony stimulating factors, also meet the criteria for designation as interleukins but for historic reasons it is unlikely that they will be redesignated.[45]

The central role played by various cytokines in immunity will mean that their measurement will become a routine in assessment of drug modulation of immune function. It is also clear that many new agents will be selected or designed on the basis of their ability to manipulate cytokines *in vivo*.

Cytokine Measurement

It is now possible to measure specific cytokines in immunoassays based on monoclonal antibodies.[46–48] These assays have greatly facilitated cytokine

Table 50.1 Previous names of interleukins

Current name	Some previous names	Abbreviation
Interleukin-1 (two distinct forms, alpha and beta, with similar affinity for IL1 receptor)	Endogenous pyrogen	EP
	Lymphocyte activating factor	LAF
	Leucocyte endogenous mediator	LEM
	Mononuclear cell factor	MCF
	B cell activating factor	BAF
	Synovial factor	SF
	Epidermal T cell activating factor	ETAF
	Haemopoietin 1	HP-1
Interleukin-2	T cell growth factor	TCGF
	B cell differentiation factor	BCDF
Interleukin-3	PAN-CSF, multi-CSF	MCGF
	Mast cell growth factor	PSH
	Pan-specific haemopoietin	
Interleukin-4	B cell stimulating factor 1	BSF-1
	Mast cell growth factor 2	MCGF-2
	T cell growth factor 2	TCGF-2
	B cell differentiation factor	BCDF
Interleukin-5	T cell replacing factor	TRF
	Eosinophil differentiation factor	EDF
	B cell growth factor	BCGF
	B cell differentiation factor	BCDF
Interleukin-6	Interferon beta-2	HGF
	Hybridoma growth factor	HSF
	Hepatocyte stimulating factor	BSF-2
	B cell stimulating factor 2	BCDF
	B cell differentiation factor	
Interleukin-7	Lymphopoietin 1 (pre-B-cell growth factor) LP-1	LP-1
Interleukin-8	Neutrophil activating peptide	NAP
	Neutrophil activating factor	NAF

studies *in vitro* and *in vivo*, because the alternative assays of biological activity are often non-specific and can be inhibited by factors present in blood and other biological fluids.

Immunoassays (ELISA or RIA) are available in kit form for a wide range of cytokines at present, and it will shortly be possible to make reliable measurements of all of the characterised human cytokines by specific immunoassay. Other measurement techniques that are being developed are different forms of competition-binding assays using specific cytokine receptor proteins, and these may have the added advantage of giving results that are a true reflection of biologically active peptide.

There are some basic pitfalls in *ex vivo* cytokine measurement. Since leucocytes can be activated in blood collection tubes (or, indeed, may be activated in diseases *in vivo*), they can release cytokines during the process of clotting to make serum. Another potential problem is that proteinases in plasma, activated during clotting, can damage cytokines by proteolysis and give misleading results. For these reasons, if serum measurements are made, the blood collection and serum-preparation protocols must be completely standardised and all material that comes into contact with the sample must be free from bacterial endotoxin and other contaminants likely to activate blood monocytes. It is probably more reliable to make blood measurements in plasma (using EDTA rather than heparin) and in the presence of proteinase inhibitors such as aprotinin.[49,50]

There are already many indications that cytokine measurement in blood can give valuable information about immune activation and disease activity in immune-mediated diseases. For example, plasma interleukin-1 beta levels correlate with systemic measures of disease activity in rheumatoid arthritis[50] and measurement of the soluble form of the interleukin-2 receptor (by ELISA) appears to be a predictive marker of disease activity in rheumatoid arthritis[51,52] and other conditions such as atopic eczema.[53] It is very likely that immunoassays of these and other cytokines or their receptors will become routine in the assessment of immunomodulatory drug effects. At present, many cytokine studies are performed *in vitro*, using cells taken from animals or humans that have been treated *in vivo* with immunomodulatory agents or using normal cells or continuous cell lines and adding agents directly to the culture medium.

Since transcription of most cytokine genes is inducible and they are only expressed in activated cells, it is also possible to assess agents that alter their production by measuring specific messenger RNA.[54] This has been done on extracted mRNA (Northern analysis and slot-blotting) and is increasingly being performed by *in situ* hybridisation, which has the added advantage of being able to determine the phenotype of the producing cell, using monoclonal antibodies.[55]

Interestingly, antibodies to IL2 and its receptor are already showing promise as immunosuppressive agents *in vivo* (for example, in cardiac allograft rejection[56]) and IL2 has been used as an immunopotentiator in the treatment of several forms of cancer.[57]

ADHERENCE MOLECULES

In the immune system cell adhesion molecules enhance the efficiency of lymphocyte–accessory cell and lymphocyte–target cell interactions. They also appear critical in leucocyte–endothelial cell association which procedes leucocyte migration from the blood to tissue sites of inflammation. Monoclonal antibodies are now available which define a number of cell surface molecules associated with lymphocyte function—lymphocyte function associated antigens (LFA antigens).

LFA-1 is expressed on all leucocyte cell types and is increased following cell activation.[58] Down-regulation of LFA-1 expression may be a potential target for immunomodulatory drugs. Quantitative and qualitative studies of cells expressing the antigen, using fluoroscein-labelled mab and FACS, may be a useful assessment in the future.

Functional Assays

Monoclonal antibody-blocking of LFA function results in inhibition of killing by cytotoxic T cells.[59] The importance of LFA-1 in immunocyte interactions and the potential for immunomodulation is exemplified by the ability of LFA mab to prevent graft rejection.[60]

Intercellular Adhesion Molecule 1 (ICAM-1)

This molecule is the ligand for LFA-1 and is widely expressed on haemato-poietic cells and vascular endothelium. It is of importance in the homing of lymphocytes to sites of inflammation.[61,62] Thus, modulation of ICAM-1 expression on cell surfaces or blockade by mab could provide a target for immunomodulation and be useful in assessment of novel immunomodulators.

Several cell adhesion molecules have now been characterised, and this subject is very well reviewed in Reference 63.

REFERENCES

1. Kaplan, E. and Clark, C. (1974). Improved rosetting assay for the detection of human T lymphocytes *J. Immunol. Meth.*, **5**, 131
2. Wilson, A. B., Haegert, D. G. and Coombs, R. R. A. (1975). Increased sensitivity of the rosette-forming reaction of human T lymphocyte with sheep erythrocytes affected by papain treatment of the sheep cells. *Clin. Exp. Immunol.*, **22**, 177
3. Reinherz, E. L., Kung, P. C., Goldstein, G. and Schlossman, S. F. (1979). A monoclonal antibody with selective reactivity with functionally mature human thymocytes and all peripheral blood human T cells. *J. Immunol.*, **131**, 2–18
4. Hanly, J. and Bresnihan, B. (1985). Reduction in peripheral blood lymphocytes in patients receiving gold therapy for rheumatoid arthritis. *Ann. Rheum. Dis.*, **44**, 299–301
5. Moretta, L., Webb, S., Grossi, C., Lydyard, P. and Cooper, M. (1977). Functional analysis of two human T cell subpopulations help and suppression of B cell responses by T cells bearing receptors for IgM or IgG. *J. Exp. Med.*, **146**, 184
6. Gupta, S. and Good, R. A. (1980). Markers of human lymphocyte subpopulations in primary immunodeficiency and lymphoproliferative disorders. *Semin. Haematol.*, **17**, 1
7. Bach, M. A. and Bach, J. F. (1981). The use of monoclonal anti-T cell antibodies to study T cell imbalances in human disease. *Clin. Exp. Immunol.*, **45**, 449
8. Viera, J., Frank, E., Spira, T. J. and Landesman, J. (1983). Acquired immunodeficiency in Haitians. *New Engl. J. Med.*, **308** (3), 125
9. Veys, E. M., Harianns, P., Goldstein, G., King, R., Schudler, J. and Van Wauve,

J. (1981). Determination of T lymphocyte subpopulations by monoclonal antibodies in rheumatoid arthritis: influence of immunomodulatory agents. *Int. J. Immunopharm.*, **3**, 313–19

10. Sandes, M. E., Makgoba, M. W. and Shaw, S. (1988). Human naive and memory T cells in reinterpretation of helper-inducer and suppressor-inducer subsets. *Immunol. Today*, **9** (7 & 8), 196–9

11. Symons, J. A., di Giovine, F. S., Wood, N. C. and Duff, G. W. (1988). Soluble CD8 in rheumatoid arthritis [Abstract]. *Br. J. Rheum.*, **XXVII**, No. 180

12. Greaves, M., Janossy, G. and Doenhoff, M. (1974). Selective triggering of human T and B lymphocytes *in vitro* by polyclonal mitogens. *J. Exp. Med.*, **140**, 1–18

13. Lipsky, P. and Ziff, M. (1977). Inhibition of antigen and mitogen induced human lymphocyte proliferation by gold compounds. *J. Clin. Invest.*, **59**, 455

14. Valdviarssow, H., Higg, J. M., Wells, R. S., Yamamura, M., Hobbs, J. R. and Holt, P. I. L. (1973). Immune abnormalities associated with chronic mucocutaneous candidiasis. *Cell Immunol.*, **6**, 348

15. Kantor, T. G. (1976). Anti-inflammatory drugs. In Miescher, P. A. and Müller-Eberhard, H. J. (Eds.), *Textbook of Immunopathology*. Grune and Stratton, New York, San Francisco, London, p. 335

16. Cerottini, J. C. and Brunner, K. T. (1974). Cell mediated cytotoxicity allograft rejection and tumor immunity. *Adv. Immunol.*, **18**, 67

17. Borel, J. F. (1976). Comparative study of *in vitro* and *in vivo* drug effects on cell mediated cytotoxicity. *Immunobiology*, **31**, 631

18. Borel, J. F. (1977). Effects of the new antilymphocytic peptide cyclosporin A in animals. *Immunobiology*, **32**, 1017

19. Klaus, G. B. (1981). Cyclosporin A its influence on T and B cells. *Immunol. Today*, **2**, 83

20. Ross, G. D. (1979). Identification of human lymphocyte subpopulations by surface marker analysis. *Blood*, **53**, 799

21. Bianco, D., Patrick, R. and Nussenzweiz, B. (1970). A population of lymphocytes bearing a membrane receptor for antigen-antibody-complement complex. *J. Exp. Med.*, **132**, 702

22. Seligman, M., Preud'Homme, J. L. and Brouet, J. C. (1973). B and T cell markers in human proliferative blood diseases and primary immunodeficiencies with special references to membrane bound immunoglobulins. *Transplant*, **16**, 85

23. Mishell, R. I. and Henry, C. (1980). Cell surface markers. In B. B. Mishell and M. Shirgi (Eds.), *Selective Methods in Cellular Immunology*. Freeman, San Francisco, p. 209

24. Gottlieb, N. L., Kier, I. M., Penneys, N. S. and Scholly, D. R. (1975). The influence of chrysotherapy on serum protein and immunoglobulin levels, rheumatoid factor and anti-epithelial antibody titres. *J. Lab. Clin. Med.*, **86**, 962–72

25. Mancini, G., Carbonara, A. E. and Heremans, J. F. (1965). Immunochemical qualification of antigens by single radial immunodiffusion. *Immunochemistry.*, **23**, 235–54

26. Graber, P. and Burtin, P. (1964). *Immunoelectrophoretic Analysis*. Elsevier, Amsterdam

27. O'Sullivan, M. J., Bridges, J. W. and Marks, V. (1979). Enzyme immunoassay: a review. *Ann. Clin. Biochem.*, **16**, 221–40

28. Deaton, C. D., Maxwell, K. W., Smith, R. S. and Greveling, R. L. (1976). Use of lazer nephelometry in the measurement of serum proteins. *Clin. Chem.*, **229**, 1465–71

29. Fauci, A. S. and Baillieux, R. E. (Eds.) (1979). *Antibody Production in Man: in vitro Synthesis and Clinical Implications*. Academic Press, New York

30. Rooney, M., Feighery, C., Whelan, A. and Bresnihan, B. (1989). Changes in

lymphocyte infiltration of synovial membrane and its clinical course of rheumatoid arthritis. *Arthr. Rheum.*, **32** (4), 361–9

31. Rosenberg, S. A. and Lipsky, P. E. (1979). Inhibition of pokeweed mitogen induced immunoglobulin production in humans by gold compounds. *J. Rheum.*, **6** (Suppl. 1), 107–11

32. Olsen, N. J. and Jasin, H. E. (1984). Decreased pokeweed mitogen-induced IgM and IgM rheumatoid factor synthesis in rheumatoid arthritis patients treated with gold sodium thiomalate and penicillamine. *Arthr. Rheum.*, **27** (9), 985–94

33. Engvall, E. and Perlman, P. (1971). Enzyme linked immunoabsorbent quantitative assay for immunoglobulin G. *Immunocytochemistry*, **8**, 871

34. O'Sullivan, M. J., Bridges, J. W. and Marks, V. (1979). Enzyme immunoassay: a review. *Ann. Clin. Biochem.*, **16**, 221–4

35. Zigmond, S. H. and Hirsch, J. G. (1973). Leucocyte locomotion and chemotaxis. New methods for evaluation and demonstration of a cell derived chemotactic factor. *Imm. Exp. Med.*, **137**, 387

36. Rebuck, J. W. and Crowley, J. H. (1955). A method of studying leucocyte function *in vivo*. *Ann. N.Y. Acad. Sci.*, **59**, 757

37. Jessop, J. D., Vernon-Roberts, B. and Harris, J. (1973). Effects of gold salts and prednisolone on inflammatory cells. 1. Phagocyte activity of macrophages and polymorphs in inflammatory exudates studied by a 'skin window' technique in rheumatoid and control patients. *Ann. Rheum Dis.*, **32**, 294–300

38. Schur, P. H. (1975). Complement in lupus. *Clin. Rheum. Dis.*, **1**, 519

39. Fisscher, H. (1965). International symposium on immunological methods of biological standardization. In *Symposium Series of Immunobiological Standards*, Vol. 4. Karger, Basle, p. 221

40. Muller-Eberhard, H. J. (1976). The serum complement system. In Miescher, P. A. and Muller-Eberhard, H. J. (Eds.), *Textbook of Immunopathology*. Grune and Stratton, New York, San Francisco, London, pp. 45–73

41. Halliwell, B. (1982). Production of superoxide, hydrogen peroxide and hydroxyl radicals by phagocytic cells: a cause of chronic inflammatory disease. *Cell. Biol. Int. Rep.*, **6** (6), 529

42. Roisman, F. R., Walz, D. T. and Finkelstein, A. E. (1982). Inhibitory action of auranofin on superoxide production by phagocytic cells and blockade of the inhibition by thiol protecting agents. *Arthr. Rheum.*, **25** (Suppl.), 5130 (Abs) D56

43. Weening, R. S., Wever, R. and Roos, D. (1975). Quantitative aspects of the production of superoxide radicals by phagocytosing human granulocytes. *J. Lab. Clin. Med.*, **85**, 245

44. O'Gara, A. (1989). Peptide regulatory factors. Interleukins and the immune system 1 and 2. *Lancet*, **1**, 943–6, 1003–6

45. Duff, G. W. (1988). Interleukins and clinical medicine. In Shepherd, M. (Ed.), *Advanced Medicine*, Vol. 24. Royal College of Physicians, Baillière Tindall, Philadelphia, pp. 237–46

46. di Giovine, F. S., Meager, A., Leung, H. and Duff, G. W. (1988). Immunoreactive tumour necrosis factor alpha and biological inhibitors in synovial fluids from rheumatic patients. *Int. J. Immunopathol. Pharm.*, **1** (1), 17–26

47. di Giovine, F. S., Poole, S., Situnayake, R. D., Wadwha, M. and Duff, G. W. (1989). Absence of correlations between indices of systemic inflammation and synovial fluid interleukin 1 (alpha and beta) in rheumatic diseases. *Rheum. Int.* (in press)

48. Rooney, M., Symons, J. and Duff, G. (1989). Local interleukin 1 beta concentrations is related to local disease activity in rheumatoid arthritis. Submitted

49. Cannon, J. G., Van Der Meer, J. U. M., Kwaitkowski, D., Endres, S., Lonneman, G., Burke, J. G. and Dinarello, C. A. (1988). Interleukin 1 beta in

human plasma: optimization of blood collection, plasma extraction and radioimmunassay methods. *Lymphokine Res.*, **7**, 457–67
50. Eastgate, J. A., Wood, N. C., di Giovine, F. S., Symons, J. A., Grinlinton, F. M. and Duff, G. W. (1988). Correlation of plasma interleukin 1 levels with disease activity in rheumatoid arthritis. *Lancet*, **1**, 706–9
51. Symons, J. A., Wood, N. C., di Giovine, F. S. and Duff, G. W. (1988). Soluble IL2 receptor in rheumatoid arthritis. Correlation with disease activity, IL1 and IL2 inhibition. *J. Immunol.*, **141**, 2612–18
52. Wood, N. C., Symons, J. A. and Duff, G. W. (1988). Serum interleukin 2 receptor in rheumatoid arthritis: a prognostic indicator of disease activity? *J. Autoimmun.*, **1**, 353–61
53. Colver, G. B., Symons, J. A. and Duff, G. W. (1989). Soluble interleukin 2 receptor in atopic eczema. *Br. Med. J.*, **298**, 1426–8
54. Duff, G. W., Dickens, E. M., Wood, N. C., Manson, J. C., Symons, J. A., Poole, S. and di Giovine, F. S. (1988). Immunoassay bioassay and in situ hybridization of monokines in human arthritis. In Oppenheim, J. J., Dinarello, C. A. and Kluger, M. (Eds.), *Progress in Leucocyte Biology*. Alan R. Liss, New York, pp. 387–92
55. Duff, G. W. (1989). Interleukin 1 in arthritis. In Bomford, R. and Henderson, B. (Eds.), *Interleukin 1 in Inflammation and Disease*. Elsevier, Amsterdam (in press)
56. Smith, K. A. (1988). Interleukin-2 inception, impact and implication. *Science, N.Y.*, **240**, 1169–76
57. Rosenberg, S. A., Packard, B. S., Aebersold, P. M. *et al.* (1988). New approaches to the immunotherapy of cancer using interleukin 2. *Ann. Int. Med.*, **108**, 853–64
58. Kurzunger, R., Reynolds, T., Germain, R. N., Davignon, D., Matz, E. and Springer, T. A. (1981). A novel lymphocyte function associated antigen (LFA-1) cellular distribution, quantitative expression and structure. *J. Immunol.*, **127**, 596–602
59. Sanchez-Madrid, F., Krensky, A. M., Ware, C. F., Robbins, E., Stromuger, J. L., Burakoff, S. J. and Springer, T. A. (1982). Three distinct antigens associated with human T lymphocyte-mediated cytolysis: LFA-1, LFA-2 and LFA-3. *Proc. Natl Acad. Sci. USA*, **79**, 7489–93
60. Fischer, A., Blanche, S., Veber, F., Le Deist, F., Gerota, I., Lopez, M., Dunardy, A. and Griscelli, C. (1988). Correction of immune disorders by HLA matched and mismatched bone marrow transplantation. In Gale, R. P. (Ed.), *Recent Advances in Bone Marrow Transplantation*. Alan R. Liss, New York
61. Rothlein, R., Dustin, M. L., Marlin, S. D. and Springer, T. A. (1986). A human intercellular adhesion molecule ICAM-1, distinct from LFA-1. *J. Immunol.*, **137**, 1270–4
62. Dustin, M. L., Rothlein, R., Shaw, A. K., Dinarello, C. A. and Springer, T. A. (1986). A natural adherence molecule (ICAM-1): induction by IL1 and interferon gamma; tissue distribution, biochemistry and function. *J. Immunol.*, **137**, 245–54
63. Springer, T. A., Dustin, M. L., Kishimoto, T. K. and Marlin, S. (1987). The lymphocyte function associated LFA-1, CD2 and LFA-3 molecules; cell adhesion receptors of the immune system. In Paul, W. E., Fallman, C. G. and Metzger, H. (Eds.), *Ann. Rev. Immunol.*, Ann. Rev. Inc., California, pp. 223–52

51
Anti-inflammatory Drugs

P. S. Helliwell and V. Wright

The Rheumatism and Rehabilitation Unit, University Dept of Medicine, General Infirmary, Leeds, UK

INTRODUCTION

Non-steroidal anti-inflammatory drugs (NSAIDs) are one of the most widely prescribed drugs in general practice. They also head the list of drugs whose side-effects are reported to the Committee on Safety of Medicines. Many of their therapeutic effects and side-effects result from inhibition of the enzyme (cyclo-oxygenase) responsible for the production of prostaglandins from arachidonic acid, as originally suggested by Vane (1971). NSAIDs have little effect on cell migration, unless they also inhibit the enzyme lipo-oxygenase (as did benoxaprofen; see Leader, 1982), when an effect on cell migration may be seen. In this chapter it will be assumed that the novel NSAID inhibits cyclo-oxygenase and that it has been shown to have anti-inflammatory activity in animal models such as the rat adjuvant arthritis and/or carrageenin paw oedema model.

Prostaglandins are important in inflammation. PGE_2 is a potent vasodilator and enhances vascular permeability induced by bradykinin and histamine. Furthermore, PGE_2 causes a potent and long-lasting potentiation of pain induced by bradykinin and histamine. Therefore, prostaglandin inhibition results in analgesia and reduction in inflammation, but only in the presence of pre-existing tissue destruction and inflammation. Usually it is impossible to separate the analgesic from the anti-inflammatory effect of these drugs.

EVALUATION IN NORMAL VOLUNTEERS

In the absence of tissue damage or inflammation, it is impossible to test the analgesic, anti-inflammatory properties of these drugs. Therefore, studies in normal volunteers are only useful for generating information on the tolerability and pharmacokinetics of a new chemical entity tested for the first time in humans. In this way useful information on dosage, duration of action and pharmacokinetic data may be obtained while screening for any untoward and dangerous side-effects. Measurement of the *in vivo* antiprostaglandin effect may be obtained by measuring inhibition of malonyldialdehyde (MDA) production by platelets.

However, there are a number of precautions to be observed in carrying out and interpreting such studies.

(1) There are few data relating serum concentration of NSAID to clinical effect and, similarly, tolerability is not easily related to serum concentration. The reason for this is unclear. The methodology of many of the studies attempting to relate serum concentrations to clinical effect has been criticised (Brookes and Day, 1987). Furthermore, it may be that even small doses of NSAID may produce trough levels sufficient to suppress prostaglandin production, so that no additional effect is seen at higher doses. It may be that the plasma concentration of the drug is not relevant: synovial fluid concentrations are much more appropriate in terms of anti-inflammatory action in arthritis, and the pharmacokinetics of drug in the synovial fluid may be markedly different from the kinetics of the drug in plasma. Furthermore, some NSAIDs, particularly the aryl acetic acids, exhibit optical isomerism, only one of the enantiomers possessing active inhibition of cyclo-oxygenase (Lee *et al.*, 1985). Some conversion of inactive to active enantiomer occurs *in vivo* and this may vary from patient to patient. Finally, despite adequate serum concentrations, a certain percentage of patients with inflammatory conditions will remain 'non-responders' for reasons which are not entirely clear (Day *et al.*, 1982).

(2) The timing of administration of the drug is important, since single-dose oral pharmacokinetic data may change according to the time of day of administration of the drug (Surrall *et al.*, 1986).

(3) Pharmacokinetic data obtained in healthy volunteers may differ markedly from the pharmacokinetics of the drug in the presence of disease and other pharmacological agents. Ideally, the drug needs investigating in a population of similar age and sex to the intended target population. This means that if a new drug is intended for rheumatoid arthritis and osteoarthritis, then the initial studies of the drug should be in elderly female volunteers. This rarely happens in normal volunteers, but data must be obtained on a similar group at an early stage in efficacy studies. Similarly, information is necessary on drug interaction between NSAIDs and other drugs that are highly protein-bound, such as anticoagulants and hypoglycaemic agents. This is initially obtained in animal studies. Other commonly prescribed pharmacological agents with which NSAID interaction must be closely monitored are analgesics and antacids.

(4) If an elderly non-patient group is required for tolerability data, it is worth noting that there are three different groups of elderly people. First, those in their homes, who represent the 'survivors': a very resilient group. Second, those in local authority homes or private residential homes. Third, those in hospital. The latter group are the most relevant: they are lighter in weight, have a multiplicity of diseases, receive numerous drugs, are less mobile, and usually have impaired renal function.

ASSESSMENT IN PATIENTS

A number of inflammatory musculoskeletal conditions occur which have potential for initial testing of a new NSAID. These include rheumatoid arthritis, seronegative polyarthritis, ankylosing spondylitis, juvenile chronic arthritis and crystal deposition disease. Undoubtedly the most commonly used human model is the inflammation of rheumatoid arthritis (RA). Why should this be so? RA is a good example of musculoskeletal rheumatism which is not self-limited, is unresponsive to placebo and is less variable from day to day than other diseases. Furthermore, RA is prevalent in many outpatient clinics and established NSAIDs have a good clinical effect. In our clinic we see 1500 new patients, and 8500 old patients annually, of whom half have rheumatoid arthritis. Diagnostic criteria are well defined and standardised, as are criteria of disease activity (see Table 51.1).

Although the other inflammatory arthritides may respond well to NSAIDs, for the purpose of evaluating a new drug it must be remembered that diagnostic and activity criteria may not be as well defined as in RA and the conditions may be less common. For example, acute gout is seen infrequently, and unpredictable numbers of patients may present from week to week, thus playing havoc with any investigational plan. With other diseases, such as ankylosing spondylitis, measures of disease activity are not well defined and objective criteria may be insensitive over a short assessment period. NSAIDs are effective in osteoarthritis, yet this effect may be largely related to their analgesic action, since clinical signs of inflammation in osteoarthritis are usually absent. Therefore, in osteoarthritis assessment of the effect of an NSAID is largely subjective. For these reasons RA is usually chosen as the disease in which the initial evaluation of a new NSAID is undertaken.

However, it must be remembered that any drug evaluation must be carried out in parallel with normal patient care but quite separate from it, in line with the Helsinki declaration (Herxheimer, 1988). Investigators ought to know that clinicians often have a cohort of patients in their clinics who are suitable for trials of new drugs. These patients are partly self-selected and partly selected by the physician for such attributes as intelligence, co-operation, mobility, mild-to-moderate level of disease activity or poor tolerance of previous drug therapy. Extrapolating trial results to the general arthritic population may not always be appropriate.

Rheumatoid arthritis is a chronic inflammatory condition of the synovial joints which is characterised by natural variation in disease activity. This natural variation causes problems with baseline measurements and requires carefully controlled studies in adequate numbers of patients, using precise and reproducible assessments of change in order to evaluate different treatments and, in particular, new forms of treatment.

A further problem occurs with respect to side-effects. Patients who are HLA DR3 positive are more likely to develop renal problems on treatment

Table 51.1 Criteria used to define active rheumatoid arthritis

Number of joints painful or tender on motion	6 or more
Number of swollen joints	3 or more
Duration of morning stiffness	more than 45 min
ESR (Westergren)	more than 28 mm/h

with gold or penicillamine. Sulphoxidation and acetylator status may also be relevant: the former in respect to penicillamine side-effects, the latter in respect to sulphasalazine. It is possible that intolerance to and/or lack of response to NSAIDs is also related to genetic factors. At the moment we have not yet reached the position of tissue typing for patients entering studies, but this may be necessary in the future in order to obtain a homogeneous sample.

In practice, assessment of disease activity is based on a number of different clinical and laboratory measures which reflect disease activity (Table 51.2). Some of these measures are 'objective', but not necessarily relevant. Most of the measures are subjective, relevant but liable to idiosyncratic change. An ideal measure is both relevant, objective and easy to perform with little discomfort to the patient: such an index is as yet unavailable.

METHODS OF ASSESSMENT OF INFLAMMATION IN RHEUMATOID ARTHRITIS

Assessment of Pain

The appreciation of pain is a cerebral phenomenon personal to each individual. The experience of pain intensity does not necessarily relate to the peripheral stimulus causing excitation in the pain pathways and is affected by such factors as mood and personality. Attempts to measure pain using physiological correlates of fear, such as pulse rate and sweating (with concurrent lowering of peripheral skin resistance), have proved unreliable. Similarly, standardised painful stimuli such as those imposed by clinical algometers have proved irrelevant because of the different way in which individuals respond to those stimuli.

Furthermore, response to a standardised painful stimulus can change as a result of unrelated factors; the studies of Moldofsky *et al.* (1975) clearly showed that particular forms of sleep disturbance can change clinical algometer readings at specified sites.

Asking the patient exactly how much pain he/she has at the present time is the method of assessment employed by most investigators. Methods of quantification, as will be discussed below, may differ but cannot detract from the fact that the patients' response will depend on a number of factors unrelated to inflammation. These include mood, their relationship with the assessor, their concept of the disease, and how they think they ought to respond.

The less complicated scales offer the patient a choice of adjectives. Descriptive words such as 'slight', 'moderate', 'severe' or 'agonising', where each word is appointed a numerical equivalent, are available. Such a scale is simple to use, but subjects may have trouble in deciding which word best describes their pain and it may well be that individuals interpret descriptive terms in different ways (Hill and Bird, 1986). Numerical progression scales,

Table 51.2 Measures of efficacy of non-steroidal anti-inflammatory drugs in rheumatoid arthritis

Measurement of pain using a visual analogue scale
Measurement of stiffness as duration of morning stiffness
Grip strength
PIP joint circumference
Ritchie Articular Index
Functional index
Overall patient evaluation
Overall physician evaluation

where each end of a numerical range (e.g. 1–5) is given a descriptive term such as 'no pain' and 'extreme pain', are also employed, but these have been criticised on the grounds that people prefer to choose certain numbers irrespective of the pain they are experiencing.

The visual analogue scale is currently in widespread use in clinical trials of anti-inflammatory drugs. The principle is to present to the patient a line of fixed length with descriptive terms at either end and to ask the patient to mark which point along the designated line represents the intensity of his/her symptom. The performance of the visual analogue scale is profoundly affected by its design (Table 51.3). The scale can be either vertical or horizontal and, although there is a good relationship between the two, scores on the vertical scale tend to be higher than those on the horizontal scale (Hinchcliffe *et al.*, 1985). It is important to have the scale presented at a uniform position relative to the patient because of distortion, and it is also important to ensure that the patient understands correctly what he/she has

Table 51.3 Important points to remember when using visual analogue scales

Vertical or horizontal presentations in front of patient
Keep instructions clear, precise and consistent
Define end stops
Higher in-trial scores produce greater changes

been requested to do. This point has been well illustrated by the use of visual analogue scales to measure low back pain, where some patients interpreted the vertical visual analogue scale as a representation of their spinal column and thus marked the position of pain rather than the degree of pain as intended. Other points relevant to visual analogue scales are:

(1) Scales should have defined end-stops, otherwise patients may mark beyond the defined limits.

(2) A photocopy of an original 10 cm line may not be exactly 10 cm, causing variation in the results.

(3) In serial assessments higher initial scores produce greater changes.

(4) When assessing joint pain, it is important to define the difference between pain at rest and pain on movement.

There is good correlation between repeated measurements of pain on the visual analogue scale (Scott and Huskisson, 1979), although this has been challenged (Dixon and Bird, 1981; Hinchcliffe *et al.*, 1985). A major question is whether patients should be allowed to see their previous scores when making judgements: since patients tend to overestimate pain severity without knowledge of their previous scores, access to these scores tends to remove this bias.

Studies involving the use of visual analogue scales generate a lot of paper and, unless each measurement is noted at the time the patient is assessed, each piece of paper needs to be accurately marked with the name of the patient and the time of the assessment. To overcome this problem plastic scales, looking rather like slide rules, have now been introduced. The patient runs a plastic pointer along the rule between the two marked extremes; on the reverse side of the rule is a 100 mm scale which can be read directly once the patient has made his/her assessment. The plastic double-sided scale has recently been improved by the use of a graded colour scale in an attempt to help patients discriminate between different grades of symptom.

Despite their obvious limitations, visual analogue scales of pain and other symptoms (including morning stiffness) are still widely used in clinical trials of anti-inflammatory drugs. As long as their limitations are recognised, they are useful tools. Statistical analysis of the results obtained with visual analogue scales must be made with non-parametric tests.

A further dimension in pain evaluation is provided by the McGill Pain Questionnaire, which attempts to assess the qualitative as well as the quantitative aspects of pain. This questionnaire is well validated but administration is time-consuming, although a shorter version is available (Jamieson, 1988).

Assessment of Stiffness

Early morning stiffness is one of the cardinal symptoms of RA. The duration of this morning stiffness, in minutes, is frequently used as an indication of disease activity. It is unlikely that there is a single point in time when morning stiffness is relieved, so it would be surprising if the duration of morning stiffness did not vary from day to day. However, this figure can be remarkably consistent; most investigators use an average duration over a fixed period of a week. The more recently diagnosed arthritics may need further prompting and to be specifically asked what time they rise and what time they feel the joints have 'loosened up'. The onset of fatigue later in the day has also been used as an indicator of disease activity. Both of these symptoms have been assessed with visual analogue scales in an attempt to measure severity rather than duration. Unless this is clearly stated, confusion may occur between duration and severity of the symptoms. Duration is usually expressed in minutes, although occasionally defined periods are used and the duration is classed accordingly on a simple numerical scale.

Occasionally confusion occurs between morning stiffness and articular gelling, which is stiffness experienced in the joints after a period of inactivity during the day. This latter stiffness is usually relieved quickly on exercising the joint.

Over the last 30 years a number of attempts have been made to quantify stiffness, employing a variety of devices. The original studies appeared to show an increase in stiffness either directly or indirectly in rheumatoid arthritis (Scott, 1960; Wright and John, 1960; Ingpen, 1968). Later studies using more sophisticated and precise equipment have been unable to confirm this (Helliwell *et al.*, 1988a). However, this symptom remains a useful indicator of disease activity and still heads the list of diagnostic criteria for rheumatoid arthritis (Arnett *et al.*, 1988). Clearly, further studies are needed to quantify exactly what patients are describing when they refer to their joints as 'stiff'.

Assessment of Joint Tenderness

In the main, two systems are in use, reflecting North American and European practice. The index of the Co-operating Clinics of the American Rheumatism Association (Co-operating Clinics, 1967) uses a count of 66 joints, counting one for each joint showing active disease defined as tenderness, pain on passive movement or inflammatory swelling. The Ritchie Articular Index (Ritchie *et al.*, 1968) is a similar system which relies on assessing the grade of response to firm pressure in a similar number of joints, but also includes the cervical spine, hips, and subtalar and midtarsal joints, which are assessed by passive movements. Maximum score for the Co-operating Clinics Index is 66 and that for the Ritchie Articular Index is 78. Both tests take only a few minutes to perform, correlate highly with each other and have low intraobserver variation, but somewhat erratic interobserver variation (Ritchie *et al.*, 1968). The Ritchie Articular Index is in common use in the UK and forms an integral part of most clinical trials. However, it is important to use the same observer in serial assessments.

Assessment of Grip Strength

Methods for assessing strength are widely used in clinical trials of antirheumatic drugs. The popularity of this measure using a pneumodynamometer is largely due to its ease and rapidity of use and to its reported reproducibility. However, grip strength is not an entirely objective measure of muscle power; the large interobserver error suggests a significant physician–patient interaction (Lee *et al.*, 1974). Furthermore, grip strength assesses function in several different anatomical systems, including muscles, joints, tendons, ligaments and skin, and ultimately may be a function of pain experienced while gripping.

Although the pneumodynamometer is cheap, portable and acceptable to most patients with RA, the device has certain limitations. Intraobserver variation is low only with experienced observers, suggesting that they unconsciously smooth the results obtained. This is not hard to understand.

When patients are asked to squeeze the bulb or bag of the pneumodynamo-meter, the peak value is only achieved for a fraction of a second, following which there is a period of sustained grip. During sustained grip the mercury column or manometer needle is flickering and rarely is a steady sustained grip produced, even in normal subjects. This effect can probably be overcome to a certain extent by the use of a peak-hold facility, as suggested by Fernando and Robertson (1982).

Another problem is the relationship between force and pressure within this system. The mercury column is displaced by an increase in pressure within the enclosed air-filled bag, which in turn is manipulated by the patient. The pressure within the closed system is a function of the force exerted and the area over which it is applied; this means that the same pressure can be achieved by the use of a small force over a large area as by the use of a large force over a small area. In other words, the result would depend on the type of grip the patient applies to the bag or bulb. Many grip strength assessments are also made using an air-filled bag attached to an aneroid manometer, which has a tendency to become inaccurate after a certain time in use and should be checked periodically against a standard mercury column.

Partly as a result of theoretical uncertainties of the pneumodyanamometer, electronic strain-gauge devices were introduced for the assessment of strength. These devices are adaptable so that not only can total grip strength be measured, but also pinch grip and individual finger strength. On the whole, these devices are a much more precise measure of force and have enabled an assessment of the relevant contribution of different movements to total hand strength.

Whichever device is used, it is difficult to relate absolute strength measure-ments to the functional capability of the hand. This in part results from the fact that we do not know the minimal force required to perform certain tasks. For example, a person with severe rheumatoid deformity of the hand can still drive a car. An attempt to relate hand strength to functional capability was made recently by Jones *et al.* (1985), in which a variety of strain-gauge devices were arranged in such a manner as to measure applied forces in a number of everyday activities. These included lifting a pan and kettle and twisting a key.

The information obtained from electronic strain-gauge devices is ideal for further analysis by microprocessor, so that analysis of the relationship between grip and time can be obtained (Helliwell *et al.*, 1987). Although useful information may be obtained, such as time taken to reach maximum grip, fatigue and release rate, this information does not appear to provide any particular additional benefit in patients with painful arthritic joints (Helliwell *et al.*, 1988b).

Electronic strain-gauge devices, if necessary linked to a microprocessor, are expensive and less portable than the more commonly employed pneumodyanamometer. They may provide a more precise measure of force and allow adaptability in design for measuring strength of different move-ments. However, the problem of physician–patient interaction still applies to these devices, and unless they can offer significant advantages over the cheaper and more portable pneumodynamometers, their future is limited by cost.

Measurement of Joint Circumference

By the use of a plastic spring-loaded flexible loop, or arthrocircometer, the circumference of finger joints can be readily measured. More recently other devices for measuring circumferences of larger joints have been introduced. Although this is a purely objective assessment, the measure has proved particularly insensitive in assessment of the effect of non-steroidal drugs on the rheumatic hand (Deodhar *et al.*, 1973). Changes in joint circumference can occur over a much longer period than is usual for trials of anti-inflammatory drugs, and some joints are incapable of change (Boardman and Hart, 1967). Intraobserver error is small, but interobserver error is unacceptably high (Webb *et al.*, 1973).

Many authorities still recommend measuring the circumference of the three most swollen proximal interphalangeal joints in trials of NSAID efficacy, but the method is not popular with clinical metrologists and probably ought to be abandoned.

Assessment of Joint Range of Motion

Measurement of joint range of motion is traditionally by the angle goniometer, which can be adapted to most joints. A new spirit gravity goniometer, designed originally by Loebl (1967), is now widely available and has added to the accuracy and ease of measurement of joint range of motion. Since joint motion decreases with age, the normal values for each age group need to be established.

There is an important distinction between active and passive joint range. The active range may well be dependent on such factors as pain and stiffness in the joints. The passive range may well be dependent on the assessor's zeal. One method of overcoming this latter problem is to use a fixed-torque goniometer (Cantrell and Fisher, 1982), but such devices are unlikely to be applicable to a wide range of joints. Furthermore, fixed-torque goniometers are unpopular with patients, since they frequently cause pain at the limit of the joint range (Helliwell, 1987).

Functional Assessment

Many clinical trials in rheumatic diseases include some form of functional assessment, and improvement in functional ability must be a major objective in treatment. The original scale for assessing functional state was the Steinbrocker grade (Steinbrocker *et al.*, 1949). This is a simple 5-point scale indicating the degree of disability which the patient experiences, ranging from total dependence to full independence. Although widely used to express the function of a patient at any one time, the scale is too insensitive for use in the short term.

More recently the Stanford Health Assessment Questionnaire has been adapted for use in British arthritis patients (Young and Chamberlain, 1987).

This scale is fairly easy to use and covers such areas as personal care, walking and function around the house. It has been shown to be more sensitive than the Steinbrocker Scale (Kirwan and Reeback, 1986).

Regional assessments designed to assess, for example, the function of the hand have been designed (Clawson *et al.*, 1977; Evans and Lawton, 1984). Both these indices comprise measures of strength of both grip and pinch, and include tests of manual dexterity such as fastening buttons and tying knots. However, these assessments are time-consuming and on frequent use becoming uninteresting for the patient and assessor alike. They are seldom used in short-term trials of NSAIDs.

Laboratory Assessment

Since NSAIDs have no effect on interleukin-1 production they have little effect on the acute phase response as reflected by such measures as ESR, plasma viscosity, C-reactive protein and haptoglobin. However, full blood count and plasma viscosity are usually recorded at regular intervals as an index of underlying disease activity.

Thermography

Infrared radiation with a wavelength of approximately 2–5 μm is emitted from human skin. In the knee joint a raised intrasynovial temperature (i.e. synovial inflammation) is associated with a high skin surface temperature over the joint. This provides the basis for thermography, which essentially is the mapping of isotherms over a joint; the derived integral of these isotherms over a standard area is described as the thermographic index. Early reports on this technique were promising (Bacon *et al.*, 1976). The test is simple to administer, and is reproducible, relevant and an objective index of joint inflammation. Furthermore, the index appears sensitive to changes in inflammation as a result of intra-articular steroid injections and oral anti-inflammatory drugs. However, this technique has not been widely incorporated in clinical trials, most probably because of the prohibitive cost of the thermographic equipment and the need for a constant-temperature room in which to make the observations.

More recently a less expensive system has become available, using a pyroelectric camera linked to a microprocessor, but this system has yet to be fully evaluated (Black *et al.*, 1986). Development of a system for measuring microwave radiation with a wavelength of approximately 100 μm is under way in Glasgow, but no studies using this technique have yet appeared (Fraser *et al.*, 1987).

Radioisotope Studies

Original studies using ^{99m}Tc suggested that this isotope would be a relatively quick and easy method of making an objective global assessment of joint inflammation. Since uptake of the isotope into joints appears to be largely dependent on synovial blood flow, this technique is likely to give the same information as thermography. As the equipment is already available, the same cost restrictions should not apply, but the procedure is time-consuming and requires a dose of radioactivity. Possibly for this reason and because of the time involved in obtaining a whole-body scintiscan, this technique has received little consideration in recent trials of NSAIDs.

Conclusions

Despite the availability of truly objective indices of inflammation in rheumatic disease, most investigators prefer to continue with a few trusted, subjective and quasi-objective assessments with which they are familiar. This is mainly due to the time involved in making the objective measurements and the cost of the equipment in the more sophisticated assessments. In clinical trials it is clearly important to have the same observer making serial assessments, and this may well be more appropriately a clinical metrologist rather than a clinician (Bird *et al.*, 1985). Finally, because of circadian variation in disease, activity in RA assessments must always be made around the same time of day.

ASSESSMENT OF SIDE-EFFECTS

The evaluation of any new pharmaceutical agent should include broad-based biochemical, haematological and clinical data on all bodily systems, including and, in particular, data on elderly subjects who may have concomitant disease and renal impairment. With NSAIDs a particular problem is upper gastrointestinal inflammation due to inhibition of the cytoprotective action of prostaglandins on the gastric mucosa. Despite some claims that prostaglandin inhibition may be tissue-specific, there is little evidence to support this at the moment, and all NSAIDs which act by inhibition of cyclo-oxygenase must be regarded as potentially ulcerogenic.

Gastrointestinal System

Particular attention should be made to the presence of dyspepsia, possibly including a record of antacid usage. Since NSAIDs may cause gastric erosion and damage without actual ulceration, some measure of either blood loss or direct observation of damage is occasionally incorporated into clinical trials. However, in short-term trials (1–2 weeks) of new NSAIDS it seems unnecessary to perform endoscopic evaluation of gastric mucosa before and after the drug. An indirect measure would be to estimate gastrointestinal blood loss via ^{51}Cr-labelled red blood cells, a simple and safe technique but one which requires a lot of laboratory time. Faecal occult bloods were designed to detect blood loss from the lower gastrointestinal tract, and are of limited use in clinical trials and, indeed, in clinical practice. More recently NSAIDs have been shown to have an adverse effect on the small bowel mucosa, and if increased blood loss is detected, then it may be impossible to determine exactly where the blood is coming from in the gastrointestinal tract (Bjarnason *et al.*, 1987).

Dermatological Side-effects

NSAIDs appear to be particularly likely to cause rashes; the incidence may be as high as 10% with some established drugs. Any new NSAID may be said to have an acceptable incidence of rash at 5% or less, but clearly this needs to be given particular attention.

Method of Assessment

Daily diary cards appear to be the most successful method of assessing minor adverse events and have proved particularly reliable in practice (Bird *et al.*, 1985). An alternative method is to provide a check-list of particular symptoms which the patient can review daily; yet this method may be criticised on the grounds of suggesting to the patient symptoms which may not be apparent.

CONDUCT AND DESIGN OF TRIALS OF NEW NSAIDs

Because of the variability of the disease and the significant physician–patient interaction on many of the assessment measures, double-blind controlled studies should preferably be performed. Even so, some of the difficulties of a drifting baseline may be encountered (Co-operating Clinics, 1965). Most NSAIDs in current use have a fairly rapid onset of action and so a 1–2 week period of assessment appears satisfactory: too short and the drug may not have an optimal effect; too long and the possibility of baseline change in disease activity occurs.

Can a placebo be justifiably used in active rheumatoid arthritis? Although initial trials of a new pharmaceutical should try to establish its superiority over placebo, this is frequently impractical in RA, where without an NSAID patients often deteriorate rapidly and experience markedly increased stiffness and pain. For this reason most new NSAIDs are compared with established drugs such as naproxen, indomethacin or ibuprofen in standard doses in a double-blind crossover fashion. Despite these precautions, problems may still occur due to patient unpredictability and preference. Scott *et al.* (1982) have commented that it is impossible to rank NSAIDs on efficacy and that any attempt to assess a new NSAID by comparison with standard drugs is meaningless. It may be possible to overcome these problems by using larger numbers of patients, as recently demonstrated by Cox and Doherty (1988).

Stability of Standard Treatment

Although subjects are usually given a short run-in period for a few days on placebo to establish disease activity and baseline changes, it is assumed that standard disease-modifying therapy remains unchanged for 3 months before the start of the trial and during the trial. These drugs would include steroids, chloroquine, sulphasalazine, penicillamine and gold.

Rescue Analgesia

Analgesics such as paracetamol or a combination of paracetamol and dextropropoxyphene are supplied in case pain and stiffness are not controlled by the trial drugs. In this case a tablet count is made, to assess consumption of analgesic.

Interval of Measurement

Measurements are usually made at the start and end of each treatment period, which usually means every week during a comparative trial of a new NSAID. At the end of the trial, in addition to the standard methods of assessment discussed above, both patients and assessors are often asked for their overall assessment of each particular drug, and this is rated numerically. From the patient's point of view this is a reasonable assessment, since it may determine how acceptable the drug would be in clinical practice.

SUMMARY

For the reasons discussed above, it is unlikely that an efficacy table of NSAIDs could be constructed despite well-organised and well-conducted clinical trials. For a new NSAID the best that can be achieved by clinical trials at this stage is an assessment of equivalent efficacy to standard anti-inflammatory drugs, combined with good patient tolerability. New NSAIDs are unlikely to differ strikingly from established therapy unless they have an additional novel action, as was claimed for benoxaprofen (Meacock and Kitchen, 1979). In the absence of truly objective measures of inflammation in joints, we must rely on a number of subjective and quasi-subjective assessments and attempt to obtain a broad-based view of the anti-inflammatory properties of the new agent. Inability to respond to any NSAID despite adequate serum levels remains a problem in clinical trials, and possibly patients should be selected for their ability to respond to these drugs beforehand. The unpredictability of patient response remains a problem in most clinical trials involving anti-inflammatory drugs.

REFERENCES

Arnett, F. C., Edworthy, S. M., Bloch, D. A. *et al*. (1988). The American

Rheumatism Association 1987 revised criteria for the classification of rheumatoid arthritis. *Arthr. Rheum.*, **31**, 315–23

Bacon, P. A., Collins, A. J., Ring, F. J. and Cosh, J. A. (1976). Thermography in the assessment of inflammatory arthritis. *Clin. Rheum. Dis.*, **2**, 51–65

Bird, H. A., LeGallez, P. and Hill, J. (1985). *Combined Care of the Rheumatic Patient*. Springer-Verlag, Berlin

Bjarnason, I., Zanelli, G., Prouse, P., Smethurst, P., Smith, T., Levi, S., Gumpel, M. J. and Levi, A. J. (1987). Blood and protein loss via small-intestinal inflammation induced by non-steroidal anti-inflammatory drug. *Lancet*, **2**, 711–13

Black, C. M., Clark, R. P., Darton, K., Evans, R. and Goff, M. R. (1986). A new thermal image system for rheumatology. *Br. J. Rheum.*, **25** (Suppl. 2), 21

Boardman, P. L. and Hart, F. D. (1967). Clinical measurement of the anti-inflammatory effects of salicylates in rheumatoid arthritis. *Br. Med. J.*, **4**, 264–8

Brooks, P. M. and Day, R. O. (1987). Plasma concentration and therapeutic effects of anti-inflammatory and anti-rheumatic drugs. In Lewis, A. J. and Furst, D. E. (Eds.), *Non-steroidal and Anti-inflammatory Drugs—Mechanisms and Clinical Use*. Marcel Dekker, New York, 189–200

Cantrell, T. and Fisher, T. (1982). The small joints of the hands. *Clin. Rheum. Dis.*, **8**, 545–57

Clawson, D. K., Souter, W. A. and Carthum, C. J. (1977). Functional assessment of the rheumatoid hand. *Clin. Orthop. Rel. Res.*, **77**, 203–10

Co-operating Clinics Committee of the American Rheumatism Association (1965). A seven day variability study of 499 patients with peripheral rheumatoid arthritis. *Arthr. Rheum.*, **8**, 302–35

Co-operating Clinics Committee of the American Rheumatism Association (1967). A three month trial of indomethacin in rheumatoid arthritis with special reference to analysis and inference. *Clin. Pharm. Ther.*, **8**, 11–38

Cox, N. L. and Doherty, S. M. (1988). Out-patient audit of patient preference of NSAIDs: diclofenac, tiaprofenic acid, naproxen, magnesium choline trisalicylate. *Br. J. Rheum.*, **27** (Suppl. 2), 116

Day, R. O., Furst, D. E., Dromgoole, S. H., Kamm, B., Roe, R. and Paulus, H. G. (1982). Relationship of serum naproxen concentrations to efficacy in rheumatoid arthritis. *Clin. Pharm. Ther.*, **31**, 733–40

Deodhar, S. D., Carson, D. W., Hodgkinson, R. and Watson Buchanan, W. (1973). Measurement of clinical response to anti-inflammatory drug therapy in rheumatoid arthritis. *Quart. J. Med.*, **43**, 387–401

Dixon, J. S. and Bird, H. A. (1981). Reproducibility along a 10 cm vertical visual analogue scale. *Ann. Rheum. Dis.*, **40**, 87–9

Evans, D. M. and Lawton, D. S. (1984). Assessment of hand function. *Clin. Rheum. Dis.*, **10**, 697–725

Fernando, M. U. and Robertson, J. C. (1982). Grip strength in the elderly. *Rheum. Rehab.*, **21**, 179–81

Fraser, S., Land, D. and Sturrock, R. D. (1987). Microwave thermography—an index of inflammatory joint disease. *Br. J. Rheum.*, **26**, 37–9

Helliwell, P. S. (1987). The measurement of stiffness and strength in the rheumatoid hand. D.M. thesis, University of Oxford

Helliwell, P. S., Howe, A. and Wright, V. (1987). Functional assessment of the hand: reproducibility, acceptability and utility of a new system for measuring strength. *Ann. Rheum. Dis.*, **46**, 203–8

Helliwell, P. S., Howe, A. and Wright, V. (1988a). Lack of objective evidence of stiffness in rheumatoid arthritis. *Ann. Rheum. Dis.*, **47**, 754–8

Helliwell, P. S., Howe, A. and Wright, V. (1988b). The evaluation of the dynamic qualities of isometric grip strength. *Ann. Rheum. Dis.*, **47**, 934–9

Herxheimer, A. (1988). The rights of the patient in clinical research. *Lancet*, **2**, 1128–30

Hill, J. and Bird, H. A. (1986). Clinical assessments in rheumatoid arthritis. *Pharm. Med.*, **1**, 221–30

Hinchcliffe, K. P., Surrall, K. E. and Dixon, J. S. (1985). Reproducibility of pain measurements in rheumatoid arthritis by patients using visual analogue scales. *Pharm. Med.*, **1**, 99–103

Ingpen, M. L. (1968). The quantitative measurement of joint changes in rheumatoid arthritis. *Ann. Phys. Med.*, **9**, 322–7

Jamieson, A. H. (1988). The McGill Pain Questionnaire—thirteen years on. *J. Drug Dev.*, **1**, 8–14

Jones, A. R., Unsworth, A. and Haslock, I. (1985). A microcomputer controlled hand assessment system used for clinical measurement. *Eng. Med.*, **14**, 191–8

Kirwan, J. R. and Reeback, J. S. (1986). Stanford health assessment questionnaire modified to assess disability in British patients with rheumatoid arthritis. *Br. J. Rheum.*, **25**, 206–9

Leader (1982). Benoxaprofen. *Br. Med. J.*, **285**, 459–60

Lee, E. J. D., Williams, K., Day, R., Graham, G. and Champion, D. (1985). Stereoselective disposition of ibuprofen enantiomers in man. *Br. J. Clin. Pharm.*, **19**, 669–74

Lee, P., Baxter, A., Carson Dick, W. and Webb, J. (1974). An assessment of grip strength measurement in rheumatoid arthritis. *Scand. J. Rheum.*, **3**, 17–23

Loebl, W. Y. (1972). The assessment of mobility of metacarpophalangeal joints. *Rheum. Phys. Med.*, **11**, 365–79

Meacock, S. C. R. and Kitchen, E. A. (1979). Effects of the non-steroidal anti-inflammatory drug benoxaprofen on leucocyte migration. *J. Pharm. Pharmacol.*, **31**, 366–70

Moldofsky, H., Scarisbrick, P., England, R. and Smythe, H. (1975). Musculo-skeletal symptoms and non-REM sleep disturbance in patients with 'fibrositis syndrome' and healthy subjects. *Psychom. Med.*, **37**, 341–51

Ritchie, D., Boyle, J., McInnes, J. M., Jasani, M. K., Dalakos, T. G., Grievson, P. and Buchanan, W. W. (1968). Clinical studies with an articular index for the assessment of joint tenderness in patients with rheumatoid arthritis. *Quart. J. Med.*, **37**, 393–406

Scott, D. L., Roden, S., Marshall, T. and Kendall, M. J. (1982). Variations in responses to non-steroidal anti-inflammatory drugs. *Br. J. Clin. Pharm.*, **14**, 691–4

Scott, J. T. (1960). Morning stiffness in rheumatoid arthritis. *Ann. Rheum. Dis.*, **19**, 361–7

Scott, J. and Huskisson, E. C. (1979). Vertical or horizontal visual analogue scales. *Ann. Rheum. Dis.*, **38**, 560

Steinbrocker, O., Traeger, C. H. and Batterman, R. C. (1949). Therapeutic criteria in RA. *J. Am. Med. Assoc.*, **140**, 659–62

Surrall, K., Bird, H. A., Smith, J. A. and Dawick, D. J. (1986). Suppression of melatonin release by NSAIDs—a factor contributing to diurnal variation. *Br. J. Rheum.*, **45**, Suppl. 2

Vane, J. R. (1971). Inhibition of prostaglandin synthesis as a mechanism of action for the aspirin like drugs. *Nature*, **231**, 232–5

Webb, J., Downie, W. W., Dick, W. C. and Lee, P. (1973). Evaluation of digital joint circumference measurements in RA. *Scand. J. Rheum.*, **2**, 127–31

Wright, V. and Johns, R. T. (1960). Observations on the measurement of joint stiffness. *Arthr. Rheum.*, **3** (No. 4), 328–37

Young, J. B. and Chamberlain, M. A. (1987). Contribution of the Stanford Health Assessment Questionnaire in rheumatology clinics. *Clin. Rehab.*, **1**, 97–100

52
Analgesics

R. L. Holland

Dept of Clinical Research, Duphar BV, PO Box 900, 1380 DA Weesp, The Netherlands

INTRODUCTION

The aims of the early phase evaluation of a novel analgesic are to examine kinetics and limits to dosage by side-effects (tolerance), and to establish the therapeutic dose. Kinetics and tolerance studies are common to all novel drugs and are addressed elsewhere in this volume. This chapter will concentrate upon methods to establish efficacy, and then touch upon other pharmacodynamic properties of analgesics which can sometimes be explored.

A recent authoritative review concluded (that) 'serious problems in pain measurement theory and methodology remain' and (that) 'it is astonishing that no guidelines exist for the evaluation of analgesic interventions' (Chapman *et al.*, 1985). In this chapter some methods for studying new drugs in volunteers and patients will be described. It will be shown that although the methods may lack scientific validity, they can generate valuable information.

Ethical Considerations

Provided that consent is truly informed, that there is no duress, that permanent tissue injury is avoided and that the subject can stop the experiment at any time, it can be argued that a human volunteer pain study is more ethical than any animal experiment. However, patient studies involve more complex ethical considerations. Is it justified to use a placebo? At what stage should a treatment be regarded as a failure and pain relief be provided by other means? All protocols must take account of these questions.

STUDIES OF EFFICACY IN VOLUNTEERS

What Makes a Good Volunteer Model?

The criteria for a good volunteer model are:

(1) It should be easy to perform.
(2) It should give reliable (repeatable) results.

(3) It should be predictive: that is (a) drugs which produce pain relief should be analgesic in patients, and the clinically effective dose and duration of action should be obtainable from the model; and (b) drugs which do not produce pain relief should not be analgesic in patients.

Few models fulfil these criteria. None have been sufficiently tested to exclude non-analgesics causing artefactual pain relief, and in many models known analgesics do not cause detectable analgesia.

Volunteer Pain Models

Many methods of causing pain in volunteers have been investigated. Examples include:

(1) Electrical shocks to the finger (Seki, 1978; Bromm *et al.*, 1986); to the forearm (Buchsbaum *et al.*, 1981a,b); to the toothpulp (Gracely *et al.*, 1982); to the earlobe (Stacher *et al.*, 1982); and directly onto or into a nerve (Schady and Torebjork, 1984; Willer, 1985).
(2) Mechanical pressure on the finger (Bromm and Scharein, 1982a,b) or the interdigital web (Forster *et al.*, 1988).
(3) Hand immersion in cold water (de Jalon *et al.*, 1985).
(4) Ischaemia (Smith and Beecher, 1969; Posner, 1984).
(5) Heat on the skin (Hougs and Skoulby, 1957; Gracely *et al.*, 1988).

Pain Measurement in These Models

There are rather few methods available. They consist of either asking the volunteer to quantify subjectively pain intensity or attempting to measure some physiological correlate of the pain. Usually an attempt is made to relate the pain intensity to the magnitude of the stimulus causing the pain. Typical parameters analysed are the stimulus intensity at which pain is just perceived (threshold) and the maximum stimulus tolerated by the subjects (tolerance).

Two methods for quantifying self-reported pain have been developed.

Visual Analogue Scales

Visual analogue scales are lines, usually horizontal, anchored at both ends by terms such as 'no pain' and 'worst possible pain'. Pain intensity can be indicated by placing a mark on the line (see Sriwatanakul *et al.*, 1983, for review) or by moving a cursor along a computer-generated scale (Posner, 1984). The score is usually taken as the distance from the 'no pain' end.

Category Judgements

This is the more common technique. At its simplest, this devolves to asking whether a particular stimulus intensity is painful or not. Usually, however, several categories of painfulness are used (see, e.g., Buchsbaum *et al.*, 1981a,b; De Jalon *et al.*, 1985). Perhaps surprisingly, this methodology lends itself to some fairly sophisticated psychophysics. It is possible, for example, using the technique of cross-modality matching, to give certain categories of painfulness absolute scores which are consistent between subjects as well as within a subject (Gracely *et al.*, 1982; Gracely and Dubner, 1987).

Most research into category judgements of pain intensity has focused upon the pain threshold and upon delineating accurately the stimulus intensity at that boundary. Typically, but least accurately, the threshold is sought by use of a steadily rising stimulus intensity (see, e.g., Wolff *et al.*, 1976; Stacher *et al.*, 1982). A better technique is to use the method of limits, in which ascending and descending stimulus intensities are used. This can be improved still further with the use of random double staircases (see Gracely *et al.*, 1988). Although these techniques are usually used to delineate the prepain–pain category boundary, in principle they can be applied to any category boundary, e.g. moderate to severe pain.

Another approach to category judgement uses sensory decision theory (SDT). Statistical techniques are used to examine subject categorisations of a large number of brief, variable-intensity stimuli (usually electrical pulses). Two parameters are derived. One is an index of discrimination ability, often called sensitivity, which is obtained from accuracy and error rates. The other, often called response bias, is a measure of the conservatism with which the subject makes a judgement during that experiment (Buchsbaum *et al.*, 1981a,b).

Physiological Variables

Several physiological variables have been quantified in an attempt to obtain more objective data.

Cerebral Event Related Potentials

There have been many attempts to relate changes in the electroencephalo-gram with the presence or absence, and intensity of pain (see, e.g., Buchsbaum *et al.*, 1981b; Bromm and Scharein, 1982a; Fernandes de Lima *et al.*, 1982; Bromm *et al.*, 1986). The usual technique has been to present many brief painful stimuli, usually electrical, and then to average the cerebral potentials over the next 300 ms or so—'evoked potentials'. A negative potential is usually evident about 120–150 ms after the stimulation, and this is followed by a positive component about 100 ms later. The amplitudes of these waves are typically related to the intensity of the stimulation and to the self-reported pain intensity. However, it is by no means clear that these waves represent 'pain', as they can be evoked at low amplitude by non-noxious A delta fibre stimulation, and evoked potential responses have never been detected following pure C fibre stimulation (Chudler and Dong, 1983).

The Nociception Flexion Reflex

A painful stimulus to a limb produces a spinal reflex withdrawal of that limb from that stimulus. Willer (1985) stimulated the peroneal nerve of volunteers at the ankle and recorded electrical activity in the ipsilateral biceps femoris. This electromyogram response was quantitatively linearly related to the stimulus intensity, and to the self-reported pain intensity. However, again, an EMG response can be produced by low-amplitude (sub-pain threshold) electrical stimuli.

Other Measures

Autonomic functions have frequently been measured during volunteer pain studies. However, these measures typically relate more to the anxiety of the subjects, and to the physical procedures (e.g. cold pressor), than to the intensity of the pain experience (Chapman *et al.*, 1985).

Which Measures, in Which Volunteer Models, Respond to Which Drugs?

In essence this question can be answered as follows: in double-blind, placebo-controlled, crossover, single-dose studies: (a) a reasonable dose of an opioid will reduce the intensity of subjectively assessed pain, using practically any measure in practically any volunteer model; and (b) it is very difficult to detect effects with other types of analgesics.

Thus, therapeutic doses of opioids provide pain relief in: (a) electrically induced pain (Wolff, 1976; Buchsbaum *et al.*, 1981a,b; Gracely *et al.*, 1982; Bromm *et al.*, 1986; Stacher *et al.*, 1986, 1987); (b) cold-induced pain (Wolff *et al.*, 1976; de Jalon *et al.*, 1985; Holland *et al.*, 1988); (c) ischaemic pain (Posner, 1984); (d) thermal pain (Stacher *et al.*, 1982).

The most clear-cut effects are on tolerance and pain intensity after a constant stimulus rather than on threshold. One possible explanation for this is that the opioid effect is proportional to the pain intensity. However, a more interesting possibility is that moderate to severe pain, especially if it is increasing, more reliably represents the clinical situation with its associated anxiety and stress (Chapman *et al.*, 1985).

Evidence for pain relief by non-opioid analgesics is much more difficult to obtain.

(1) *Electrically induced pain* Some studies have found high doses of a non-steroidal anti-inflammatory drug (NSAID) to have effects on pain threshold (Wolff *et al.*, 1976; Stacher *et al.*, 1982, 1986). Occasionally, other parameters have also been affected: e.g. aspirin, on all categories of painfulness (Seki, 1978); and zomepirac, on pain intensity to constant stimulus (Schady and Torebjork, 1984).

(2) *Cold-induced pain* NSAIDs produce little if any effect (Wolff *et al.*, 1976; De Jalon *et al.*, 1985; Telekes *et al.*, 1987).

(3) *Ischaemic pain* Aspirin 600 mg produced some effects (Smith and

Beecher, 1969) but not paracetamol (Telekes, A., personal communication).

(4) *Thermal threshold* Diclofenac 75 mg and 150 mg affected this (Stacher *et al.*, 1986).

(5) *Mechanical pressure* Aspirin 1.5 mg affected category judgements (Forster *et al.*, 1988).

With the well-known bias in favour of publishing positive results, it is probable that many negative studies of NSAIDs remain unpublished. It might be, therefore, that the few positive published examples cited above represent chance findings. Two other points should also be noted. First, these studies often used very high doses of NSAIDs, which can have other (non-analgesic) CNS effects (Telekes *et al.*, 1987). Second, effects on pain threshold are the least reliable of analgesic measures (Beecher, 1957; Chapman *et al.*, 1985), as thresholds are particularly affected by placebo and instructional set.

Recommendations

If a new drug is an opioid, it is worth while investigating its efficacy in a volunteer model. Electrical stimulation and cold-induced pain are both reliable and convenient techniques. Both can predict therapeutic single doses and duration of action. However, neither has been properly explored for false-positives—i.e. drugs which might produce apparent pain relief but are not clinical analgesics. However, diazepam did not affect an electrical pain test (Gracely *et al.*, 1982) and the vasodilator nifedipine did not affect the Cold Pain Test (Holland *et al.*, 1988).

For drugs which are not opioids there are no really appropriate volunteer models. Only the electrical pain test has consistently shown pain relief with non-opioids, and even then, this effect is typically on the least reliable measure (threshold) and only occurs with high doses. The occasional positive effects of antidepressant-like drugs in this model are also worrying. It is not clear that imipramine (Bromm *et al.*, 1986) and RO15-8081 (Stacher *et al.*, 1987) are clinically effective analgesics, whereas fluradoline (rejected in the Bromm *et al.*, 1986, experiment) does seem to produce postoperative analgesia (Jones and McQuay, 1987).

EARLY STUDIES OF EFFICACY IN PATIENTS

Introduction

Testing analgesics in patients is in some ways easier than in volunteers. After all, if the patients find, on average, that the drug produces adequate relief of a diagnosed pain, then the drug is by definition an analgesic, provided that it is not acting to improve the underlying disease process.

Useful Paradigms for Investigating the Clinical Efficacy of Novel Analgesics

Any clinical situation in which pain features could, in theory, be used to assess analgesic efficacy. However, clearly: (1) it is easier to use paradigms in which the patient's physical condition is otherwise more or less stable; and (2) it is better to use conditions in which the cause of the pain has been diagnosed. Most of the studies which follow have satisfied both of these criteria.

Acute Pain

Postoperative Pain

In many ways postoperative pain represents the 'gold standard' clinical study of an analgesic, as efficacy can be reliably demonstrated in double-blind placebo-controlled parallel group single-dose studies. A typical study is described below.

The patients are assessed for suitability and informed consent is obtained preoperatively. After operation the patients are monitored until they complain of moderate or severe pain. At this point they are randomised to receive a single dose of one of the several treatments (typically placebo, two doses of the active medication and a positive control). They are then monitored frequently by a trained observer (often a nurse) for the expected duration of action of the analgesics. Observation times are usually pretreatment, then $\frac{1}{2}$ h, 1 h, 2 h, 3 h, 4 h, 5 h, and 6 h post treatment. The patients are usually asked to rate their pain intensity on a four- (or sometimes five-) point scale: $0 = $ none, $1 = $ mild, $2 = $ moderate, $3 = $ severe ($4 = $ very severe). They usually also rate their pain intensity on a 100 mm visual analogue line and their pain relief on a typical five- (or six-) point scale: ($-1 = $ worse), $0 = $ no relief, $1 = $ some relief, $2 = $ good relief, $3 = $ excellent relief, $4 = $ complete relief. Additional parameters that can be analysed include: the time at which pain is 'half gone'; pain adjectives presented randomly; and the time at which escape analgesia is required ($=$ treatment failure). It is important that the same observer be used throughout for a particular patient, and preferably for the whole study, as the patient's responses to these self-evaluations will depend upon the instructional set. It is also desirable to use a trained and experienced observer, as this allows consistent behaviour in the face of anxious, sedated or nauseated patients.

Analysis of these different category scales and analogue scales is relatively straightforward. For the pain intensity measures (category and analogue), the pretreatment measure is used as a baseline and the analysed value is usually the difference from baseline (i.e. Pain Intensity Difference—PID; or Pain Analogue Intensity Difference—PAID). Separate analyses are usually carried out at each time-point, and, in addition, a time-weighted average value is usually computed (SPID and SPAID). Patients who drop out are typically allocated their initial value for the remainder of the analysed time-points—as though the treatment had been ineffective. The pain relief scores are usually analysed directly, and once again a total time-weighted pain relief score (TOTPAR) is usually generated.

A great deal of literature has been published on the relative merits of different category and analogue scales in this postoperative situation. However, when a large number of studies were reviewed (Littman *et al.*, 1985), it was clear that intensity difference ratings, visual analogue scale (VAS) scores and pain relief scores all correlated extremely highly. There was little difference in their abilities to detect drug effects, with perhaps the pain relief scales and VAS scales being slightly more sensitive than intensity scales. The fact that the different scales all gave the same answers is hardly surprising. Patients will attempt to describe whether the drug gives effective pain relief, whatever method is used to ask this question of them. It should also be noted that the data manipulations used to compute PID and PAID essentially convert scores of intensity to scores of pain relief. Importantly, it has been shown that patients prefer adjectival descriptions to VAS, with as many as 11% failing to understand and cope with the latter (Kremer *et al.*, 1981; Jensen *et al.*, 1986).

With appropriate stratification for operation site and patient age, and with sufficient patients per group (usually 30 per treatment dose), postoperative pain studies are highly effective at showing both opioid (see, e.g. Downing *et al.*, 1981; Calimlin *et al.*, 1982) and NSAID (see, e.g. McQuay *et al.*, 1986; O'Hara *et al.*, 1987) analgesia. This technique has even been extended to investigations of analgesia produced by corticosteroids (Olstad and Skjelbred, 1986) and antidepressants (Levine *et al.*, 1986).

Another route to assessing pain relief is to analyse the numbers of patients who require additional analgesia (Sechzer, 1977). More elegantly, the total amount of additional analgesic requested can be quantified by use of a patient-controlled analgesia system (Harmer *et al.*, 1983). However, this technique may produce additional problems, given the extreme variation that occurs in analgesic demand postoperatively with such a system.

Other Acutely Painful Conditions

Techniques validated by frequent use in postoperative pain have been equally successfully applied to other acutely painful conditions. Obstetric pain is one such, with analgesia being demonstrated during labour (Frank *et al.*, 1987), and in postpartum pain, e.g. episiotomy, uterine cramp and caesarean section (Bloomfield *et al.*, 1986; Sunshine *et al.*, 1986). Similar studies have been performed equally successfully in acute renal and ureteric colic (Warren *et al.*, 1985), acute trauma, acute back pain and sciatica (Clissold and Beresford, 1987).

Chronic Pain

The assessment of an analgesic in chronically painful conditions is problematic. Clearly, the diagnosis is of fundamental importance, and not all conditions are appropriate for analgesic intervention. It is rare for patients to suffer only one pain at a time. The interplay between mental state and perceived pain intensity is crucial. Outcome measures must include more than just pain relief, with assessments of quality of life being more relevant.

Pain Due to Cancer

Deschamps *et al.* (1988) reviewed the use of category scales and VAS in studies of pain due to cancer, noting that both types of scale tended to focus only on intensity. The authors advocated the use of the McGill Pain Questionnaire (MPQ) (Melzack, 1975) as a more appropriate tool. However, there would be substantial problems in using the MPQ in a drug study. It is difficult and time-consuming to administer, and there is little consensus as to how to score it. Nonetheless, the philosophy of the MPQ is appropriate to cancer pain.

A particular problem with cancer pain is the ethical requirement for the physician to alleviate that pain. Pain control in such patients typically has two phases. The first is a titration period during which increasing doses of an analgesic are administered. The dose required at the end of this phase, for longer-term pain control, can be highly variable between patients (from 40 mg to 400 mg of oral morphine daily in one study: Hanks *et al.*, 1987). However, once patients have entered this second, relatively stable phase, it is possible to perform crossover efficacy studies—though with difficulty. For example, in the Hanks *et al.* study, 18 of 27 patients completed a randomised double-blind comparative efficacy study of 7 days of 4-hourly morphine with 7 days of slow-release morphine. Assessments of pain, alertness, nausea, mood, sleep and appetite were all made by visual analogue scales. Another approach is to regard an admission for cancer pain as equivalent to an acutely painful condition. For example, Stambaugh and McAdams (1987) performed a placebo-controlled single-dose study directly equivalent to the postoperative pain studies described above.

Chronic Arthritic Conditions

Clinical trials in these conditions are extremely complex, with multiple outcome measures. Honig (1983) presented a good example of an appropriate study on the long-term pain relief provided by zomepirac in osteoarthritis. Four separate pains were scored, each on a four-point scale: pain at rest, pain on motion, pain at night and joint tenderness (joint swelling was also scored on the same scale). Functional status was scored on at least 11 separate movements and activities related to daily living.

Other Chronic Pains

Simple studies can be performed but are usually confounded by questions about diagnosis and previous treatment. Almost by definition, patients who present to chronic pain clinics have pains which will not respond to simple treatments. Moreover, chronic pain causes low mood, but chronic pain can also be a presentation (symptom) of depression.

Discussion and Recommendations

The early phase evaluation of novel analgesics in patients is relatively easily undertaken in acutely painful conditions. Postoperative pain, particularly after orthopaedic or dental surgery, is a well-validated model sensitive to both the major classes of analgesic. Although patient numbers need to be large (30 per group), the conditions are common, patient recruitment can be rapid, and the studies are easy to analyse and have sensible outcome measures.

Chronically painful conditions are very much more complex, and rarely suitable for the early phase investigation of new drugs.

OTHER STUDIES USEFULLY PERFORMED AT AN EARLY STAGE OF ANALGESIC DEVELOPMENT

Volunteer Studies

Opioids

Opioids, in particular, have a large number of well-known side-effects relating to their specificities for particular receptor subtypes. Estimates of opioid induced sedation can be obtained from simple tests of psychomotor performance and validated visual analogue scales (e.g. Telekes *et al.*, 1987). Similarly, the likelihood of respiratory depression can be determined by looking for effects on the ventilatory response to rebreathing CO_2 (Keats, 1985; Telekes *et al.*, 1987). Abuse liability is the crucial question for an opioid. This can be addressed by giving the drug to opioid-experienced volunteers (usually ex-addicts) who can self-assess euphoria, dysphoria and 'drug liking'. In the presence of trained observers, double-blind placebo-controlled studies can give reliable and predictive results (Jasinsky and Preston, 1985; Preston *et al.*, 1987). Other effects which can be sought in volunteers include hormonal responses and gastrointestinal effects (by use of techniques to measure delay in gastric emptying, such as the H_2 breath test, or simply measuring the time until the next stool).

Other Analgesics

It is not, in general, as profitable to seek effects of non-steroidal anti-inflammatory drugs in volunteers as it is for opioids. However, occasionally CNS effects can be detected, such as self-assessed sedation and *increased* respiratory responsiveness to rebreathing CO_2 (Telekes *et al.*, 1987).

Patient Studies

Before a full test of dose response in a postoperative pain model, it is imperative to have information about possible kinetic and dynamic interactions with other drugs used in the postoperative period. These include: anaesthetics (inhalational and induction agents, e.g. barbiturates); neuromuscular blocking drugs; drugs used to reverse neuromuscular blockade; and antiemetics. This sort of information can be obtained by performing a limited rising-dose tolerance study of the potential analgesic in postoperative patients.

Later Clinical Pharmacological Studies

The safe and therapeutic dose having been established, there are many further clinical pharmacological studies to be performed. For example, drug interaction studies will be required, and dynamic/kinetic studies in particular patient populations (the elderly, impaired renal or hepatic function). However, these studies are perhaps best deferred until the later phase of drug investigation.

CONCLUSION

While some of the methodologies described above may be criticised, they do enable the development of a new analgesic. Kinetic and tolerance studies are as important as with any drug, and at least some of this work must be performed in the most likely experimental test-bed for the analgesic— postoperative pain. Volunteer pharmacodynamic models have much to offer in responding to questions about tolerance, side-effects and abuse potential, but are not predictive of efficacy for anything other than an opioid.

REFERENCES

Beecher, H. K. (1957). The measurement of pain. *Pharm. Rev.*, **9**, 59–209

Bloomfield, S. S., Mitchell, J., Cissell, G. and Barden, T. P. (1986). Analgesic sensitivity of two post-partum pain models. *Pain*, **27**, 171–9

Bromm, B., Meier, W. and Scharein, E. (1986). Imipramine reduces experimental pain. *Pain*, **25**, 245–57

Bromm, B. and Scharein, E. (1982a). Response plasticity of pain evoked reactions in man. *Physiol. Behav.*, **28**, 109–16

Bromm, B. and Scharein, E. (1982b). Principal component analysis of pain related cerebral potentials to mechanical and electrical stimulation in man. *Electroenceph. Clin. Neurophysiol.*, **53**, 94–103

Buchsbaum, M. S., Davis, G. C., Coppola, R. and Naber, D. (1981a). Opiate pharmacology and individual differences. I. Psychophysical pain measurements. *Pain*, **10**, 357–66

Buchsbaum, M. S., Davis, G. C., Coppola, R. and Naber, D. (1981b). Opiate pharmacology and individual differences. II. Somatosensory evoked potentials. *Pain*, **10**, 367–77

Calimlin, J. F., Sriwatanakul, K., Wardell, W. M., Lasagna, L. and Cox, C. (1982). Analgesic efficacy of parenteral metkephamid acetate in the treatment of post operative pain. *Lancet*, **i**, 1374–5

Chapman, C. R., Casey, K. L., Dubner, R., Foley, K. M., Gracely, R. H. and Reading, A. E. (1985). Pain measurement: an overview. *Pain*, **22**, 1–31

Chudler, E. H. and Dong, W. K. (1983). The assessment of pain by cerebral evoked potentials. *Pain*, **16**, 221–44

Clissold, S. P. and Beresford, R. (1987). Proquazone. A review of its pharmacodynamic and pharmacokinetic properties and therapeutic efficacy in rheumatic diseases and pain states. *Drugs*, **33**, 478–502

De Jalon, P. D. G., Harrison, F. J. J., Johnson, K. I., Kozma, C. and Schnelle, K. (1985). A modified cold stimulation technique for the evaluation of analgesic activity in human volunteers. *Pain*, **22**, 183–9

Deschamps, K., Band, P. R. and Coldman, A. J. (1988). Assessment of adult cancer pain: shortcomings of current methods. *Pain*, **32**, 133–9

Downing, J. W., Brock-Utne, J. G., Barclay, A. and Schwegmann, I. L. (1981). WY16225 (Dezocine) a new synthetic opiate agonist-antagonist and potent analgesic: comparison with morphine for relief of pain after lower abdominal surgery. *Br. J. Anaesth.*, **53**, 59–63

Fernandes, de Lima, V. M., Chatrian, G. E., Lettich, E., Canfield, R. C., Miller, R. C. and Soso, M. J. (1982). Electrical stimulation of toothpulp in humans. I. Relationships among physical stimulus intensities, psychological magnitude estimates, and cerebral evoked potentials. *Pain*, **14**, 207–32

Forster, C., Anton, F., Reeh, P. W., Weber, E. and Handwerker, H. O. (1988). Measurement of the analgesic effects of aspirin with a new experimental algesimetric procedure. *Pain*, **32**, 215–22

Frank, M., McAteer, E. J., Cattermole, R., Loughman, B., Stafford, L. B. and Hitchcock, A. M. (1987). Nalbuphine for obstetric analgesia. A comparison of nalbuphine with pethidine for pain relief in labour when administered by patient controlled analgesia (PCA). *Anaesthesia*, **42**, 697–703

Gracely, R. H. and Dubner, R. (1987). Reliability and validity of verbal descriptor scales of painfulness. *Pain*, **29**, 175–85

Gracely, R. H., Dubner, R. and McGrath, P. A. (1982). Fentanyl reduces the intensity of painful toothpulp sensations: controlling for detection of active drugs. *Anesth. Analg.*, **61**, 751–5

Gracely, R. H., Lota, L., Walter, D. J. and Dubner, R. (1988). A multiple random staircase method of psychophysical pain assessment. *Pain*, **32**, 55–63

Hanks, G. W., Twycross, R. G. and Bliss, J. M. (1987). Controlled release morphine tablets; a double blind trial in patients with advanced cancer. *Anaesthesia*, **42**, 840–4

Harmer, M., Slattery, P. J., Rosen, M. and Vickers, M. D. (1983). Intramuscular on demand analgesia: double blind controlled trial of pethidine, buprenorphine, morphine and meptazinol. *Br. Med. J.*, **286**, 680–2

Holland, R. L., Harkin, N. E., Coleshaw, S. R. K., Jones, D. A., Peck, A. W. and Telekes, A. (1988). Dipipanone and nifedipine in cold induced pain: analgesia not due to skin warming. *Br. J. Clin. Pharm.*, **24**, 823–6

Honig, S. (1983). Long-term therapy for the pain of ostearthritis: a comparison of zomepirac sodium and aspirin. *J. Clin. Pharm.*, **23**, 494–504

Hougs, W. and Skouby, A. P. (1957). The analgetic action of analgetics antihistaminics and chlorpromazine on volunteers. *Acta Pharm. Toxicol.*, **13**, 405–9

Jasinsky, D. R. and Preston, K. L. (1985). Assessment of dezocine for morphine like subjective effects and miosis. *Clin. Pharm. Ther.*, **38**, 544–8

Jensen, M. P., Karoly, P. and Braver, S. (1986). The measurement of clinical pain intensity: a comparison of six methods. *Pain*, **27**, 117–26

Jones, S. F. and McQuay, H. J. (1987). Letter to Editor. *Pain*, **28**, 265–6

Keats, A. S. (1985). The effect of drugs on respiration in man. *Ann. Rev. Pharm. Toxicol.*, **25**, 41–65

Kremer, F., Atkinson, J. H. and Ignelzi, R. J. (1981). Measurement of pain: patient preference does not confound pain measurement. *Pain*, **10**, 241–8

Levine, J. D., Gordon, N. C., Smith, R. and McBryde, R. (1986). Desipramine enhances opiate post operative analgesia. *Pain*, **27**, 45–9

Littman, G. S., Walker, B. R. and Scheider, B. E. (1985). Reassessment of verbal and visual analogue ratings in analgesic studies. *Clin. Pharm. Ther.*, **38**, 16–23

McQuay, H. J., Poppleton, P., Carroll, D., Summerfield, R. J., Bullingham, R. E. S. and Moore, R. A. (1986). Ketorolac and acetaminophen for orthopaedic post operative pain. *Clin. Pharm. Ther.*, **39**, 89–93

Melzack, R. (1975). The McGill Pain Questionnaire: major properties and scoring methods. *Pain.*, **1**, 277–99

O'Hara, D. A., Fragen, R. J., Kinzer, M. and Pemberton, D. (1987). Ketorolac tromethamine as compared with morphine sulfate for treatment of post operative pain. *Clin. Pharm. Ther.*, **41**, 556–61

Olstad, O. A. and Skjelbred, P. (1986). Comparison of the analgesic effect of a corticosteroid and paracetamol in patients with pain after oral surgery. *Br. J. Clin. Pharm.*, **22**, 437–42

Posner, J. (1984). A modified submaximal effort tourniquet test for evaluation of analgesics in healthy volunteers. *Pain*, **19**, 143–51

Preston, K. L., Bigelow, G. E. and Liebson, I. A. (1987). Comparative evaluation of morphine, pentazocine, and ciramadol in post addicts. *J. Pharm. Exp. Ther.*, **240**, 900–10

Schady, W. and Torebjork, H. E. (1984). Central effects of zomepirac on pain evoked by intraneural stimulation in man. *J. Clin. Pharm.*, **24**, 429–35

Sechzer, P. H. (1977). Evaluation of fenoprofen as a post operative analgesic. *Curr. Ther. Res.*, **21**, 137–48

Seki, T. (1978). Evaluation of effect of acetyl-salicylic acid using electrical stimulation on the forefinger of healthy volunteers. *Br. J. Clin. Pharm.*, **6**, 521–4

Smith, G. M. and Beecher, H. K. (1969). Experimental production of pain in man: sensitivity of a new method to 600 mg of aspirin. *Clin. Pharm. Ther.*, **10**, 213–16

Sriwatanakul, K., Kelvie, W., Lasagna, L., Calimlim, J. F., Weis, O. F. and Mehta, G. (1983). Studies with different types of visual analogue scales for measurement of pain. *Clin. Pharm. Ther.*, **34**, 234–9

Stacher, G., Bauer, P., Scheider, C., Winklehner, S. and Schmierer, S. (1982). Effects of a combination of oral naproxen sodium and codeine on experimentally induced pain. *Eur. J. Clin. Pharm.*, **21**, 485–90

Stacher, G., Steinringer, H., Schneider, S., Mittelbach, G., Gaupman, G., Abatzi, Th.-A. and Stacher-Janotta, G. (1987). Effects of graded doses of a new 5-hydroxytryptamine/noradrenaline uptake inhibitor (RO15-8081) in comparison with 60 mg codeine and placebo on experimentally induced pain and side effect profile in man. *Br. J. Clin. Pharm.*, **24**, 627–35

Stacher, G., Steinringer, H., Schneider, S., Mittelbach, G., Winklehner, S. and Gaupman, G. (1986). Experimental pain induced by electrical and thermal stimulation of the skin in healthy man: sensitivity to 75 and 150 mg diclofenac sodium in comparison with 60 mg codeine and placebo. *Br. J. Clin. Pharm.*, **21**, 35–43

Stambaugh, J. E. and McAdams, J. (1987). Comparison of intramuscular dezocine with butorphanol and placebo in chronic cancer pain: a method to evaluate analgesia after both single and repeated doses. *Clin. Pharm. Ther.*, **42**, 210–19

Sunshine, A., Zighelboim, I., Laska, E., Siegel, C., Olson, N. Z. and DeCastro, A. (1986). A double blind parallel comparison of ketoprofen, aspirin and placebo in patients with post partum pain. *J. Clin. Pharm.*, **26**, 706–11

Telekes, A., Holland, R. L. and Peck, A. W. (1987). Indomethacin: effects on cold induced pain and the nervous system in healthy volunteers. *Pain*, **30**, 321–8

Warren, M. M., Boyce, W. H., Evans, J. W. and Peters, P. C. (1985). A double blind comparison of dezocine and morphine in patients with acute renal and ureteral colic. *J. Urol.*, **134**, 457–9

Willer, J. C. (1985). Studies on pain. Effects of morphine on a spinal nociceptive flexion reflex and related pain sensation in man. *Brain Res.*, **331**, 105–14

Wolff, B. B., Kantor, T. G. and Cohen, P. (1976). Laboratory pain induction methods for human analgesic assays. *Adv. Pain Res. Ther.*, **1**, 363–7

Index